PEDIATRIC EMERGENCY NURSING

2nd Edition

PEDIATRIC EMERGENCY NURSING

2ND Edition

Susan J. Kelley, RN, PhD, FAAN
Professor
School of Nursing
Georgia State University
Atlanta, Georgia
Formerly Professor
Department of Maternal and Child Health
School of Nursing
Boston College
Chestnut Hill, Massachusetts

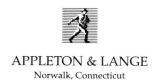

APPLETON & LANGE
Norwalk, Connecticut

Notice: The authors and the publisher of this volume have taken care that the information and recommendations contained herein are accurate and compatible with the standards generally accepted at the time of publication. Nevertheless, it is difficult to ensure that all the information given is entirely accurate for all circumstances. The publisher disclaims any liability, loss, or damage incurred as a consequence, directly or indirectly, of the use and application of any of the contents of this volume.

Copyright © 1994 by Appleton & Lange

Paramount Publishing Business and Professional Group
Copyright © 1988 by Appleton & Lange

94 95 96 97 98 / 10 9 8 7 6 5 4 3 2

Prentice Hall International (UK) Limited, *London*
Prentice Hall of Australia Pty. Limited, *Sydney*
Prentice Hall Canada, Inc., *Toronto*
Prentice Hall Hispanoamericana, S.A., *Mexico*
Prentice Hall of India Private Limited, *New Delhi*
Prentice Hall of Japan, Inc., *Tokyo*
Simon & Schuster Asia Pte. Ltd., *Singapore*
Editora Prentice Hall do Brasil Ltda., *Rio de Janeiro*
Prentice Hall, *Englewood Cliffs, New Jersey*

Library of Congress Cataloging-in-Publication Data

Pediatric emergency nursing / [edited by] Susan J. Kelley. — 2nd ed.
    p.   cm.
    Rev. ed. of: Pediatric emergency nursing / Susan J. Kelley. c1988.
    Includes bibliographical references and index.
    ISBN 0-8385-7705-9
    1. Pediatric emergencies. 2. Emergency nursing. I. Kelley,
Susan J.
    [DNLM: 1. Emergencies—in infancy & childhood. 2. Emergencies—
nursing.   WY 159 P3692   1994]
    RJ370.K45   1994
    610.73'62—dc20
    DNLM/DLC
    for Library of Congress   93-41701
                                                                CIP

Acquisitions Editor: David Carroll
Production Editor: Jennifer Sinsavich
Designer: Penny Kindzierski
Cover Designer: Elizabeth A. Schmitz

PRINTED IN THE UNITED STATES OF AMERICA

ISBN 0-8385-7705-9
90000
9 780838 577059

To my husband, Ron Verni,
for his ever present love and encouragement,
and to my mother and father, Mary Ellen and James Kelley,
for their love and support throughout the years

Contents

Contributors

Catherine R. Benson, RN, MS, PNP
Education Coordinator (Former)
Nursing Education and Research
Children's Memorial Hospital
Chicago, Illinois

Lisa Marie Bernardo, RN, PhD
Clinical Nurse Specialist
Emergency Department
Children's Hospital of Pittsburg
Adjunct Professor
University of Pittsburgh
Pittsburgh, Pennsylvania

Marianne Bove, RN, BSN, CEN
Clinical Nurse II
Emergency Department
Children's Hospital of Pittsburgh
Pittsburgh, Pennsylvania

Pamela J. Burke, PhD, RN
Associate Professor
Department of Maternal and Child Health
School of Nursing
Boston College
Chestnut Hill, Massachusetts

Martha A. Q. Curley, RN, MS, CCRN
Critical Care Clinical Nurse Specialist
Multidisciplinary Intensive Care Unit
Children's Hospital
Boston, Massachusetts

Wendy L. Daly, RN, MSN
Clinical Nurse Specialist
Shriners Burns Institute
Boston, Massachusetts

Bonnie S. Dean, RN, BSN, ABAT
Associate Director
Pittsburgh Poison Control Center
Children's Hospital of Pittsburgh
Assistant Professor
School of Pharmacy
University of Pittsburgh
Pittsburgh, Pennsylvania

Virginia L. Dodd, RNC, MS
Clinical Nurse Specialist (Former)
Neonatal Intensive Care Unit
Hartford Hospital
Hartford, Connecticut

Jan M. Frederickson, RN, MN, CPNP
Lecturer
Primary Care/Pediatrics
School of Nursing
University of California, Los Angeles
Los Angeles, California
Pediatric Clinical Nurse Specialist
Northridge Hospital Medical Center
Northridge, California

Deborah Parkman Henderson, RN, MA
Co-Director
National Emergency Medical Services for Children
    Resource Alliance
Torrance, California
Lecturer
School of Medicine
University of California Los Angeles
Los Angeles, California

Susan J. Kelley, RN, PhD, FAAN
Professor
School of Nursing
Georgia State University
Atlanta, Georgia

Catherine Knox-Fischer, MSN, RN
Clinical Nurse Specialist for Mental Health
Children's Hospital of Philadelphia
Philadelphia, Pennsylvania

Patricia Kraepelien-Bartels, RN, MS, CS
Nurse Practitioner/Nurse Manager
Comprehensive Child Health Program
Children's Hospital
Boston, Massachusetts

Linda K. Manley, RN, BSN, CEN, CCRN, EMT-P
Emergency Medical Services Coordinator
Emergency Services
Children's Hospital
Flight Nurse
Skymed
Columbus, Ohio

Mary E. McClain, RN, MS
Project Coordinator
Massachusetts Center for Sudden Infant
   Death Syndrome
Pediatrics
Boston City Hospital
Instructor in Pediatrics
Boston University School of Medicine
Boston, Massachusetts

Joan Meunier-Sham, RN, MS
Assistant Director of Nursing
Shriners Burns Institute
Boston, Massachusetts

Sandra Mott, RNC, MS
Associate Professor
Department of Maternal and Child Health
School of Nursing
Boston College
Chestnut Hill, Massachusetts

Beth S. Nachtsheim, RN, BSN
Clinical Educator/Acting Clinical Nurse Manager
Emergency Pediatric
Children's Memorial Hospital
Chicago, Illinois

Anne Phelan, MS, RN
Clinical Coordinator
Emergency Department
Children's Hospital
Boston, Massachusetts

Ann Powers, RN, MS, CS
Clinical Nurse Specialist,
   Pediatrics and Pediatric Critical Care
Hartford Hospital
Hartford, Connecticut

Laurette Quinn, RN, MS, CDE
Instructor/Practitioner-Teacher
Department of Medical Nursing/Department of
   Medical Endocrinology
Rush University/Presbyterian-St. Luke's
   Medical Center
Chicago, Illinois

Ellen Reynolds, MS, RN, CEN
Clinical Research Nurse Specialist
Ambulatory Care
General Academic Pediatrics
Children's Hospital of Pittsburgh
Adjunct Faculty
Parent-Child Nursing Program
University of Pittsburgh
Pittsburgh, Pennsylvania

Judith Schurr Salzer, RN, MS, CPNP
Pediatric Nurse Practitioner
Health Screening and Maintenance Clinic
Children's Memorial Hospital
Adjunct Instructor
Public Health Nursing
University of Illinois at Chicago
Chicago, Illinois

Reneé Semonin-Holleran, RN, PhD, CEN, CCRN
Chief Flight Nurse/Emergency Clinical
   Nurse Specialist
University Air Care
University of Cincinnati Hospital
Cincinnati, Ohio

Patricia A. Southard, RN, MN, JD
Associate Hospital Director
Oregon Health Sciences University and Clinics
Instructor
Community Health
Oregon Health Sciences University
School of Nursing
Portland, Oregon

Rachel E. Spector, RN, PhD, CTN
Associate Professor
Department of Community Health
School of Nursing
Boston College
Chestnut Hill, Massachusetts

Arlene M. Sperhac, PhD, RNC, PNP
Director, Nursing Education and Research
Children's Memorial Hospital
Adjunct Faculty
Rush University
Loyola University
University of Illinois
Chicago, Illinois

Barbara Woodring, RN, EdD
Associate Professor and Chair
Parent-Child Nursing Department
School of Nursing
Medical College of Georgia
Augusta, Georgia

Preface

Emergency nursing care of children has emerged as a specialty area of nursing practice during the past decade. Simultaneously, our knowledge of the unique emergency nursing care needs of children has grown exponentially. Since publication of the first edition of *Pediatric Emergency Nursing* in 1988, several other texts devoted to emergency nursing care of children have followed, as have standardized curricula for courses preparing nurses for the emergency care of children.

The material in this second edition of *Pediatric Emergency Nursing* reflects this increase in knowledge and incorporates the suggestions of colleagues who used the first edition. Chapters from the first edition have been revised and expanded. Eight new chapters have been added. They include Emergency Medical Services for Children; Triage; Physical Assessment; Developmental Considerations; Sociocultural Issues Related to Child Health Care; Legal Issues; Transportation of Critically Injured or Ill Children; and Care of the Pediatric Organ Transplant Recipient.

Pediatric Emergency Nursing has been written for nurses practicing in a variety of settings, including emergency departments treating both children and adults; emergency departments in children's hospitals; transportation care; and pre-hospital care. This book also serves as a reference for nurses practicing in any setting where they may encounter an acutely injured or ill child.

Pediatric Emergency Nursing, 2nd edition, has been written from the perspective that nursing expertise is essential to the successful treatment of an acutely ill or injured child in an emergency department or other emergency setting. Each chapter provides a comprehensive approach to the nursing care of the child and family, organized within the nursing process framework. The nursing diagnoses included were selected from those approved by the North American Nursing Diagnosis Association and are meant to serve as examples of nursing diagnoses and defining characteristics that may, upon patient assessment, be appropriate for the clinical entity discussed.

The book is organized into five major areas: Foundations of Emergency Nursing Care of Children; Psychosocial Emergencies; Cardiorespiratory Emergencies; Trauma and Environmental Emergencies; and Medical Emergencies. Topics were selected according to their importance and prevalence in emergency settings. Although emphasis is placed on true emergency conditions, select nonemergency disease entities and injuries of an urgent nature are also included.

A major strength of the second edition is contributors who are recognized experts in their specialized areas of pediatric emergency nursing. Extensive use of tables throughout the text facilitates quick access to vital information. Numerous illustrations enhance the reader's understanding of disease processes, mechanisms of injury, and nursing interventions. Appendices include teaching instructions for parents for select illnesses and injuries; normal pediatric laboratory values; recommended immunization schedules; and growth charts.

Susan J. Kelley

Acknowledgments

The completion of the second edition was made possible by the efforts and talents of many people. I am especially grateful to the contributing authors for sharing their expertise and giving so generously of their time.

I express my sincere appreciation to the staff of Appleton & Lange, especially David Carroll, Senior Editor; Sally Barhydt, Editor-in-Chief of Nursing; Jennifer Sinsavich, Production Editor; and John Williams, Senior Managing Editor.

I am especially grateful to Elaine Boyle of Boston College for her outstanding secretarial support and good nature. I also acknowledge the assistance of Stephen Vedder of the Boston College Audiovisual Department for preparation of artwork for the book. Special thanks go to Suzanne DeBenedetto, Katherine Ladetto, and Anne Lippman of Boston College for their library assistance.

Thank you to Lorna Grazio, RN, BS, for providing several of the drawings by sexually abused children;

Seth Asser, MD, and Barton Schmitt, MD, for photographs in the child abuse chapter; Richard DeNise, MD, for x rays in the respiratory emergencies chapter; and Kate Feinstein, MD, for the x ray in the Gastrointestinal Emergencies chapter.

Thank you to Annette Grace, RN, MS, and Diane Limbo, RN, MS, for their assistance to Patricia Kraepelein-Bartels on the nursing diagnosis sections in the ENT chapter.

Many individuals have generously given me their collegiality, advice, and friendship during this project. Special thanks to Pamela Burke, Joellen Hawkins, Sandy Mott, Barbara Hazard Munro, Lisa Bernardo, Anne Phelan, and Jan Fredrickson.

To my mother and father, Mary Ellen and James Kelley, my brother, Jim, and sister, Linda, thanks for all of your love and support through the years. And finally, my warmest appreciation to my husband, Ron Verni, for your unending love and encouragement.

Foreword

"Pediatric emergency"—two words that cause even the most experienced emergency nurse to develop a knot in her or his stomach—and that's a good thing. It's OK to be a little scared. It keeps your senses astute and your mind open. It means that you are honest. When I think about the very first pediatric emergency patient I ever cared for, I can remember feeling very frightened and saying lots of prayers asking for help to do the right things. When I think about the last pediatric emergency patient I cared for, I still have some of those same feelings, and I still say the same prayers. No matter how prepared we think we are to deal with a sick or injured child, we can never be prepared enough . . . because *it's a child*.

In the past, little focus was placed on the care of the ill or injured child in the emergency care setting by emergency nurses. Emergency nursing textbooks included chapters on pediatric emergencies, but not enough. Emergency departments developed policies and procedures for the care of the pediatric emergency patients, but not enough. Emergency nursing courses included sections on the pediatric emergency patient, but not enough. That is why this book is important.

Susan Kelley has done a marvelous job of bringing together experts in pediatric emergency care to write chapters for this book. Experts who are willing to share their knowledge with us. Experts whose willingness to share this information will enhance our ability to deliver the highest level of care possible. We owe it to the children who are entrusted to our care to know as much as we can about how to care for them. We owe it to ourselves to be as prepared as we can possibly be and to be able to be a functional and proficient member of the emergency care team.

Of all of the blessings that one can receive in a professional nursing career, perhaps the most profound is to be able to care for an ill or injured child. It is a blessing that brings us to the heights and depths of emotion. It is a gift that gives much meaning to what we do. And it is the ultimate challenge.

Susan Budassi Sheehy, RN, MSN, CEN
1995 President, Emergency Nurses Association
Trauma Clinical Nurse Specialist
Dartmouth-Hitchcock Medical Center
Lebanon, New Hampshire

PEDIATRIC EMERGENCY NURSING

2nd Edition

Part 1

Foundations of Emergency Nursing Care of Children

Chapter 1

Emergency Medical Services for Children

DEBORAH PARKMAN HENDERSON

"It is well known that half of our children die before the age of eight. That is Nature's Law. Why try to change it?"

Jean-Jacques Rousseau, 1762

INTRODUCTION

Today it is hard to imagine how the deaths of half of children younger than 8 years could have been accepted with such equanimity. Fortunately, the health care of infants and children has undergone remarkable transformations in recent history, and very sophisticated and effective methods of treating most serious childhood illnesses and injuries are now available. In pediatric emergency care, as knowledge and technology have become more advanced, access to organized systems of care has become increasingly important in saving the lives of children. All levels of providers and facilities caring for ill and injured pediatric patients should have the staffing, equipment, and education to recognize and stabilize the conditions of children with life-threatening illnesses and injuries. Once these patients have entered the emergency medical services (EMS) system, prompt access to definitive care is possible only through effective mobilization of community resources.

DIFFERENCES BETWEEN ADULTS AND CHILDREN

The need for specialized care for children in emergency settings has been recognized and documented

within the last decade (Ramenofsky et al, 1984; Seidel et al, 1984). Problems in the care of critically ill and injured children were generally attributed to: (1) lack of access to specialized care centers; (2) lack of understanding of the severity of illness or injury; and (3) improper care of pediatric patients. It is now universally acknowledged that there are clear differences between the emergency care of children and that of adults, and that these differences should be reflected in all aspects of prehospital and in-hospital care. Some of the most important differences are in

- General assessment of a critically ill or injured child
- Airway management and ventilation
- Treatment of head injuries
- Vascular access
- Fluid administration

There are also considerable differences in the management of fractures, metabolic imbalances, and psychosocial issues. Child abuse and neglect, injury prevention, and developmental problems are additional areas in which children have unique needs. These differences must be considered in developing a system of pediatric emergency care and in organizing a network of community resources for pediatric patients.

HISTORY OF EMS SYSTEMS

The earliest EMS systems in the United States—one in Los Angeles, California, the other in Dade County, Florida—were organized and implemented in 1969

(Boyd, 1983). These early EMS systems were largely designed by cardiologists, anesthesiologists, and surgeons. They were developed primarily for adult cardiac and trauma patients. To increase access to emergency care, the Emergency Medical Services Act of 1973 (PL 93-154) provided funding for the development of comprehensive EMS systems. Fifteen necessary components of EMS were recognized in this law, and funding was directed to improve all aspects of prehospital care. During this period, grants from the Robert Wood Johnson Foundation also helped to organize EMS systems and to improve field communication.

INCIDENCE OF PEDIATRIC ILLNESS AND INJURY

The developers of the early EMS systems did not anticipate the tremendous growth in the scope of and demand for their services, nor did they anticipate the use of the systems for the care and transport of pediatric patients. Although children are seen less frequently than adults in the prehospital setting, research has shown that 10% of prehospital responses are for children younger than 18 years and that at least 20–35% (in rare cases up to 50%) of emergency department (ED) visits involve pediatric patients (Tsai and Kallsen, 1987; Seidel et al, 1991). Children are transported most frequently between noon and midnight and are most likely to require emergency medical care on weekends. The EMS system is used less frequently for the transport of children in rural areas than in urban areas; children are often transported by family vehicles in rural areas. In both rural and urban areas, however, pediatric emergencies are divided almost equally between medical and traumatic emergencies, although slightly greater percentages of traumatic injuries are seen by prehospital personnel in rural areas (Seidel et al, 1991).

The most common traumatic complaints for pediatric patients in the prehospital setting are head trauma, lacerations, and abrasions; the most common medical complaints are seizures, ingestions, and respiratory distress. More field procedures are used for traumatic injuries than for medical problems, and medications are infrequently used for children younger than 14 years (Seidel et al, 1991). When pediatric patients are assessed in the field, vital signs are taken less frequently for children than for adults, especially for children younger than 2 years. It has been shown that prehospital personnel are less confident in assessing children; many cite lack of cooperation on the part of pediatric patients as being a barrier to assessment (Gausche et al, 1990).

EMERGENCY MANAGEMENT FOR PEDIATRIC PATIENTS

Early research focused attention on problems in the emergency treatment of pediatric patients. The findings indicated that morbidity and mortality were greater for children when the patients did not have access to well-organized, regionalized care (Ramenofsky et al, 1984; Seidel et al, 1984). The essential issues in emergency care, described by Ramenofsky et al (1984), are: (1) initial identification of injured patients; (2) field care, which initiates treatment of the patient and sustains life until definitive care is reached; (3) triage of patients to appropriate facilities; (4) transport of critically injured patients to definitive care; (5) definitive care at a level equal to the needs of the patient; and (6) rehabilitation. Each component is an important factor in the care of pediatric patients and has the potential to affect the outcome.

Identification
Identification of ill and injured children requires an educated public with knowledge of how and when to gain access to the emergency care system. It also requires prehospital care providers with education and expertise in assessing pediatric patients. The general public must be aware of what constitutes an emergency, some first aid procedures, and the fastest way to obtain emergency care. Providers of prehospital and emergency health care should be able to identify critical illness and injury in pediatric patients and should be especially aware of the early signs of pediatric respiratory distress, respiratory failure, and shock (Chameides, 1988).

Field Care
Field treatment protocols are necessary to address the needs of pediatric patients. When on-line medical control is unavailable, prehospital care providers should have clear guidelines for the treatment of pediatric patients, including per-kilogram dosages of medications. Knowledge of methods of accurately assessing the weight of children, such as the Broselow tape method, should limit error (Lubitz et al, 1988). Lists of equipment for prehospital use in age-appropriate sizes are helpful in organizing pediatric kits to be carried by transport providers and first responders; they are being used in many EMS regions.

Triage
An important aspect of the development of EMS for children (EMSC) is the design of efficient and effective regional systems of triage. Field triage requires awareness of community levels of pediatric care, knowledge

of available transport systems, and skills in pediatric assessment on the part of the prehospital care providers and base hospital personnel. Specific pediatric triage criteria must be addressed in prehospital and base station protocols for critically ill and injured pediatric patients. In some areas, it may be desirable for prehospital providers to perform triage and request air transport directly from the field (Henderson, 1992).

Transport

Transport systems vary greatly in accessibility, availability, and personnel. Personal preference on the part of personnel arranging transfers may have considerable influence when a transfer is being arranged, so a coordinated approach is necessary (Foltin and Tunik, 1992). The development of EMSC may require comprehensive agreements for helicopter and air transport of patients across county, city, and state lines so that providers are able to transport in a timely manner. Both ground and air transport personnel must have equipment and training to care for pediatric patients (Foltin and Tunik, 1992).

Definitive Care

A tiered approach to definitive care is often advisable to coordinate pediatric emergency care in a region; critically ill and injured pediatric patients are categorized and transported to facilities equipped to meet their needs. Community-wide standards for levels of care can assist in assuring the availability of staffing and equipment in hospitals receiving pediatric patients through the EMS system. An example of this is Los Angeles County's pediatric emergency care system, which is two-tiered: pediatric critical care centers (PCCCs) constitute the higher level of care, and emergency departments approved for pediatrics (EDAP) are used for less critically ill or injured patients. This model has been used by many states in the process of development of EMSC. In some areas, especially in rural and semi-rural areas, where transport times may be an hour or more, an additional level of care may be required to stabilize a patient's condition before transport to definitive care. An intermediate level of care may be required for children in communities that lack intensive care units (Pediatric Rural Emergency Systems and Education Project, 1991).

The characteristics and requirements of the levels of pediatric care may vary considerably depending on the population base and the facilities and resources available. A community-based effort to develop standards has been used successfully in many regions, and may help to assure cooperation. In all cases, EMSC must include access to tertiary care facilities, sometimes out of state, for the small number of the critically ill and injured pediatric patients who need the highest level of care. Both prehospital care providers and hospital personnel must have information about the types of care available at all levels and about the transport and transfer protocols.

Rehabilitation

The development of EMSC includes comprehensive care of pediatric patients through the rehabilitation phase of care and return to the community. There are many repercussions of hospitalization, both physical and psychological, for the child and for the family (Leahey and Wright, 1987). In addition to the obvious stresses of illness, injury, and hospitalization, regionalization of care brings with it the additional stress of displacement. Regional centers that care for seriously ill and injured children should address the long-term effects of the disease on patients from the moment of their entry into the system. In addition, traveling to regional centers may pose problems for families, and the absence of familiar support systems may weaken customary coping mechanisms. The needs of hospitalized children and their families for support and rehabilitation mandate the development of programs to meet these needs (Seidel and Henderson, 1991e).

ADDITIONAL COMPONENTS

Several other components of pediatric emergency care are involved in reducing mortality and morbidity among children in emergency care systems. These components include prevention, education, quality improvement, and research.

Prevention

It is well known that trauma is the leading cause of death in children from 1 to 14 years of age. Motor vehicle crashes are the leading cause of traumatic deaths in children, followed by submersion incidents (Micik et al, 1987). Almost all childhood injuries are preventable, and any regionalized care system must involve comprehensive injury prevention programs, including community education and outreach. Hospitals are an obvious resource to assist in developing community injury prevention programs, such as car seat lending programs, instruction in the use of seat restraints, and drowning prevention programs. Prevention programs that bring about a reduction in motor vehicle crashes and submersion injuries can greatly reduce deaths from childhood trauma (National Committee for Injury Prevention and Control, 1989). In recent years, more attention has been focused on injury prevention. Two national centers for dissemination of information about childhood injury prevention form the Children's Safety Network.* Several other more specialized centers are funded through the Department of Health and Human Services, Maternal Child Health Bureau. Other national campaigns such as the Coalition for America's Children (1710 Rhode Island Ave. NW 4th Floor, Washington DC 20036) and the National SAFE KIDS Campaign (111 Michigan Ave. SW, Washington DC 20010-2970), are working to increase public awareness of childhood injury and to develop national coalitions and injury prevention programs.

A disproportionate amount of time and resources is often spent on the care of illnesses when prevention programs may offer great benefits to large numbers of children. Pediatric morbidity and mortality also may be reduced by community education in the early treatment of illnesses and by immunization programs. Regionalized pediatric care systems are responsible for providing leadership in promoting prevention of illness and for serving as resources for information about illness prevention programs.

Education

Education and training of health care personnel are major concerns in improving pediatric emergency care. With the leadership of the American Academy of Pediatrics (AAP), pediatric emergency medicine became recognized as a medical subspecialty. A board examination was offered for the first time in 1992. Several programs for continuing education in pediatric emergency care are also available. In the last three years, two national courses have been developed: (1) the Pediatric Advanced Life Support (PALS) course developed by the American Heart Association and the American Academy of Pediatrics (Chameides, 1988) and (2) the Advanced Pediatric Life Support (APLS) course developed by the AAP and the American College of Emergency Physicians (Bushore et al, 1990). The PALS course lasts 2 days and focuses on early recognition of respiratory distress and shock in pediatric patients and on resuscitation. This course is designed primarily for health care providers who work in acute care areas. The course is offered nationally through the American Heart Association. The APLS course lasts several days longer than PALS and includes recognition and medical treatment of a wide variety of acute illnesses and injuries; it is designed primarily for physicians. Programs in pediatric emergency care targeted specifically for a nursing audience

*Children's Safety Network Education Development Center, Inc., 55 Chapel St., Newton MA 02160; Children's Safety Network National Center for Education in Maternal and Child Health, 2000 N. 15th St. Suite 701, Arlington VA 22201.

are less available, but several are under development (Seidel and Henderson, 1991b).

Because prehospital care began with adult cardiac and trauma care, training for prehospital personnel often does not have a strong pediatric component. Paramedics and emergency medical technicians (EMTs) should have specific instruction in pediatric emergency care, and they should continue to have didactic and clinical education in pediatric emergency care on an ongoing basis. Several prehospital programs have been developed and are becoming more widely used (Washington State EMSC, 1988). The Department of Transportation provides national guidelines for the various levels of EMT training. The department will be revising the guidelines for the basic curriculum to include greater emphasis on pediatric emergency care.

Quality Improvement

An ongoing, timely, and thorough assessment of services rendered in emergency care systems can assist in maintaining and improving the level of health care provided to pediatric patients. Each component of EMSC from injury prevention through rehabilitation should be reviewed. A criteria-based quality assurance program is essential in a regionalized system of pediatric emergency care to ensure compliance with the system, to review care, to identify problem areas, and to improve services (Seidel and Henderson, 1991d). Objective review, using proven methods of evaluation, should be used whenever possible. Problem areas can be discussed and improved through cooperative arrangements such as the Pediatric Liaison Nurse (PdLN) groups in Los Angeles and in San Francisco, in which nurses representing the EDAP facilities meet on a regular basis to share information, to review quality improvement issues, and to provide education. Pediatric registries, collaborative studies, and individualized quality improvement and risk management programs enable efficient and effective systems to prove their worth. They also provide the opportunity for systems that are not functioning well to define areas for improvement. Health care providers must learn to accept review of care at all levels and to see this type of self examination as beneficial to patients and providers alike.

Data Collection and Research

In the early days of EMS systems, research about the care of pediatric patients was instrumental in documenting the need for improvement (Seidel et al, 1984). All phases of pediatric emergency care continue to invite study. The field is still new and exciting and the potential to affect system development and national decision-making is high. To date, there is little agreement as to what data should be collected by EMS systems, and there is much variability in the definitions of data components (Seidel and Henderson, 1991a). At the national level, pediatric trauma registries are beginning to provide some data, but there is still little information about pediatric patients with medical problems. An important and unanswered research question is whether time-consuming procedures, such as attempts at venous access, should be performed when transport times are short and whether the potential benefit of prehospital procedures is clearly worth the additional time in the field. Some focused research is currently underway to determine the effectiveness and usefulness of endotracheal intubation and intravenous line placement (New York City Targeted Issues Grant, 1992). This type of research is essential to assist in the development of useful guidelines and protocols for prehospital providers of care.

Most important, there are no available comparative data on the outcomes of pediatric patients cared for before and after the integration of EMSC components into EMS systems. The number of variables involved, including varieties of prehospital care response, distances traveled, range of ages, and types of illnesses and injuries makes an accurate evaluation extremely difficult. Perhaps the greatest obstacle in conducting research in this area is the difficulty of tracking individual patients from the moment of identification and the dispatch of trained providers through the entire system of care and back into the community. Persisting in this effort is important, however. With limited health care resources, information is needed to determine the most essential interventions and to assure continued funding for necessary programs (Seidel and Henderson, 1991c).

THE EMSC INITIATIVE

Once the problems in caring for pediatric patients in EMS systems were well recognized, federal legislation was drafted to provide funding for demonstration projects in pediatric emergency care. Because of the determined efforts of Cal Sia, MD, and Senator Daniel Inouye (D-HI) and his staff assistant Patrick DeLeon, PhD, JD, federal funding was made available in 1985 through the Department of Health and Human Services, Health Resources and Services Administration, Maternal and Child Health Bureau, for four EMSC demonstration projects. The first grants were awarded to Alabama, California, New York, and Oregon. Funding for eight additional grants was provided in 1987, and four new grants have been awarded each year since then. As of 1993, 35 states had received EMSC funding (Emergency Medical Services for Children, 1993).

The EMSC initiative is an ongoing effort to improve pediatric emergency care in EMS systems. Applicants for EMSC funding are encouraged to address all areas of pediatric emergency care from injury prevention through rehabilitation (Figure 1–1). Some of the areas addressed by EMSC projects include the following.

Prehospital Triage and Transport
Many of the EMSC projects developed protocols for triage and transport. Some of these protocols are for urban areas (New York City, Los Angeles) and some are for more rural areas (California, Idaho, Wisconsin). In Santa Cruz County, California, an algorithm was developed to assist prehospital providers in coordinat-

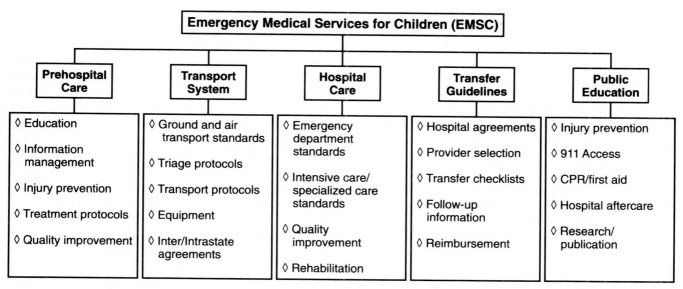

Figure 1–1. Components of emergency medical services systems to be considered in EMSC development.

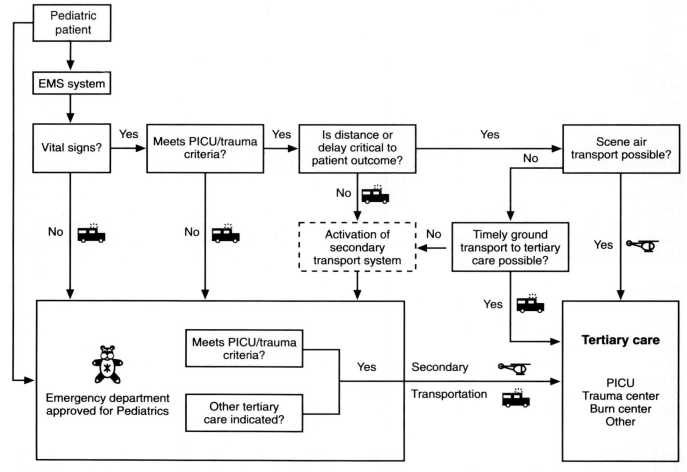

Figure 1–2. Santa Cruz County EMS Agency Pediatric Transport Protocol. PICU, pediatric intensive care unit; EDAP, emergency department approved for pediatrics.

ing transport of pediatric patients from the field directly to definitive care (Figure 1–2). A goal of the Utah EMSC Project has been to develop a regionalized system of air transport covering the tri-state area of Montana, Wyoming, and Utah. Regional protocols and educational programs are being developed throughout this intermountain region.

Education for Emergency Personnel

Eleven comprehensive prehospital curricula have been developed with EMSC funding. Some of these training programs are designed for basic EMTs, and others are for advanced levels of care. The length of these courses varies from 4 hours to 1 week long. The courses include a variety of educational approaches. Idaho EMSC developed a sophisticated interactive video learning program that is taken by a mobile training unit to rural areas. Training programs for emergency physicians have been developed by the Arkansas EMSC Project. Several nursing education programs also resulted from EMSC funding. The most

comprehensive nursing program, developed as a collaborative effort of 12 EMSC grantees, is the Pediatric Emergency Nursing Collaborative Curriculum, a self-learning modular course providing continuing education credit through the Emergency Nurses Association. This course was especially developed to meet the needs of nurses in rural areas, who often do not have access to national courses or other continuing education in pediatric emergency care. Florida EMSC (1990) used a lecture and seminar format in developing the PED-NIC course, which has been adapted and given in many states. The Arkansas EMSC Project developed a program in pediatric emergency care for physicians, and many EMSC projects have adopted standards that include completion of the PALS or APLS course.

Rehabilitation

Several EMSC Projects developed programs for children with long-term disabilities caused by critical illness or injury. The Washington, DC EMSC Project (1990) developed materials to help emergency personnel identify head-injured pediatric patients with potential for long-term disability, and to assist parents of children with head injuries in adapting to the disabilities.

Research
Some useful research has been performed by EMSC grantees. A study conducted by the EMSC project in Oregon showed that critically ill pediatric patients cared for in non-tertiary-care facilities have poorer outcomes. This would indicate that a system that assures identification and transport of critically ill and injured pediatric patients to appropriate facilities can improve outcomes (Pollack et al, 1991). Research by Quan et al (1991) showed that pediatric patients with submersion injuries have improved outcomes with endotracheal intubation in the field.

Specialized Programs
Programs developed through EMSC address such areas as minority access to emergency care, farm injury prevention, suicide prevention, cultural sensitivity training, Native American health issues, and emergency care of children with disabilities (Shaperman and Backer, 1991).

National Centers
A national EMSC network was established in 1990; it includes the National EMSC Resource Alliance (NERA) and the National Resource Center (NRC). The NERA (1124 W. Carson St. Building N-7, Torrance CA 90502) is responsible for dissemination of information about EMSC, coordinating the evaluation and distribution of EMSC products, and providing consultation and information to agencies and individuals interested in improving pediatric emergency care. The NRC (111 Michigan Ave. NW, Washington, DC 20010) is available to assist new and continuing EMSC grantees in public policy issues, developing coalitions, and continued funding of EMSC components.

To date, 35 states have received EMSC funding to improve pediatric emergency care (Emergency Medical Services for Children, 1993). EMSC should be designed to fit the unique needs and resources of each state or region. Agencies, organizations, and institutions that provide care for critically ill and injured children in each region should continue to be actively involved in the review, operation, and improvement of these systems.

The Future of EMSC
The movement to improve the care of ill and injured children is continuing and expanding. There is rarely any argument with the goal of improving health care for children; when this goal is consistently kept in

focus, EMSC development and integration into EMS systems is more readily accepted. Regionalized systems that are developed collaboratively and implemented with the support of an educated community have the best chance of improving the care of children in the emergency medical system. To assure that critically ill and injured children receive appropriate services and are rapidly transported to appropriate facilities, regionally organized systems of care should be available in all states.

With the growing awareness that EMS systems need to address the needs of children comes the responsibility of health care providers to conduct research that documents the effects of EMSC implementation. To date, little research has been done; it will be essential to demonstrate the need for improvements in pediatric emergency care and to assist in obtaining funding for these improvements. Although it seems reasonable to suppose that improved education, training, equipment, and management will ultimately result in improved care for pediatric patients and in reduced morbidity and mortality for ill and injured children cared for in EMS systems, there is a continued need to document the usefulness of such improvements.

The most important element in implementing any type of coordinated care for ill and injured pediatric patients is commitment; commitment on the part of civic leaders, public agencies, health care providers, and the general public. Once this commitment is assured, the collaborative effort should include concerned individuals from many disciplines. Planning groups may include prehospital care providers, nurses, physicians, lawyers, representatives from public and private agencies, hospital administrators, and consumers. Involvement of health care providers at all levels from the inception greatly facilitates implementation of protocols and standards that meet the needs of a community. Improving pediatric emergency care is not necessarily expensive, but it does require reorganization of resources and a community-wide effort. This effort, however, will have long-lasting effects: Our children are our future.

REFERENCES
Boyd DR (1983). The history of emergency medical services in the United States of America. In Boyd DR, Edlich RE, Micik S (eds), *Systems approach to emergency medical care.* Norwalk: Appleton-Century-Crofts

Bushore M, Fleisher G, Seidel JS, Wagner D (1990). *Course Curriculum, Advanced Pediatric Life Support.* Dallas: American College of Emergency Physicians, American Academy of Pediatrics

Chameides L (ed) (1988). *Textbook of Pediatric Advanced Life Support.* Dallas: American Heart Association

Emergency Medical Services for Children. (1993). *Abstracts of active projects FY 1993.* Arlington, Va: National Center for Education in Maternal and Child Health, pp 1–102

Florida EMSC Project and University Medical Center, Jacksonville. (1990). *Emergency nursing–advanced pediatric management course.* Jacksonville, Fla: University Medical Center

Foltin GL, Tunik MG (1992). Transport systems. In Dieckmann RA (ed), *Pediatric emergency care systems: Planning and management.* Baltimore: Williams and Wilkins, pp 220–229

Gausche M, Henderson DP, Seidel JS, Ward P, Wayland B, Ness B (1990). Vital signs as part of the prehospital assessment of the pediatric patient. *Annals of Emergency Medicine,* 19:173–178

Henderson DP (1992). Rural EMSC development. In Dieckmann RA (ed), *Pediatric emergency care systems: Planning and management.* Baltimore: Williams and Wilkins, pp 450–461

Leahey M, Wright LM (1987). *Families and life-threatening illness.* Springhouse, Pa: Springhouse Corporation, pp 29–41

Lubitz DS, Seidel JS, Luten RC, Zaritsky AL, Campbell FW (1988). A rapid method for estimating weight and resuscitation drug dosages from length in the pediatric age group. *Annals of Emergency Medicine* 17:576–581

Micik S, Yuwiler J, Walker C (1987). *Preventing childhood injuries.* San Marcos, Calif: North County Health Services

The National Committee for Injury Prevention and Control (1989). Injury prevention: Meeting the challenge. *American Journal of Preventive Medicine* 5 Suppl: 1–303

New York City EMSC Targeted Issues Grant (1992). U.S. Department of Health and Human Services, Maternal and Child Health Bureau.

Pediatric Rural Emergency Systems and Education Project (1991). *Emergency medical services for children: Development and integration of pediatric emergency care into EMS systems.* Washington, DC, and Princeton, NJ: U.S. Department of Health and Human Services, Health Resources and Services Administration, Maternal and Child Health Bureau, and the Robert Wood Johnson Foundation

Pollack MM, Alexander SR, Clarke N, Ruttimann UE, Tesselaar HM, Bachulis AC (1991). Improved outcomes from tertiary center pediatric intensive care: A statewide comparison of tertiary and nontertiary care facilities. *Critical Care Medicine* 19:150–159

Quan L, Wentz KR, Gore EJ, Copass MK (1989). Outcome and predictors of outcome in pediatric submersion victims receiving prehospital care in King County, Washington. *Pediatrics* 86;4:586–593

Ramenofsky M, Lutterman A, Quidlen A, et al (1984). Maximum survival in pediatric trauma: The ideal system. *Journal of Trauma* 24:818–823

Seidel J, Henderson DP (1991a). Data collection and analysis: A collaborative effort. In Seidel J, Henderson DP (eds), *Emergency medical services for children: A report to the nation.* Washington, DC: National Center for Education in Maternal and Child Health, pp 131–141

Seidel J, Henderson DP (1991b). Education. In *Emergency medical services for children: A report to the nation.* Washington, DC: National Center for Education in Maternal and Child Health, pp 49–62

Seidel J, Henderson DP (1991c). Financing EMSC. In *Emergency medical services for children: A report to the nation.* Washington, DC: National Center for Education in Maternal and Child Health, pp 143–154

Seidel J, Henderson DP (1991d). Quality assurance. In *Emergency medical services for children: A report to the nation.* Washington, DC: National Center for Education in Maternal and Child Health, pp 109–129

Seidel J, Henderson DP (1991e). Rehabilitation. In Seidel J, Henderson DP (eds), *Emergency medical services for children: A report to the nation.* Washington, DC: National Center for Education in Maternal and Child Health, pp 63–82

Seidel JS, Henderson DP, Ward P, Wayland BW, Ness B (1991). Pediatric prehospital care in urban and rural areas. *Pediatrics* 88:681–690

Seidel JS, Hornbein M, Yoshiyama K, et al (1984). Emergency medical services and the pediatric patient: Are the needs being met? *Pediatrics* 73:769–772

Shaperman J, Backer TE (1991). *Emergency medical services for children innovation bank.* Washington, DC: National Center for Education in Maternal and Child Health

Tsai A, Kallsen G (1987). Epidemiology of pediatric prehospital care. *Annals of Emergency Medicine* 16:284–292

Washington State EMSC (1988). *Pediatric prehospital care.* Seattle: Washington EMSC Project

Washington D.C. EMSC Project (1990). *EMSC assessment battery for the brain injured child.* Washington, DC: Washington DC EMSC Project

CHAPTER 2

Triage

JAN M. FREDRICKSON

INTRODUCTION

Triage is a French word that means to pick, choose, sort, or select. The term was originally used in a medical context by the French during World War I. It referred to a place where wounded soldiers were triaged, or sorted, to appropriate hospitals. Triage, or sorting, has been used to prioritize care in the United States military since World War I (Rund and Rausch, 1981).

After World War II, the number of patient visits to emergency rooms increased dramatically. Patient triage in the emergency department (ED) was initially performed by physicians, but now it is usually done by registered nurses. As early as 1966, specific pediatric triage systems were in place.

Triage is used in EDs to categorize patients into groups based on the seriousness of their illness or injury. Pediatric patients account for approximately 25–35% of general ED visits nationally each year (Seidel and Henderson, 1991). Infants and children may present to the ED in a well, acutely ill, chronically ill, or critically ill condition. Minor complaints may sometimes indicate serious illness. Children are also labile, and their condition may rapidly improve or deteriorate. Consequently, children require careful triage to prevent increased morbidity or mortality.

GOALS OF TRIAGE

The most crucial component of a pediatric triage system is rapid identification of a serious illness or injury. Other goals include prioritization of care for all pa-

tients and control of patient flow in the ED. The triage assessment also must be documented in a consistent and expedient manner. In some triage systems, diagnostic or therapeutic measures such as x rays or antipyretics are initiated. Children with highly contagious diseases and immunosuppressed children should be isolated by the triage nurse. Finally, the triage nurse should promote good consumer relations with patients and parents.

PRE-HOSPITAL TRIAGE

In several areas of the country, pediatric pre-hospital care has become regionalized to transport children to facilities specially equipped to care for them. A prototype system developed in 1984 in Los Angeles utilizes Emergency Departments Approved for Pediatrics (EDAPs) and Pediatric Critical Care Centers (PCCCs) (Seidel and Gausche, 1992).

Hospitals that meet basic pediatric standards are designated EDAPs. Hospitals with a pediatric intensive care unit (PICU), trauma center designation, and specified pediatric medical subspecialists, equipment, and ancillary services can apply for PCCC status. Critically ill or injured pediatric patients are transported by paramedics to the nearest PCCC (Table 2–1). All other pediatric patients are transported to the nearest EDAP. There are currently approximately 70 EDAPs and nine PCCCs in Los Angeles County. Pediatric ED guidelines are now being developed for all California hospitals through an Emergency Medical Services for Children (EMSC) grant.

To qualify as an EDAP, a hospital must meet spe-

TABLE 2–1. GUIDELINES FOR PATIENT REQUIRING TRANSPORT TO A PEDIATRIC CRITICAL CARE CENTER (PCCC)

Trauma	Medical
Hypotension	Unstable vital signs
Abnormal capillary refill	Severe respiratory distress
No spontaneous eye opening	Cyanosis
Penetrating cranial injury	Profuse bleeding
Penetrating thoracic injury between the midclavicular lines	Altered mental status
Gunshot wound to abdomen or thorax	Cardiac dysrhythmias
Blunt injury to chest with unstable chest wall (flail chest)	Status epilepticus
Penetrating injury to neck	Severe dehydration
Diffuse abdominal tenderness (following blunt or penetrating trauma)	Near drowning
Falls from a height > 15 feet	Moderate to severe burns
Intrusion of motor vehicle into passenger space	Suspected child abuse

Los Angeles Pediatric Society. *Information handbook for emergency departments approved for pediatrics and pediatric critical care centers.* Los Angeles: Los Angeles Pediatric Society, 1984.

cific requirements for pediatric equipment and physician coverage. Each facility must also have a designated pediatric liaison nurse (PdLN), who acts as a clinical resource, coordinates pediatric emergency nursing education, and administers a pediatric nursing quality improvement program for ED patients. The role of the PdLN can be modified for use in almost any ED setting. The goal of the PdLN is to promote optimal care for pediatric patients in the ED (Fredrickson, 1988).

THE TRIAGE NURSE

A triage nurse must have excellent assessment, communication, and organizational skills (Kitt & Kaiser, 1990). Nurses should attend a formal education program before being assigned to triage. This program should include both didactic information and clinical practice with an experienced triage nurse. The ED should have written triage guidelines. Because of the expertise required for the triage of children, nurses should have a strong foundation of ED experience, including care of pediatric patients, before functioning in this role.

THE TRIAGE SETTING

The triage area should allow visibility of both the waiting area and the entrance to the ED. The child and

parents' privacy should be protected as much as possible during the triage interview and assessment. Unfortunately, the question of personal safety for the triage nurse must be addressed. The triage area should be equipped with a telephone for immediate access to hospital security or the police department in the event that a patient or a visitor is armed or potentially violent.

TRIAGE SYSTEMS

The most common triage system divides patient's conditions into three categories (Weinerman, 1966).

Triage Level

1. Emergent. The condition requires immediate medical attention; time delay is harmful to patient; disorder is acute and potentially threatening to life or function.
2. Urgent. The condition requires medical attention within the period of a few hours; there is possible danger to the patient if medical attention is not given; disorder is acute but not necessarily severe.
3. Non-urgent. The condition does not require the resources of an emergency service; referral for routine medical care may or may not be needed; disorder is nonacute or is minor in severity.

Table 2–2 includes a list of emergent and urgent pediatric triage criteria.

EMERGENCY DEPARTMENT TRIAGE

Pediatric triage ideally begins when the patient first enters the ED waiting area. This "across the room assessment" (Soud, 1990) facilitates the earliest identification of conditions requiring emergent treatment.

Factors Assessed from Across the Room

1. State of health—Does the child appear well, mildly ill, or seriously ill?
2. Presence of respiratory distress—Is breathing rapid or labored? Is wheezing or stridor audible?
3. Color—Is the child cyanotic, dusky, mottled, or pale?
4. Level of consciousness—Is the child alert, active, and responsive to the environment? Is he or she listless, lethargic, or comatose?

Emergently ill children should be sent to the treatment area immediately. Patients who have highly contagious diseases or who are immunocompromised should be isolated. The triage nurse should monitor

TABLE 2–2. MAJOR PEDIATRIC TRIAGE CATEGORIES

■ **Emergent**

Abnormal vital signs

Age	Systolic BP (mm Hg)	Pulse (beats/min)	Respirations (breaths/min)
0–2	<60	<80	<15 or >40
2–5	<70	<60	<10 or >30
>5	<90	<50	<5 or >25

Respirations
  Irregular
  Apneic
  Labored
Pulse
  Irregular
  Dysrhythmic
Coma
Cyanosis
Status epilepticus
Multiple or major trauma
  Head
    Loss of consciousness
    Altered mental status
    Changing neurologic or asymmetric neurologic findings
    CSF leak
    Depressed fracture
  Neck or spinal injury
  Chest
  Abdomen

Orthopedic
  Two or more long bone fractures
  Pelvic fracture
  Potential neurovascular compromise
  Amputation
Major burn
  Bleeding: acute and significant

■ **Urgent**[a]
Abuse, child
Abuse, sexual
Acute symptoms in child <2–3 months
Behavioral alteration
Bite, poisonous snake
Bleeding, moderate
Dehydration
Drowning (near)
Eye: alkali, acid, or chemical burn
Fever ≥ 40°C
GI hemorrhage
Headache: acute and severe
Hypertension
Hyperthermia
Hypothermia
Neck pain or stiffness
Pain: acute and severe
Poisoning
Rash (isolate patient)
SIDS (near)

[a] May be emergent, depending on patient's condition.
[a] If none of these emergent or urgent conditions is present, the patient should be appropriately screened and treated according to normal facility flow patterns unless there is a complicating condition. Repeat visits or very anxious parents may require that the visit be categorized as urgent.
BP, blood pressure; CSF, cerebrospinal fluid; GI, gastrointestinal.
Barkin R, Rosen P (1994). Emergency pediatrics (4th ed). St. Louis: Mosby, p. 7

patient flow and periodically use the foregoing criteria to re-assess patients who remain in the waiting area. Patients should always be seen by the triage nurse before registration procedures are initiated.

Once in the triage area, all pediatric patients should be quickly evaluated for signs and symptoms of serious illness or injury. If the child's condition permits, triage-area assessment should include taking a brief history, taking vital signs, and a quick physical examination.

Pediatric History

A history is composed of subjective data obtained from the pediatric patient or the parent, since children cannot always speak for themselves. The history should include a note about whether or not the parent seems to be a reliable historian and the parent's level of concern about the illness or injury.

The history begins with the chief complaint. This is a brief description of the reason for the visit and should include the duration of the problem.

The triage nurse must elicit additional information about the chief complaint. Questions about the onset, location, duration, timing, associated symptoms, aggravating or relieving factors, and treatment of the problem may be asked. The nurse should inquire about allergies, immunizations, and any clinically significant past medical history. This includes a history of medications taken, trauma, serious illnesses, or hospitalizations. Any history of prematurity or chronic illness, especially an illness that may cause immunocompromise, such as cancer or AIDS, should be noted. The nurse also should ask about exposure to others with symptoms similar to the child's.

Finally, the patient and the parent should be asked how the child's behavior seems to them, what they think may have caused the problem, and if they have any other questions or concerns. A simple method for remembering key components of the history is to take an AMPLE history

Allergies
Medications
Past medical history
Last meal
Events surrounding illness or injury

Vital Signs

The triage nurse should have a general knowledge of normal ranges of pediatric vital signs (Table 2–3). Whenever possible, vital signs should be assessed when the child is quiet. They should always be evaluated with the child's general appearance and other assessment data.

Fever is one of the body's natural ways of fighting infection. Febrile illnesses are common in children, and the degree of temperature elevation is not necessarily proportional to the severity of illness. Mildly ill children may present with high fevers, and critically ill children may have a slight fever or be afebrile. Fever or hypothermia may indicate a serious illness in infants younger than 3 months. These infants' immunologic systems are immature and less able to localize an infection. These infants usually require a full septic work-up to determine the cause of the fever.

Vital signs may deviate from normal for a variety of reasons. Both heart rates and respiratory rates can increase because of fever, respiratory distress, and shock. They can also increase with pain, crying, anxiety, or exercise.

Bradycardia can occur with hypothermia, cardiac disease, and certain medications. It can also occur in athletes, with vagal stimulation, and during sleep.

Decreased respiratory rates or apnea may indicate impending respiratory failure. However, slower respiratory rates also can be seen in athletes, during sleep, and with hypothermia.

Accurate measurement of blood pressure in pediatric patients depends on using the correct cuff size. The blood pressure cuff width should cover approximately two-thirds of the child's upper arm or thigh (Seidel et al, 1991). Using a cuff that is too large gives a falsely low reading, and using a cuff that is too small gives a falsely high reading. It is frequently difficult to auscultate an accurate blood pressure reading in children. Using a Doppler device or Dinamapp can solve this problem.

Hypotension is a late sign of shock in children. *Minimum* acceptable systolic blood pressures are as follows (American Heart Association and American Academy of Pediatrics, 1991).

> Younger than 1 month = 60 mm Hg
> 1 month–1 year = 70 mm Hg
> Older than 1 year = 70 + (2 × age in years) mm Hg

Because blood pressure can be normal in a pediatric patient in a state of shock, the triage nurse must assess other parameters to determine if the child is in a state of cardiovascular compromise. These parameters can be thought of as a fifth vital sign in infants and children (see "Circulation").

Brief Physical Examination

The triage nurse should perform a brief examination of the child to identify any conditions that necessitate emergent treatment. This is called the primary survey. It includes assessment of the ABCs (airway, breathing, circulation), a quick neurological examination, and exposure of the child. The primary survey should be completed in a few minutes or less.

Airway—Assess for Patency and Signs of Distress, which May Include

- Patency—Is the airway open and maintainable, or is it unmaintainable?
- Adventitious airway sounds—stridor, wheezing, or grunting
- Preferred posture—tripoding or holding head to maintain open airway
- Drooling or dysphagia

Breathing—Assess for Signs of Respiratory Distress or Failure, which May Include

- Poor air exchange
- Tachypnea
- Bradypnea or apneic periods
- Retractions, nasal flaring, or head bobbing
- Anxiety
- Altered level of consciousness
- Cyanosis, a late sign

A child with respiratory distress should be given supplemental oxygen *stat*. If respiratory arrest has occurred, rescue breathing should be initiated (see Chapter 13 for a discussion of pediatric basic life support [BLS] and pediatric advanced life support [PALS] techniques).

Circulation—Assess for Signs of Impaired Circulatory Status, which May Include

- Tachycardia
- Abnormal skin signs
  Decreased capillary refill (normal = 2 seconds or less)

TABLE 2–3. VITAL SIGNS BY AGE

Age	Respiration (breaths/minute)	Pulse (beats/minute)	Systolic Blood Pressure (mm Hg)
Newborn	30–60	100–160	50–70
1–6 weeks	30–60	100–160	70–95
6 months	25–40	90–120	80–100
1 year	20–30	90–120	80–100
3 years	20–30	80–120	80–110
6 years	18–25	70–110	80–110
10 years	15–20	60–90	90–120

Seidel J, Henderson D (eds) (1989). Prehospital care of pediatric emergencies. Los Angeles: Los Angeles Pediatric Society, p. 10.

Decreased peripheral pulses
Cool extremities
- Decreased level of consciousness
- Decreased urine output (< 1–2 ml/kg/hr)
- Cyanotic, dusky, mottled, or pale skin color
- Hypotension, a late sign

Neurologic Assessment (Disability)—Assess for Signs of Neurologic Abnormalities, which May Include

- Pupils unequal or nonreactive to light
- Decrease in level of consciousness
    Lethargy
    Decreased response to the environment
    Poor eye contact
    Failure to interact with parents
- Irritability
    May be normal in a sick child
    Primary neurologic problems (eg, meningitis, head trauma, brain tumor) must be ruled out
- Paradoxical irritability (irritable when held and lethargic when left alone) may be seen in infants and small children with neurologic infections
- Abnormal cry—moaning or a high-pitched or unusual cry may be heard with central nervous diseases
- Flaccidity—generalized decreased muscle tone
- Abnormal fontanel
    Bulging may indicate increased intracranial pressure
    Sunken fontanel may be seen in dehydration
- A Pediatric Glasgow Coma Scale score may be obtained using the Pediatric Glasgow Coma Scale (see Chapter 18).

Exposure—Undress the Child to Perform a Thorough Assessment.

Red Flags in Pediatrics
The following warning signs may indicate serious illness or injury.
- Hypothermia
- Fever
    In infants younger than 3 months
    Temperature over 104–105°F (any age)
- Petechiae, purpura
- Indications of child abuse or sexual abuse
- Hypoglycemia
- Dehydration
    Dry mucous membranes or tongue
    Decreased tearing
    Decreased urine output
    Decreased skin turgor
    Sunken fontanel
    Tachycardia
    Decreased peripheral perfusion

- Pain
- History of chronic illness
- Return ED visit within 24 hours
- Sixth sense: A subjective feeling or intuition that a child is more seriously ill than objective data indicate

MEDICOLEGAL ASPECTS OF TRIAGE

Triage is a potentially litigious patient care area because rapid decisions must be made in a stressful environment, sometimes with little information. The patient may be placed at risk and negligence may occur during triage when appropriate patient assessments are not performed, communication between the triage nurse and the patient is poor, or adequate treatments and instructions are not given (Anderson, 1991).

Triage policies, procedures, and protocols should be developed and strictly followed. Emergency departments should have a procedure for care of pediatric patients in the ED. Urgently and non-urgently ill and injured children must be reassessed periodically and triaged to a higher level if necessary.

A patient care record should be initiated for every child who presents to triage area. All patients should be seen by a physician (or a nurse practitioner or physician's assistant if applicable). Patients cannot be denied care for financial reasons. Referrals to other hospitals or clinics must adhere to Consolidated Omnibus Budget Reconciliation Act (COBRA/OBRA) regulations. Inappropriate transfer puts the hospital at increased risk for liability (Anderson, 1991; Singer, 1989).

TELEPHONE TRIAGE

Another potential area of liability is telephone triage in the ED. It is difficult, if not impossible, to adequately evaluate patients over the telephone. Some exceptions occur. For example, patients or parents who call regarding a life-threatening emergency should be instructed to call for help (911 where available) and begin emergency measures. Also, if the patient or parent was seen in the ED within the past 24 hours, questions about treatment or return to the hospital can be discussed. If telephone triage is done, protocols should be followed, and all calls should be logged, recorded, or both.

A continuous quality improvement (CQI) program to monitor the quality of pediatric triage should be developed. Criteria for evaluation may include documentation of the triage visit, appropriate triage level based on history and physical assessment, and comparison of triage level on presentation to the ED and condition at discharge from the ED or admission to the hospital. Educational programs should be developed on the basis of the results of chart reviews; new indicators should be evaluated periodically.

CONCLUSION

Although most children seen by a triage nurse are not critically ill or injured, those who are often cause more anxiety than any other type of patient. Following the guidelines discussed in this chapter will assist the nurse in performing appropriate assessment and triage for all pediatric patients.

REFERENCES

American Heart Association and American Academy of Pediatrics (1988). *Textbook of pediatric advanced life support.* Dallas: American Heart Association

Anderson S (1991). Triage. In Henry G (ed) *Emergency medicine risk management: A comprehensive review.* Dallas: American College of Emergency Physicians

Fredrickson J (1988). The pediatric liaison nurse: A new specialist in the emergency department. *Journal of Emergency Nursing* 15:129

Kitt S, Kaiser J (1990). *Emergency nursing: A physiologic and clinical perspective.* Philadelphia: Saunders, p 31

Rund D, Rausch T (1981). *Triage.* St. Louis: Mosby, pp 1–7

Seidel H, Ball J, Dains J, Benedict W (1991). *Mosby's guide to physical examination,* 2nd edition. St. Louis: CV Mosby, p 31

Seidel J, Gausche M (1992). Standards for emergency departments. In Dieckmann R (ed), *Pediatric emergency care systems: Planning and management,* Baltimore: Williams & Wilkins, pp 267–275

Seidel J, Henderson D (eds) (1991). *Emergency medical services for children: A report to the nation.* Washington, DC: National Center for Education in Maternal and Child Health

Singer L (1989). Review and analysis of federal "antidumping" legislation. Practical advice and unanswered problems. *Journal of Health and Hospital Law* 22:145–149

Soud T (1990). Pediatric triage. In *Emergency nursing; Advanced pediatric management.* Jacksonville: University Medical Center, pp 21–28

Weinerman E, Ratner RS, Robbins A, Lavenham MA (1966). Yale studies in ambulatory medical care: Use of hospital emergency services. *American Journal of Public Health* 56:1037

SUGGESTED READING

American Academy of Pediatrics and American College of Emergency Physicians (1989). *Textbook of advanced pediatric life support.* Elk Grove Village, Ill: AAP, Dallas: ACEP

Barkin R, Rosen P (eds) (1994). *Emergency pediatrics* (4th ed) St. Louis: Mosby

Beach L (1981). Pediatric emergency services triage. *Journal of Emergency Nursing* 7:50–55

Dieckmann R (ed) (1992). *Pediatric emergency care systems: Planning and management.* Baltimore: Williams & Wilkins

Emergency Nurses Association (1991). *Trauma nursing core course (provider) instructor manual* (3rd ed) Chicago: Award Printing Corporation, pp III-1–III-20

Fleisher C, Ludwig S (eds) (1988). *Textbook of pediatric emergency medicine.* Baltimore: Williams & Wilkins

Greene M (1991). *The Harriet Lane handbook* (12th ed) St. Louis: Mosby–Year Book

Grossman M, Dieckmann R (eds) (1991). *Pediatric emergency medicine: A clinician's reference.* Philadelphia: JB Lippincott

Hall M (1987). Assessment and priority setting. In Rea R, Bourg P, Parker J, Rushing D, *Emergency nursing core curriculum* (3rd ed). Philadelphia: Saunders, pp 9–25

Hazinski ME (1992). Children are different. In Hazinski M, *Nursing care of the critically ill child* (2nd ed). St. Louis: Mosby

Henderson D (1988). The Los Angeles pediatric emergency care system. *Journal of Emergency Nursing* 14:96

Hoekelman R (1991). The physical examination of infants and children. In Bates B, *A guide to physical examination and history taking.* Philadelphia: Lippincott, pp 561–633

McCaffery M, Beebe A (1989). *Pain: Clinical manual for nursing practice.* St. Louis: Mosby, pp 264–306

Nichols D, Yaster M, Lappe D, Buck J (1991). *Golden hour: The handbook of advanced pediatric life support.* St. Louis: Mosby–Year Book, pp 1–8

Rivara F, Wall HP, Worley P, et al (1986). Pediatric nurse triage. *American Journal of Diseases of Children* 140:205–210

Sacchetti A, Carracio C, Warden T, Gazak S (1984). Community hospital management of pediatric emergencies. *American Journal of Emergency Medicine* 4:10–14

Seidel J, Henderson D (eds) (1987). *Prehospital care of pediatric emergencies.* Los Angeles: Los Angeles Pediatric Society

Simon J, Goldberg A (1989). *Prehospital pediatric life support.* St. Louis: Mosby, pp 1–13

Thomas D (1988). The ABCs of pediatric triage. *Journal of Emergency Nursing* 14:154–159

Thomas D (1991). Triage of the pediatric patient and pediatric physical assessment. In Thomas D (ed), *Quick reference to pediatric emergency nursing.* Rockville: Aspen, pp 25–37

Tsai A, Kallsen G (1987). Epidemiology of pediatric prehospital care. *Annals of Emergency Medicine* 16:284

Weibe R, Rosen L (1991). Triage in the emergency department. *Emergency Medicine Clinics of North America* 9:491–505

Wong D, Whaley L (1990). *Clinical handbook of pediatric nursing* (3rd ed). St. Louis: Mosby, pp 280–282

Zwick H (1989). Initial assessment and stabilization of the critically injured child. In Joy C (ed), *Pediatric trauma nursing.* Rockville: Aspen, pp 9–22

CHAPTER 3

Physical Assessment

JUDITH SCHURR SALZER

INTRODUCTION

Physical assessment provides an objective means of obtaining information. The prerequisite to physical assessment is a carefully taken, detailed history. For a healthy child, the history provides information on risk factors, complaints, and concerns. For an ill or injured child, the history provides the sequence, timing, and relationship of events. The history points the way to areas on which to focus the physical assessment and to possible diagnoses.

Performing an accurate physical examination on a child presents challenges not encountered with adults. The approach to the patient, use of techniques, and range of normal findings are different for children, and they vary with the child's age. Because the physical examination is a tool for differentiating between normal variations and abnormal states, familiarization with variations among children of various ages is imperative. Table 3–1 provides a summary of how children differ physically from adults.

As in any physical examination, the examiner and the environment must be prepared. The examiner must have a knowledge of anatomy and physiology to understand physical findings. A clear, receptive mind enhances the examiner's observational abilities.

A quiet environment with good lighting provides privacy and maximizes the examiner's ability to make observations. Interruptions are distracting and convey an attitude of limited attention. Only true emergencies should be allowed to interrupt an examination. Taking notes during an examination assures accuracy, but care must be taken to avoid extensive note taking that limits eye contact or interferes with observations. Notes should be limited to descriptions of unusual findings. The findings of the examination are recorded in a logical order immediately after the examination.

Every physical examination should be approached in a systematic, almost compulsive manner. Through repetitive practice, the system of examination becomes automatic, freeing the examiner to focus on observations. Although the same basic techniques and skills are always used, the system's order varies for the situation and the age of the child.

Knowledge of child development provides a foundation for developing a repertoire of approaches to children of various ages (see Chapter 4). Infants are usually quieted by being held or talked to during an examination. Often, steady eye contact and a smile can achieve cooperation. Toddlers do not like being touched, manipulated, or restrained. No cooperation can be expected, but the examiner should never fail to try. Toddlers quickly make it known whether or not they have any intention of cooperating. When lack of cooperation is evident, the best approach is to calmly and efficiently perform the examination. Preschoolers usually cooperate if a few props are used. Having the child touch instruments and try them out on a doll or puppet is helpful. It is important to explain what will be done at each step of the examination, because preschoolers truly want to cooperate. Once the child has to lie down, however, fear and apparent loss of control may overwhelm the desire to cooperate. Older children are generally cooperative, but still need explanations and reassurance.

A "head-to-toe" examination is performed; however, with children it rarely begins at the head and ends at the toes. The sequence of each examination

TABLE 3–1. HOW CHILDREN DIFFER PHYSICALLY FROM ADULTS

Difference	Clinical Significance	Nursing Intervention
■ VITAL SIGNS Higher heart and respiratory rates, lower blood pressure	Smaller quantitative changes may be more significant	Obtain vital signs with child at rest because stress, fright, pain, may affect findings
Weight considered a "fifth" vital sign	Medication calculated according to child's weight in kilograms	Weigh all children on admission
■ TEMPERATURE REGULATION Temperature-regulating mechanism less stable (the younger the child, the less stable the mechanism)	Hypothermia may occur rapidly, leading to acidosis, hypoxemia, and hypoglycemia	Keep infants warm
Larger surface area–to–volume ratio	Heat lost through convection, evaporation, conduction	Control environment and keep infants warm
Infants younger than 6 months cannot shiver; they break down fat to conserve heat	Breaking down fat requires energy, which increases oxygen consumption	Keep infants warm; observe infants who are uncovered for procedures for signs of respiratory distress
■ ELECTROLYTE BALANCE More total body water; a larger proportion is extracellular	Rapid dehydration from fluid loss through vomiting or diarrhea or decreased intake	Monitor intake and output; frequently assess for signs of dehydration if vomiting or diarrhea occurs
Higher metabolic rate and greater insensible and evaporative water losses	High daily fluid requirement per kilogram body weight, although the absolute amount of fluid required is small	Individualize fluid administration rate according to calculated requirements; control all fluids through use of IV burette and pump; monitor intake and output
■ HEAD AND NECK Skull is not rigid in infants; bones softer, more pliable	Head injury may be present without fracture; skull expansion may occur to accommodate increased intracranial pressure or tumor growth	Take careful head circumference measurements on all children younger than 2 years; monitor anterior fontanelle for bulging
Head larger in proportion to torso; center of gravity is shifted toward the head	Children most often fall head first, resulting in high percentage of head injuries	Suspect head injury in any young child who has fallen or been thrown; observe for symptoms
Sinuses, except for ethmoid, underdeveloped	Facial bones more resistant to injury; severe direct trauma necessary to produce fracture	In facial trauma, observe for injury to underlying structures even if fracture not present
Greater percentage of blood in head	Heavy bleeding may come from scalp lacerations	Observe for signs of hypovolemia, especially in infants younger than 1 year
Eustachian tubes shorter and straighter	Children are prone to ear infections because of easy entrance of bacteria through eustachian tube	Teach parents about anatomy and related risk factors, such as the infant's drinking a bottle lying down and upper respiratory infections
Muscle support of neck weak	Hyperextension or hyperflexion can cause cervical fractures or bleeding around the spinal cord	Teach families that shaking babies can cause severe damage or death; support the heads of infants
Cricoid cartilage narrowest portion of infant's trachea	Cuffed endotracheal tubes in children younger than 8 years can damage trachea	Ensure that cuffed endotracheal tubes are not used in children younger than 8 years
■ CARDIOVASCULAR SYSTEM Heart rate greater and stroke volume less; blood volume larger per unit body weight but absolute blood volume remains relatively small	Because stroke volume depends on heart rate, a decrease in stroke volume due to loss in blood volume increases heart rate in an attempt to compensate	Monitor all sources of blood loss, including phlebotomy

(continued)

TABLE 3–1. (Continued)

Difference	Clinical Significance	Nursing Intervention
■ RESPIRATORY SYSTEM		
Infants breathe through the nose for the first 2–4 months of life	Nasal obstruction can cause respiratory distress	Keep nose cleared of mucus and vomitus
Airways smaller and have increased resistance	Small amounts of mucus can cause major airway obstruction	Observe for distress in children with asthma or bronchiolitis
Thorax more pliable	Rib cage and sternum resist fracture but provide little protection to heart and lungs; injuries can cause contusions and laceration of the heart or lungs	Observe trauma victims closely even if no external injury is apparent
Lungs have fewer alveoli	Tendency for small airways to collapse	Observe children with asthma for rapid onset of distress
Intercostal muscles poorly developed	With decreased lung compliance and increased intrathoracic pressure during inspiration, chest wall moves in instead of out	Observe for retraction, which indicates increased respiratory effort and distress
■ ABDOMEN		
Liver and spleen larger and have poor muscle protection	Severe internal injury may result from blunt trauma	Observe trauma victims for signs of injury to internal organs
■ NERVOUS SYSTEM		
Central nervous system immature in young children	Reflexes present in adults may be absent normally in children; reflexes present in infants may be absent normally in adults	Know normal neurologic findings and how to elicit them in infants and young children

depends on the child's age and level of cooperation. Most examiners experienced in assessing children take advantage of quiet moments to listen to the heart and lungs. This part of the examination may be accomplished while the child is held by a parent. Examinations of the ear, nose, mouth, and throat are most often left until last because they are frequently upsetting to young children. The examination of older school-aged children and adolescents may be approached in a head-to-toe sequence.

ASSESSMENT TECHNIQUES

The techniques used for pediatric physical assessment are the same techniques used in adults: inspection, palpation, percussion, and auscultation. In addition, the examiner often uses her or his sense of smell to identify normal from abnormal odors.

Inspection
The most useful of the techniques is inspection, which includes observations made with the naked eye and those aided by instruments such as an otoscope and an ophthalmoscope. Developing skill in inspection requires concentration and attention to detail.

Palpation
Palpation—using touch to obtain information—generally follows inspection. It includes assessing temperature, vibration, size, shape, position, and movement. Different parts of the hands are used to assess various sensations. Fine tactile details are best assessed by using the fingertips; the backs of the fingers are most sensitive to temperature; and the flat of the palm or ulnar side of the hand perceives vibration, such as cardiac thrills. All parts of the body, including skin and hair, are palpated thoroughly.

Percussion
Percussion is tapping the skin with short, sharp strokes and interpreting the resulting sound. Percussion, direct or indirect, produces vibrations heard as sound tones described as resonant, hyperresonant, tympanic, dull, or flat. Direct percussion involves striking the body directly with the finger; it is useful in assessing an infant's thorax or an adult's sinuses. Indirect percussion is used more frequently. The middle finger of each hand is used; the tip of the striking finger firmly taps the middle finger of the stationary hand, which is hyperextended and placed firmly against the skin. Medium loud, low-pitched resonance

is heard over normal adult lung tissue. Hyperresonance is very loud and low-pitched; it is heard normally over a child's lung. The loud, high-pitched sound heard over gas-filled organs, such as the stomach or intestines, is tympanic. The soft, high-pitched sound produced over a relatively dense organ like the liver or spleen is dull. A flat sound is very soft and high-pitched; it is heard over bone, muscle, or solid tumor.

Auscultation

Auscultation refers to listening to sounds produced by the body with and without a stethoscope. A stethoscope helps focus sound and blocks out room noise. The flat-surfaced diaphragm held firmly against the skin is used to hear high-pitched sounds, such as breath, bowel, and normal heart sounds. The cup-shaped bell of the stethoscope held lightly against the skin allows the examiner to hear low-pitched sounds produced by extra heart sounds or murmurs. Grunting respirations, stridor, the sound of a child's voice, and the pitch of an infant's cry are important sounds heard without the assistance of any tools.

Smell

The sense of smell can be very useful in evaluating health status. A foul odor may help identify a source of infection, as in omphalitis. Odors from the breath, sputum, vomitus, feces, or urine can point the way for further evaluation.

Vital Signs

Clinical measurement of vital signs, height, weight, and head circumference are important aspects of physical assessment and must be accurately obtained. The examiner is responsible for ensuring the accuracy of measurements and determining whether or not the results are within normal range.

GENERAL APPEARANCE

Assessing general appearance provides an overall impression of the child's general state of health and outstanding characteristics. Observing physical appearance, body structure, mobility, and behavior may point to problems that require further investigation. In addition to noting obvious abnormalities, the examiner observes whether the child appears well and comfortable, has any signs of unusual respiratory effort, and is clean or dirty. One side of the body is compared with the other to assess symmetry.

Measurements

Measurements help assess body structure. Plotting height, weight, and head circumference on appropriate charts provides some indication of appropriate growth. The measurements must be evaluated in relation to each other. Is the weight appropriate for height and age? Is the height appropriate for age, and is the head circumference appropriate for height and age? Single measurements are of limited value in determining deviations from normal. A single measurement of weight that falls significantly above or below the child's height percentile may be considered abnormal. A single head circumference measurement falling above the 95th percentile or below the 5th percentile is suspect. Serial measurements provide a more accurate assessment because they demonstrate the child's rate of growth. When available, the child's medical record provides comparison measurements. If no documentation of previous measurements is available, parents may be able to provide a height and weight from a recent health care visit.

Mobility

Mobility is assessed as the child walks around the room and participates in or reacts to the examination. Smoothness of motion, steadiness, use of all limbs, tremors, limping, and favoring one side are noted. Activities such as crawling are assessed for appropriateness in relation to the child's age. The examiner must be familiar with the normal range of developmental expectations to make an accurate assessment.

SKIN, HAIR, AND NAILS

Skin

Valuable information about the child's general health and state of nutrition may be obtained by careful examination of the skin. Clues may be provided to identify systemic disease or reveal specific problems of the skin.

The skin of the entire body is both inspected and palpated. Assessment of the skin is usually integrated throughout the physical examination as each area is uncovered. Attention must be focused on the condition of the skin while the organ systems underneath are assessed. All skin folds must be spread; the chin of an infant is gently lifted to show the neck folds. Intertrigo, a bright pink, moist excoriation sometimes with a foul odor, results from continuous approximation of skin in deep folds like those of the neck or groin.

General Condition. The examiner notes the general condition of the skin, including the texture, consistency, and color. Does the skin feel dry or moist? Is it firm, flabby, or soft? Is there peeling of the hands or feet? Peeling hands may be seen after scarlet fever (strep throat with a body rash) or with Kawasaki disease, a febrile disease of children notable for the occurrence of vasculitis of the large coronary blood vessels with potential myocardial ischemia. Peeling feet occurs in children who wear sneakers all day and sleepers with feet at night. Athlete's foot is rarely seen in children before adolescence.

Color. The color of the skin is noted. Circumoral cyanosis or slight peripheral cyanosis may be seen in infants during the first few weeks of life, especially if they are chilled. Infants with coarctation of the aorta may show striking cyanosis of the lower extremities. Cyanosis in older infants and children is indicative of inadequate oxygenation and may indicate respiratory distress or cardiac anomalies. Jaundice, a yellowing of the sclera and skin, is best seen in sunlight. Because jaundice develops from the head down, a careful assessment of the entire body is important. Pressing gently on the nose and abdomen and noting the color when the skin is blanched assists in assessing the degree of jaundice. Physiologic jaundice appears about 24 hours after birth and disappears by the second week of life. Although this condition is usually normal, other causes of the jaundice, such as ABO incompatibility, sepsis, hepatitis, and bile duct obstruction should be considered. Jaundice sometimes occurs in breastfed infants after the third day of life and may continue for several weeks. Carotenemia, a yellowing of the skin caused primarily by excessive intake of yellow vegetables such as carrots, is sometimes mistaken for jaundice. However, in carotenemia the sclera remains clear.

Generalized pallor may be indicative of shock, circulatory failure, or chronic disease. Mild pallor may be detected by examining the nail beds, conjunctivas, and oral mucosa. Pallor is not an accurate estimate of hemoglobin level and may be an inherited trait in some children. Generalized erythema may be seen in children with fevers, and defined areas of redness are present in infection or sunburn. Bright red cheeks are often the result of windburn or cold exposure; they are also seen in children with fifth disease (erythema infectiosum), a mildly contagious childhood disease with lacy body rash and a "slapped cheek" appearance.

Birthmarks. The size, color, shape, and location of birthmarks are noted. Café-au-lait spots, flat light brown patches, may be an early indication of neurofibromatosis, a developmental disease characterized by multiple tumors of the peripheral and cranial nerves and skin. One or two café-au-lait spots are normal, whereas five or more are suspect. Mongolian spots are flat, blue areas usually found on infants or young children of African-American, Hispanic, Asian, or Native American descent. Although usually located on the buttocks or sacral area, these spots may be found anywhere on the body. These spots gradually fade and may disappear by adulthood. It is imperative that examiners of children learn to recognize Mongolian spots and differentiate them from bruising. Too often children with these birthmarks are erroneously identified as victims of child abuse. Superficial or simple hemangiomas (stork bites) are flat vascular lesions present at birth. Frequently located on the eyelids, midforehead, or base of the neck, these hemangiomas fade during the first several years. Capillary hemangiomas often appear as flat, pink lesions soon after birth, become raised and red during the first year, then gradually recede. They may be anywhere on the body, small or large, external or cavernous. Cavernous hemangiomas, which enlarge inside the body, may require treatment to avoid damage to underlying structures.

Bruising. Children past infancy often have some bruises. Examiners must be aware of areas of common bruising and ask questions about all bruises in unusual locations or of an unusual shape. Bruises are common on the anterior lower legs and are usually round or oval. Bruising on the face and trunk should raise questions, as should any linear bruises. Child abuse must be in the back of the mind of every examiner of children. Bite marks, burns, and any unusual skin lesions must be thoroughly investigated.

Lesions. Skin rashes, a common problem in infants and children, are worrisome to parents and often present a challenge to diagnosticians. The examiner must be able to accurately describe the type, size, color, distribution, and configuration of the lesions that merge into a rash.

Common Primary Skin Lesions

- Macule—flat, circumscribed discoloration less than 1 cm in diameter, such as freckles and viral exanthems
- Papule—raised, circumscribed, superficial solid lesions less than 1 cm in diameter, such as elevated nevi and warts
- Vesicle—sharply defined blister-like lesion less than 1 cm in diameter, as in varicella, herpes simplex, or poison ivy
- Bullae—vesicles larger than 1 cm in diameter, as in second-degree burns

- Pustule—elevated, circumscribed lesion less than 1 cm in diameter containing pus, as in impetigo or acne
- Wheal—elevated, edematous, transitory lesion seen in hives, insect bites, or urticaria
- Petechiae—reddish purple, circumscribed, superficial lesions smaller than 2 mm in diameter, as seen in severe systemic disease such as meningococcemia
- Ecchymoses—deposits of blood larger than 1 cm in diameter; bruises

Secondary lesions result from some type of change to a primary lesion. They may be scales, crusts, excoriations, ulcers, or lichenification (diffuse thickening and scaling due to chronic scratching or rubbing).

Nails
While examining the skin, it is important to observe the nails. The nail beds should be pink. Nails should be convex with the edges covering the edges of the fingers. The cleanliness and condition of the nails are noted. Scratching with dirty fingernails commonly precipitates impetigo. Paronychia, an infection around the nail, often occurs in children who bite their nails. Toenails are inspected for any areas that may tend to become ingrown. A serious infection may result from an ingrown toenail of an infant.

Hair
Examining the hair is another important aspect of evaluating the skin. The hair should be clean and shiny, be generally the same color all over, and should cover the head. Young infants may normally have areas of baldness on the back and sides of the head. The hairline and distribution of hair over the body are noted. The examiner parts the hair to expose and examine the scalp for excoriation, bald spots, seborrhea, and evidence of pediculosis. The hair shaft is examined for pediculotic nits (head lice), which are not uncommon in school-aged children. Nits may be mistaken for dandruff flakes, but nits adhere to the hair shaft. Brittle or coarse hair is abnormal. The eyebrows and lashes are examined for texture, shape, and length of hair. The presence, distribution, and texture of body hair are noted. Most children do not have pubic or axillary hair before puberty, but they may have fine body hair. Tufts of hair along the spinal column may be indicative of an underlying abnormality, especially in the sacral area, where spina bifida occulta, a defect of closure in the laminae of one or more vertebrae, may be found.

LYMPHATIC SYSTEM

The lymphatic system provides a defensive network against the invasion of microorganisms; it is a very sensitive indicator of health or illness. Enlarged lymph nodes are most frequently used as indicators of localized or generalized infection, but they may also provide clues to certain hypersensitivities or metabolic and lymphoid diseases. Although lymph nodes are scattered throughout the body, those most accessible to examination are found in the head and neck, axillae, arms, and groin (Figure 3–1).

Inspection
Examination of the lymphatic system, like that of the skin, involves inspection and palpation. The examination is integrated throughout the physical examination. During inspection, any visible lymph nodes are noted.

Palpation
The lymph nodes are palpated using both hands and the findings are compared. The examiner uses a gentle, circular motion of the fingerpads. The location, size, mobility, consistency, and tenderness of palpable nodes are noted. Are the nodes discrete or matted together? Cervical and inguinal nodes up to 1 cm in diameter that are discrete, movable, and non-tender are normal in children up to 12 years of age. Enlarged or tender nodes require further examination of the area drained by the nodes. Lymph nodes that respond to systemic and local infections become enlarged and tender. They are usually 2 cm or less in diameter, discrete, slightly firm, and mobile. When nodes are markedly enlarged with pronounced inflammation, adenitis is present. This condition, in which the lymph node itself is infected, is evident on inspection.

Interpretation of Findings
Scalp infections may cause inflammation of occipital, posterior cervical, preauricular, and postauricular lymph nodes. The submental and submandibular nodes drain areas of the teeth, gingivae and tongue and may become enlarged with a dental abscess, gingivitis, or herpetic stomatitis, which causes painful vesicular lesions of the oral mucosa. Infections of the ear canal and auricle may be accompanied by enlargement of the preauricular or postauricular nodes. Axillary nodes become enlarged in response to wounds, skin infections, or cellulitis of the upper chest, hand, or arm. Inguinal nodes react to infections of the external genitalia, anus, lower abdomen and back, buttocks, and upper thigh.

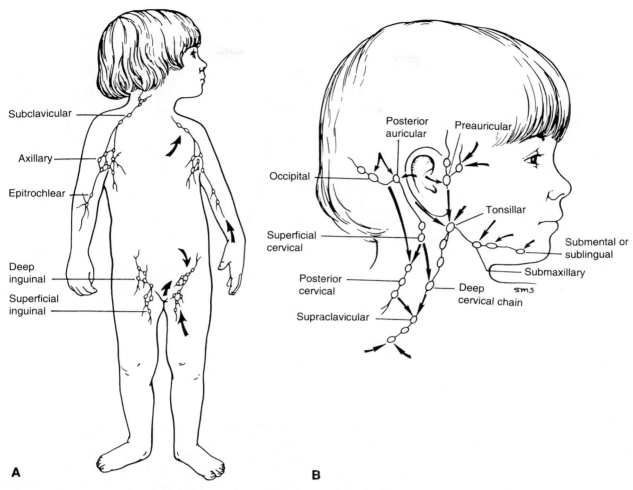

Figure 3–1. A. Location of lymph nodes. **B.** Directions of flow of lymph. (From Mott SR, James SR, Sperhac AM [eds] [1990]. Nursing care of children and families [2nd ed]. Menlo Park, Calif: Addison-Wesley, p 357.)

Certain infectious diseases have a characteristic distribution of lymphadenopathy. Rubella (German measles) is often accompanied by enlarged occipital, posterior cervical, and postauricular nodes. Cervical adenitis is usually present in children with scarlet fever.

HEAD, FACE, AND NECK

The head, face, and neck are vital areas of the pediatric physical assessment. The skull and face provide a protective vault for the brain and other vital centers of the central nervous system. The neck must support the relatively large head; it contains major blood vessels, the trachea, esophagus, and thyroid. Careful inspection, palpation, and head circumference measurement at regular intervals assure early identification of ab-

normal growth and early intervention for improved outcomes. It is important to remember to integrate the examinations of the skin and lymphatic system when assessing the head, face, and neck.

Inspection

Inspection of the head and face is best accomplished with the infant or child sitting. Infants and young children may be held on a parent's lap. By the age of 3 years, many children are happy to sit on the examining table with a toy. The examination begins with a general inspection then proceeds to the specifics. The head is observed from the front, top, sides, and back. The shape, symmetry, movement, control, and position are noted. In infants, the appearance of the anterior fontanelle is noted (Figure 3–2). Is the fontanelle bulging, sunken, or pulsating? The infant or child's facial features are seen as a whole, individually, and in

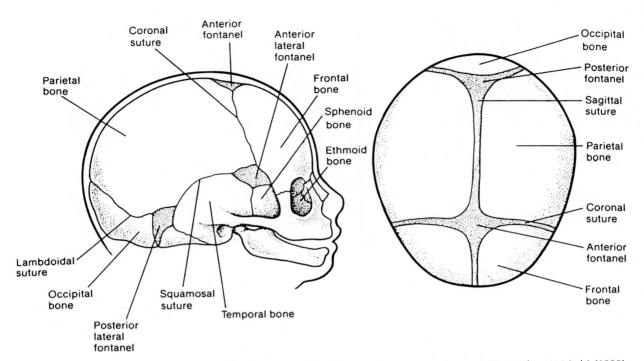

Figure 3–2. The bones of the skull showing the fontanelles and suture lines. (From Mott SR, James SR, Sperhac AM [eds] [1990]. *Nursing care of children and families* [2nd ed]. Menlo Park, Calif; Addison-Wesley, p 360.)

relation to each other. One side is compared with the other for symmetry. Are the eyes level, the nostrils the same size, the lips symmetric, and the ears set at the same level on both sides? Low-set ears may be associated with mental retardation or renal abnormalities. Normally the top of the pinna of the ears crosses an imaginary line from the lateral corner of the eye to the most prominent protuberance of the occiput. Placing a thumb at the lateral corner of the eye and spreading the index finger to the occipital prominence provides an estimation of the imaginary line.

The facial expression is noted. Is the child bright-eyed and smiling, crying with or without tears, angry, terrified? Asymmetry, weakness, or paralysis in facial movements is noted. How the child holds the head at rest is important. Is it held straight or tipped to one side? How much head control is evident? Infants normally have good head control by 3 months of age. The examiner gently moves the infant's head in all directions and notes any limitation of movement. Older children are asked to watch a toy as it is moved to the right, left, up, and down. Any jerking movements, tremors, or limitation of movement are noted.

Palpation

The examiner palpates the head by gently placing both hands on the head and feeling it all over in a systematic manner. For infants, each of the suture lines is felt

and any separation or overriding is noted. The examiner feels the posterior fontanelle area to determine if the fontanelle is open and notes the size of the opening. The fontanelle normally closes by 2 months of age. With the infant quiet and in an upright position (supported in a sitting position or held against a parent's shoulder), the anterior fontanelle is palpated. The anterior fontanelle of most infants closes between 7 and 19 months of age. It is normally slightly concave, may have slight pulsations, and varies greatly in size. The size of the fontanelle is recorded in centimeters using a horizontal and a vertical measurement (eg, 2.5 × 3 cm). The face is palpated gently, and any unusual consistency or reaction to pain is noted.

Interpretation of Findings

During infancy rapid growth of the skull and the structures it incases makes the skull vulnerable to developmental abnormalities and allows for a wide range of normal findings. Infants born prematurely often can be identified by their long, narrow heads throughout infancy. In the first few days of life some infants have a large, edematous mass of the scalp called caput succedaneum. This variation of normal, which results from birth trauma, generally crosses the suture line and lasts only a few days, but it alters the infant's appearance and is of great concern to parents. Cephalhematoma, also the result of birth trauma, presents a similar appearance. Unlike caput succedaneum, a cephalhematoma is the result of subperiosteal hemorrhage, is normally restricted to one bone, and takes several weeks or longer to reabsorb. An abnormal head shape may be the result of infant positioning or craniosynostosis, premature closure of a cranial suture. Further evaluation is indicated because the two conditions may appear identical depending on the suture involved. Suture lines may be palpable as ridges in infants up to 6 months of age, and they may be overriding in early infancy since during the birth process, edges of the cranial lines overlap to accommodate passage of the head through the birth canal.

Palpating the fontanelle may yield information of critical importance. A bulging anterior fontanelle, perhaps with marked pulsations, is seen in infants with increased intracranial pressure due to meningitis, hydrocephalus, or other life-threatening conditions. Infants with hydrocephalus may have separated sutures, an open posterior fontanelle, a bossing forehead, sunset eyes, and an abnormally large head. A depressed anterior fontanelle is found in dehydrated or malnourished infants. Microcephalic infants have a small head with a small or nonpalpable anterior fontanelle.

A consistent head tilt to one side may indicate torticollis (wryneck, contraction of the neck muscles pulling the head to one side) or vision or hearing problems. When torticollis is suspected, an associated flattening of one side of the head and face is sought. Facial palsy may also give the appearance of a flattened face.

Because the neck of an infant is so short, inspecting it requires gently tipping the head back while the child is supine and tipping it forward when the infant is prone. The neck is observed for symmetry, size, shape, control of movement, and pulsations. Retracting in the suprasternal area at the upper edge of the sternum may indicate respiratory distress. The neck is palpated and assessed for pulsations, movement, strength, and masses. Pain or resistance to flexion may indicate meningeal irritation; lateral resistance is present with torticollis or injury. The trachea is located; it normally feels like cartilaginous rings in the midline. Lung problems may cause the trachea to shift from the midline. The thyroid is often difficult to palpate in infants, but in older children the gland is normally a firm, smooth mass that moves up with swallowing. The thyroid may be palpated from the front or the back in the same manner as in an examination of the thyroid of an adult.

EYES

Regular eye assessment provides early identification of eye abnormalities and protects a child's vision. Un-identified visual problems can interfere with an infant's or child's ability to respond and learn, leading to developmental delay. Although newborns see unclearly, they fixate best on objects 8–12 inches away, such as a mother's face when holding her infant in her arms. Visual acuity develops gradually during the first years of life, reaching 20/20 in 5–6 years. Visual acuity should be tested regularly starting at 3 or 4 years of age. An infant's vision is evaluated by having the infant fixate on and follow a bright object.

Inspection is the primary method used in evaluating the eyes. The eyes are evaluated together, in relation to each other, and separately in an organized sequence. Infants may be examined on a parent's lap or lying on an examining table. Toddlers are more cooperative sitting with a parent, and preschool and older children usually do well on an examining table.

General Survey

The general survey of the eyes includes the eyebrows and eyelids. One side is compared with the other. The shape, size, and thickness of the eyebrows are noted. Do they meet in the middle? Do they have an unusual shape or color? Are they thick or thin? The placement of the eyes is noted. Are the eyes close together or set wide apart? Are they set straight across or slanted up or down? Eyes slanting upward are seen in children with Down syndrome. Do the eyes appear the same or different? If different, how do they differ?

Eyelids

The lids are inspected and palpated. Ptosis—drooping of the lid—may be congenital or acquired. If ptosis is present, does the lid cover the pupil and obstruct vision? Amblyopia, loss of vision in the covered eye, may result if ptosis is not corrected. The lid is examined for red, scaly, crusted edges, which may be seen in children with seborrhea. Excessive blinking or squinting is noted. Does the upper lid fully cover the eye when closed? The examiner gently palpates the lids, feeling for cysts and noting any edema.

Continuous tearing or a discharge may indicate infection, allergy, or a blocked lacrimal duct. Unilateral clear tearing from a young infant is indicative of a blocked lacrimal duct. An infected conjunctiva with or without discharge may be an allergic reaction or a viral or bacterial infection. It is important to note the color and character of any discharge.

Ocular Muscles

Examination of ocular muscle movement is an essential part of the eye examination. The full range of motion of the eyes is checked by having the child watch a toy such as a finger puppet as it is moved through all visual fields. Transient strabismus, an imbalance of the extraocular muscles, may be normal in infants younger than 6 months. Consistent strabismus or strabismus that persists after 6 months is not normal. This condition may not be readily apparent and must be tested for during the eye examinations of all children older than 6 months. If strabismus is not identified and treated during the first few years of life, amblyopia results. Two easily conducted tests for strabismus should be done during every examination. The Hirschberg test involves shining a light into the eyes and observing the reflection on the pupil. The reflection should be in exactly the same spot on each pupil. Strabismus is present if the reflections are not identical. The cover-uncover test involves having the child focus on an object held about 12 inches from the eyes. The vision of one eye is occluded by holding a hand or card in front of it but not touching the eye. The eye is quickly uncovered after a few seconds, and the examiner watches it for movement. Any movement indicates strabismus. The test is repeated on the second eye.

The eyes are observed for nystagmus, which are tremorous movements that may be horizontal, vertical, or rotary. Occasional nystagmus may occur in healthy infants, but continuous nystagmus is abnormal at any age.

Sclera

The sclera is examined for color, hemorrhage, or lesions. A yellow-tinged sclera indicates jaundice. The sclera of newborns often appears slightly blue. Scleral hemorrhages, which may occur with birth trauma, severe vomiting, or severe coughing, resolve spontaneously.

Ophthalmoscopic Examination

The iris is inspected for irregularities. The pupils are observed for size, equality, and direct and consensual reaction to light. Although some people have pupils that normally differ in size (anisocoria), unequal pupils are indicative of a central nervous system abnormality.

An ophthalmoscopic examination is difficult in infants and is not usually part of the routine examination until a child is old enough to cooperate by fixing his or her eyes on a distant object. Becoming comfortable and developing expertise with an ophthalmoscope requires determination and practice. The room is darkened, and the child is asked to focus on a distant object such as a light switch across the room. The examiner uses her or his right eye to examine the child's right eye and her or his left eye to examine the child's left eye. Initially the ophthalmoscope is set on the black positive numbers +8 to +10. The examination begins about 12 inches from the child, when the

examiner looks for the red reflex and any opacities. The absence of a red reflex is abnormal. Opacities are indicative of cataracts or other serious conditions. The examiner then slowly comes to within a few inches of the child, turning to the smaller plus numbers then through the red negative numbers to about −5. The higher black positive numbers are used to examine the cornea, iris, and lens. The red negative numbers are used to examine the optic disc and retina. The disc should be clear, the veins and arteries should be identified, and abnormalities such as retinal hemorrhages should be noted. If a thorough examination cannot be performed and an eye abnormality is suspected, an ophthalmologist should be consulted immediately.

EARS

Ear problems are common during infancy and early childhood. Ear disorders may cause delays in language, speech, and social development. Although often difficult for an inexperienced examiner, a thorough ear examination is an essential component of any pediatric assessment.

Examination of the ear involves inspection and palpation of the outer ear (Figure 3–3) and surrounding structures and inspection of the inner ear and canal with the aid of an otoscope (Figure 3–4). Infants and toddlers generally require some degree of restraint for examination of the inner ear. When necessary, restraint should be accomplished in a calm and matter-of-fact manner. The examiner speaks to the child using a quiet, reassuring tone and explains what is being done regardless of the child's age. Talking to

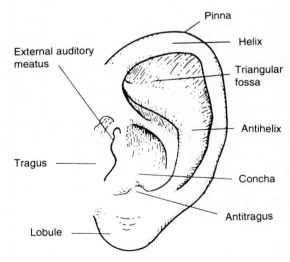

Figure 3–3. Structures of the external ear. (From Mott SR, James SR, Sperhac AM [eds] [1990]. Nursing care of children and families [2nd ed]. Menlo Park, Calif; Addison-Wesley, p 366.)

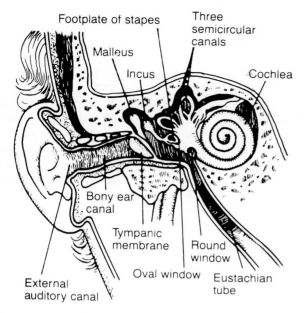

Figure 3–4. External auditory canal, middle ear, and inner ear. (From Mott SR, James SR, Sperhac AM [eds] [1990]. Nursing care of children and families [2nd ed]. Menlo Park, Calif; Addison-Wesley, p 367.)

an infant reassures the parent. Apprehensive preschoolers may be given a choice whether to sit on a parent's lap or on the examining table, if they can hold still, or to lie on the examining table with help holding still. If the child is unable to control his or her apprehension enough to be still for the examination, he or she is calmly restrained supine on the examining table.

Approach

Each examiner develops an approach that she or he finds comfortable, efficient, and effective. Often the examiner approaches from the child's chest with the parent holding the child's arms above the child's head tightly enough to restrain the head. An alternative is to approach from the head of the examining table with the parent leaning over the child's chest, gently holding the child's hands and having eye contact with the child. The examiner controls the movement of the head with both hands in conducting the examination. In examinations of children, the otoscope is held underhand, or as a pencil, allowing the lateral palm and little finger to have constant contact with the child's head. Therefore, if the head moves, the otoscope moves with it and does not cause injury to the ear canal. The examiner's free hand helps hold the head and positions the auricle.

Pneumatic Otoscopy

It is essential that an examiner of children become comfortable using the pneumatic bulb (insufflator) to assess the mobility of the tympanic membrane. A thorough examination is not possible without this element. The pneumatic bulb attaches to the otoscope and is either held in the same hand as the otoscope and depressed against the otoscope or held in the free hand and gently squeezed. Only with consistent practice and perseverance does the examiner become comfortable with this procedure. Again, because no examination of a child's ear is complete without this component, it is well worth taking the time to develop the skill.

Inspection

The examination of the ear begins with inspection of the structure, placement, and position of the ears. Normally the ears are vertically placed with the top of the auricle at an imaginary line drawn from the lateral eye to the occipital prominence. Newborns' ears may be flat against the head. Protruding ears may indicate swelling behind the ear or congenital lop ears. Both ears are checked for normal skin folds, skin tags, and any noticeable difference in structure, position, or placement. The area in front of the ear is inspected for any sinus or pit, which is a normal variation. Any discharge from a sinus may indicate infection. The outer ear is palpated for consistency. It should feel like firm cartilage. The ears of premature infants may have the feel of thin tissue. If a gentle pull on the auricle, exacts pain, there is a problem in the ear canal. The mastoid process, the protuberance behind the ear, is palpated for abnormal swelling or tenderness. Any wax or discharge in the outer ear canal is noted, as are the color, consistency, and smell of the wax or discharge.

Otoscopy

Examination of the structures of the canal and inner ear requires an otoscope with various sized specula and a pneumatic bulb. The speculum must fit into the canal easily but must form a seal when inserted ¼ to ½ inch. Occasionally a different sized speculum is required for each ear. The examiner straightens the ear canal by pulling the pinna gently down and out for children younger than 3 years and up and back in older children. The examiner places the hand holding the otoscope in contact with the child's head before beginning to insert the speculum. The speculum is inserted slowly into the canal. The canal is inspected for foreign bodies, lesions, edema, discharge, and cerumen as the speculum is inserted. Cerumen blocking the canal may be removed with a curette by an experienced examiner. Some foreign bodies also may be removed with a curette; others may require more extensive intervention.

The tympanic membrane (Figure 3–5) is normally

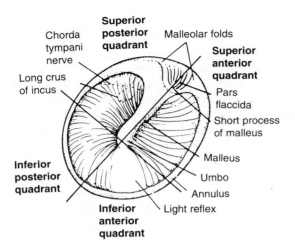

Figure 3–5. Anatomic landmarks of the right middle ear. (From Mott SR, James SR, Sperhac AM [eds] [1990]. Nursing care of children and families [2nd ed]. Menlo Park, Calif; Addison-Wesley, p 369.)

pearly gray, but it may be erythematous in a crying or febrile child. Any bulging or retraction is noted. Lesions or bubbles on the surface may indicate trauma or myringitis. Any fluid level or bubbles behind the tympanic membrane may indicate serous otitis media. The location of a perforation should be sought if there is purulent discharge in the canal. The bony landmarks are the incus, the short process of the malleus, the handle of the malleus, and the umbo. The cone of light is noted. Normally it is sharply defined and meets the umbo. In otitis media the cone of light may be diffuse, split, wide, or short. The examiner depresses the pneumatic bulb and notes the movement of the tympanic membrane. Normally it is seen "flapping" or moving well. Fluid or pus behind the tympanic membrane impedes movement.

NOSE AND SINUSES

The nose is the beginning of the respiratory system; it may give clues to how the rest of the system is functioning and about the overall health of the child. Sinuses, air-filled spaces lined with mucous membranes, develop throughout childhood. Both the nose and sinuses are frequent sites of disease in children.

Infants are usually examined lying supine; preschoolers and older children are usually sitting. Inspection and palpation are used to examine the nose and sinuses.

Nose

Inspection of the nose begins with the observation of its shape, placement, symmetry, and proportion in re-

lation to other facial features. An unusual shape, deformity, asymmetry of the nose and nares, inflammation, and lesions are noted. The nose should be straight and placed in the midline. Nasal flaring, an indication of increased respiratory effort or distress in infants, is noted. Infants breathe through their noses up to the age of about 3 months. This predisposes them to compromise of the upper airway. The amount, color, smell, and consistency of any discharge are noted. Unilateral discharge, often with a foul smell and sometimes with unilateral swelling, is a clue to a foreign body in the nose. A thin, watery discharge may indicate an upper respiratory infection or allergic rhinitis. A thick yellow-green or green discharge is associated with infection. A clear nasal discharge following a head injury may be cerebrospinal fluid. If the child is breathing through the mouth, there may be a nasal obstruction. The nose is palpated for irregularities and tenderness. For infants the examiner presses each naris closed to evaluate the patency of the nares. Smell is not usually tested during a routine examination.

An otoscope with a short, broad speculum is used to evaluate the inside of the nose. Lifting the nose slightly by placing mild pressure on the tip, the examiner gently inserts the speculum into the rim of the naris. It is not necessary to proceed past the rim to visualize the naris adequately. Any foreign body is noted, as are the color and condition of the mucous membrane and turbinate bones. Normally they appear pink and moist. Bright red, edematous turbinate bones are seen in infection, whereas pale, boggy, gray turbinate bones are indicative of an allergy. Any polyps visible on the turbinate bones are noted. The septum is inspected for deviation to one side, perforation, lesions, or areas of bleeding.

Sinuses

Assessment of the sinuses requires knowledge of their development. Only the maxillary and ethmoid sinuses are present at birth. Maxillary sinuses reach full size only after all the permanent teeth have erupted. The ethmoid sinuses are made up of numerous small cavities and are located behind the frontal sinus near the anterior part of the nasal cavities. The ethmoid sinuses grow rapidly between 6 and 8 years of age and after puberty. The ethmoid sinuses are the most common site of sinusitis in infants and young children. The sphenoid sinus is a minute cavity at birth and develops after puberty. The frontal sinuses are fairly well developed by 8 years and develop fully after puberty (Figure 3–6).

Because the sinuses are poorly developed in infancy, the examination is limited to evaluating nasal discharge as a possible indication of infection. In older

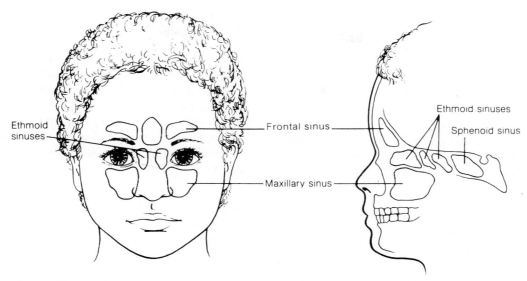

Figure 3–6. Front and lateral views of the facial sinuses. (From Mott SR, James SR, Sperhac AM [eds] [1990]. Nursing care of children and families [2nd ed]. Menlo Park, Calif; Addison-Wesley, p 370.)

children the areas over the sinuses are inspected for any swelling. The examiner evaluates the frontal sinuses by pressing with thumbs below the eyebrows and evaluates the maxillary sinuses by pressing below the cheekbones. Tenderness is indicative of sinusitis.

MOUTH AND THROAT

Examination of the mouth and throat requires thorough knowledge of normal structures and quick observational skills. Infants and young children are rarely cooperative for this portion of the examination, which is best done last. Because critical information may be obtained about health status, illness, and congenital defects, perseverance in developing skill in examining the mouths and throats of children is well worth the trouble.

Inspection and palpation are used to assess the mouth and throat. Smell is used to detect odors associated with poor hygiene, infection, or systemic disease. A tongue depressor, penlight, and gloves are usually required. Infants and young children are usually examined lying with some restraint. Older children who are cooperative in opening their mouths are examined sitting.

Mouth

Proceeding from the outside to the inside, the examiner notes the color, symmetry, moisture, and condition of the lips. Any dryness, swelling, sores, fissures,

or cyanosis are noted. Using a tongue depressor, the examiner gently retracts the lips and cheeks away from the gums and observes every surface of the mucous membrane. Normally the membrane is pink, firm, smooth, and moist with no lesions. In dehydration the mucous membranes are dry and tacky. White, ulcerated sores may be the result of trauma or viral infections. White, curdy patches that are not easily scraped off are present in thrush. Thrush is common in infants, especially when antibiotics are given. It is not common in older children and may indicate an immune deficiency. Bruising or evidence of trauma in an infant's mouth is seen in child abuse as a result of forced feeding. The tongue is evaluated for color, surface characteristics, movement, and size. The examiner looks under the tongue to inspect the frenulum and to note any lesions. A protruding tongue is seen in children with Down syndrome or cerebral palsy. A red tongue with prominent papilla (strawberry tongue) is sometimes seen in children with scarlet fever or strep throat. Older children are asked to stick their tongues out so that the examiner may note any deviation or tremor indicative of nerve damage. The gums and teeth are evaluated for color, condition, and hygiene. Red, swollen, bleeding gums may indicate poor oral hygiene, poor nutrition, or infection. The teeth are counted, and their color and condition are noted. By 30 months of age most children have twenty temporary teeth. Caries of the upper central and lateral incisors usually indicate prolonged use of a baby bottle. A temporary gray discoloration may be seen in children taking liquid iron.

The hard palate should appear intact with a mild arch. The palate is palpated and an infant's sucking assessed. A high arch may interfere with adequate sucking. The appearance of a thin membrane in the midline may indicate an underlying cleft. The soft palate and uvula are inspected. They should rise with crying or when the child says "ahh." Deviation or lack of movement is indicative of nerve damage. Petechiae may be seen on the soft palate of a child with strep throat. A bifid or split uvula requires further evaluation because it may indicate a submucosal cleft of the palate.

Throat

The tonsils and posterior pharynxes of cooperative children are examined without a tongue depressor. Many school-aged children become upset and uncooperative at the sight of a tongue depressor. When using a tongue depressor to assess other areas of the mouth, the examiner should explain to the child that its use will be limited to looking at the teeth and cheeks. If the child is still upset about the tongue depressor, a gloved finger is used to view the mouth. In young children who clamp their mouth shut, the examiner can gently slide the tongue depressor between the cheek and gums, rotate it to slip between the back teeth, and then depress the tongue. A quick look is obtained as the child gags. A tongue depressor is never used for a child believed to have epiglottitis because the depressor may cause total laryngeal obstruction. The tonsils are evaluated for size, position, and condition. Tonsils are usually not visible in newborns, but they are quite large in pre-school and school-aged children. They recede at about the age of 12 years. Normal tonsils may have crypts that look like linear pits. The crypts may trap white debris, which should not be confused with the exudate associated with infection and found on the tonsilar surface. The anterior tonsilar pillars are inspected for lesions or ulcers. The posterior pharyngeal wall is inspected and the color and character of any postnasal discharge are noted.

CHEST AND LUNGS

Accurate assessment of the chest and lungs requires knowledge of the normal physical findings in children of various ages. The nearly round thoracic cage of a newborn gradually grows in transverse diameter, achieving the elliptic adult shape at about 6 years of age. The infant's thoracic cage is also relatively soft, allowing it to pull in during labored breathing. In infants and children younger than 6 or 7 years, respirations are primarily diaphragmatic or abdominal. Breathing is less regular during infancy than in later childhood.

Inspection, palpation, percussion, and auscultation are all used in assessing the chest and lungs. The entire chest from neck to abdomen, front to back including the sides and under the arms must be examined. Only by undressing the child to the waist can an accurate assessment be made. Young infants may be examined lying or held upright in their parents' arms. Infants old enough to sit alone and older children are best examined sitting. Every attempt should be made to quiet the child because abnormal findings may be masked by crying.

Inspection

The chest is evaluated for shape, movement, symmetry, and abnormalities. Any protuberance or depression of the sternum indicates pectus carinatum (pigeon chest) or pectus excavatum (funnel chest); either deformity may compromise lung expansion. Asymmetry may indicate scoliosis (lateral curvature of the spine), underlying deformity, or a mass. Movement should be symmetric. Note the respiratory depth, rate, and effort. Rapid respirations are seen in infants and children with fever and respiratory or general illness. Retracting, a "pulling in" during inspiration, may be supraclavicular, suprasternal, substernal, or intercostal; it is seen in children with increased respiratory effort. A prolonged expiratory phase is seen in obstructive respiratory problems such as asthma. The shape, color, and placement of nipples are noted. Occasionally supernumerary nipples occur along the milk line; they are considered normal.

Palpation

The examiner palpates the chest to evaluate chest expansion, swelling, pain, and respiratory vibrations. To evaluate expansion, the examiner places a palm with fingers spread on each side of the chest. Expansion, which is normally symmetric, is noted. Asymmetric expansion indicates a unilateral abnormality of the lung. The entire chest is palpated for lumps, irregularities, or pain. The nipple area is palpated for breast tissue. The size of the breasts in relation to the age of the child is noted. Both male and female infants often have some breast tissue because of maternal hormonal influences. Breast tissue in young children may indicate precocious puberty. Normal breast development may begin as early as 8 or 9 years of age and is most often unilateral. When breasts are present, they are evaluated by Tanner staging, and a full adult breast examination is done. Gynecomastia, breast tissue in a pubertal boy, is also often unilateral. Although usually normal and temporary, gynecomastia may indicate a hormonal imbalance.

Fremitus is respiratory vibrations felt through the

chest wall; it is evaluated by having an older child repeat "ninety-nine" while the examiner's hands are placed all over the chest. Distinct vibrations of equal intensity should be felt on corresponding areas of each side of the chest. The intensity of the fremitus is diminished over areas of lung collapse or pleural effusion. It is enhanced over areas of consolidation.

Percussion

Percussion requires a cooperative child and is therefore used primarily in older children. Moving symmetrically and systematically and comparing one side with the other, the examiner evaluates the front, sides, and back of the chest using indirect percussion over the intercostal spaces. Resonance is heard normally over the lung surfaces. Dullness is heard normally over the heart and liver, but it is abnormal over the lungs and may indicate fluid or a mass.

Auscultation

Auscultation begins by listening with the ear for any sounds associated with breathing. Grunting respirations in an infant indicate respiratory distress. Coughing should be evaluated for its character—dry, moist, hacking, choking. Audible wheezing (a continuous, high-pitched, musical squeaking) and whether or not it is associated with a cough are noted. Stridor, a crowing sound, indicates a compromised upper airway. Auscultation with the diaphragm of the stethoscope should be systematic, symmetric, and proceed from apex to base (top to bottom). By listening in a specific spot on one side then in the same spot on the other side, the examiner can compare air exchange, character of breath sounds, and adventitious sounds. Because they have thin chest walls, infants and young children have breath sounds that are louder and harsher than adults. Breath sounds are generally vesicular throughout the lung field. Transmitted upper airway sounds from mucus in the nose or throat may be confused with adventitious sounds. Upper airway sounds may be differentiated by holding the stethoscope near the nose and mouth and listening for the sounds. Rales (fine crackles) are heard in children with pneumonia or congestive heart failure. Rhonchi (continuous, low-pitched musical snoring) and wheezes that clear with coughing are indicative of bronchiolitis. Scattered expiratory wheezing is heard in children with asthma, although it must be kept in mind that an absence of wheezing may indicate that an asthmatic child has considerably diminished air exchange and is in distress. Unilateral wheezing, usually occurring on the right side, is indicative of foreign body aspiration. The right bronchus is shorter and wider and is angled less sharply than the left, allowing foreign bodies easier entry.

CARDIOVASCULAR SYSTEM

The cardiovascular system is evaluated for indications of normal or abnormal heart functioning. Pulse and blood pressure measurements are integral parts of the assessment and are covered in detail in Chapter 2. Because the child must be quiet for accurate assessment, listening to the heart is often done as the first part of the examination. Infants and children should be examined in both sitting and lying positions. Examiners of children quickly learn to take advantage of any quiet moments to listen to the heart.

Inspection, palpation, percussion, and auscultation are used to assess cardiovascular function. The child is undressed to the waist before the examination is begun. The chest is observed for visible pulsation, and the location of the pulsation is noted. The apical impulse is often visible in children with thin chest walls. Any obvious bulge or heave is noted. A precordial bulge to the left of the sternum signals cardiac enlargement. The bulge occurs because the cartilaginous rib cage of children is more compliant than that of adults.

Palpation

Palpation of pulses in all extremities for rate, rhythm, and strength is part of the cardiovascular assessment (Figure 3–7). Normal pulse rates vary with the age of the child, but pulses should be strong and equal throughout. Palpation of the femoral pulses is especially important for children. Absent or diminished femoral pulses suggest coarctation of the aorta. The chest is palpated gently with the fingers to locate the apical impulse or point of maximal impulse (PMI). The PMI in children younger than 4 years is normally felt in the fourth intercostal space just to the left of the midclavicular line. The PMI gradually changes location with growth; it is found in the fourth intercostal space at the midclavicular line between 4 and 6 years and in the fifth intercostal space at the midclavicular line by about 7 years. In cardiac enlargement, the PMI moves laterally. The examiner palpates the chest with the surface of the ulnar hand feeling for a thrill—a "purring" sensation—and noting the location and timing. A thrill indicates organic heart disease.

Percussion

Percussion to determine heart size is sometimes used for older children, but it is of limited value in infants and young children. The indirect scratch method of percussion is often more useful in determining cardiac borders. In this method the stethoscope is placed over the heart and longitudinal "scratches" are made with a finger beginning in the axillary line and moving toward the heart in 1-cm increments. As soon as the scratches

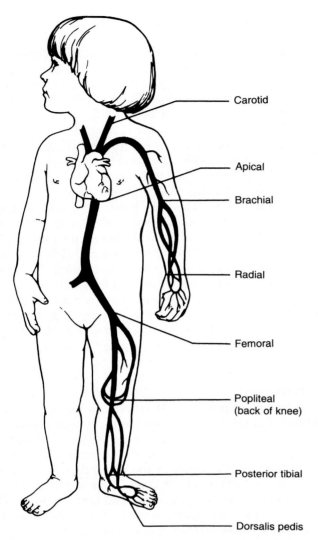

Figure 3–7. Location of pulses. (From Mott SR, James SR, Sperhac AM [eds] [1990]. Nursing care of children and families [2nd ed]. Menlo Park, Calif; Addison-Wesley, p 350.)

are over the heart, a change in the intensity of the scratch sound is detected through the stethoscope.

Auscultation

Auscultation provides the most important information about cardiac status. A quiet environment and child are required. The examiner must learn to attend completely to what is being heard. Closing the eyes while listening blocks some environmental distractions and is a tool some examiners find helpful. Adhering to a rigid system of examination frees the examiner to focus on listening. One system for examining the heart is as follows.

With the child sitting, the examiner places the stethoscope diaphragm firmly on the chest at the aor-

tic listening area at the second right intercostal space (Figure 3–8). The heart rate and rhythm are noted. The examiner then identifies and listens to the first heart sound (S1) and notes its strength, character, and any split. She or he identifies and listens to the second heart sound (S2) making the same observations. The examiner listens to the systole for any murmurs, clicks, or snaps and listens to the diastole for any murmurs, clicks, snaps, or third or fourth heart sounds (S3, S4). The stethoscope is inched along to the pulmonic area at the second left intercostal space, and the examiner notes the same observations at each stop. The examiner continues inching along and listening to the tricuspid area at the fourth and fifth left intercostal spaces and to the mitral area at the apex. The entire examination is repeated with the bell of the stethoscope placed lightly on the chest. The examiner listens to the back for any radiating murmurs. The child is laid down, and the entire examination is repeated with the diaphragm then the bell. Regardless of the sequence, the stethoscope should be inched along to all listening areas, and the S1, S2, systole, and diastole should be focused on individually throughout the examination.

Interpretation of Findings

Sinus arrhythmia, when the heart speeds up with inspiration and slows down with expiration, is normally heard in children of all ages; the greatest degree is heard in adolescents. Children's heart sounds are higher pitched and of shorter duration than those heard in healthy adults. Heart sounds are also louder in children because their chest walls are thin. The S1 is loudest at the apex and S2 is loudest at the base (aortic and pulmonic areas). Splitting of the S2 can be heard in most young children at the second left intercostal space. Some children have a physiologic S3, which is best heard at the apex.

Venous Hum. A venous hum is commonly heard in children, is not pathologically significant, and needs to be differentiated from a murmur. A continuous, low-pitched sound that is loudest in diastole, the venous hum originates in the internal jugular vein and is heard above or below the clavicles. It is accentuated when the child is sitting, but disappears when he or she lies down.

Murmurs. A murmur is the sound of turbulent blood flow. Many children have murmurs without heart disease, but the significance of a murmur is often difficult to determine. The examiner must learn to hear and describe murmurs to differentiate those requiring referral. Murmurs are described by their timing (early, middle, late systole or diastole), pitch (high,

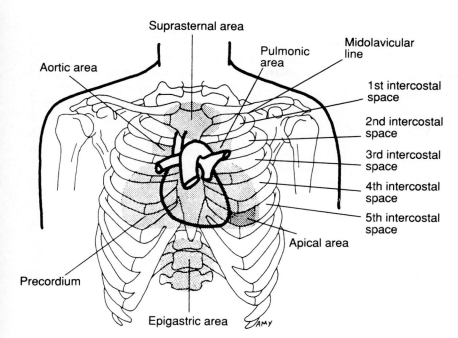

Figure 3–8. Sites for auscultation of the heart. (From Berger KJ, Fields WL [1980]. Pocket guide to health assessment. Reston, VA; Reston Publishing Co.)

medium, low), location, radiation, quality (musical, vibratory, blowing), and grade of intensity. Murmur intensity is graded on a scale of 1 to 6. Grade 1 is barely audible; grade 2 is soft but easily audible; grade 3 is moderately loud but not accompanied by a thrill; grade 4 is louder and associated with a thrill; grade 5 is audible with the stethoscope barely on the chest; and grade 6 is audible with the stethoscope off the chest.

Innocent murmurs are characteristically systolic, vibratory, short, medium pitched, grade 1–2 in intensity, do not radiate, and are usually heard along the left sternal border. Murmurs of grade 3 or louder, those associated with a thrill, and those heard during diastole almost always indicate heart disease.

ABDOMEN

The abdomen is examined for abnormal masses and enlargement or tenderness of the vital organs it contains. Inspection, palpation, percussion, and auscultation are used, but auscultation follows inspection because palpation and percussion may disturb normal abdominal sounds.

Inspection
The contour and movement of the abdomen are observed. Any localized fullness is noted. Young children normally have a potbelly that appears flat when lying down. A protuberant abdomen in infants or a concave appearance in older children may indicate malnutrition. A midline protrusion is seen in diastasis recti abdominis when the two halves of the rectus abdominis muscle are separated; it may be a normal variant. Distention may indicate pregnancy in older girls, organomegaly, feces in the intestine, or tumor. Peristaltic waves indicate obstruction or, in young infants, possibly pyloric stenosis. The umbilicus should be clean and dry. An umbilical hernia may cause umbilical protrusion in children up to the age of 6 years and require no intervention. Umbilical discharge in a young infant may indicate a granuloma or infection. The appearance of the discharge and any associated odor are noted. A foul smell usually accompanies infection.

Auscultation
Auscultation follows inspection. The stethoscope is placed firmly on the abdomen, and the examiner listens for peristalsis in all four quadrants. Bowel sounds are usually heard every 10–30 seconds and have a gurgling sound. The examiner must listen for a full 5 minutes before determining that bowel sounds are not heard. Absence of bowel sounds is indicative of paralytic ileus. High-pitched tinkling sounds are heard in children with diarrhea or obstruction.

Percussion
All areas of the abdomen are systematically percussed by the indirect method. The scratch method may be used to further define organ borders. Tympany is heard over most of the abdomen and dullness over the liver margin at or 2–3 cm below the right costal margin. Dullness also may be heard over a full bladder or large masses of feces.

Palpation

The abdomen is palpated twice, first superficially then deeply. The same sequence is used for both, except in the presence of pain, when the painful area is palpated last. For a crying child palpation should be done during inspiration. Cooperation may be increased if the child participates in the examination by placing his or her hand over the examiner's. Beginning at the lower left abdomen, the examiner palpates lightly using the fingers of one hand, inching up to the left costal margin. The procedure is repeated on the right and in the midline; tenderness, lesions, and muscle tone are noted. Deep palpation is conducted in the same manner, but one hand is placed on top of the other. The spleen is not usually felt. When enlarged the spleen feels like the tip of a nose or a thumb below the left costal margin. The liver may normally be palpated as a superficial mass a few centimeters below the right costal margin. Feces may occasionally be palpated as a firm mass in the left lower quadrant and must be differentiated from a pathologic condition. All other masses require further evaluations.

GENITALIA

Evaluation of the genitalia involves thorough inspection and palpation of the external structures. Because children are often modest, only the area to be examined is uncovered. Parents should be present during the examination of prepubertal children. Table 3–2 describes the developmental stages of the secondary sex characteristics.

Girls

The child's genitalia are inspected for the presence and distribution of hair. The labia majora are spread gently for inspection of the mucous membrane, clitoris, and urethral and vaginal openings. Any edema, erythema, discharge, or lesions are noted. Labial adhesions may obscure the vaginal and urethral openings. A foul-smelling discharge may indicate a foreign body or infection. The mons pubis and labia majora are palpated to check for masses. In pubertal girls, the stage of development is rated by the Tanner staging system.

Boys

The examiner inspects the genitalia and notes penis size, scrotal size, the presence of testes in the scrotum, and whether or not a circumcision has been done. The urinary meatus, which is normally a slit-like opening at the tip of the penis, is inspected, and any discharge is noted. The quantity and distribution of any hair are noted. The stage of development of pubertal boys is rated by the Tanner staging system. A gentle attempt is made to retract the foreskin. The foreskin of an uncircumcised boy is not expected to retract if the child is younger than 3 years. It is never appropriate to forcibly retract the foreskin at any age. Any adhesions on circumcised boys are noted. The testes are palpated for size, consistency, shape, and mobility. The testes are normally small, smooth, and moveable. Testes not in the scrotum can usually be milked down into the scrotum from the inguinal canal, where they often ascend. If the testis is not easily brought down into the scrotum in a child older than 3 years, an evaluation for an undescended testis is required. The continuous

TABLE 3–2. SEQUENTIAL DEVELOPMENT OF SEXUAL MATURITY

Tanner Stage	Female Breast Development	Male Genital Development	Pubic Hair Development
Stage 1	No breast tissue	Preadolescent	No pubic hair
Stage 2	Breast buds; small elevated mound of breast and papilla	Testes and scrotum begin to enlarge; reddening and texture change of scrotal skin	Sparse, lightly pigmented straight hair at base of penis or along labia
Stage 3	Breast and areola enlarge with continuous round contour	Penis increases in length and breadth; further growth of testes and scrotum	Darker, coarser, more curled hair; spreads over pubic symphysis
Stage 4	Areola and papilla further enlarged and form a secondary mound	Penis length and breadth increase further; glans has developed, testes and scrotum further enlarged; scrotal skin darkens	Adult character; thick and curly covers a larger area
Stage 5	Adult stage; smooth rounded contour	Adult size and shape	Adult quantity and type; hair spread to medial thighs

presence of fluid in the scrotum of an infant is likely a hydrocele, which reabsorbs over time. Intermittent fluid, usually unilateral, in the scrotal sac of an older infant or child is indicative of an inguinal hernia.

ANUS

The anal area is inspected with the child prone or lying on his or her side. The examiner spreads the buttocks to fully view the anal area. Hygiene is evaluated, and the presence of stool, which may be associated with encopresis (fecal incontinence without an organic cause), is noted. Any marks, fissures, tears, scars, hemorrhoids, polyps, or skin tags are noted. Evidence of scratching is suggestive of pinworms. Fissures are commonly seen in children with hard stools. Irregular tears or scars may be an indication of sexual abuse. The examiner strokes the anal area to elicit the anal reflex. The absence of an anal reflex also may indicate abuse. A rectal examination is not generally part of a routine examination.

MUSCULOSKELETAL SYSTEM

Assessment of the musculoskeletal system begins by observing the child move, walk, crawl, and play before the examination. Knowledge of gross motor developmental milestones is required to make an accurate assessment. Every joint, muscle, and bony structure is inspected and palpated. The child's movement is evaluated for symmetry. The lack of use of a limb or the favoring of one side is noted. Inspection and palpation are integrated as the examiner moves down the child's body.

Upper Body
The clavicles are observed and palpated to note any irregularities. A clavicular fracture resulting from birth trauma may be recognized by a hard, fixed mass on the clavicle. The surrounding muscles are observed and palpated; symmetry and strength are noted. The arms, hands, and fingers are moved, and the range of motion and symmetry are noted. The muscles of both arms are palpated from shoulder to hand. Transverse palmar creases are seen in some healthy children, but they may be an indication of Down syndrome. The muscles of the chest and abdomen are palpated; consistency and symmetry are noted.

Back
The back is evaluated for symmetry. The scapulae, vertebrae, and muscles are palpated. The backs of school-aged children and adolescents are examined while they are standing straight. The scapulae and hips should be at the same level and the spine should be straight. The child is asked to bend at the waist so that the examiner may look for any unilateral fullness or obvious lateral curvature of the spine, which is indicative of scoliosis.

Hips
The hips are inspected, palpated, and moved. Any pain, limitation, or asymmetry is noted. With infants, unequal gluteal skin folds may indicate congenital dislocation of the hips. Infants are tested for the Ortolani sign: With the infant supine the examiner places her or his thumbs on the inside of both the infant's thighs with the fingertips resting over the trochanter muscles. The examiner flexes both the hips and knees and fully abducts each knee. A click is heard or felt if an infant has congenital dislocation of the hip. The Ortolani sign is most reliable in infants younger than 4 months.

Lower Limbs
The thighs, knees, lower legs, and feet are inspected and palpated. The range of motion of all joints is tested. Young infants often have turned-in ankles and feet as a result of fetal positioning. The examiner manipulates the ankles and feet to assure that they correct to neutral. Stiffness or failure to correct is a reason for referral to a specialist.

NERVOUS SYSTEM

The extent of the neurologic assessment of a child depends on the reason for the examination and age of the child. A thorough assessment is required of any child who has fallen, sustained a head injury, complains of headache, or for whom developmental delay or a neurologic disorder is suspected. Much of the routine neurologic assessment can be integrated with other areas of the examination.

Mental Status
Mental status in infants and young children is observed as the child responds to the mother and to the examination. The child's ability to understand and follow directions is noted. Is behavior appropriate for the child's age? Evidence of a short attention span, impulsivity, or hyperactivity is noted. The child's speech should be easily understood by about 3 years of age. Comprehensive developmental assessment may be accomplished in young children by administering a standardized screening test.

Motor Function

Motor function is assessed during the musculoskeletal examination and developmental screening test. Deep tendon reflexes (biceps, triceps, brachioradialis, patellar, and Achilles) are tested on children after infancy. During infancy they yield variable results.

Cranial Nerves

Evaluation of the cranial nerves is part of a thorough neurologic evaluation, although infants and young children are not able to adequately participate in some of the tests. The function of many of the cranial nerves is part of the routine assessment of other systems. Cranial nerves II (optic), III (oculomotor), IV (trochlear), and VI (abducens) are tested during assessment of the eye. Cranial nerves X (vagus) and XII (hypoglossal) are evaluated during examination of the mouth. Cranial nerve I (olfactory) is tested by having the child identify smells such as lemon or coffee with eyes closed and one nostril occluded. Cranial nerve V (trigeminal) is tested by palpating the temple and jaw for strength and symmetry as the child bites down. The examiner notes if the child can feel light touch to the cheeks. The corneal reflex is tested by lightly touching the eye from the side with a twist of cotton. Cranial nerves VII (facial) and IX (glossopharyngeal) require the child to identify the taste of solutions placed on the anterior and posterior tongue. Cranial nerve XI (accessory) is tested by having the child attempt to turn the head against the examiner's hand and by having the child shrug his or her shoulders while the examiner applies pressure.

Infant Automatisms

Infant automatisms or reflexes are a good indication of neurologic function during the first months of life. Table 3–3 summarizes infant reflexes. The infant's sucking and rooting reflexes are assessed during the examination of the mouth. The Moro or startle reflex is best elicited at the end of the examination because it may cause an infant to cry. The grasp reflex is easily elicited as part of the musculoskeletal examination. The Babinski sign is also elicited during the musculoskeletal examination by stroking the outer edge of the sole. The toes are observed as they fan and the great toe dorsiflexes. The stepping reflex is elicited by holding the infant with his or her feet lightly touching a firm surface.

CONCLUSION

Developing expertise in pediatric physical assessment requires each examiner to develop a system that is

TABLE 3–3. INFANT REFLEXES

Reflex	Description	Clinical Significance	When Normally Observed
Blinking (dazzle)	Eyes close in response to bright light	Absence of reflex suggests blindness	During first year
Babinski sign	Toes fan and big toes dorsiflex in response to stroking sole of foot along outer edge, beginning from heel	Suggests lesion in extrapyramidal tract after 2 years	During first 2 years
Extrusion	Tongue extends outward when touched with tip of tongue blade	Persistent extension of tongue after 4 months may indicate Down syndrome	Until 4 months of age
Galant (trunk incurvation)	Back moves toward side that is stimulated when infant's back is stroked along side of spine from shoulder to buttocks	Absence may indicate transverse spinal cord lesions	First 4–8 weeks
Moro reflex	In response to abrupt change of position or jarring, arms extend, fingers fan, head is thrown back, legs may flex weakly; arms return to center with hands clasped; spine and lower extremities extend	Asymmetry is indicative of hemiparesis, clavicle fracture, or injury to brachial plexus; persistence beyond 4 months suggests brain damage	Strongest during first 2 months; disappears at 3–4 months
Palmar grasp	Infant's fingers curve around finger placed in infant's palm from ulnar side	Asymmetric flexion is indicative of paralysis; persistence is indicative of cerebral disorder	Disappears by 3–4 months
Stepping	Infant's feet move up and down as if walking when feet lightly touch firm surface	Persistence is abnormal	Disappears by 4–8 weeks
Tonic neck	Infant assumes fencing position when head is turned to one side; arm and leg extend on side to which head is turned and flex on opposite side; does not occur each time head is turned	Abnormal if response occurs each time head is turned; persistence indicates major cerebral damage	Appears at about 2 months; disappears at 6 months

comfortable, systematic, thorough, and adaptable for children of various ages. Experience sharpens observational skills and allows the examiner to integrate the various components of the examination with ease.

SUGGESTED READING

Athreya B, Silverman B (1985). *Pediatric physical diagnosis.* Norwalk: Appleton-Century-Crofts, 1985

Barness L (1991). *Manual of pediatric physical diagnosis* (6th ed). St. Louis: Mosby, 1991

Bates B (1991). *A guide to physical examination and history taking.* (5th ed). Philadelphia: Lippincott, 1991

Engle J (1989). *Pocket guide to pediatric assessment.* St. Louis: Mosby, 1989

Jarvis C (1992). *Physical examination and health assessment.* Philadelphia: Saunders, 1992

Malasanos L, Barkauskas V, Stoltenberg-Allen K (1990). *Health assessment* (4th ed). St. Louis: Mosby, 1990

Park M (1991). *The pediatric cardiology handbook.* St. Louis: Mosby, 1991

Tanner JM (1962). *Growth at adolescence* (2nd ed). Oxford, England: Blackwell Scientific, 1962

CHAPTER 4

Developmental Considerations

PAMELA J. BURKE

INTRODUCTION

Emergency departments (EDs) hold different meanings for people. The connotation of an ED depends on the person's role in the visit and on his or her expectations, previous experiences, and developmental level. To an ED nurse, the hustle and bustle of a busy ED holds excitement, professionally challenging opportunities, and personal satisfaction from life-sustaining and well-coordinated interventions. For a parent, an ED represents a safe haven or a place where tragedy strikes. To a child, an ED is a place with funny smells, bright lights, noisy machines, cold surfaces to lie on, and strangers who do things that hurt. Nurse, parent, child—each with a perception of an emergency hospital experience—work interdependently to make the experience a growth-fostering one.

Caring for a child in an ED demands specialized knowledge and skills, not only about the physiologic differences between children and adults but also about children's psychosocial needs. This chapter focuses on developmental considerations for pediatric emergency nursing. The discussion is organized around the following periods of development: infancy and toddlerhood; early childhood; school age; and adolescence. Discussing a developmental issue during one age period does not preclude its importance during other periods. Issues are discussed within the context of what I believe to be the most salient developmental period. For example, fear of strangers is a concern for most hospitalized children, yet a discussion of stranger anxiety is most salient to the discussion of infancy and toddlerhood. The chapter concludes with a brief discussion on children with special health care needs.

An in-depth discussion of child development is beyond the scope of this chapter. Table 4–1 presents an overview of growth and developmental considerations for children seen in an ED. Before a discussion of specific developmental periods, there are some general points to consider about caring for children in an ED, including pediatric pain management and changing family lifestyles.

GENERAL CONSIDERATIONS

A child's size and appearance do not necessarily reflect the child's chronological age. A number of factors can influence a child's appearance, including nutritional status, growth pattern, chronic conditions, and acquired characteristics, such as speech pattern, dress, hair style, and general grooming. Nevertheless, the nurse should be alert to noticeable discrepancies between a child's chronological age and his or her general appearance, because such a discrepancy may indicate that the child is failing to thrive. Conversely, some children dress provocatively to look older, which might indicate lack of parental supervision or that the child is a runaway.

An ED visit is usually an unplanned event in a family's day. Parents, especially those who are already sleep deprived, become quite fatigued by the long ED wait, and they can easily loose patience with their children, staff, and each other. Likewise children away from their familiar surroundings and usual daily routine become bored, fidgety, and irritable. Expecting children to act their age or sit still and be quiet while they wait in an ED is rather unreasonable; yet this is a

TABLE 4–1. OVERVIEW OF GROWTH AND DEVELOPMENTAL CONSIDERATIONS FOR CHILDREN SEEN IN THE EMERGENCY DEPARTMENT

Age	Developmental Milestones	Common Fears	Injury Prevention
Infancy (birth to 18 months)	Newborns regain birthweight by 3 weeks of age, birthweight doubles by 5 months, and triples by 12 months. Average monthly weight gain is 900 g (birth to 6 months) and 450 g (6 to 12 months); average monthly length gain is 2.5 cm (birth to 6 months). Head circumference increases 2 cm per month (birth–2 months) and 1 cm/month (3–6 months). Head circumference equals chest circumference by 12 months of age. ■ **4–5 MONTHS** Reaches for objects; when prone rests on forearms to elevate head; with truncal support sits with head steady; babbles ■ **6–8 MONTHS** Transfers objects hand to hand; holds own bottle; sits independently; rolls from back to stomach; babbles and laughs ■ **10–12 MONTHS** Has neat pincer grasp; creeps and crawls; starts to walk; climbs stairs; imitates speech; is "Mama" and "Dada" specific ■ **15–18 MONTHS** Has a sense of object permanence; walks up stairs with help; can use eye contact to get an adult's attention; makes one word utterances	As infants learn to recognize their parents and other family members, they become increasingly anxious if separated from their primary caretakers or if they are approached by strangers. Environmental stressors include bright lights, sudden or jerky movements, loud or unpleasant sounds (eg, crying and shouting), and excessive temperatures (cold or hot). Some infants go through a phase when they are afraid of tub baths. Likewise they may struggle while being undressed, especially when undressing is associated with something traumatic, like a medical exam. Once infants become accustomed to the sights, sounds, and smells of their own home environment, they may be wary of unfamiliar surroundings (eg, a different bed).	Use car seats, sturdy furniture, safe toys, and smoke detectors; keep infants from wandering off or falling from high places (eg, use playpens, window screens, gates, door locks); avoid leaving unattended on high surfaces (eg, beds, tables, sofas, counter tops) Electrical safety (eg, monitor plugs in outlets, avoid loose cords); keep hot liquids out of reach; monitor stoves and fireplaces Prevent ingestions (eg, keep drugs and poisons in locked cabinets and monitor handbags that may contain medicines); supervise infants eating and be alert to food substances that are too big for them to chew (eg, hot dogs) or small enough for them to stick up their nose (eg, round oat cereal, coated chocolate pieces); monitor access to other substances that could cause choking and aspiration (eg, nuts, pins, gum, balloons, popcorn) Prevent drowning and promote water safety (eg, use caution around bath tubs, buckets, toilet bowls, ponds, beaches, and swimming pools)
Toddlerhood (18 months–3 years)	During the second year the average monthly weight gain is 200 g and the average monthly height gain is 1 cm ■ **2 YEARS** Turns book pages one at a time; develops right or left handedness; runs well; goes up and down stairs (one step at a time); jumps off floor with both feet; capacity for symbolic thought coincides with language development; uses 2 word sentences; likes saying no ■ **3 YEARS** Goes up and down stairs (alternating feet); pedals tricycle; stands on one foot momentarily; speaks in three word sentences; is able to engage in pretend play	Being left alone and interacting with strangers; interruptions to their usual routine or an unusual event (eg, seeing their parent dressed in a hospital gown); people who have masks on or who are dressed in clown costumes; getting hurt (falls, cuts, skin abrasions); losing control or having to revert to baby things (eg, wearing diapers when they are used to wearing underpants)	Prevent injuries and poisonings as with infants; teach street safety

(continued)

TABLE 4–1. (*Continued*)

Age	Developmental Milestones	Common Fears	Injury Prevention
Early Childhood (4–6 years)	During early childhood the average yearly weight gain is 2 to 3 kgs and the average yearly height gain is 6 cm ■ **4 YEARS** Throws ball overhand; uses scissors; well defined concept of external body (draws people with 2–4 parts); goes down stairs alternating feet; likes to imitate other children ■ **5–6 YEARS** Draws people with bodies; may be able to skip; can run fast; stands on one foot for 10 seconds; is very curious; pretend play peaks	Vivid imaginations invent invisible friends or imagine that monsters are hiding under beds and in closets; may need a light left on so that they can fall asleep; being lost or abandoned; adults who look or act mean, even if that is not the adult's intent; vomiting, lacerations, and blood tests seen as a threat to a young child's sense of body integrity	Promote bicycle safety, including the use of helmets; prevent car occupancy injuries by using seat belts; supervise play and anticipate risks for falls, ingestions, drowning, and burns
School Age (7–12 years)	During the elementary school years the average yearly weight gain is 1–2 kgs and the average yearly height gain is 1.25 cm. Puberty begins with development of breast buds in girls (9–11 years) and with scrotal enlargement and lengthening of the penis in boys (10–12 years). Menarche 10–16 years. Greater variation in physical development among children of the same chronologic age. The growth spurt for girls can start as early as age 7½ and as late as age 11½. The growth spurt for boys can start as early as age 10½ and as late as age 16. Has increased gross motor ability and strength; masters reading, writing, and arithmetic; capable of cooperative play; likes competitive games; engages in concrete thinking; is aware of bodily functions and internal organs	Being unable to compete in school, sports, or play; interruptions to daily routine; concerned about how others view them; being rejected by peers; they work hard to make friends and follow rules; hero worship is very common; try to please authority figures (eg, parents, teachers, coaches, health care providers); even minor surgery can trigger fear of disfigurement or death; need to appear strong may spawn a false bravado and denial of pain	Promote sports safety (eg, proper conditioning and use of equipment); avoid overexertion; avoid false bravado of "playing with pain," and foster good sportsmanship Encourage use of seat belts and helmets (eg, for bicycle riding, in-line skating, and skate boarding) Reinforce water safety (eg, swimming with a buddy, avoiding deep water, proper diving techniques); caution against skating on inadequately frozen ponds or lakes Properly supervise after school and weekend time
Adolescence (13–17 years)	Female growth spurt begins at about age 10½, lasts for about two years, and results in a gain of about 8¾ cm per year. Male growth spurt begins at around age 12½, also lasts for about two years, and results in a gain of about 10 cm per year. Tanner staging (I–V) used to categorize secondary sexual characteristic maturation. Skin becomes oily. Apocrine glands begin to secrete. Changes in body fat and musculature occur. Has a sense of invulnerability; is self-conscious and self-centered; has a need for belonging and a desire for independence or freedom to do what he or she wants and with whom; becomes logical, abstract, and idealistic in thinking	Overriding concern about being normal; need to belong; being left out or socially isolated; sexuality (gender role identity and sexual preference); prospects for future happiness and well being; as teens become more aware of their own parents' shortcomings, they may fear that they will inherit some of these same problems (eg, alcoholism and mental illness); as today's youth witness the increasing rate of adolescent homicide, suicide, and motor vehicle accidents, more teens are faced with the ever present fear of an early and violent death	Promote responsible decision-making and moderation of risk-taking by helping adolescents recognize that for every action there is a consequence (intended or unintended) Help adolescents recognize the dangers of premature and unprotected intercourse, drugs and alcohol, speeding, riding without seat belts, carrying weapons, and fighting Encourage adolescents to talk about their feelings rather than "suffering in silence"

(Adapted from Dixon SD, Stein MT (1992). Encounters with children: Pediatric behavior and development (2nd ed). St. Louis: Mosby) common source of conflict between parents and children. Dixon and Stein (1992) noted that "developmental regression symbolizes both a stress and a protective maneuver to defend against the loss of parent or parents and settle into the hospital experience" (p 405). The nurse can help parents to understand the impact of a visit to an ED on a child's behavior and to select appropriate strategies for distracting or calming the child. Thus the ED should be stocked with child-safe, washable toys and books so that children who are well enough can pass the time away with play.

Parents expect to protect and nurture their child. They may feel obstructed in this caretaking role when they stand helplessly by watching their frightened child experience pain or wait outside a treatment room as a team of strangers works on the child. Nurses can promote adaptive coping by keeping parents informed about the child's condition, by attending to the parents' verbal and nonverbal anxiety cues, and by conveying a sense of empathy. Nervous pacing, hand-ringing, and tense postures are obvious signs of anxiety. Parents who shyly and quietly sit by, reluctant to ask questions or verbalize concerns, need to be encouraged to share their thoughts and feelings. It is important, however, that what is told to parents and the tone in which it is said not frighten the child. This may require the nurse's taking the parents aside for a private conference.

In the absence of available babysitters, parents may have had to bring their other children with them. As necessary and when possible, parents should be encouraged to find appropriate supervision for their other children so that they are not needlessly exposed to the chaos of an ED and parents can concentrate on the ill child. Family members and friends who have good intentions but who are anxious may accompany parents to the ED. Sometimes these companions are helpful, but at other times they bring more stress than support. The nurse can help parents delegate tasks to the companions as a way to help parents while maintaining crowd control. Furthermore, a visit to the ED may culminate in hospitalization or an emergency operation. Some parents become immobilized in a crisis and unable to concentrate. The nurse plays a key role in helping parents to process information and make critical decisions. Problem-solving in the midst of a crisis involves prioritizing needs, identifying social supports, and mobilizing resources.

Pediatric Pain Management

"Pain is determined by many factors, including the medical condition, developmental level, emotional and cognitive state, personal concerns, meaning of pain, family issues and attitudes, culture and environment" (Agency for Health Care Policy and Research [AHCPR] 1992a, p 38). A number of invasive and painful procedures are performed in an ED. Nurses in an ED use both pharmacologic and nonpharmacologic measures to manage children's pain. The AHCPR (1992b) recommends the following guidelines for nonpharmacologic management of children's procedure-related pain.

Nonpharmacologic Management of Pain

- For infants, sensorimotor strategies include pacifiers, swaddling, holding, and rocking.
- Cognitive or behavioral strategies include hypnosis; relaxation; distraction; music, art, and play therapy; preparatory information; and positive reinforcement. Rehearsal before the procedure may be helpful.
- Child participation strategies focus on involving children in age-appropriate decisions about the procedure and in activities related to its conduct.
- Physical strategies include the application of heat or cold, massage, exercise, rest, and immobilization.
- Older children and adolescents who find nonpharmacologic strategies helpful may prefer these strategies over pharmacologic agents for procedures that are not excessively painful.

It is vital that ED pain management protocols incorporate developmental considerations and that all members of the team regularly discuss strategies for managing children's pain and factors that precipitate alterations in comfort.

Changing Family Lifestyles

A final note should be made about changing family realities. Twenty percent of children live in a single-parent family and 10% of American children live away from their parents—with relatives, neighbors, friends, or in institutions (Annie E. Casey Foundation, 1992). Such changes in family composition, to say nothing of the confounding effects of childhood poverty, connote the stress under which many of today's families are living and the impact that this stress has on a child's health and development. Emergency department nurses frequently encounter children who are not receiving routine primary health care, who are incompletely immunized, and who are uninsured or underinsured. It is understandable that repeatedly seeing families who are in crisis and children who are deprived provokes anger and frustration on the part of nurses. Nurses need to be aware that their feelings about a family's living conditions could be misinterpreted by parents as blame for their child's illness or injury. Emergency department nurses have the difficult task of trying to be nonjudgmental and sensitive to caregivers' feelings while carrying out a careful assessment of the child's condition and being alert for the possibility of neglect or abuse. In addition to attending educational programs and reading current publications, ED nurses benefit from group discussions about their personal reactions to working with critically ill children and distressed families.

INFANCY AND TODDLERHOOD

Many psychological activities are just beginning during infancy, such as language development, sensorimotor coordination, and social learning. The primary task during the first 18 months of life is for infants to engage in consistent and positive relationships with their primary caregivers, thereby establishing a sense of trust and a secure base from which to explore their environment. Growth patterns are cephalocaudal (ie, from top to bottom or head to toe) and proximodistal (ie, starting at the center and moving toward the extremities).

Cognitive Development: Sensorimotor Stage
Cognitive development proceeds through six substages, which Piaget described as the sensorimotor stage of cognition. Sensorimotor thought begins with simple reflexes during the first month and culminates with internalization of schemes between 18 and 24 months of age, when the infant can internalize a sensory image or word to represent an event (Santrock and Yussen, 1992). This primitive symbolic thinking accounts for one of the most important accomplishments in infancy, object permanence, whereby infants can understand that objects and events continue to exist even when they cannot directly be seen, heard, or touched.

Stranger Anxiety and Separation Anxiety
Wariness of strangers begins at around 6 months of age and peaks at about 12–18 months (Schuster and Ashburn, 1992). Most children between 8 and 24 months of age cry and protest if they are separated from their parents. The terms *stranger anxiety* and *separation anxiety* have been used interchangeably, but they are not the same. "Separation anxiety is the insecurity experienced by a young child when removed from a familiar person, object, or environment. . . . Stranger anxiety is the tension felt by the young child when introduced to an unfamiliar person" (Schuster and Ashburn, 1992, p. 175). Infants take their cues from their parents when approached by strangers. This has been termed social referencing. Thus parental anxiety is easily transmitted to infants by parents' facial expressions and body language.

To the extent possible, infants should not be separated from their parents in the ED. Rather, parents should be incorporated into examinations and procedures. Nurses should approach the infant positively, capitalizing on the novelty of the situation to distract the infant. Even if wearing a mask, the nurse can use gentle eye contact, soothing voice, and sensitive touch to comfort a fearful infant. If separation is unavoidable, then transitional objects, such as the parent's keys, a security blanket, or an article of clothing with the parent's familiar scent can help to decrease the infant's anxiety.

Assessing Infant Behavior
Because an infant is so small and vulnerable, illness—no matter how benign it may seem to the health care provider—is a major concern to the parents. They desperately want reassurance that their infant is all right and, by implication, that their parenting is all right too. It takes time for parents to get to know their infant's cues and to adapt to their infant's individual behavioral style or temperament. During the first 6 months of life, infants are most concerned with the effects of an altered schedule, such as hunger, lack of warmth, and inconsistent care giving, and with noxious stimuli that interfere with their state regulation, such as pain, loud noises, rough handling, and lack of non-nutritive sucking (Dixon and Stein, 1992).

Interpreting infants' cues and assessing parent-child interaction has been aided by the use of global observational measures. Barnard (1990) categorized cues as engagement or disengagement. Engagement cues, such as smiling or eyes widening, signal an infant's readiness for interaction. Disengagement cues, such as gaze aversion or hiccoughs, signal the need for a break from the interaction. Infants use these signaling devices to regulate their interaction with the environment. Nurses need to know what is typical infant behavior so that they can read infants' cues, assess parent-infant interaction, and provide anticipatory guidance to parents. Each visit to an ED offers an opportunity for enhancing parents' infant-care knowledge and skills, especially for recognizing signs of illness, seeking timely medical care, and managing routine illnesses at home.

An infant's excessive crying, inconsolability, or changes in feeding, elimination, and sleeping patterns may be the presenting complaint on arrival to the ED, thus nurses should be able to assess an infant's sleep and awake states. These include two sleep states (deep sleep and light sleep) and four awake states (drowsy, quiet alert, active alert, and crying (Blackburn and Loper, 1992). In addition, the nurse should note the degree to which the infant responds to visual and auditory stimuli; in other words, the nurse observes how easily the infant can be aroused and the degree to which the infant habituates (shuts out) the stimuli. How active is the infant and how smoothly and evenly does she move her extremities? What is the quality of the cry and can the baby be consoled? When held, does the infant cuddle and mold to the caregiver or does she stiffen, arch her back, and thrash about hysterically? Furthermore, how does the behavior observed in the ED compare with what the parent describes as typical behavior in the home?

Parents' concerns should not be dismissed just because they appear to be acting like "over anxious" or "typical" new parents. After all, parents know their children best and are often the first to notice subtle though vital clinical signs and symptoms. Parents need to believe that health care providers are listening to them and not judging them. Some parents enter an ED having had an unpleasant experience in the health care system. These parents may appear aggressive or even hostile toward health care professionals. However, if professionals are able to show empathy and respect to these parents, then the parents will be more receptive to medical and nursing interventions.

TODDLERHOOD

Toddlers (approximately 18 months–3 years of age) are especially threatened by strangers and fear being separated from their parents and losing control. Their attention span is limited and their sense of time is the here and now. They are very ritualistic and so even the slightest break from their routine (eg, having to drink fluids from a paper cup instead of their own tippy cup) could trigger a protest. Regressive behavior, such as temper tantrums, listlessness, and refusal to eat or drink, are considered adaptive and appropriate for toddlers in a crisis situation (Dixon and Stein, 1992). Some parents, however, are so concerned about trying to control their child's behavior that they mistake their toddler's protest as a personal rejection. This presents an opportunity for the nurse to talk with parents about how toddlers cope with stressful situations and to model developmentally sensitive approaches, such as using simple explanations, letting them play with the equipment, and incorporating security objects, into the procedures.

Toilet Training

Even though the focus of a visit to an ED is treatment of an illness or injury, routine parenting concerns almost always surface. Parents regard health care providers as knowledgeable about child care and may use this contact as an opportunity for advice on childrearing. A major childrearing challenge during toddlerhood is toilet training. This is the classic issue over which all parents struggle as they attempt to promote their child's independence and shift the burden from themselves as trainers to themselves as loving facilitators of their children's development. "The current consensus in our society is that children should be at least 18 months of age and walking well when one introduces the potty chair in a gradual fashion. Training efforts should be postponed if a family has recently moved, if a sibling has just been born, or other potentially upsetting family events have occurred" (Committee on Psychosocial Aspects of Child and Family Health, 1988, p 128). Nurses who find themselves in such a teachable moment may find the guidelines suggested by Powell (1981) helpful to reinforce with parents how to assess a child's readiness for toilet training, which is a *process*.

Toddlers who have achieved some degree of toilet training may perceive the application of a urine collection bag as a threat to their independence. Similarly, their parents may be reluctant to have the child use diapers because they fear backsliding or lost progress. Thus the ED nurse, armed with the knowledge of the developmental considerations for toilet training, can reassure the parents that any change to the toddler's elimination pattern is temporary and that some regression is expected as a result of illness and a stressful hospital experience.

Limit Setting

Another developmental issue commonly played out between toddler and parents involves discipline or limit setting. When a toddler's striving for mastery and autonomy is met with rigid parental control and unrealistic expectations, a power struggle is bound to ensue. Parental beliefs about how their child should behave may differ from what nurses expect. Yelling at a hysterical toddler only escalates the child's anxiety and causes the situation to go further out of control. Hitting a child back is likewise inappropriate and is an abuse of power. In such a situation nurses need to stay calm and assume an authoritative role as they attempt to redirect the toddler's behavior while encouraging the parents to soothe and support the child. Frightened toddlers may exhibit physically aggressive behavior, such as biting, kicking, and hitting. Sometimes simply trying to restrain a toddler for a procedure triggers an explosive and desperate struggle. Physical aggression, whether directed toward others or toward oneself, can be injurious. Toddlers who become out of control need gentle yet firm limits so that they will feel safe and secure.

Preparing Toddlers for Procedures

Keeping explanations and instructions simple—telling toddlers they are going to be all right and praising them for coping—fosters a supportive environment.

When possible, toddlers should be allowed to sit on their parent's lap for procedures. Attention must be paid to the parent's level of comfort, and a parent's individual needs and capabilities must be considered.

When multiple procedures need to be performed, the advantages and disadvantages of clustering care are weighed against spacing procedures out. Toddlers should not be prepared for procedures too far in advance; otherwise their anxiety will increase prematurely. Phrases with double meanings, such as "I'm going to give you a *shot*"; "Let me *take* your temperature"; or "We're going to *fix* your broken leg" should be avoided (Mott et al, 1990). Toddlers may be encouraged to play with the equipment before it is used on them. It must be kept in mind that what may seem non-threatening to an adult can be terrifying to a toddler. Routine procedures such as checking vital signs and looking in ears can feel very intrusive. Toddlers have a poorly defined concept of bodily integrity, and therefore the problem with routine procedures is not pain but fear of injury (Hazinski, 1992).

The role of parent normally includes that of protector. Not surprisingly then, many parents feel torn between wanting to help the ED staff with procedures and removing themselves from a painful situation to avoid guilt by association. If a parent chooses to leave the room while a procedure is done, the care provider should keep in mind that toddlers' sense of immediacy and limited sense of time may make it difficult for them to appreciate their parent's promise that they "will be back in a few minutes."

EARLY CHILDHOOD

Between the ages of 4 and 6 years, children learn to become more self-sufficient and to care for themselves. They develop school readiness skills and spend many hours in play and with peers. They have an active imagination, a burgeoning vocabulary, and an increased tolerance of separation experiences. Of course, the latter depends on their past experiences, attachment relationships, and environmental supports.

Cognitive Development: Preoperational Thought

Cognitive development during the early childhood period was described by Piaget as the preoperational period. Children between the ages of 4 and 7 years exhibit what Piaget termed the intuitive thought substage. During this substage children use primitive reasoning and ask a barrage of questions. Piaget called this time period intuitive because young children seem sure about what they know yet they are unaware of how they know what they know (Santrock and Yussen, 1992). The characteristics of intuitive thinking are described below.

Precausal or Transductive Thinking. Cause and effect relationships are ascribed to events linked together in time and space. For example, a child who is injured at play may believe that this is punishment for something she or he did wrong earlier in the day.

Animism. Inanimate objects are believed to have animate or life-like capabilities. For example, to a young child, an x ray machine may look like a monster; rubber tourniquets and blood pressure tubing may feel like a snake; and oxygen flowing through water may sound like someone is whispering.

Egocentrism. The child is unable to distinguish between his or her own perspective and that of someone else. For instance, when a father helps hold a child still for an injection, the child may view this cooperation as betrayal; ie, the father hurt the child because the father let the nurse give the injection rather than make her or him go away.

Symbolic Thought. The child uses one object (animate or inanimate) to represent another. Pretend play is a good example of this phenomenon. Medical or therapeutic play can help children work out their fears and frustrations around hospitalization and traumatic events. When children's anxiety levels are lowered they are better able to tolerate invasive procedures. For example, a child with asthma who has made numerous trips to the ED may bring her or his superhero dolls to the ED and pretend that they came along to get special power medicine. Reenacting treatments on a doll decreases anxiety and increases tolerance of the procedures.

Childhood Safety

"Nearly half of all childhood deaths are due to unintentional injuries, and about half of these stem from motor vehicle crashes" (United States Department of Health and Human Services [DHHS], 1990, p 13). It is ironic that injuries are the most preventable causes of childhood death. For example, the rate of childhood deaths from motor vehicle crashes has been reduced by the use of car seats and seat belts (DHHS, 1990). There are, however, still many children who ride in motor vehicles without proper restraints. Nurses in the ED are all too familiar with the tragic results of such crashes, and thus they are credible advocates of the use of car seats and seat belts. Nurses in the ED have a unique opportunity to screen all families for seat belt or car seat use. They can be a source of information about the proper use of car seats and seat belts for children and about how parents can use car seat loan programs in their communities. Another concern related to car safety is the practice of leaving children unattended in a car while the parent runs in "for a minute" to a store or back into the house for a forgotten article. It does not take a child very long, especially when unrestrained, to get behind the wheel of the car and imitate mommy or daddy driving.

Other types of injuries in childhood include drownings, falls, poisonings, and fires. From a developmental perspective, these all reflect the result of a young child's normal curiosity for exploring the environment and, in some instances, a lack of appropriate adult supervision. The latter might be due to a family crisis that leaves the parent less attentive to the child's activities. For example, one mother journeyed out of state for a family funeral and stored her antidepressant medication in her handbag. While the mother was engrossed in conversation with her relatives, her bored 4-year-old son rifled through the purse and ingested the pills. He thought they were candy.

Environmental safety requires parental vigilance and recognition of children's seemingly limitless abilities to acquire things for play, including matches and weapons. Children at play can be fearless and imaginative, as exemplified by children who test their ability to fly by jumping off a second-story porch. Living in impoverished and unsafe neighborhoods increases the risk of unintended injuries for a number of reasons. For one thing, there may be fewer safe places and less child-safe equipment for play. Second, parents who are struggling to make ends meet may need to relegate child care responsibilities to older children or adolescents. Third, undersupervised young children who are exposed to older children might try to imitate some of the risk-taking behavior they have observed.

There is no shortage of literature on injury prevention. A number of organizations have produced educational materials for parents. This information should be displayed in all ED waiting areas. More important, an ED encounter offers a unique opportunity for nurses to reinforce with parents the importance of minimizing environmental risks to children's safety and preventing access to poisons, matches, weapons, and equipment that is unsafe or is inappropriate for a child's age.

Preparing Four-to-Six-Year-Olds for Procedures

By the age of 4 years, children have a well-defined concept of their external bodies and the relationships among their body parts; however, their concept of the inner body is primitive (Vessey et al, 1990). Children between the ages of 4 and 8 years can recall about three to six internal body parts (most commonly the brain, heart, bones, and blood) (Vessey et al, 1990). Children in this age group, however, often misrepresent the size, shape, position, and consistency of these parts, such as drawing the heart in the shape of a valentine. Young children tend to be quite literal. They understand explanations if familiar words are used. Analogies are helpful, for example, the brain acts as the "boss" of the body; lungs fill up with air like "balloons"; and the heart keeps the body running like a car's "motor."

Explanations should be honest and age appropriate. If the child asks "Is it going to hurt?" he or she should be given a truthful answer, "It will hurt for just a moment." When a child asks "Why do you have to do that?" she or he should be given a simple answer, "To make you better." As with infants and toddlers, parents of young children should be involved in their child's care; the ED staff should take into consideration the parents' needs, fears, and capabilities. Adhesive bandages symbolize healing and protection of bodily integrity, so they should be used liberally. The child is allowed to participate in procedures when possible. For example, before drawing blood, the nurse could ask, "Which arm would you like the blood test from?" Never imply that a child has a choice when this is not so. For example, saying "I'm going to do a blood test now, OK?" denotes a question. An astute child will respond with an emphatic "No!" leaving the nurse struggling to regain the child's trust.

Letting children know what a procedure is going to feel like is another way of helping them cope. Most children 4–6 years of age fear imaginary creatures, the dark, being alone, and bodily injury (Dixon and Stein, 1992). Routine occurrences in an ED may seem harmless to an adult, but to an imaginative young child, these events are very threatening. Such things include the tight squeeze of an inflated blood pressure cuff; the pinch of a tourniquet; the blood-like appearance of povidone-iodine; the caustic smell of rubbing alcohol; the gush of fluid into an ear canal; gagging from a tongue blade; the sight of blood backing up an intravenous line or trickling from the site of a blood test; the shedding of one's own clothes for the impersonal hospital gown; the claustrophobic feeling of being papoosed or held down by a bunch of strangers; and the sense of suffocation when an oxygen mask covers the face. To an adult these things may seem harmless, but to an imaginative young child, the meaning holds no bound. A number of techniques can be used to lessen preschoolers' fears, including story-telling, use of imagery, puppetry, and relaxation breathing.

SCHOOL-AGED PERIOD

Children of school age (ages 7–12 years) master skills of reading, writing and arithmetic, and they are formally exposed to the larger world and its culture. Achievement becomes a more central theme of the child's world, and self-control increases. These children lead very busy lives; school, peers, and extracurricular activities such as sports, music lessons, or clubs take up much of their day. Social involvement and social acceptance are very important during the school-aged years. This gives nurses a variety of topics to converse about with a school-aged child, thereby focusing on the child's strengths and abilities, while taking some of the attention away from stressful ED events.

Gross motor abilities and strength increase during this age period. With new-found athletic abilities and independence come increased risks for unintentional injuries, especially with bicycle riding, roller skating, and in-line skating. In addition to the physical pain associated with trauma, the child may experience some emotional pain or guilt, especially when the injury resulted from violating their parents' proscriptions, for example, riding a bicycle with no hands or running out into the street for a ball. Parents may voice anger and disappointment over their child's disobedience. This a point where the nurse can intervene by encouraging the parent to focus on helping the child cope and avoiding the disconfirming "I told you so." Discussions about safety and injury prevention are better left to when the child is more comfortable and over the initial shock and fear from getting hurt and coming to the ED.

Cognitive Development: Concrete Operational Thought

School-aged children are able to reason about things and can appreciate several characteristics of an object rather than focusing or centering on a single property. Piaget described this stage of cognitive development as one of concrete operational thought (Santrock and Yussen, 1992). Increased verbal skills and understanding of causality enable school-aged children to participate more in their own care. Between the ages of 7 and 12 years, children become increasingly aware of their body and internal organs; they fear bodily harm and annihilation (Hurley and Whelan, 1988). Thus with a stressful hospital experience, there is the potential for feeling out of control.

Preparing School-aged Children for Procedures

Increased anxiety can hinder a child's ability to comprehend what under less stressful circumstances would be readily understood. Because they are so concerned about competency and projecting a brave self-image, school-aged children may suffer in silence rather than verbalize their fears or cry. Nurses need to consider all these possibilities as they assess a child's understanding of an event, and offer the child simple, clear, and truthful explanations. School-aged children love to impress one another with personal tales of prowess and may exaggerate events in favor of a more interesting story. Therefore, it is important to listen to what a child has been told about hospitals and to clear up any misconceptions. Nurses may decrease school-aged children's fears by providing them with reassurance, support, and praise for their efforts to cope. They need to know that they need not be ashamed about feeling afraid or crying. These children should be offered choices when appropriate and encouraged to take part in procedures. Cooperating with staff contributes to a personal sense of mastery and provides distraction from the discomfort. Hero worship is quite common with this age group. Nurses and doctors can capitalize on children's admiration and take the opportunity to teach them about healthy behaviors.

School-aged children look to those whom they admire to show knowledge and competence in getting things done. Helping parents feel in control and knowledgeable of what is transpiring in the ED ultimately helps allay their children's fears. Parents may share their own worries and concerns with staff and ask for suggestions on how to discuss certain concerns with the child. Parents often hope that they can protect their children from worry by holding back information. However, school-aged children are quite good at reading between the lines and interpreting their parents' nonverbal cues. In some situations, children may feel more afraid about what they have not been told, because they assume that all of the remote possibilities are true and that their parents are holding back information because they cannot deal with these issues (Dixon and Stein, 1992). Nevertheless, each child's case should be considered individually. Parents and children have different styles of coping, and clinicians should respect these differences.

ADOLESCENT PERIOD

Adolescence is a time of tremendous growth and discovery. This period of development begins with rapid physical changes—dramatic gains in height and weight; changes in body contour; and the development of secondary sex characteristics. During adolescence, reasoning becomes more logical, abstract, and idealistic.

Pursuit of independence (interdependence) and identity are prominent. Part of this discovery process entails risk-taking, which is fueled by adolescents' sense of invulnerability, their need for a positive self-image, and their desire for acceptance by peers. Today's adolescents have grown up in a culture in which they have been exposed regularly to graphic displays of guilt-free sex and violence, predictions of economic gloom and doom, forecasts of ecologic disaster, and the threat of nuclear war. Thus, there is an increasing concern that hopelessness about the future and disappointment in adult role models will result in more adolescents engaging in excessive risk-taking behavior.

Cognitive Development: Formal Operational Thought

Although formal operational thought or abstract reasoning is generally attributed to the adolescent's stage of cognitive development, not all adolescents reach this stage at the same time or to the same degree. Piaget believed that formal operational thought came into play between the ages of 11 and 15 years (Santrock and Yussen, 1992). Adolescents vary in their cognitive style, so it is perhaps more appropriate to think about adolescent cognition on a continuum of concrete to abstract thinking. Indeed, some adolescents may not advance beyond concrete operations. Elkind (1984) aptly described behavioral characteristics of egocentric thinking in adolescence: self-consciousness (imaginary audience); self-centeredness (personal fable); and a profound sense of invulnerability.

Adolescent Health Issues

Adolescents present unique challenges to professionals given the developmental, ethical, and legal issues that arise in adolescent health care (English, 1990). The primary objectives of nursing care are to promote adaptation, to enhance family functioning, and to foster communication between and among health care providers and families. Adolescents sometimes use an ED visit to gain access to health care. In other words, although they may present with one type of complaint, abdominal pain for example, adolescents may actually be concerned about another possibility, such as a sexually transmitted infection or pregnancy. Adolescents who have a hidden agenda are not trying to misuse the ED system. Rather, they are trying to find help and treatment for a condition they may believe to be both embarrassing and frightening.

Contemporary adolescent health problems are all preventable. The consequences of excessive risk-taking are reflected in contemporary adolescent health problems, the so-called social morbidities, which include violence, injuries, substance use, sexually transmitted diseases, and unintended pregnancies (Gans, 1990). Many youths manage to cope with the stresses of adolescence and are able to avoid or resolve situations that threaten their well-being. However, adolescents who suffer from poverty, abuse, depression, social isolation, and negative self-image are at higher risk for health problems.

It is still possible for adolescents who engage in excessive risk-taking to learn to become less impulsive and more responsible. Intervention requires assessment of the biopsychosocial factors associated with an adolescent's excessive risk-taking behavior; collaboration with other providers in the health care, social service, and educational systems; and participation in grass roots, community-based efforts toward youth development programs. Planning and evaluating nursing interventions should take into consideration not only adolescents' perceptions of the problem but also their ideas for change (McClelland, 1987).

Another issue germane to adolescents revolves around their right to know about their diagnosis and to be involved in decisions about their medical care. Parents and health care providers may disagree about what to tell an adolescent and about who should authorize testing and treatments. Each case should be considered on an individual basis while the health care providers endeavor to foster a trusting and open relationship with the adolescent and her or his parents. Rather than passing judgments on parents or the adolescent, the nurse should try to learn what is motivating parental decision-making, for example, fear, uncertainty, previous experience, or intuition (Worell and Danner, 1989). How are decisions normally made in this family and who, if anyone, usually takes charge? An adolescent may disagree with parents over the plan of care or about who should know about the diagnosis. Family mediation may be necessary to unravel the feelings of anger, resentment, and control that polarize family members. Whose best interest is at stake and what compromises are acceptable? Communication among family members is critical.

Preparing Adolescents for Procedures

Each adolescent is unique in terms of her or his level of cognitive development, health beliefs, and previous health care experiences. All adolescents deserve honest, straightforward, and clear explanations about ED treatments and procedures. Even though most adolescents are able to understand verbal explanations, using pictures, diagrams, and anatomic models enables them to grasp the meaning of what is being done. Because adolescents learn much of what they know from their peers, they may have misconceptions about their bodily functions or medical care. The ED nurse should probe for misinformation and myths but do so without making adolescents feel inferior for what they know or believe.

One issue that frequently arises for health care providers is that of balancing an adolescent's need for privacy with the parents' need for information. When parents are present, adolescents may refrain from asking questions for fear of divulging personal information or feeling embarrassed. Providing an opportunity for adolescents to discuss their care without their parents being present allows them to talk confidentially and to ask personal questions.

Adolescent Parents*

Adolescent pregnancy is regarded as a major health and social problem. However, the experience of becoming a mother holds special meaning for an adolescent depending upon her personal history, developmental maturation, and sociocultural context. Assuming the role of parent during one's adolescence means that the responsibility of caring for a helpless infant coincides with a time when an adolescent is struggling with her own developmental needs and is striving for greater independence and positive self-regard. The birth of a child places stress on the family system, which must realign as the adolescent's parents adapt to their new role. During the early months after delivery, family members and friends may rally around an adolescent mother, who in turn enjoys what has been referred to as the honeymoon phase. Ultimately the demands of parenting place the adolescent in a dependent position as she relies on family and other sources of support for child care.

Many adolescent mothers use the ED for their child's care, which is not surprising for a number of reasons. Adolescents are present oriented, and, generally speaking, they are also concerned about their child's welfare. So when adolescent mothers suspect that their child is ill, they want instant action. Adolescent mothers are also more apt to be unmarried, poor, and inexperienced in child care. Calling to schedule an appointment with their child's pediatrician or nurse practitioner, is not simple. Young mothers have little preparation in how to recognize and report children's symptoms of illness or about how to respond to triage questions. Therefore a trip to the ED may seem like a more direct way of dealing with the uncertainty. For those who are able to make an appointment (ie, for non-emergent or non-urgent health care needs), the thought of waiting, even for a day, may be so anxiety-producing that they opt for an ED visit instead. Transportation is another factor. Obtaining a ride to an ED may be more feasible if an otherwise uninvested family member believes that the child is "really sick." Likewise, taxi vouchers are usually available only for emergencies. All this is not to argue for inappropriate use of the ED by adolescent mothers, but rather to put adolescent behavior into perspective.

Adolescent mother-child interactions have been

---

*The author recognizes the importance of incorporating adolescent fathers into the plan of care. However, this discussion focuses on adolescent mothers because they are more likely to be seen in the emergency department.

rated as less effective than those of older mothers. Crockenberg (1987) found that adolescent mothers were more likely to be angry and punitive toward their 2-year-olds if they recalled feeling rejected as a child and were experiencing low partner support. The availability of social support is especially important for adolescent mothers, given the direct and indirect effects that stress can have on their children's development. A mother who feels supported in the day-to-day responsibilities of childrearing is more apt to function effectively as a parent than a mother who feels isolated and dissatisfied (Crnic and Greenberg, 1987).

A number of factors influence an adolescent's ability to be a parent—stress, coping, social support, childrearing attitudes, knowledge of child development, characteristics of the infant, and the adolescent mother's cognitive development. Socioeconomic factors such as income, education, housing, and access to health care are also important factors (Brooks-Gunn, 1990; Panzarine, 1989). Living with their own mothers, although it provides tangible and emotional support, may generate conflict over child care. It is not uncommon for this conflict to spill over into the ED, where grandmother and daughter openly disagree over the child's care. The nurse must avoid siding with one over the other. Instead she or he focuses on the child's needs and gives factual information. The nurse helps the mother and daughter see that although they might disagree about some childrearing practices, they both have the child's best interest at heart.

The resources available to a young mother may not be what she thinks she needs or wants, and there is often a cost-to-benefit ratio to social support. For example, an adolescent mother who herself needs to be admitted to the hospital from the ED may expect that her parents will care for their grandchild. The grandparents in turn may feel angry and overburdened. In such a situation the ED nurse should consult with the hospital social worker, who can help the family explore existing child care options and available resources.

Working with adolescent mothers can be difficult because they require patience, understanding, and a nonjudgmental approach. It is common to hear health care professionals ventilate about children raising children. However, it is not acceptable to let personal feelings like frustration, anger, and resentment interfere with a therapeutic, helping relationship. If an ED staff member feels inadequately prepared to work with adolescent mothers she or he can consult with other colleagues who specialize in working with this population. Often, recognizing one's own feelings of inadequacy or aversion for working with a particular group provides the stimulus for staff development, which in turn leads to improvement of care.

CHILDREN WITH SPECIAL HEALTH CARE NEEDS

Approximately 7.5 million children in the United States have a chronic condition; 10–15% of these conditions are considered to be severe (Jackson and Vessey, 1992). The prevalence rate of chronic conditions has been estimated at 10–20% of the pediatric population. Technologic and medical advancements have contributed to a greater survival rate for children, especially infants born prematurely, and thus there has been an increase in the proportion of children with special health care needs (Revell and Liptak, 1991). Given that children with chronic conditions are more likely to have higher health care utilization rates, it is not inconceivable that at least one of every five pediatric ED encounters involves a child with a chronic condition. Revell and Liptak (1991) described the many factors that characterize a child's chronic condition, including unpredictable course (eg, exacerbation of an asthmatic condition); complication of an ongoing condition (eg, shunt malfunction); increased susceptibility to infection (eg, in premature infants); pain (eg, sickle cell crisis); and problems associated with pharmacologic management of a condition (eg, subtherapeutic levels of phenytoin).

Parents of children with chronic conditions are invested in and knowledgeable about their children's care. Their protective roles may take on the characteristics of a broker or gatekeeper. Parents expect ED staff to pay heed to what they specify as their child's needs and wants. When ED staff are not familiar with a particular child's case or at least with the child's condition, the parent may fear that the child will receive substandard care. This can trigger a series of negative interactions between parent and provider. If the parent challenges the competency of the ED staff, the staff may respond defensively. Ultimately the person who suffers most from parent-provider conflict is the child.

Caring for children with special health care needs in an ED demands that a parent-provider partnership be formed. The parent really is the first and foremost source of information on the child. Old medical records, if available to the ED, take time to retrieve and, for children who have had multiple hospitalizations, are tedious to review. Therefore, if the child's primary provider can be contacted, the information that she or he provides will further enlighten staff and reassure parents. Coordination and continuity of care are vital for children with chronic conditions. Likewise, nurses (in-patient, home care, outpatient) who are involved with the child's ongoing care can contribute valuable information about a child's typical response patterns to acute exacerbations of the chronic condition.

Just because a child has a chronic condition does not mean he or she is comfortable with hospital treatments and invasive procedures. With each new experience, the child is struggling to make sense of what is happening now and is reminded of previous painful or frightening encounters. Thus children with chronic conditions need just as much, if not more, support and preparation as children without a chronic condition. Furthermore, children with a chronic condition may have impaired cognitive development or some other developmental disability as a result of the condition, so nurses need to adjust their preparation to each child's level of understanding. A child with a chronic condition is a child first and foremost, not a condition.

Terminally ill children may arrive at the ED for palliative measures (for example, hydration or pain management) or when parents have changed their minds about their child's dying at home, opting instead for the hospital environment. On arrival to the ED, there may be some debate among staff as to what measures ought to be carried out and about whether or not to resuscitate the child. Parents are already feeling devastated by their child's impending death; they do not need to suffer the added burden of fighting with ED staff. This is an example of why EDs need linkages with community providers and need established policies and procedures for the care and support of terminally ill children and their families.

CONCLUSION

Emergency department nurses can enhance their ability to meet children's psychosocial needs through (1) learning as much as they can about typical child development; (2) networking with pediatric primary care providers and community programs serving families; (3) joining forces with their colleagues (physicians, social workers, psychologists, respiratory therapists, child life workers, clerks, laboratory technicians, emergency medical technicians, porters, and hospital volunteers) to promote a nurturing, developmentally sensitive, and family friendly ED environment.

REFERENCES

Agency for Health Care Policy and Research (1992a). *Acute pain management in infants, children, and adolescents. Operative and medical procedures: quick reference guide for clinicians* (AHCPR Publication No. 92-0020). Rockville, Md: Agency for Health Care Policy and Research, Public Health Service, United States Department of Health and Human Services

Agency for Health Care Policy and Research (1992b). *Acute*

pain management. Operative or medical procedures and trauma: Clinical practice guideline (AHCPR Publication No. 92-0032). Rockville, Md: Agency for Health Care Policy and Research, Public Health Service, United States Department of Health and Human Services

Annie E. Casey Foundation (1992). *Kids count data book.* Washington, DC: Center for the Study of Social Policy

Barnard KE (1990). Assessment of parent-child interaction. In Meisels SJ, Shonkoff JP (eds), *Handbook of early childhood intervention.* New York: Cambridge University Press, pp 278–302

Blackburn ST, Loper DL (1992). *Maternal, fetal, and neonatal physiology: A clinical perspective.* Philadelphia: Saunders, pp 560–564

Brooks-Gunn J (1990). Adolescents as daughters and as mothers: A developmental perspective. In Siegel IE, Brody GH (eds), *Methods of family research.* Hillsdale, NJ: Lawrence Erlbaum Associates, pp 213–248

Committee on Psychosocial Aspects of Child and Family Health (1988). *Guidelines for health supervision II.* Elk Grove Village, Ill: American Academy of Pediatrics

Crnick K, Greenberg M (1987). Maternal stress, social support and coping: Influences on the early mother–infant relationship. In Boukydis CFZ (ed). *Research support for parents and infants in the postnatal period.* Norwood, NJ: Ablex Publications, pp 25–40

Crockenberg S (1987). Predictors and correlates of toddlers by adolescent mothers. *Child Development* 58:964–975.

Dixon SD, Stein MT (1992). *Encounters with children: Pediatric behavior and development* (2nd ed). St. Louis: Mosby, pp 2–6; 401–409

Elkind D (1984). *All grown up & no place to go.* Reading, Mass: Addison-Wesley, pp 23–43

English A (1990). Treating adolescents: Legal and ethical considerations. *Medical Clinics of North America* 74:1097–1112

Gans JE (Ed) (1990). *America's adolescents: How healthy are they?* Chicago: American Medical Association, pp x–xii

Hazinski MF (1992). *Nursing care of the critically ill child* (2nd ed). St. Louis: Mosby, pp 30–33

Hurley A, Whelan EG (1988). Cognitive development and children's perception of pain. *Pediatric Nursing* 14:21–24

Jackson PL, Vessey JA (1992). *Primary care of the child with a chronic condition.* St. Louis: Mosby Year Book

McClelland DC (1987). *Human motivation.* New York: Cambridge University Press, pp 508–510

Mott SR, James SR, Spherac AM (1990). *Nursing care of children and families* (2nd ed). Menlo Park, Calif: Addison Wesley, pp 812–858

Panzarine S (1989). Interpersonal problem solving and its relation to adolescent mothering behaviors. *Journal of Adolescent Research* 4:63–74

Powell ML (1981). *Assessment and management of developmental changes and problems in children* (2nd ed). St. Louis: Mosby

Revell GM, Liptak GS (1991). Understanding the child with special health care needs: A developmental perspective. *Journal of Pediatric Nursing* 6:258–268

Santrock JW, Yussen SR (1992). *Child development.* Dubuque: Wm. C. Brown, pp 255–286

Schuster CS, Ashburn SS (1992). *The process of human development: A holistic life-span approach* (3rd ed). Philadelphia: Lippincott, pp 166–185

United States Department of Health and Human Services (1990). *Healthy people 2000* (DHHS Publication No. PHS 91-50212). Washington, DC: United States Government Printing Office

Vessey JA, Braithwaite KB, Wiedmann M (1990). Teaching children about their internal bodies. *Pediatric Nursing* 16:29–33

Worell J, Danner F (1989). *The adolescent as decision-maker.* New York: Academic Press, pp 3–12

CHAPTER 5

Sociocultural Issues Related to Child Health Care

RACHEL E. SPECTOR

Why do parents bring their children to the emergency depart-ment when all they have is a fever? Or a cough? Or a sore throat? They could go to a pediatrician or clinic. Why do parents wait so long to bring their children to the emergency department when they have an acute abdomen? When they have a fractured arm? When they have a dangerously high fever? Are they unaware of the context of the problem? Why do so many people come together? Why did that mother be-come so abusive and hysterical when her son died? I thought I did the right thing by keeping her outside the room.

INTRODUCTION

All too often situations such as these occur in emer-gency departments (EDs) throughout the United States. Parents bring their children to the ED with problems best handled in a pediatrician's office (Woodwell, 1992), or they delay seeking treatment—sometimes until it is too late. Many family members may accompany parents when they seek emergency services. They may do so for pragmatic reasons, such as transportation, or they may come to provide kin-ship, support, and consolation. The needed cultural rituals that accompany death may be overlooked and omitted by ED personnel in the intensity of the mo-ment. These events, and countless others, are fre-quently observed among the families of children who are victims of triple jeopardy (Kunitz and Levy, 1991). They are young, they are poor, and they are most often members of a minority community.

Emergency nurses are perched on the edge of enormous demographic, social, and cultural change. Many of these changes play a dramatic role in both observed health care beliefs and practices, and the use of the ED by a family. This chapter addresses the de-mographic changes that are occurring in the United States and the sociocultural factors that serve both to facilitate and to hinder the provision of both primary and acute care services to children and their families in the ED. Nurses must give consideration to sociocul-tural issues and beliefs that vary from the dominant norms of health care beliefs and practices that have an impact on nursing care. This chapter is an overview of the rapidly growing field of transcultural nursing as it interfaces with the other specialty areas in profes-sional nursing.

DEMOGRAPHIC ISSUES

It has been said that "demography is destiny" (Hodg-kinson, 1986, p 273). Evidence of demographic change is seen in two ways—a comparison of the census of 1990 with that of 1980 and a comparison of immigra-tion profiles.

One need only analyze the 1990 census and com-pare it with the 1980 census to see how the population of the US is changing. The data from these two sources may be viewed in two ways. The commonly presented way is to look at the census that includes Hispanic origin without breaking down people of non-Hispanic origin. When this method is used, the comparison is as follows. In 1980, the overall population of the US (226.5 million) was 83.2% white; 11.7% black; 0.6% Na-tive American; 1.5% Asian/Pacific Islander; and 3% other. That is, 16.8% of the population comprised peo-ple of color. It may also be noted that 6.4% of the population claimed Spanish origin but could have been of any race. In 1990, despite an estimated shortfall of 5.3 million people in the head count, many of whom were non-white and Hispanic city dwellers (Sege and Mashek, 1991), the overall population of the US (248.7 million) was 80.3% white; 12.1% black; 0.8% Native American; 2.9% Asian/Pacific Islander, 3.9% other. That is, 19.7% of the population comprised people of color. Nine percent of the population claimed Spanish origin, but could have been of any race (Barringer, 1991). By 1990 the European majority had shrunk by about 3% (Figure 5–1). When the two sets of data are compared by taking Hispanic and non-Hispanic origin into account, the results are 79.7% white; 11.5% black; 0.6% Native American; and 1.5% Asian/Pacific Islander for 1980 (US Bureau of the Census, 1983) and 75.6% white; 11.7% black, 0.7% Native American; and 2.8% Asian/Pacific Islander for 1990 (US Bureau of the Census, 1991a) (Figure 5–2). Another example of demographic change was seen in New York, a city with a population of more than 7 million people. In New York the racial breakdown is white 43.2%; black 25.2%; Asian/Pacific Islander 6.7%; American Indian and other 0.5%; and Hispanic 24.4%, people of Hispanic origin being of any race (Basaden, 1992). The white majority population is shrinking and there is an emerging majority population composed of people of color and new immigrants from the Americas and Asia.

Most of the people who make up the population of the US are immigrants or their ancestors were immigrants. The early waves of immigrants were predominantly European, subsequent waves coming from Asia (1970s and 1980s) and from the Americas, especially Mexico and Central America (Lefcowitz, 1990). Every immigrant group has brought with them their own culture, beliefs, and attitudes (Castillo, 1979). This construct holds for beliefs and practices related to the prevention and treatment of illness. It is expected that a family learns from its heritage how to prevent and treat an episode of illness, including an acute episode. The relevance of these population changes to the study of the sociocultural aspects of illness prevention and treatment is readily understood when one realizes that much of the "American norm" regarding the prevention and treatment of illness is predicated on European-heritage philosophies, predominantly those of an allopathic nature.

There are differences in beliefs about health and illness both between and within groups. These differences occur not only between specific ethnic groups but also between the nurse and a child and his or her family. In addition, there are other differences to which the nurse must be sensitive to be both safe and

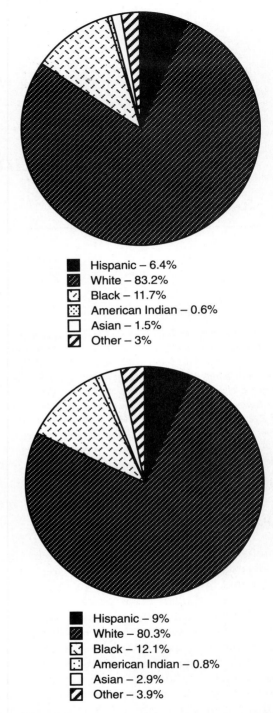

Hispanic – 6.4%
White – 83.2%
Black – 11.7%
American Indian – 0.6%
Asian – 1.5%
Other – 3%

Hispanic – 9%
White – 80.3%
Black – 12.1%
American Indian – 0.8%
Asian – 2.9%
Other – 3.9%

Figure 5–1. A. Census of the United States, 1980. (From United States Bureau of the Census [1983]. *Census of Population* [vol 1]. Characteristics of the population, section C, United States: Summary general social and economic characteristics, part 1. Washington, DC: US Government Printing Office, pp 1–13). **B.** Census of the United States, 1990. (From United States Bureau of the Census [1990]. Current population reports: 1990 census of population and housing. *Current population reports: 1990 census of population and housing.* Summary population and housing characteristics, United States. Washington, DC: Government Printing Office, p 59).

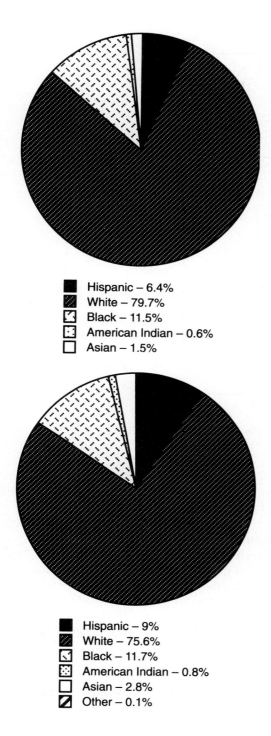

Hispanic – 6.4%
White – 79.7%
Black – 11.5%
American Indian – 0.6%
Asian – 1.5%

Hispanic – 9%
White – 75.6%
Black – 11.7%
American Indian – 0.8%
Asian – 2.8%
Other – 0.1%

Figure 5–2. A. Census of the United States of Hispanic origin and not of Hispanic origin. (From United States Bureau of the Census [1983]. *Census of population* [vol 1]. Characteristics of the population, section C, United States: Summary general social and economic characteristics, part 1. Washington, DC: US Government Printing Office, pp 1–13). **B.** Census of the United States of Hispanic origin and not of Hispanic origin, 1990. (From United States Bureau of the Census [1990]. *Current population reports: 1990 census of population and housing.* Summary population and housing characteristics, United States. Washington, DC: US Government Printing Office, p 59).

effective in the delivery of emergency nursing care. These differences include social issues, such as poverty; biologic issues, such as susceptibility to disease; and psychological issues, such as emotional and mental health problems.

SOCIAL BARRIERS TO CHILD HEALTH CARE

Innumerable barriers of a social nature, including poverty, language, and transportation, restrict families from using emergency services in an ordinary, expected manner. The major factor is poverty because it restricts a person's access to these services.

Poverty

The federal government has defined *poverty* as living below the poverty threshold. The poverty threshold is based on pre-tax income only, excluding capital gains, and does not include the value of non-cash benefits such as employer-provided health insurance, food stamps, or Medicaid. The average poverty threshold for a family of four was $12,674 in 1989 and $13,359 in 1990. The average poverty thresholds in 1990 varied from $6,652 for a person living alone to $26,848 for a family of nine or more members. (US Bureau of the Census, 1991b). The number of people living below the official government poverty level in 1990 was 33.6 million; this represented 13.5% of the nation's population. This figure represents the first statistically significant rise in poverty since 1982. Nearly half the nation's poor (40%) were children younger than 18 years. The poverty rate for children continues, as it has since 1975, to be higher than that for any age group. (US Bureau of the Census, 1991b). Overall, the poverty rates for whites and people of Hispanic origin increased in 1990; the rate for blacks did not change, remaining 30.7%. In 1990 the poverty rate for children younger than 18 years was 15.9% for white children; 38.4% for children of Hispanic origin; and 44.8% for black children (US Bureau of the Census, 1991b).

Cycle of Poverty

Poverty means more than the absence of money. One way of analyzing the phenomenon is by observing the effects of the cycle of poverty as illustrated in Figure 5–3. In this cycle, the child and family live in a situation that may lead to poor intellectual and physical development, poor economic production, and a high birth rate. Poor production leads to insufficient family salaries and a subsistence economy that forces the family to reside in densely populated areas or in remote rural areas, where there is often a lack of shelter and potable water and where the family members suf-

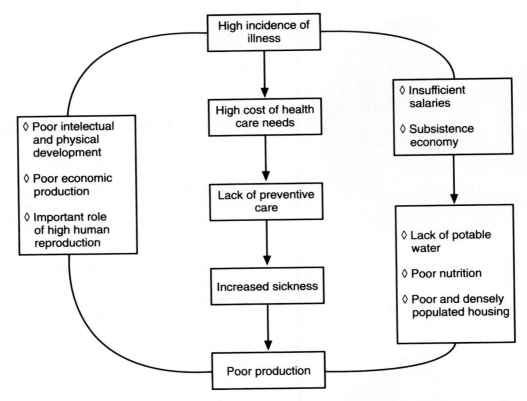

Figure 5–3. The cycle of poverty and poor health. *(From Spector M [1979]. Poverty: The barrier to health care. In Spector R [ed] [1979]. Cultural diversity in health and illness. New York: Appleton-Century-Crofts, p 150).*

fer from chronically poor nutrition. These phenomena all too often lead to high morbidity and accident rates which precipitate high health care costs, which prevent the family members from seeking health care services. This leads to an increase in sickness and poor production—a cycle that has yet to be broken (Spector, 1979). Other barriers related to this cycle are the lack of access to health care services, language barriers, and transportation problems.

Access
Several factors limit a family's access to the health care delivery system. They include availability, location, transportation, and whether or not the family has health insurance. The lack of insurance, be it public (Medicaid) or private, is a rapidly increasing problem. In Massachusetts alone, more than 600,000 people— 11% of the population—do not have health insurance (Kong, 1992).

Language
Because many new Americans tend to retain their native language (AnthroSight, 1992), there is a need for interpreters. As more and more immigrants arrive in the US, the need for adequate interpreters increases. All too often, however, these services are not available.

Communication and language are discussed later in this chapter.

Transportation
Families often are not able to get to emergency services because of geographic distance, and they may have to depend on other family members or friends for transportation. Many hospitals responsible for providing free care are not in the same area as the families needing this care. Public transportation may be expensive and, in some locations, unavailable.

CULTURAL BARRIERS TO PREVENTIVE HEALTH CARE

There are numerous ways of analyzing the role that culture plays in child health care practices. It is discussed in the contexts of heritage consistency and environmental factors, such as the ongoing use of traditional preventive and therapeutic practices. *Heritage consistency* is a theory that was originally developed in 1980 by Estes and Zitzow to develop a means of assessing and counseling within a cultural context Native Americans with alcoholism. The theory describes the degree to which one's lifestyle reflects his or her tribal culture. The theory has expanded in an attempt to study to what degree any person's lifestyle reflects his or her traditional culture. The value characteristics, such as spoken language of preference, food preferences, name, schools attended, neighborhood ties, and social activities, that indicate heritage consistency exist on a continuum. Any person can possess value characteristics of both a heritage-consistent (traditional) and a heritage-inconsistent (acculturated) nature. The concept includes a determination of one's cultural, ethnic, and religious background (Spector, 1991). This theory encompasses three broad concepts—culture, ethnicity, and religion.

Culture

Culture is the sum of socially inherited characteristics of a human group that comprises everything one generation can tell, convey, or hand down to the next (Fejos, 1959).

Ethnicity

Ethnicity is the condition of belonging to a particular ethnic group. Included in the characteristics of an ethnic group are common language; migratory status; race, language and dialect; religious faith or faiths; ties that transcend kinship, neighborhood, and community boundaries; shared traditions, values, and symbols; literature, folklore, and music; food preferences; settlement and employment patterns; special political interests; an internal sense of distinctiveness; and an external sense of distinctiveness. There are at least 106 different ethnic groups in America and more than 170 Native American tribes, or nations (Thernstorm, 1980).

Religion

Religion is the belief in a devine or superhuman power or powers to be obeyed and worshipped as the creator(s) and ruler(s) of the universe; and a system of beliefs, practices, and ethical values (Abramson, 1980). Religion provides a person with a frame of reference and a perspective with which to organize information. Religious teachings in regard to prevention, health, and illness help to present a meaningful philosophy and system of practices. This is done in a system of beliefs, practices, and social controls that have specific values, norms, and ethics and that vary among religious groups. Ethnicity and religion are related, and one's religion is quite often the determinant of his or her ethnic group.

TRADITIONAL EPIDEMIOLOGY

Numerous beliefs about the prevention and treatment of illness *may* be found among families from different

backgrounds who are members of the various ethnic communities of the US. The word *may* is used to prevent any kind of stereotyping, for the range of definitions of health and illness, beliefs, and practices is infinite. There are individual differences both within a group of people and between groups. There are also, however, discernible commonalties in the connotation of the terms *health* and *illness*. These commonalties *within* various ethnic groups are listed in Table 5–1 to sketch an image of the diversity that exists *among* groups.

Among families who have maintained traditional belief systems, there tend to be culturally based or folk beliefs that determine the definitions of health and illness. Folk medicine is related to other types of medicine. It has coexisted, with increasing tension, with modern medicine, but it was derived from earlier theories of academic medicine. There is ample evidence that the folk practices of ancient times have only in part been abandoned in modern belief systems; many of these beliefs and practices continue to be observed today. There are two varieties of folk medicine.

Varieties of Folk Medicine

1. Natural folk medicine—the use of the natural environment, including herbs, plants, minerals, and animal substances, to prevent illness
2. Magicoreligious folk medicine—the use of charms, holy words, and holy actions to prevent illness (Yoder, 1972).

There are also traditional healers within a given cultural community with whom parents may consult before they seek health care services or whom they may consult in the course of treatment.

The traditional or folk methods of prevention and treatment of illness rest in the family's ability to understand the cause of a given illness. Beliefs regarding the cause of illness differ vastly from the modern model of epidemiology. To more fully appreciate the richness of the methods used to prevent illness, it is important to have an awareness of what may be deemed the causation of illness, that is, traditional epidemiology. This model may be seen as having traditional agents, traditional hosts, and traditional environmental factors.

Traditional agents include hexes, spells, and the evil eye. The evil eye is a concept that manifests itself among numerous cultural, religious, and ethnic populations. Belief in the evil eye is one of the oldest held beliefs. It asserts that there is a power that emanates from the eye or mouth that strikes a victim, usually a child, with an injury, illness, or other misfortune. This belief helps explain misfortune (Spector, 1991). Illness also may be caused by people, such as witches, who have the ability to make others, again usually children, ill. Believers consider it necessary to avoid these peo-

TABLE 5–1. CROSS-CULTURAL EXAMPLES OF CULTURAL PHENOMENA

Place of Origin	Environmental Control	Health/Illness Beliefs	Methods of Prevention	Methods of Treatment	Traditional Healer

■ ASIA
China
Hawaii
Philippines
Korea
Japan
Southeast Asia
  Laos
  Cambodia
  Vietnam
	Traditional beliefs about health and illness
	Use of traditional medicines
	Traditional practitioners, Chinese doctors and herbalists
		Health is the balance of yin and yang
		Illness is an imbalance of yin and yang
			Diet
			Exercise
			Jade amulets
			Religion
			Ancestors
			Maintenance of body's balance
				Diet to rebalance yin and yang
				Acupuncture
				Herbal teas
					Chinese physician
					Acupuncturist

■ AFRICA West Coast (as slaves) Many African countries West Indies Dominican Republic Haiti Jamaica	Traditional beliefs about health and illness Folk medicine tradition	Health is harmony with nature Illness is disharmony with nature	Avoidance of evil spirits or demons Wearing bangles or a talisman Practice of voodoo Religious observances	Prayer Laying-on of hands Traditional remedies	Minister or priest Voodoo practioner
■ EUROPE Germany England Italy Ireland Other European countries	Primary reliance on modern health care system Traditional beliefs about health and illness Some remaining folk medicine tradition	Health is feeling all right Illness is feeling bad	Cleanliness Faith in God Wearing of amulets Prayer	Homeopathic remedies Prayer and faith Herbal teas	Priest or other religious leader Powwow person
■ NORTH AMERICA 170 Native American tribes Aleuts Eskimos	Traditional beliefs about health and illness Folk medicine tradition Traditional healers, medicine man	Health is living in harmony with nature Illness is disharmony with nature	Avoidance of witches Respect for the earth	Restoration of body's balance Conjuring and star-gazing Sand paintings	Medicine man
■ HISPANIC COUNTRIES Spain Cuba Mexico Central and South America	Traditional beliefs about health and illness Folk medicine tradition Traditional healers, Curandero	Health is a reward for good behavior, a balance of hot and cold Illness is a punishment for bad behavior, an imbalance of hot and cold	Proper diet Use of candles Wearing of amulets Avoidance of harmful people	Restoration of balance of hot and cold Herbal teas Prayer and faith	Herbalist Curandero Santero

(continued)

TABLE 5–1. (*Continued*)

Place of Origin	Variations/High Morbidity	Social Organization	Communication	Space	Time Orientation

▪ ASIA
China
Hawaii
Philippines
Korea
Japan
Southeast Asia
  Laos
  Cambodia
  Vietnam
	Liver cancer
	Stomach cancer
	Coccidioido-
	  mycosis
	Hypertension
	Lactose intol-
	  erance
		Family—Hierar-
		  chial structure,
		  loyalty
		Devotion to
		  tradition
		Many religions,
		  including Tao-
		  ism, Buddhism,
		  Islam, and
		  Christianity
		Community so-
		  cial organiza-
		  tions
			National and lo-
			  cal languages
			Cantonese
			Pidgin
			Tagalog
			Korean
			Haragei
			French and na-
			  tional lan-
			  guages
				Avoidance of
				  contact
					Present

▪ AFRICA
West Coast (as slaves)
Many African countries
West Indies
Dominican Republic
Haiti
Jamaica
	Sickle cell
	  anemia
	Hypertension
	Cancer of the
	  esophagus
	Stomach cancer
	Coccidioido-
	  mycosis
	Lactose intol-
	  erance
		Family—many
		  female, single
		  parent
		Large extended
		  families
		Strong church af-
		  filiation with
		  community
		Community so-
		  cial organiza-
		  tions
			National
			  languages
			Dialect
			Pidgin
			Creole
			Spanish
			French
				Close personal
				  space
					Present over fu-
					  ture

▪ EUROPE
Germany
England
Italy
Ireland
Other European coun-
  tries
	Breast cancer
	Heart disease
	Diabetes mellitus
	Thalassemia
		Nuclear families
		Extended families
		Judeo-Christian
		  religions
		Community so-
		  cial organiza-
		  tions
			National
			  languages
			Many learn En-
			  glish imme-
			  diately
				Avoidance of
				  contact
				Aloof
				Distant
				In Southern
				  countries,
				  closer contact
				  and touch
					Future over pres-
					  ent

▪ NORTH AMERICA
170 Native American
  tribes
Aleuts
Eskimos
	Accidents
	Heart disease
	Cirrhosis of the
	  liver
	Diabetes mellitus
		Most extremely
		  family oriented
		Biologic and ex-
		  tended families
		Children taught
		  to respect
		  traditions
		Community so-
		  cial organiza-
		  tions
			Tribal languages
			Silence and body
			  language
				Space is very im-
				  portant and
				  has no bound-
				  aries
					Present

▪ HISPANIC COUNTRIES
Spain
Cuba
Mexico
Central and South
  America
	Diabetes mellitus
	Parasites
	Coccidioido-
	  mycosis
	Lactose intol-
	  erance
		Nuclear families
		Extended
		  families
		Compadrazzo
		  (godparents)
		Community so-
		  cial organiza-
		  tions
			Spanish or
			  Portuguese
			Native languages
			  and dialects
				Tactile
				  relationships
				Touch
				Handshakes
				Embracing
				Physical pres-
				  ence valued
					Present

ple. When the person is successful in causing illness, the illness can best be cured by physically removing the person's influence from the vulnerable child.

Traditional host factors include such phenomena as soul loss; spirit possession; the ability to provoke the envy, hate, and jealousy of a friend, acquaintance, or neighbor; and the religious and social behavior of the person. Health is often viewed as the reward for good behavior, illness the punishment for bad behavior.

Traditional environmental factors include air quality—*mal aire* (bad air)—and such natural events as a solar eclipse.

TRADITIONAL PRACTICES

Traditional practices of prevention developed from the folk beliefs about the causes of illness. People avoided those who were known to cause or transmit hexes and spells, and many elaborate methods were developed to prevent the envy, hate, and jealousy of others. Countless methods evolved over generations and exist today to protect people from the evil eye. Every effort is made by the host to avoid situations in which behavior, be it social or religious, is compromised. In many traditions people take extra precautions to protect themselves from *mal aire*. Pregnant Hispanic women are not allowed to go outside during an eclipse.

The following are examples of traditional practices used in the prevention and treatment of illness.

Protective or Religious Objects
Various protective objects may be worn, carried, or hung in the home. Amulets are objects with magical powers, such as charms, worn on a string or chain around the neck, wrist, or waist to protect the wearer from the evil eye or evil spirits. These spirits can be transmitted from one person to another, or they may have supernatural origins. Amulets have been found to exist in societies all over the world; they are associated with the protection of mankind from trouble (Budge, 1978). In addition to amulets is a talisman, a consecrated religious object believed to posses extraordinary powers (Spector, 1991). A talisman may be worn on a rope around the waist or carried in a pocket or purse. The evil eye also may be avoided by touching a baby when it is admired, a Puerto Rican belief, or by drawing a circle around a baby's bed and spitting on the child three times, an Eastern European belief.

Illness is frequently treated by the use of religious beliefs, practices, and objects. The wearing of religious medals, carrying of prayer cards, and performance of sacrifices are not unusual practices.

Substances
The use of substances employs the use of diet, which consists of many different observances. It is believed that the body is kept in balance or harmony by the type of food that is eaten. There are numerous food taboos and combinations that are prescribed in traditional belief systems. People from many ethnic backgrounds eat raw garlic or onion in an effort to prevent illness. Garlic or onions may also be worn on the body or hung in the home.

A wide variety of substances may be ingested for the treatment of maladies. Frequently, the active ingredients of these traditional remedies are unknown. If a child is believed to have been given these remedies, an effort must be made to determine what the child has taken and the active ingredients of the remedy. Often the active ingredients can be either antagonistic or synergistic to prescribed medications. When this is the situation, the medication may have no effect, or a severe overdose may occur. When children are assessed and it is found that parents are not adhering to a pharmacological regimen, an effort must be made to determine if they are giving the child traditional remedies. Substances may also be used to restore the body's balance, and they may be introduced into the body in other ways. An example of this is the Asian practice of coining, in which a substance, usually tiger balm, is rubbed over the body in certain areas, such as the back or arms, with a coin to release wind and restore the body's balance.

Religious Practices
Religion strongly affects the ways in which people choose to prevent and treat illness. It plays a strong role in rituals associated with prevention, therapy, death, and dying. It dictates social, moral, and dietary practices designed to keep a person in balance and healthy; it plays a vital role in a person's perception of the prevention of illness and restoration of health. Many people believe that illness is prevented and treated by strict adherence to religious codes, morals, and practices. They view illness as a punishment for breaking a religious code. There are strong beliefs in religious healing and there continues to be an active use of traditional healers. There are countless rituals that must be adhered to during the dying process, such as the Catholic ritual of the anointing of the sick (Spector, 1991) when they are extremely ill or at the moment of death. Numerous other religious practices must be performed at the moment or just before death that require the active participation of family members. In some ethnocultural groups, ritual anointing of the body and washing is necessary. Some groups, such as gypsies, believe that a person should die close to the

earth; the family requests that their loved one be placed on the floor to die. The practice of isolating a family member from the rest of the group is not necessary; it may cause more harm than good.

TRADITIONAL HEALERS

In the traditional context, healing is the restoration of a person to a state of harmony among body, mind, and spirit—the restoration of holistic health. Within a given community there are specific people who are known to the members of the community to have the power to heal (Table 5–1). The healer may be male or female and is most often a person who is thought to have received the gift of healing from a divine source.

In many instances, a person who is heritage consistent may consult a traditional healer before, instead of, or during the use of a modern health care provider. The relationship between the person and the healer is quite often much closer than that of the person and the health professional. The person sees in the healer one who understands the problem within his or her cultural context, who speaks the same language, and who shares a similar worldview. The following are examples of traditional healers.

Traditional Healers

- Medicine man—the traditional healer of Native Americans
- Señora—a Puerto Rican woman knowledgeable in the treatment of illness
- Esperitista—a woman who possesses more sophisticated skills than a señora
- Curandero—a man who has the God-given ability to heal; he uses a religious psychiatric approach
- Partera—a Mexican-American midwife
- Root-worker—a black person who is able to determine the cause of an illness and the treatment

It must be remembered that traditional healers have been a part of human cultures for as long as the cultures have existed. The methods used to heal have been developed over the generations by trial and error, and religious beliefs and social circumstances contribute to the methods. The effective methods have been preserved and adapted to meet the needs of the present time. A traditional healer is aware of the needs of the child and the family, and is able to understand them within the cultural context of the problem in today's world.

OTHER CONSIDERATIONS

Several other factors (Table 5–1) vary among cultural groups and are related to the delivery of emergency care.

Biological Variations and High Morbidity

Countless physiological differences exist in respect to the susceptibility to disease, dermatologic conditions, and food and eating habits. Susceptibility to disease varies because of genetic or life-style differences. Some ethnic groups are more susceptible to certain diseases than others. In general, ethnic groups of lower socioeconomic status are more susceptible to acquired diseases and conditions, such as malnutrition and infections. Table 5–1 displays selected diseases and the ethnic groups that have high rates of the diseases. There also may be differences between the nurse's expectations and the client's perceptions of emotional and mental health, emotional expression, and reactions to pain, gender role behaviors, and attitudes toward the family.

Communication

Differences in communication are manifested in the following ways.

Manifestations of Differences in Communication

- Use of English as the common language
- Various connotations and denotations for a given word
- Verbal as opposed to nonverbal communication
- The use of body language (Giger and Davidhizar, 1991).

Culture also may be defined as a metacommunication system, in which not only words but also how one handles oneself has meaning. This system includes how people handle time commitments and conversation (Hall, 1988). For example, a given person may not arrive at the time specified for an appointment. It is common for nurses to ask questions, but in many cultures people do not ask questions directly and they do not answer probing questions. In many cultures, true communication is implemented nonverbally.

Space

The distances that people prefer to keep from one another is a legendary problem; the dimensions of acceptable spatial distances vary among cultural groups. The use of touch, a source of communication with a spatial relationship, also differs across cultures. In some Hispanic cultures, one is expected to shake hands, and it is permissible to embrace a person with whom one has a limited acquaintance. In Northern European cultures such behavior is taboo, and a touch can do more harm than good. Eye contact is common among people of a European background, and it is expected; people may think the worst when a person does not look them in the eye. Among black Americans, however, eye contact is quite often taboo (Giger and Davidhizar, 1991).

Time Orientation

Time has countless sets of meanings, two of which are important in that they focus either on specific points in time (clock time or future orientation) or on duration (social time or present orientation). People who are oriented to future time tend to adhere strictly to clock time, whereas, those who are present-oriented tend not to adhere to rigid time boundaries (Giger and Davidhizar, 1991).

Social Organization

The ways in which a child and his or her family are organized as a unit and the manner in which they interact with the larger community also are structured within a cultural context. Families may depend on a particular person or group, and through this affiliation acquire their health-seeking practices and behaviors. There are numerous ways in which a family is structured and there are multiple functions for this unit.

IMPLICATIONS FOR EMERGENCY NURSING

Practitioners of emergency nursing must continuously expand their awareness of and sensitivity to the cultural needs of children and their families. The ongoing awareness of changing demographic and immigration trends; the continuous monitoring of social and political responses to issues such as poverty; a sensitivity for culture-based health traditions in respect to prevention and treatment; an ability to communicate in another language, either by speaking the language or by using competent interpreters; and an awareness of the person's beliefs in regard to space and time orientation are several of the ongoing activities that will enhance the cross-cultural practice of emergency nursing. The following are a list of cultural assessment points and recommendations for providing culturally sensitive care.

Cultural Assessment Points

- Cultural Background—Obtain a brief history of the parents' ethnic, religious, and racial origins and heritage level

- Values Orientation—Explore the attitudes of the family based on their cultural concepts of health and illness
- Cultural Sanctions and Restrictions—Know the rules in this family's cultural background in respect to exposure of body parts, for example
- Communication—Determine what language the family speaks and if competent interpreters are available
- Health- and Illness-Related Beliefs and Practices—Determine what cultural factors the family associates with the health problem. Find out what types of traditional healers are known to be available to the family
- Nutrition—Find out if there are specific dietary restrictions to consider
- Socioeconomic Considerations—Investigate what social and economic resources are available to the family
- Educational Background—Ask the parents about their level of education. Determine if they are able to read and to understand and follow instructions
- Religious Affiliation—Explore the role religion plays in the life of the family. Determine if a mem-

TABLE 5–2. NURSING RESOURCES IN CULTURAL DIVERSITY

Transcultural Nursing Society
Journal of Transcultural Nursing

Membership information available from
Donna Barnes, Executive Assistant
Transcultural Nursing Society
Madonna University Office
College of Nursing and Health
36600 Schoolcenter
Livonia, MI 48150
(313) 541-8320

Transcultural Nursing Certification available from
Dr G Roessler
8401 Munster Dr
Huntington Beach, CA 92646

Council on Nursing and Anthropology
c/o Millie Roberson
Coordinator, Graduate Program
Nursing Department
Southwest Missouri State University
Cape Girardeau, MO 63701
(314) 651-2955

Anthropological Perspectives
PO Box 1721
Richland, WA 99352
(509) 627-2944
Several publications, including *AnthroSight: Anthropology for Decision Makers.*

ber of the clergy of their background is available. Explore the mandates of the religion in respect to death and dying and emergency care (Jarvis, 1992)

A careful patient assessment and an awareness of the family's unique cultural heritage enhance the delivery of culturally sensitive nursing care in the pediatric emergency setting. Table 5–2 presents a number of resources on this topic.

REFERENCES

AnthroSight (1992). January, p 5

Abramson P (1980). Religion. In Thernstorm S (ed), *The Harvard encyclopedia of American ethnic groups*. Cambridge, Mass: Harvard University Press, pp 869–875

Barringer F (1991). Census shows profound change in racial makeup of nation. *New York Times*, 11 March, p 1

Basaden A (1992). Census Bureau, Webster Encyclopedia, World Almanac, NY '92. *Boston Herald*, 7 July, p 6

Budge EAW (1978). *Amulets and superstition*. New York: Dover, pp 10–12

Castillo LJ (1979). Keynote address. Communicating with Mexican Americans: *Pour su bueno salud*. Houston: Baylor College of Medicine

Estes G, Zitzow D (1980). Heritage consistency as a consideration in counseling Native Americans. Presented at the National Indian Education Association Convention, Dallas, Texas, November 1980

Fejos P (1959). Man, magic, and medicine. In Goldstone I (ed), *Medicine and anthropology*. New York: International University Press, p 43

Giger JN, Davidhizar RE (1991). *Transcultural nursing assessment and intervention*. St. Louis: Mosby Year Book, pp 7–26; 42–48; 78–79

Hall ET (1988). Introduction. To Matsumoto M, *The unspoken way*. New York: Kodansha International, pp 14–15

Hodgkinson HL (1986). Reform? Higher Education? Don't be absurd! *Higher Education*, December: 271–274

Jarvis C (1992). *Physical examination and health assessment*. Philadelphia: Saunders, pp 98–99

Kong D (1992). Access to care. *Boston Globe*, 15 July, pp 1;13

Kunitz SJ, Levy JL (1991). *Navajo aging: The transition from family to institutional support*. Tucson: University of Arizona Press, p 146

Lefcowitz E (1990). *The United States immigration history timeline*. New York: Terra Firma Press

Sege I, Mashek J (1991). Census total will stand despite undercounting. *Boston Globe*, July 16

Spector M (1979). Poverty: The barrier to health care. In Spector R, *Cultural diversity in health and illness*. New York: Appleton-Century-Crofts, pp 141–162

Spector R (1979). *Cultural diversity in health and illness (3rd ed)*, Norwalk: Appleton & Lange, pp 50–58;126;144;

Thernstorm S (ed) (1980). *The Harvard encyclopedia of American ethnic groups*. Cambridge, Mass: Harvard University Press, p vii

US Bureau of the Census (1983). *Current Population Reports*.

1980 General Social and Economic Characteristics. Part 1, United States Summary, PC80-1-C1, United States. Washington, DC; US Government Printing Office, pp 1–13

US Bureau of the Census (1991a). *Current Population Reports*. 1990 Census of Population and Housing: Summary Population and Housing Characteristics, United States. Washington, DC; US Government Printing Office, p 59

US Bureau of the Census (1991b). *Current Population Reports*. Series P-60, No. 175. Poverty in the United States: 1990, Washington, DC; US Government Printing Office, p 1

Woodwell D (1992). Office visits to pediatric specialists, 1989. Advance data from *Vital and health statistics, #208*. Hyattsville, Md: National Center for Health Statistics

Yoder D (1972). Folk medicine. In Dorson RH (ed), *Folklore and folklife*. Chicago: University of Chicago Press, pp 191–193

SUGGESTED READING

Books

Becerra RM, Shaw D (1984). *The elderly Hispanic: A research and reference guide*. Lanham, Md: University Press of America

Bienvenue RM, Goldstein JE (1981). *Ethnicity and ethnic relations in Canada (2nd ed)*. Toronto: Butterworth

Blattner B (1981). *Holistic nursing*. Englewood Cliffs, NJ: Prentice-Hall

Boyle JS, Andrews MM (1989). *Transcultural concepts in nursing care*. Glenview, Ill: Scott, Foresman / Little, Brown

Bryant CA (1985). *The cultural feast: An introduction to food and society*. St. Paul: West

Carnegie ME (1987). *The path we tread: Blacks in nursing 1854–1984*. Philadelphia: Lippincott

Carson VB (1989). *Spiritual dimensions of nursing practice*. Philadelphia: Saunders

Comas-Diaz L, Griffith EEH (eds) (1988). *Clinical guidelines in cross-cultural mental health*. New York: Wiley

Curry MA (1987). *Access to prenatal care: Key to preventing low birthweight*. Kansas City: American Nurses' Association

Delaney J, Lupton MJ, Toth E (1988). *The curse: A cultural history of menstruation*. Chicago: University of Chicago Press

Dinnerstein L, Reimers DM (1988). *Ethnic Americans*, 3rd Edition. New York: Harper & Row

Fuentes C (1985). *The old gringo*. New York: Farrar, Straus, Giroux

Gibbs JT, Huang LN (1983). *Children of color*. San Francisco: Jossey-Bass

Gonzalez-Wippler M (1985). *Tales of the Orishas*. Bronx: Original Publications

Gonzalez-Wippler M (1987). *Santeria: African magic in Latin America*. Bronx: Original Publications

Hammerschlag CA (1988). *The dancing healers: A doctor's journey of healing with Native Americans*. San Francisco: Harper & Row

Hirsch ED (1987). *Cultural literacy: What every American needs to know*. Boston: Houghton Mifflin

Kalish RA, Reynolds DK (1976). *Death and ethnicity: A psycho-*

cultural study. Los Angeles: Ethel Percy Andrus Gerontology Center

Lawless EJ (1988). *God's peculiar people.* Lexington: University of Kentucky Press

Lesnoff-Caravaglia G (ed) (1987). *Realistic expectations for long life.* New York: Human Sciences Press

Meyer CE (1985). *American folk medicine.* Glenwood, Ill: Meyerbrooks

Morrison T (1981). *Tar Baby.* New York: Alfred A. Knopf

Morrison T (1987). *Beloved.* New York: Knopf/Random House

Murray P (1987). *Song in a weary throat: An American pilgrimage.* New York: Harper & Row

Stoll RI (1990). *Concepts in nursing: A Christian perspective.* Madison, Wis: InterVarsity Christian Fellowship

Strange H, Teitelbaum M (eds) (1987). *Aging and cultural diversity.* South Hadley, Mass: Bergin & Garvey

Walker A (1989). *The temple of my familiar.* New York: Harcourt, Brace, Jovanovich

Zahler D, Zahler KA (1988). *Test your cultural literacy.* New York: ARCO

Zambrana RE (ed) (1982). *Work, family, and health: Latina women in transition.* New York: Fordham University

Articles

Airhihenbuwa CO (1989). Health education for African Americans: A neglected task. *Health Education* 20:9–14

Bartlett EE (1989). Learning from special populations. *Patient Education and Counseling* 13:87–89

Bashshur R, Steeler W, Murphy T (1989). On changing Indian eligibility for health care. *American Journal of Public Health* 77:690–693

Bernal H, Froman R (1987). The confidence of community health nurses in caring for ethnically diverse populations. *Image: Journal of Nursing Scholarship* 19:201–203

Capers CF (ed) (1985). Cultural Diversity in Nursing Practice. *Clinical Nursing* 7:1–84

Conway FJ, Carmona PE (1989). Cultural complexity: The hidden stressors. *Journal of Advanced Medical Surgical Nursing* 1:65–72

DeSantis L (1989). A profile of cultural diversity in nursing practice. *Florida Nurse* 37:15

DeSantis L, Thomas J (1990). The immigrant Haitian mother: Transcultural nursing perspective on preventive health care for children. *Journal of Transcultural Nursing* 2:2–15

Douglass T (1989). A real case for non-verbal communication in nursing practice. *Washington Nurse* 19:12–14

Fleming J (1989). Meeting the challenge of culturally diverse populations. *Pediatric Nursing* 15:566, 634, 648

Foreman JT (1985). Susto and the health needs of the Cuban refugee population: Symptoms of depression and withdrawal from normal social activity. *Topics in Clinical Nursing* 7:40–47

Frye BA (1990). The Cambodian refugee patient: Providing culturally sensitive rehabilitation nursing care. *Rehabilitation Nursing* 15:156–158

Gann P, Nghiem L, Warner S (1989). Pregnancy characteristics and outcomes of Cambodian refugees. *American Journal of Public Health* 79:1251–1256

Herndon TR (1990). Cultural factors play a role in pediatric assessment. *Florida Nurse* 38:11

Hobus R (1990). Living in two worlds: A Lakota transcultural nursing experience. *Journal of Transcultural Nursing* 2:33–36

Holtz C, Bairan A (1990). Personal contact: A method of teaching cultural empathy. *Nurse Educator* 15:13,24,28

Horn B (1990). Cultural concepts and postpartal care. *Journal of Transcultural Nursing* 2:48–51

Huttlinger K, Wiebe P (1989). Transcultural nursing care: Achieving understanding in a practice setting. *Journal of Transcultural Nursing* 1:17–21

Johnston JB (1987). Giving effective emergency care to patients from differing cultures. *Emergency Nursing Reports* 2:1–7

Lawson LV (1990). Culturally sensitive support for grieving parents. *American Journal of Maternal Child Nursing* 15:76–79

Leduc E (1989). The healing touch. *American Journal of Maternal Child Nursing* 14:41–43

Leininger M (1989). Transcultural nurse specialists and generalists: New practitioners in nursing. *Journal of Transcultural Nursing* 1:4–16

Leininger M (1989). Transcultural nursing: Quo vadis (where goeth the field?) *Journal of Transcultural Nursing* 1:33–45

Leininger M (1989). The transcultural nurse specialist: Imperative in today's world. *Nursing and Health Care* 10:250–256

Leininger M (1990). The significance of cultural concepts in nursing. *Journal of Transcultural Nursing* 2:52–59

Luna L (1989). Transcultural nursing care of Arab muslims. *Journal of Transcultural Nursing* 1:22–26

Oneha MF, Magyary DL (1992). Transcultural nursing considerations of child abuse/maltreatment in American Samoa & Federated States of Micronesia. *Journal of Transcultural Nursing* 4:11–17

Pasquale EA (1984). The evil eye phenomenon: Its implications for community health nursing. *Home Health Care Nurse* 2:19–21

Pasquale EA (1986). Santeria: A religion that is a health care system for Long Island Cuban-Americans. *Journal of the New York State Nurses' Association* 17:12–15

Phillips S, Lobar S (1990). Literature summary of some Navajo child health beliefs and rearing practices within a transcultural nursing framework. *Journal of Transcultural Nursing* 1:13–20

Pickwell S (1989). The incorporation of family primary care for Southeast Asian refugees in a community-based mental health facility. *Archives of Psychiatric Nursing* 3:173–177

Poss JE (1989). Providing health care for Southeast Asian refugees. *Journal of the New York State Nurses' Association* 20:4–6

Ray M (1990). Transcultural caring: Political and economic visions. *Journal of Transcultural Nursing* 1:17–21

Reinert BR (1986). The health care beliefs and values of Mexican-Americans. *Home Healthcare Nurse* 4:23,26–27

Rosenbaum JN (1989). Depression: Viewed from a transcultural nursing theoretical perspective. *Journal of Advanced Nursing* 14:7–12

Sobralske MC (1985). Perceptions of health: Navajo Indians, *Topics in Clinical Nursing* 7:32–39

Tripp-Reimer T (1989). Cross-cultural perspectives on patient teaching. *Nursing Clinics of North America* 24:613–619

Valente SM (1989). Overcoming cultural barriers. *California Nurse* 85:4–5

Wallace G (1979). Spiritual care: A reality in nursing education and practice. *The Nurses Lamp* xxxi:1–4

Wenger AF (1992). Transcultural nursing & health care issues in urban & rural contexts. *Journal of Transcultural Nursing* 4:4–10

Wilson DA (1989). My trips over the language barrier. *American Journal of Nursing* 89:17–18

Wissow LS, et al (1988). Poverty, race, and hospitalization in childhood asthma. *American Journal of Public Health* 78: 777–782

CHAPTER 6

Legal Issues

PATRICIA A. SOUTHARD

INTRODUCTION

Health care providers are often overwhelmed with the abundance of apparent legal considerations present in the provision of medical care to adult patients. Medical personnel who practice in the field of pediatrics find different and to some extent greater legal considerations that must be taken into account in the medical care of a child. This chapter explores medicolegal considerations for children, including assent as opposed to consent, refusal of treatment, the responsibilities of health care providers to report child abuse and neglect, a child's ability to terminate life support, minors as organ donors, the application of COBRA laws to childrens' hospitals, and participation in research by minors.

Each state has enacted laws that address medicolegal issues relative to children. This chapter is designed to provide the reader with the basic concepts involved in pediatric medicolegal concerns. To obtain specifics on state law, the reader must contact the state in question or hospital legal counsel.

CONSENT

In 1914, Justice Cardozo provided the ruling that is considered the essence of consent principles for the delivery of medical care.

> Every human being of adult years and sound mind has a right to determine what shall be done with his own body and a surgeon who performs an operation without his patient's consent commits an assault, for which he is

liable in damages (*Schloendorff v. Society of the New York Hospital,* 211 NY 125, 129–30, 105 NE 92.93, 1914).

The choice of the term *adult* in this ruling reflects the legal reality that minors were and are held incapable of making legally binding decisions. This legal incapability of minors is present throughout various areas of the law, such as entering into contracts. Because minors were deemed to be incapable of entering into such agreements because of their inability to understand all the potential ramifications of their decisions, the common law provided that someone must be able to speak for the minor. From the common law in England and America, children were determined to be the property of the father, who was considered, beyond doubt, the head of the family (Wilkins, 1973).

The vast legal authority of parents over their children has been carried forth into modern law. The legal presumption is that parents will make choices for the child that reflect the best interest of the child.

A child is allowed to make decisions in some legal areas irrespective of the wishes and, in some cases, the knowledge of the parents. These decisions are based in state law and cover such topics as the ability to consent to treatment for a sexually transmitted disease (Oregon Revised Statute 109.610, 1977), the right to donate blood (Oregon Revised Statute 109.670, 1977), and the right to the diagnosis or treatment of a mental or emotional disorder (Oregon Revised Statute 109.675, 1985). Louisiana has perhaps the most permissive law; it allows any minor who is either ill or believes himself or herself to be ill to consent to medical treatment (Louisiana Revised Statute Annotated Section 40:1095, 1984).

A Colorado statute allows physicians and hospital personnel to examine and treat minors who have the human immunodeficiency virus (HIV) without contacting a parent or guardian. In some limited instances under the Colorado statute, medical professionals may inform the parents or guardian. The health care workers are required to counsel the minor regarding the importance of advising their parents or guardians of the condition (Colorado Revised Statute Section 25-4-1401–1409, 1991).

RESTRICTIONS ON PARENTS' AUTHORITY

Although parents and guardians have been given immense legal authority to make decisions for their children and wards, the court will intervene when the welfare of the child appears to be threatened by the decision of the parent or guardian. A 1944 case illustrates the court's approach to parental decisions that may be harmful to a child.

In Prince v. Massachusetts, a Jehovah's Witness was accused of violating child labor laws by allowing her ward to sell religious material on a public street. The guardian was found guilty in trial court, and she appealed to the United States Supreme Court. The Supreme Court agreed with the finding of the trial court. The ruling read in part, "parents may be free to become martyrs themselves. But it does not follow they are free, in identical circumstances, to make martyrs of their children before they have reached the age of full and legal discretion when they can make that choice for themselves" (*Prince v. Massachusetts*, 321 U.S. 158, 1944).

In 1987, the California Appellate court ruled on a case involving the provision of medical treatment to a 3-year-old child (*In re Eric B.* 189 Cal. App. 3d 996, 235 Cal. Rptr. 22, 1987). The child, Eric, had an enucleation for carcinoma and his physicians wanted him to have follow-up care with chemotherapy. The parents, who were Christian Scientists, had agreed to the surgical procedure but refused to allow the follow-up care because they viewed it as a violation of their religious beliefs. The initial court ordered the family to assure that the child received the prescribed medical treatment. The parents agreed to follow the court order.

After the chemotherapy, Eric's physicians ordered an additional 2 years of monitoring the child's condition. The parents appealed the decision because the child was receiving Christian Science therapy at the time. The appeals court ordered the parents to comply with the monitoring regimen prescribed by the physicians. The court's decision was based on several factors: "The seriousness of the harm the child is suffering or the substantial likelihood that he will suffer serious harm; the evaluation for the treatment by the medical profession; the risks involved in medically treating the child; and the expressed preferences of the child (Id at 1005, 235 Cal. Rptr. at 27 quoting *In re Phillip B.*, 92 Cal. App. 3d 796, 802, 156 Cal. Rptr. 48, 51 [1979], cert. denied, 445 U.S. 949, 1990).

The foregoing cases reflect the balancing test the court uses when parents' decisions regarding their children could result in harm to the children. Whereas the court has an abiding interest in the integrity of the family relationship, that interest will be overridden if it appears the child will be put at risk by the parental decision.

MINORS AS DECISION-MAKERS

All states have statutory exceptions for minors who meet certain criteria to give consent. The exceptions include emancipated minors, mature minors, and minors in an emergency condition.

Emancipated minors are allowed to give consent for medical treatment without the need for parental notification or agreement. The original criteria of an emancipated minor are that the minor is living on his or her own, is self supporting, and is not subject to parental control. These criteria have been expanded to include college students who still rely on their parents to provide financial support, unmarried minor mothers, minors in the military, and married minors (Holder, 1987).

The mature minor rule provides that if a minor 14 years of age or older can understand the components of informed consent (procedure, alternatives, and risks), the minor is allowed to consent. This type of consent would be sought in conditions in which the risk of the procedure was not great and the parents or guardians were not able to be contacted. The application of the mature minor rule has three components in common.

Components of the Mature Minor Rule

1. The treatment provided is for the benefit of the minor rather than of a third party
2. The minor in question is near the age of majority and is thought to have the ability to understand the nature and importance of the medical steps proposed
3. The proposed medical procedure could be described as minor or not serious (Holder, 1985)

The mature minor rule places the responsibility on the health care workers to determine that the minor in question possesses the necessary characteristics to be able to provide consent. Factors that may assist the

TABLE 6–1. RULE OF SEVENS: AGE GUIDELINES FOR DETERMINING A MINOR'S CAPACITY TO GIVE CONSENT

Under the age of 7 years, there is no capacity to give consent

Between the ages of 7 and 14 years, it is presumed that there is no capacity to give consent; however, that presumption can be rebutted with evidence to the contrary

Between the ages of 14 and 21 years, it is presumed that there is a capacity to give consent; however, that presumption can be rebutted with evidence to the contrary

caregiver in making the determination include age, ability, experience, educational background, and the degree of maturity evidenced in the minor's behavior (*Cardwell v. Bechtol*, 724 S.W. 2d 739, Tennessee, 1987). The Tennessee Supreme Court provided some age-related guidelines for the determination of *mature minor*. These guidelines, known as the rule of sevens, are listed in Table 6–1 (Id at 747).

In cases in which minors do not fit any of the exceptions yet may require emergency medical treatment, the courts have been willing to utilize an implied consent theory. This theory postulates that if a child is in a medical emergency situation and the parents cannot be reached, consent for treatment is implied because parents would want what is best for the child. The urgency of the medical emergency is proportional to the court's willingness to find implied consent (Rozovsky, 1990).

It is clear that there are many exceptions to the common law rule that minors are incapable of giving consent for medical treatment. These exceptions create ambiguity for health care providers, who must decide whether or not the minor in question fits into one of the articulated exceptions. In response to this predicament faced by medical personnel, many of the state legislatures have passed statutory laws of consent. Oregon Revised Statute 109.675 (1985) is an example of such a statute

(1) A minor 14 years of age or older may obtain, without parental knowledge or consent, outpatient diagnosis or treatment of a mental or emotional disorder or a chemical dependency, excluding methadone maintenance. . . .

When a statute is passed that gives minors the ability to give consent, it is important for health care providers to have a parallel statute passed that removes civil liability for providing treatment to minors. Without this statutory protection, there would be an unwillingness to follow the provisions of the minor consent law.

The concepts of *consent* versus *assent* are important in the area of providing health care to minors. Consent is an active agreement following the presentation of the facts of the procedure. To assent is to concur with the proposed procedure. This distinction is important when dealing with minors who are determined to lack capacity to give consent. The role of assent is discussed more completely in the section on medical research involving children.

CHILD ABUSE AND NEGLECT

Every state in the US has statutes that direct identified groups of health care professionals to report suspected or confirmed cases of child abuse to specified authorities. These statutes generally extend protection from civil liability for reporting suspected child abuse, as long as the report is made in good faith. Many of the states have extended the obligation for reporting to practitioners of other disciplines such as law enforcement officials, social workers, teachers, and members of other occupations who have routine contact with children.

Health care workers may be reluctant to report child abuse for a variety of reasons, including concern that their suspicion is not correct and a report would put blameless parents in an awkward position. Other concerns include unsubstantiated fear of personal liability and worries that reporting the parents may cause them to be even more abusive to the child. Actually, the threat of legal action is greater for failure to report; several states have statutes with associated legal penalties for failure to report. In addition, if a child is permanently injured or killed in an abusive situation, the health care professional may be negligent for failure to report the abuse in a timely manner that may have removed the child from the situation before the near lethal or fatal injury occurred.

The 1976 California case of Landeros v. Flood is one of the few examples in the legal literature of a malpractice claim against a physician for failure to report child abuse (*Landeros v. Flood*, 17 Cal. 3d 399, 131 Cal. Rptr. 69, 551 P.2d 389, 1976). In this case, an 11-month-old child was brought to a hospital emergency department (ED); a comminuted spiral fracture of the tibia and fibula was diagnosed and treated. Upon physical examination, the child was found to have numerous bruises and abrasions. In addition, the child had a nondepressed skull fracture that was not diagnosed at the time of the hospital visit. The child was released to the care of her parents, and no report was made of possible child abuse.

After the child was returned to her parents, she was further physically abused with human bites and second- and third-degree burns. The child was ultimately removed from her parents' care and went to live with foster parents. The foster parents filed a lawsuit against the original treating physician for failure to report the suspicion of child abuse.

The abuse and neglect statutes are often used to allow the state to remove a child from the control of the parents. When the child is removed from the parents' home, the state places the child in protective custody, which varies from a foster home to a state or county facility that provides shelter and temporary care for these children. The law has a strong interest in maintaining the family integrity, so the parents are given an opportunity to correct the situation so as to allow the child to return to the home of the biologic parents. Traditionally, the child has not had the ability to direct actions that would impact his or her destiny in these situations.

A 1992 precedent-breaking case in Florida may provide the spark to re-evaluate the scope of parental authority over children. The case of Gregory K. was brought by a 12-year-old child who sought to have his parents' parental rights terminated so that he could be adopted by his foster family. It is not uncommon to have parental rights terminated because of abuse or neglect, but it is uncommon for a child to be the party requesting the termination.

Gregory K. alleged that his parents neglected him in a variety of ways during the period of time he lived either with both of them or with his mother or father separately. He was ultimately placed in a children's shelter by his mother when she believed she was unable to financially provide a home for Gregory K. After more than a year at the shelter, Gregory K. was placed with a foster family. It was with that family that Gregory described the first feelings of happiness and stability in his life. He wanted to become a permanent part of the foster family by having that family adopt him. This desire prompted Gregory K. to consult an attorney with the ultimate goal of obtaining termination of the relationship from his biologic parents.

On September 25, 1992, an Orlando, Florida, judge ruled that the legal parental relationship with Gregory K.'s biologic parents was terminated and Gregory could be adopted by his foster family (Levenson, 1992). This decision could potentially have a dramatic impact on the rights of minors as viewed by the legal system.

MEDICAL RESEARCH INVOLVING MINORS

The role of children in medical research raises both legal and ethical issues. There are some who would argue that parents do not have the authority to grant consent for their minor children to participate in experimental medical research. On the contrary, others would argue that if children do not participate in medical research, there will be no technologic advances in the field of pediatrics (Langer, 1984).

Before accepting a child as a research subject, the investigator should address a number of concerns. First, a risk-to-benefit analysis of the proposed research study should be done; participation by a minor should take place only if the potential benefits are greater than the potential risks. It needs to be recognized that the participation of a child in a research project carries greater concerns than that of a consenting adult. A child's perception of pain and invasive procedures is often greater than an adult's.

In the assessment of the potential risk to the child in medical research projects, several factors should be taken into consideration. The age of the child is a critical component for consideration. How will the child fare with disruption of normal routines and separation from the parents? What type of pain or discomfort will the child feel?

All medical research involving children should be brought to an Institutional Review Board (IRB) for approval before implementation. The role of an IRB is to assure that the research has scientific merit and is significant, that risks to the child are minimized, that adequate safeguards are in place to assure the child's privacy is protected, that data from the study will be kept confidential, and that the research subjects will be selected in an equitable manner (Beauchamp, 1982).

Once the research project has been approved through all the appropriate institutional channels, consent for the child's participation must be obtained. Written consent for the child's participation must be obtained from a person who is legally qualified to provide consent, usually a parent or guardian. For any child who is 7 years of age or older, the child's assent to participate in the research should be sought. Children who display emotional maturity and an ability to comprehend information should be given the opportunity to give informed consent for participation in a research study. If a child objects to participation, coercion cannot be used to obtain the child's consent.

MINORS AND DEATH ISSUES

Since the landmark legal decision in the Karen Ann Quinlan case, there has been controversy over right-to-die or death-with-dignity issues. These difficult issues apply to children as well as to adults. A child's parents are given the authority to agree to or refuse treatment for a terminally ill child unless there is some reason to believe the decision is not being made in the child's best interest.

There are many fewer legal cases involving the foregoing of life-sustaining treatment for children than there are for adults. This discrepancy can probably best be explained by the fact that the legal authority of parents to make that kind of decision is clearer than for relatives of an adult in the same situation (Meisel, 1989). The laws governing decision-making by children emanate from the same legal precedents that apply to adults.

The first right-to-die case, *In re* Quinlan, was decided in New Jersey in 1976. In the past, courts generally held that the right to die is based on a constitutional right to privacy. The court in Quinlan stated:

> Although the Constitution does not explicitly mention a right of privacy, Supreme Court decisions have recognized that a right of personal privacy exists and that certain areas of privacy are guaranteed under the Constitution . . . Presumably this right is broad enough to encompass a patient's decision to decline medical treatment under certain circumstances (*In re* Quinlan, 355 A.2d 647, 663).

In more recent right-to-die cases, courts have attempted to find other bases for the right to choose rather than relying on the right to privacy. Strict constitutional interpretists see the right-to-privacy argument as vulnerable because it has to be interpreted from the Constitution rather than being listed as a specific right. The most common basis for the current right-to-die rulings is from the common law of autonomy of self-determination.

Most right-to-die cases involve incompetent patients. The question before the court is what these patients would want if they could speak for themselves. The incompetency of these adult patients makes the decisions easily applicable to children who are also considered legally to be incompetent.

The ability to determine death by brain death as opposed to cessation of respiratory and circulatory function raised some interesting legal issues for children who were on life support after episodes of child abuse. Parents, who often committed the abuse, would petition the court to forbid the removal of life support from the child. As long as the child was alive, the parents could not be charged with murder. Dority v. Superior Court of San Bernardino County contains such a situation.

A 19-day-old infant was admitted to a local hospital for evaluation of a seizure disorder. After evaluation at the local hospital, the child was transferred to Loma Linda University Medical Center. Diagnostic tests revealed the presence of increased intracranial pressure. The child's condition deteriorated, and a brain flow study and an electroencephalogram (EEG) were ordered and repeated 1 month after admission. The EEG indicated electrocerebral silence; brain death was the conclusion.

The hospital petitioned the court to have life sup-port terminated. Soon after the child was admitted to Loma Linda, the parents were arrested and charged with felony child neglect. The parents were present for the hearing, and they chose to withhold consent for removal of the life support device.

When the parents refused to grant consent for the termination of life support, the court appointed the Department of Public Social Services as temporary guardian of the child, but the parents appealed to seek prohibition against the removal of the life support device. Before the court could act on the parent's petition, the child's vital functions ceased, and the child was removed from life support. The death of a person critical to litigation normally renders the case moot, but the California court opted to proceed with this case because of the likelihood that the same situation would arise again and the court wanted to have a precedent on record.

The court ruled that brain death was a medical determination and health care personnel do not have to come to court to obtain judicial approval for removal of life support devices. When important decisions must be made regarding a child and the parents have demonstrated an inability to make decisions in the child's best interest, it is proper to appoint a guardian to be a spokesperson for the child. If the court appoints a legal guardian to speak for the child, that guardian has the same legal authority as a parent having legal custody of the child (*Dority v. Superior Court of San Bernardino County*, 145 Cal. App. 3d 273, 1983).

In the Dority case, the parents became unavailable as decision-makers for their child by reason of their actions. When a guardian is appointed in this type of situation, it would not be unexpected for that appointee to seek guidance from the court because of the gravity of the decision to be made on termination of life support.

It is the usual case that parents acting as decision-makers for their children do so with the child's best interest at stake. When there are no apparent conflicts in the decisions made by the parents, those decisions are controlling in regard to the care provided or withdrawn.

In 1990, Congress passed the law which became the Patient Self Determination Act (PSDA). This law was introduced by Senators John Danforth (R-Mo) and Daniel Moynihan (D-NY). Senator Danforth is from Missouri, the state where the Cruzan family fought a successful legal battle to have Nancy Cruzan's tube feedings withdrawn.

The PSDA requires hospitals, skilled nursing facilities, home health agencies, hospice programs and health maintenance organizations (HMOs) that participate in Medicare and Medicaid programs to maintain written policies and procedures guaranteeing that every adult receiving care in that facility must receive written information concerning the patient's involvement in their treatment decisions (Omnibus Budget Reconciliation Act, 1990). The provisions of the PSDA apply only to adults.

MINORS AS ORGAN DONORS

When a child is being considered as an organ donor, associated legal issues must be taken into account. The organ donation procedure has no therapeutic benefit to the minor donor; however, parents and guardians do have the authority to authorize this type of surgical procedure, which is performed for the benefit of another.

Even if parents agreed to a child's being a donor, it would not be uncommon for the physicians and hospitals involved to seek court approval of the decision. It is clear that when these cases arise, the minor child is often being asked to provide a donor organ for a sibling. The hospital and physician must be assured that the parents' decision is being made considering the best interest of the potential minor donor. When the court receives this type of case, it must balance the interest the state has in the welfare of its citizens against the decision made by the parent or guardian. When faced with this balancing test, the courts have used three tests. These tests are the best interest test, the substitute judgment test, and a court's review of the parents' decision.

The *best interest test* is an analysis performed by the court to determine if the organ donation by the child is in the best interest of that child. That determination is made by weighing the psychological benefits the minor donor would receive in contrast to the physical harm from the operative procedure. The donation is ordered if the psychological benefits outweigh the physical harm.

In 1979, the Texas court reviewed a case that demonstrates the judicial application of the best interest test. In Little v. Little, the potential minor donor was a 14-year-old child with Down syndrome. Her brother required a kidney transplant and the 14-year-old child was the only family member who had the compatible tissue type. The parents sought court approval for the organ donation from the minor. The court performed comprehensive interviews with the child, the child's parents, physicians, and psychologists to determine the harm as opposed to the benefits of the proposed procedure. The court ruled that the child could be a donor; it based its decision on the finding that the child was upset during the time her brother was away at the hospital. The court determined that the organ donation procedure was in the best interest of the

child because of the severe psychological effects that would result from the loss of her brother (*Little v. Little,* 576 S.W. 2d 493, Texas, 1979).

The *substitute judgment test* requires a surrogate decision-maker to place himself or herself in the position of the incompetent patient to determine what the incompetent person would choose if he or she were competent to make the decision. In the substitute judgment test, the court is allowed to consider what the overall benefits would be to all involved. This test is the most difficult to apply when the incompetent person in question has never been competent. Without the historical background of knowing what this patient's values were, the substitute judgment becomes more a subjective determination than a formulated decision that is in congruence with the patient's previously expressed thoughts and wishes (Huna, 1992).

The third and final test that may be used to determine whether or not a minor may be an organ donor is *court review* of the parents' decision. The primary focus of the judicial review is to assure that the parents' decision to make the minor child an organ donor was made in a fair and objective manner and to assure that no conflict of interest existed. In this type of review, the best interests of the donor are not considered. This lack of consideration of the potential donor's interest probably renders this test the weakest of the three.

The three tests are imperfect in their application. It is critical to devise guidelines that can be used more easily by the legal system with the emphasis on doing what is best for the child. Huna (1992) proposed the following guidelines: consent from the guardian; demonstrated need by the recipient that there is a strong probability of benefit to him or her; the absence of an acceptable alternative to the donation procedure; minimal risks to the donor both at present and in the future; strong evidence of a psychological benefit to the donor; and the presence of an independent physician for the donor.

The foregoing proposal provides direction to courts, who have the difficult task of making the decision regarding organ donation. The concerns for the donor and the recipient are adequately addressed with the proposal.

COBRA AND ITS APPLICATION TO CHILDREN

The Consolidated Omnibus Budget Reconciliation Act (COBRA) (1985) is federal legislation passed by Congress in response to concerns raised regarding the inappropriate transfer of uninsured people seeking medical care. The federal law defined penalties, primarily monetary, against hospitals and physicians participating in Medicare who violated the antidumping provisions of COBRA.

COBRA provides protection for any person, child or adult, with an emergency medical condition or pregnancy with contractions who goes to an ED seeking care. The ED is legally obligated to provide a screening examination to the person irrespective of that person's ability to pay for the treatment. When the decision is made to transfer the patient who has an emergency medical condition, the patient or the patient's family, after being advised of the risks and benefits of the transfer, must agree to the transfer before it can be consummated. If the transfer is accepted, COBRA specifies the requirements that must be met for the transfer. These requirements are: there must be a physician at the receiving hospital who has agreed to accept the patient; the receiving hospital must have adequate space and qualified personnel to provide the necessary care; the transport agency must have adequately trained personnel and equipment appropriate to the level of care required by the patient; and copies of all relevant medical records must be sent with the patient.

One section of COBRA has particular relevance for any specialized facilities such as trauma centers, neonatal intensive care units, burn units, or rural regional referral centers. A specialized facility is one that holds itself out to the community as providing a special type of care not available at other hospitals. Under COBRA, those specialized facilities are required to accept appropriate transfers of patients who need the type of care the receiving hospital provides.

It is probable that this section of COBRA would apply to children's hospitals. Those hospitals would be required to accept transfers of appropriate pediatric patients from transferring hospitals that do not have the distinctive capabilities of providing care to the pediatric population.

The major question in these cases will be what constitutes an appropriate transfer? Each hospital must be proactive in determining what type of illnesses or injuries would fit into that category. There should be policies and procedures in place that describe the specialized facilities available and the process for accepting patients who meet the defined criteria.

CONCLUSION

Pediatric patients provide special challenges to health care professionals. These professionals must have not only a specialized knowledge of children's needs but also knowledge of the legal and ethical aspects of providing care to children, who are often not able to speak for themselves.

It is imperative for all hospitals to have specific policies and procedures that address the unique aspects of providing care to children. The procedures should include the statutory mandates regarding consent and reporting requirements. Information should be available to describe the process for obtaining court intervention for children whose parents refuse life- or limb-saving treatment.

A minimum of an annual in-service education program should be presented in the ED to address the legal issues specific to the pediatric population. Orientation to the ED should include the aspects of care that are particular to children, including the process of reporting infectious diseases and the documentation required for cases of suspected child abuse.

The rights of children are receiving renewed attention from the legal system. Greater latitude is being given to the ability of children to participate in decisions about their physical well-being. It is incumbent that hospital administration and legal counsel provide hospital personnel with current information as the law evolves in this important area. Each person providing care to children has an obligation to understand the legal responsibilities attendant with this role.

REFERENCES

Beauchamp TL, Walter L (1982). *Contemporary issues in bioethics*

Consolidated Omnibus Budget Reconciliation Act (COBRA) of 1985 (42 USC 1395 dd), as amended by the Omnibus Budget Reconciliation Acts (OBRA) of 1987, 1989 and 1990

Holder AR (1987). Minors' rights to consent to medical care. *Journal of the American Medical Association* 24:3400–3402

Holder AR (1985). *Legal issues in pediatrics and adolescent medicine* (2nd ed). New Haven: Yale University Press

Huna P (1992). Infants as organ transplant donors: Should it happen? *The Health Lawyer* 6:24–27

Langer DH (1984). Medical research involving children: Some legal and ethical issues. *Baylor Law Review* 36:1–39

Levenson B (1992). Gregory wins a new life. *Orlando Sentinel*, 26 September

Meisel A (1989). *The right to die*. New York: Wiley, pp 171–201

Rozovsky FA (1990). *Consent to treatment: A practical guide* (2nd ed). Boston: Little, Brown, pp 256–360

Omnibus Budget Reconciliation Act of 1990 (Suppl 1991). Public Law 101-508, sections 4206, 4751 (OBRA), 42 U.S.C. section 1395cc(f)(1) & 42 U.S.C. section 1396a(a)

Wilkins LP (1975). Children's rights: Removing the parental consent barrier to medical treatment of minors. *Arizona State Law Journal* 31:41, citing H. Bevan, The Law Regarding Children 256, 257 (1973)

CHAPTER 7

Transportation of Critically Injured or Ill Children

LINDA K. MANLEY

INTRODUCTION

Critically ill and injured children often present to an emergency department (ED) miles from a pediatric definitive care center. Preparation for and planning of transportation of a child allows for a smooth transition between facilities and optimizes outcome. This chapter briefly explores the history of transport, legal considerations, key personnel, methods of transport, and roles and responsibilities of the referring facility and transport team.

HISTORY OF PATIENT TRANSPORT

The concept of a rapid transportation system for critically ill and injured patients has been recognized for centuries. Ground transportation systems were first developed during the 1790s by French surgeon Baron Dominique Jean Larrey (1766–1842). Larrey, appalled by the long time a wounded soldier lay on the battlefield, developed the *ambulance volante,* or flying ambulance, a light-weight, horse-drawn wagon used for emergency transportation (Chou and MacDonald, 1989; Haeger, 1988; Howell, 1988). Larrey is also credited with inventing a system for triage and with advancing surgical techniques in the field, particularly amputations. Ground transport programs were refined during World War II and are currently the backbone of the patient transportation system in the United States.

Medical air transport also has been in existence for some time. The first air medical transfer reportedly took place in Paris in 1870, when 160 injured soldiers were air-lifted by hot air balloon (Chou and MacDonald, 1989; Howell, 1988). Hot air balloons were a fascinating development. Five years later, three French scientists ascended to 26,000 feet in a hot air balloon, but they were profoundly affected by the effects of hypoxia and hypothermia; two died (Parsons and Bobechko, 1982). With the advent of fixed-wing transport in the early 1900s, airplanes were planned to be used for patient transfers. The first air ambulance service, though, ended in disaster in 1910, when the only medically configured plane crashed (Chou and MacDonald, 1989).

Current transport systems are largely the outcome of the Korean and Vietnam Wars. These systems have resulted in a marked decrease in death and disability rates, particularly from trauma. The first hospital-based helicopter program was established in 1972 at St. Anthony's Hospital in Denver (Merrill, 1988). Currently, more than 200 air medical programs, both rotary-wing and fixed-wing, are in operation nationwide (Merrill, 1988).

Although transport systems have become more sophisticated over time, uniform standards for pediatric critical care transport are just beginning to emerge (Aoki and McCloskey, 1992; Brink et al, 1993; Continenza and Hill, 1990; Day et al, 1991; McCloskey and Orr, 1992). Abundant information exists in the literature pertaining to adult and neonatal transport, yet the same cannot be said for pediatric transport systems. Critically ill or injured children are often transported by adult-oriented or regional perinatal systems. It is rare to find a totally dedicated and specially designed pediatric transport program, even though the clinical skills and knowledge required to transport critically ill children are unique. The wide range of patient ages, developmental levels, diagnoses, medications, and therapeutic modalities demand expertise in pediatric emergency care, resuscitation, and stabilization.

Several organizations are working to establish guidelines for interhospital transportation. Comprehensive pediatric critical transportation standards are currently being addressed by the American Academy of Pediatrics (AAP) Section on Transport Medicine (Day et al, 1991).

LEGAL IMPLICATIONS

General Considerations

Several medicolegal issues are raised by interhospital transportation. Although applicable laws vary from state to state, the responsibilities of each person involved in a pediatric transport should be defined and reviewed. Health care professionals involved in pediatric transportation need to practice what some authors refer to as defensive medicine (Ginzburg, 1989). This concept is simply a conscious effort to recognize that medical transportation is an inherently dangerous enterprise.

For a pediatric transportation system to function optimally, there must be a strong communications network, expertly trained team members, committed leadership, financial resources, and safety-conscious personnel. Failure to incorporate any of these essential components may result in less than optimal care and initiation of a malpractice claim (Ginzburg, 1989). Occasionally, optimal medical and nursing care is not possible because of the inappropriate selection of patients for transport, undertrained or inadequately supervised transport team members, inordinate delays, poor weather-related decisions, and the inability to maintain patient stability in the transport environment (Ginzburg, 1989). The legal ramifications of such care are dramatic.

Consent

Informed consent requires that sound, reasonable, comprehensible, and relevant information be provided to a competent parent or patient, if older, by a health care professional for the purpose of eliciting a voluntary, educated decision by the parent about the advisability of permitting one course of action as opposed to another (Ginzburg, 1989). In emergency situations, most parents do not question the need for air or ground transportation. Even more rarely do they question the qualifications of those executing the transport. Informed consent should clearly reflect that the risks and benefits of the recommended mode of

transportation were discussed and documented. Some authors advocate that the transport team obtain parental consent for the transport as well as a written order from the referring physician (Aoki and McCloskey, 1992).

COBRA

In the early to middle 1980s, a phenomenon known as dumping became widespread in the United States. Dumping was said to occur when a hospital refused to accept patients at the ED or transferred financially undesirable patients (Frew et al, 1988; Rhee and Burney, 1986; Southard, 1989). Until 1986, the only deterrent to poor transfer practices was voluntary adherence to ethical standards of responsibility and care (Rhee and Burney, 1991).

In 1986, the Consolidated Omnibus Budget Reconciliation Act (COBRA) (Public Law 99-272) was implemented to address the medical, legal, and ethical issues of medical transportation for all hospitals receiving Medicare reimbursement. COBRA has had a profound effect on the actions and legal responsibilities of some hospitals, emergency physicians and nurses, and prehospital emergency medical service (EMS) providers. Although COBRA does not specifically address the mechanics of pediatric transportation, many of the recommendations are applicable. In brief, COBRA requires that the following standards be met (Frew et al, 1988; Rhee and Burney, 1991; Southard, 1989).

COBRA Standards

- All hospitals must provide qualified personnel to examine all patients presenting to an ED, even if doing so requires the involvement of an on-call physician.
- If an emergency exists, the hospital must provide stabilization or provide for an appropriate transfer to another facility. Exceptions to the stabilization rule include patients who do not consent to further treatment or who leave without being discharged.
- If a patient is transferred, the patient's condition must be stabilized before transport. The physician must certify in writing that the benefits of transfer outweigh the risks.
- Transfer criteria that must be satisfied include that the receiving facility have available space and qualified personnel, that the receiving hospital agrees to accept the patient before transport, that the transferring hospital provide appropriate medical records.
- The transfer is effected by qualified personnel and equipment. For pediatric patients, it is essential that the transport team be proficient at pediatric

advanced airway and venous access skills and carry appropriate equipment.

Failure to comply with COBRA has a direct economic impact on both hospitals and physicians. Hospitals may be fined $50,000 for each violation and be suspended or terminated from the Medicare program. In addition, individual physicians may be fined $25,000 per violation and be prohibited from providing services under Medicare.

In 1990, the American College of Emergency Physicians (ACEP), also concerned about unethical transfer decisions, developed guidelines to ensure access to emergency care and patient safety when transfer is necessary (American College of Emergency Physicians, 1990).

TRANSPORT CONSIDERATIONS

Transport of a critically ill or injured child to a definitive care center is indicated when the needs of the patient have exceeded local expertise or when specific subspecialties are required. It is not logical to impose on the transferring hospital the added responsibility of transporting such a patient, and indeed, this practice could pose additional problems (Harris et al, 1975). The transferring and receiving hospitals have a joint responsibility to ensure appropriate, safe transport. Several considerations must be taken into account, including the child's hemodynamic stability, the distance between the two hospitals, the experience of the personnel, the mode of transport, the quality of communication, and the roles and responsibilities of both the transferring and receiving hospitals.

Personnel

The key to a successful pediatric transport service is a well-organized system and transport personnel who are meticulously trained and experienced. The critical issue is not how long it takes a child to arrive at the regional pediatric center but rather how long it takes the center's expert care to arrive to the child (Black et al, 1982).

Various team compositions are used throughout the US, and team composition is a controversial issue (Continenza and Hill, 1990; Day et al, 1991; McCloskey et al, 1989; Rhee et al, 1986). In general, team composition depends on the type and size of the transport program, personnel available within the receiving hospital, and the philosophy of the receiving institutions involved. Cost, distance, and the type of patient to be transported are major factors. Clearly, transport team members must meet certain standards and be able to function independently in the transport environment.

Expertise in pediatric assessment, documented proficiency with clinical skills, and a flexible, adaptable attitude are imperative.

Each transport team member has designated responsibilities and functions under the direction of a team leader. The team leader usually reports to an attending-level medical director at the base station, who assumes individual responsibility for the transport. The medical director often takes the initial transport call, determines team composition, offers stabilization advice while mobilizing the team, and facilitates communication throughout the transfer.

Transport team configurations usually include a combination of two or three medical professionals. Formal pediatric training for all transport teams must be available, whether it is an adult-, perinatal-, or pediatric-oriented team. It should not be assumed that teams with a high degree of expertise and experience with adults have comparable training and skills for children (Aoki and McCloskey, 1992; Day et al, 1991).

The initial training of any transport team caring for children should include courses covering topics related to pediatric critical care, pediatric emergency care, clinical intervention, transport theory and physiology, and the use of specialized pediatric equipment. Transport training should also include clinical rotations through pediatric EDs, pediatric critical care units, and the operating room for advanced airway intervention. In addition, maintaining mandatory competency certifications, such as Pediatric Advanced Life Support (PALS) or Advanced Pediatric Life Support (APLS), and regular pediatric in-service training sessions are equally as important. Clinical skill alone, however, is not the only requirement. Diplomacy, collaboration, and cooperation are also essential skills and are often overlooked. Transport teams must be able to function in stressful situations and under adverse conditions. Consideration must be given to physical abilities, such as loading patients into a vehicle and weight restrictions of an aircraft.

Transport teams may include physicians, nurses, respiratory therapists, and emergency medical technician-As (EMT-As) or paramedics. Ideally, the team composition is based on the needs of the child. Flexible team compositions, incorporating subspecialties when necessary, is optimal. In general, transport team member roles are as follows.

Transport Physician. In general, when a physician accompanies the team, he or she acts as the team leader and is responsible for patient assessment and diagnosis, plans for treatment, directs the team, and anticipates problems that may arise en route. The role of a physician during transport, however, is a highly debated issue (Baxt and Moody, 1987; Day et al, 1991; McCloskey et al, 1989; Rhee and Burney, 1991; Rhee et al, 1986; Smith and Hackel, 1983). Some authors advocate employing physicians for their judgment and skill (Smith and Hackel, 1983). After much discussion, the AAP has recommended that there needs to be a shift away from titles of team members toward the skills required for the patients being transported (Day et al, 1991). The presence of a physician alone does not always guarantee that an appropriate level of care is being given, because the spectrum of physician expertise is very broad, ranging from junior residents to critical care or emergency medicine attending level (Rhee and Burney, 1991).

Transport Nurse. Nurses are considered the core of a transport team. An experienced nurse who undergoes rigorous training and testing can maintain a high skill level. The AAP recognizes that there are numerous benefits to having a free-standing nurse transport team (Day et al, 1991). Patient care is not interrupted by pulling a nurse off a unit; the logistics of planning and executing the transport are managed by personnel who do it frequently; equipment is maintained consistently; clinical and quality assurance programs are formally integrated; and communication systems are enhanced, often through outreach efforts.

The transport nurse may function as a team leader in the absence of a physician, coordinating all aspects of care. He or she may collaborate with the transport physician under established protocols to provide and direct the delivery of nursing care.

Respiratory Therapist, EMT or Paramedic. Respiratory therapists and paramedics are often included on transport teams to assist with the assessment and management of specific problems, such as airway maintenance. These team members are highly skilled in advanced life support procedures and are knowledgeable about the logistics of transport, especially equipment and vehicle operations. These team members complement both the nurse and physician crew.

Mode of Transportation

The mode of transportation, ground or air, should be based on the child's physiologic status, the distance to be traveled, existing weather conditions, and the availability of an appropriate transferring service. The goal is to provide a safe, efficient transport. The AAP has recommended that the optimal pediatric transport system have both ground and air capabilities available in a flexible, coordinated system.

Ground. Ground transportation is available virtually everywhere in the US, although with varying degrees of organization and skill. Ground transportation is thought to be the most efficient method for transports up to 20–30 miles, assuming good road conditions. If road conditions are poor (heavy traffic, construction, difficult terrain), helicopter transport may be considerably faster. Ground transportation, though, must be available in the event of poor weather conditions, when the helicopter service is grounded, or simultaneous helicopter requests exist.

In general, ambulances are considered safer than helicopters, are more cost efficient, and carry a larger payload, that is, additional equipment and personnel. Departure response time for a pediatric ground transport unit should be within 15 minutes of receiving the call from the referring facility, with the capability of mobilizing a full team in less than 10 minutes, if necessary (Continenza and Hill, 1990).

In rural areas, some hospitals may prefer to make their own transportation arrangements, using their local EMS ground units in an effort to expedite the transportation of a critically ill or injured child. This type of transport is sometimes referred to as a one-way transport. Local EMS units are often minimally equipped and do not have personnel trained to deal with the pediatric life-threatening complications that may develop en route. Clearly, the use of local EMS units can be a hazardous practice. The transferring and receiving hospitals must discuss the qualifications of the transport crew selected and the legal ramifications of the decision. Nurses from the transferring hospital who accompany the child should not be expected to perform interventions they would not perform unsupervised in their hospital (McCloskey and Orr, 1992). If a transferring hospital refuses a transport team after it has been recommended, the receiving hospital should document this in writing, because doing so decreases the level of legal liability (Aoki and McCloskey, 1992; Day et al, 1991). Another issue to consider when dispatching a local EMS unit to transport a patient to a tertiary care center is the risk of little or no EMS coverage in the community should an emergency arise.

Air. Medical air transportation is a rapidly expanding and integral component of modern health care networks. Air transportation provides a benefit by linking the patient with appropriate, timely medical care. Despite the popularity of medical air transportation, there are surprisingly few data available documenting effectiveness, especially for pediatric patients. Air transportation systems are expensive and potentially dangerous. The safety of the crew and patients should never be jeopardized by bad weather conditions. The likelihood of an accident is a remote, yet real, risk. Air transportation is by either a rotary-wing (helicopter) or fixed-wing craft.

Helicopters are most efficient for trips of 30–150 miles, or 1 hour of flight time. Helicopters can land at a hospital or respond directly to an accident scene (Figure 7–1). Depending on the size and type of the helicopter, a landing area as small as 60 × 60 feet may be adequate for the aircraft.

Although helicopters are extremely versatile, they have a limited amount of room, are inherently noisy, and have a considerable amount of vibration. All of these factors must be taken into consideration while preparing the child for the flight.

If the transport distance is greater than 150 miles, a fixed-wing aircraft provides the most rapid method of transport, although there is a time delay in lift-off. Fixed-wing aircraft may be able to fly in more adverse weather conditions than are helicopters, but they require a suitable airport and ground transportation within a reasonable distance of the hospital. Fixed-wing aircraft generally have more room, require less maintenance, are quieter, and often provide a pressurized cabin.

Concerns regarding flights in fixed-wing aircraft involve the airplane's acceleration and deceleration forces and altitude. All can affect neurologic, cardiac, and pulmonary disorders. For example, accelerational forces on takeoff may decrease cerebral blood flow and perfusion depending on the patient's position (Brink et al, 1993). Children with increased intracranial pressure should be positioned with their head to the front of the aircraft to prevent a potential increase in intracranial pressure. Similarly, hemodynamically compromised children should be loaded with their head to the rear of the aircraft during takeoff and acceleration to prevent compromised cerebral perfusion (Brink et al, 1993).

The adverse effects of altitude must be considered with fixed-wing transports. The partial pressure of oxygen falls as altitude increases. Children with mild undiagnosed hypoxia at ground level may have a catastrophic event at high altitudes in a nonpressurized cabin (Kissoon, 1992). Gas expands as atmospheric pressure falls, mandating careful attention to pressures in endotracheal tube cuffs and air splints. Some disease entities, such as a pneumothorax or eye injury, may be a contraindication to air transport. Finally, for every 1,000 foot increase in altitude, the temperature decreases 3°F. Children, particularly infants, are at a much greater risk for hypothermia, thus their temperature should be carefully monitored. Despite these concerns, most air transports should be uneventful if the emphasis is placed on preflight stabilization and careful monitoring (Harris et al, 1975; Kissoon, 1992).

Equipment. The limits of weight, space, and vehicle chosen dictate how much equipment accompanies the transport team. The more thought that goes into planning for equipment needs, the better prepared the team will be. Each piece of medical equipment should be durable and be evaluated by a biomedical engineer before it is used, especially if used aboard an aircraft. Vibration, thermal, and barometric and electrical stress can damage or severely limit the capabilities of sensitive medical gear. All equipment must be stored and properly secured for both air and ground transport.

Pediatric equipment should be available and committed to transport, as opposed to rented or shared. Air, oxygen, and electrical capabilities are essential for both air and ground transport. Batteries should be able to supply power for twice the expected duration of the transport. Additional equipment should be lightweight, portable, and easily cleaned and maintained. In general, it is a good practice to have the same equipment available for all pediatric transports. On occasion, what appears initially to be a medical diagnosis may actually be caused by trauma, necessitating specific trauma equipment, such as a cervical spinal immobilization device or pneumatic antishock garment. Standardized pediatric equipment eliminates the possibility of being unprepared (Table 7–1).

Communication Network. A rapid, reliable communication network is essential for interhospital transports. As noted in the COBRA guidelines, communication between the transferring and receiving agencies must be initiated before the transport. Ideally, the communication network should include a central dispatch center available to transferring hospitals at all times (Day et al, 1991). Programs advertising a hot line that is often inaccessible may have an associated legal liability. The staff of the communication center must be trained to handle emergency calls, to operate under updated protocols, and to be active in a quality assurance program to monitor the strengths and weaknesses of the system.

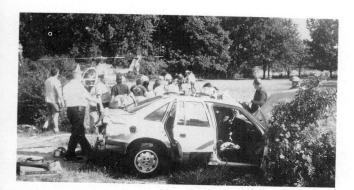

Figure 7–1. The mechanism of an injury may reveal clues to the nature of the injury.

TABLE 7–1. RECOMMENDED PEDIATRIC TRANSPORT EQUIPMENT

■ **AIRWAY AND VENTILATION EQUIPMENT**
Non-rebreather infant, pediatric, and adult masks
Infant, pediatric, and adult airway adjuncts (oral airways, naso-pharyngeal airways)
Disposable 0.5 and 1-L bag-valve mask device with assorted clear infant, pediatric, and adult masks
Uncuffed endotracheal tubes, sizes 2.5–6.0 mm; cuffed endotracheal tubes, sizes 6.0–8.0 mm
Laryngoscope and laryngoscope blades, straight no. 0–3 blades, curved no. 2–3 blades
Suction device and assorted sterile catheters, sterile gloves
Pulse oximetry unit and assorted sensors
Colorimetric end-tidal CO_2 detector or capnography
Needle chest decompression equipment (angiocatheter, syringe, one-way flutter valve)

■ **CIRCULATION EQUIPMENT**
Assorted intravenous catheters (14–24 gauge)
Assorted intravenous administration sets (blood tubing, pediatric volumetric set)
Adult pediatric pneumatic antishock garment
Assorted needles and syringes
Assorted intravenous fluids
Intraosseous needles

■ **MISCELLANEOUS EQUIPMENT**
Resuscitation medications, sedatives, paralytic agents, antibiotics, steroids, inhalants
Blood pressure cuffs (premature infant to adult sizes)
Nasogastric tubes (6–14F)
Cervical spine immobilization devices and splints
Noninvasive blood pressure unit
Restraints
Isolation equipment
Warming equipment

The ability to communicate in transit by either radio or cellular phone must be available for both ground and air transportation. The medical control physician must be able to talk with the transport team at all times to gather patient information and disseminate medical advice. Times and key conversations should be documented.

ROLES AND RESPONSIBILITIES DURING A TRANSPORT

Emergency care providers have distinct responsibilities during each phase of care. The primary goal is to resuscitate the patient and stabilize his or her condition as quickly as possible.

Even before the decision to transport has been reached, the severity of the child's injury or illness should be determined as soon as the child reaches the emergency department, if not earlier. In pediatric trauma, as the local EMS describes the mechanism of injury, their report may reveal subtle clues as to the need for a pediatric tertiary care center. For example, a child in a motor vehicle crash who responds only to deep pain stimuli and has unequal pupils most likely requires care by a pediatric neurosurgeon. Communication with the pediatric definitive center can be initiated, even before the child is admitted to the transferring ED.

For trauma patients, guidelines have been developed by the American College of Surgeons to assist with the difficult decisions of triage and transport to a Level I trauma center (Table 7–2). For an injured child, a pediatric trauma score has been developed, which may be helpful (Table 7–3). Unfortunately, little information exists on transfer guidelines for pediatric patients.

Teamwork among the transferring and receiving institutions and the transport team expedites the child's transfer and improves outcome. The following are guidelines that define the responsibilities of each institution.

TABLE 7–2. GUIDELINES FOR FIELD TRIAGE TO A TRAUMA CENTER

■ **VITAL SIGNS AND LEVEL OF CONSCIOUSNESS**
Glasgow Coma Scale ≤ 14
Blood pressure < 90 mmHg systolic
Respiratory rate < 10 or > 20 breaths per minute
Pediatric Trauma Score < 9
Revised trauma score < 11

■ **MECHANISM OF INJURY**
Falls > 20 feet
High speed auto crash (> 40 mph)
Extrication time > 20 minutes
Ejection from automobile
Death of another occupant
Auto–pedestrian injury with significant impact
Pedestrian thrown or run over
Motor cycle crash (> 20 mph)
Roll over

■ **ANATOMIC CONSIDERATIONS**
2 or more proximal long bone fractures
All penetrating injuries to head, neck, torso, and extremities proximal to elbow and knee
Combination trauma with burns
Flail chest
Amputation proximal to wrist and ankle
Limb paralysis
Pelvic fractures

■ **OTHER CONSIDERATIONS**
Age < 5 or > 55
Cardiac disease, respiratory disease
Insulin-dependent diabetes, cirrhosis, or morbid obesity
Pregnancy
Immunosuppressed patients
Patient with bleeding disorder or patient on anticoagulants

Adapted with permission from Committee on Trauma, *Resources for Optimal Care of the Injured Patient,* Chicago: American College of Surgeons, 1993.

Responsibilities of the Transferring Hospital

The most important goal for the transferring hospital is to perform a rapid initial assessment while instituting resuscitation. Other goals include documenting care, obtaining informed consent, and establishing timely communication with the pediatric definitive care center (Table 7–4).

Initial Evaluation and Resuscitation.

The initial assessment of an injured or ill child is often divided into the primary survey and resuscitation phase and the secondary survey. During the primary survey, the ABCs (airway, breathing, circulation) are carefully assessed. The emphasis is on early identification of respiratory failure, cardiovascular collapse, and life-threatening injuries. As each area is assessed, appropriate resuscitative actions are implemented if a problem is found. When the primary survey is complete and the patient's condition stabilized, a secondary survey is per-

TABLE 7–4. GUIDELINES FOR THE REFERRING HOSPITAL

Perform primary survey and rapid cardiopulmonary assessment and treat life-threatening problems:

Airway—Establish patent airway with cervical spinal control if indicated

Breathing—Administer supplemental oxygen to maintain oxygen saturation of 100%

Circulation—control blood loss; establish two intervenous or intraosseous lines; initiate fluid therapy if indicated (20 mL/kg)

Deficit, neurological—Evaluate neurologic status carefully for signs of increased intracranial pressure

Expose—Assess for other injuries; take temperature; keep warm

Perform secondary survey; obtain necessary x rays; order laboratory tests. Send copies with transport team

If indicated, place Foley catheter and orgastric tube

Obtain history of immunization status, past medical illness, recent meal, drug allergy status, current medications

Have O-negative or type-specific blood available for transport if indicated

Notify pediatric definitive care center of referral early. Document communications

TABLE 7–3. PEDIATRIC TRAUMA SCORE: CATEGORY DEFINITIONS

Component	Score		
	+2	+1	−1
Size	Child or adolescent < 20 kg	Toddler 11– 20 kg	Infant < 10 kg
Airway	Normal	Assisted O₂; mask; cannula	Intubated ETT, EDA, Cric
Consciousness	Awake	Obtunded; lost consciousness	Coma; unresponsive
Systemic blood pressure	90 mmHg; good peripheral pulses and perfusion	51–90 mmHg; Carotid/femoral pulses palpable	< 50 mmHg; weak or no pulses
Fracture	None seen or suspected	Single closed fracture anywhere	Open, multiple fractures
Cutaneous	No visible injury	Contusion, abrassion or laceration < 7 cm not through fascia	Tissue loss, any GSW/stab through fascia

The Pediatric Trauma Scale is primarily designed to function as a checklist. Each component can be assessed by basic physical examination. Airway evaluation is designed to reflect intervention required for effective care. An open fracture is graded −1 for fracture *and* −1 for cutaneous injury. As clinical observation and diagnostic evaluation continues, further definition and reassessment will establish a trend that predicts severity of injury and potential outcome. **A score of 8 or less suggests admission to a pediatric trauma center.**
Abbreviations: ETT, endotracheal tube; EOA, esophageal obturator airway; GSW, gunshot wound; Cric, cricothyroidotomy.
(Adapted from Tepas JJ, Mollitt DL, Talbert JL, Bryant M (1987). The pediatric trauma score as a predictor of injury severity in the injured child. Journal of Pediatric Surgery 22:14)

formed. The secondary survey is a more complete head-to-toe evaluation. It includes a review of pertinent laboratory data, x rays, and the patient's history.

All EDs that admit pediatric patients must have adequate equipment and supplies for the wide spectrum of pediatric emergencies. Estimating appropriately sized pediatric equipment is a difficult task in adult-oriented facilities. Equipment must be available in a variety of sizes and be readily accessible. Typically, selection of pediatric equipment is based on estimated age or weight. Studies have shown, however, that a length-based system for selection of pediatric emergency equipment, such as the Broselow resuscitation tape (BRT), is simple, useful, and accurate (Luten et al, 1992). The BRT is fairly inexpensive and is highly recommended for EMS units and EDs (Figure 7–2).

Perhaps the most difficult part of a pediatric resuscitation is obtaining control of the airway. Most pediatric patients can be ventilated with a bag-valve-mask (BVM) for a period of time, unless there is direct tracheal or laryngeal injury or the patient has aspirated. This technique, however, is not without complications. If done incorrectly, BVM ventilation can worsen an airway obstruction, cause gastric distention, and induce vomiting and subsequent aspiration. Practicing BVM ventilation on infant and pediatric mannequins is highly recommended and should be done at routine intervals.

Endotracheal intubation is the ideal method of securing a child's airway if the child is at high risk for an airway obstruction or if respiratory failure occurs. Endotracheal intubation should be accomplished before transfer; it can be a difficult procedure in a noisy, moving environment. Correct placement of an endotra-

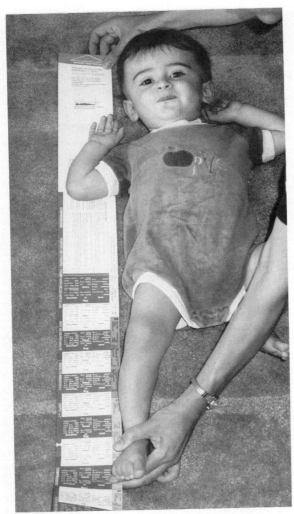

Figure 7–2. Use of length-based resuscitation tape for an infant (Vital Signs, Inc., Totowa, NJ.)

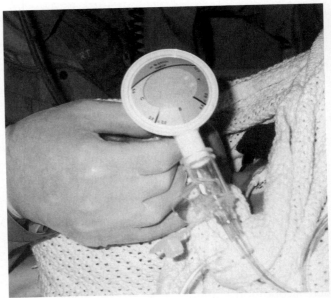

Figure 7–3. Use of colorimetric end-tidal carbon dioxide device for evaluation of endotracheal tube placement in a child.

cheal tube must be confirmed before the transfer by a chest x ray, an arterial blood gas determination, capnography, or an end-tidal carbon dioxide (CO_2) detector. The end-tidal CO_2 detector is a disposable, colorimetric device; it has been found reliable in verifying endotracheal tube placement in infants and children (Figure 7–3) (Bhende et al, 1992; Todres, 1993). With correct placement of the endotracheal tube, the diaphragm of the detector changes from purple to yellow. The manufacturer cautions against use of this device in children weighing less than 15 kg; however, it can be used safely to confirm placement of an endotracheal tube in children as small as 2 kg for a brief period of time. Regardless of the means used to protect the airway and provide for airway maintenance, adequacy of ventilation and oxygenation must be assessed continuously.

Oxygenation is maximized by the administration of supplemental oxygen. One need not worry that supplemental oxygen will be detrimental to a pediatric patient. Children require twice as much oxygen as adults because children have a higher metabolic rate. Pulse oximetry should be initiated and documented; this technology has proved to be a sensitive indicator of hypoxia. In the presence of anemia or carboxyhemoglobin, however, pulse oximetry may not reflect tissue oxygenation. Oxygenation also may be maximized by early placement of an orogastric or nasogastric tube. Decompression of the stomach allows for improved diaphragmatic excursion and may minimize vomiting and aspiration.

Early detection and control of shock are the next priority in the ED. Detection of shock in children may be difficult. The early, subtle signs of hypovolemic shock in children are tachycardia, tachypnea, poor perfusion (capillary refill in more than 2 seconds), decreased level of consciousness (anxiety, restlessness, lethargy), and decreased urinary output (< 1 mL/kg/hour). A child does not become hypotensive until late shock, that is, loss of 30–35% of the circulating blood volume. At this point, resuscitation is extremely difficult. Control of external bleeding, rapid intravenous or intraosseous access, and fluid resuscitation with a 20 mL/kg bolus of an isotonic fluid can be life-saving. Type-specific or O-negative blood should be available if necessary for transport.

As noted, the secondary survey consists of a thorough head-to-toe assessment in which other injuries or conditions are evaluated and treated. In general, laboratory and radiologic studies are done in this

SKYMED TRANSFER FORM

(Please have a copy of all the patients records - including x-rays)

Name:		Age:	Weight:	Sex:
Address:			DOB:	
SS #:	Insurance:			
Referring MD:		Receiving MD:		

History of Illness/Injury:
_____
_____
_____
_____
_____

Past Medical History:
_____
_____
_____

Allergies:

Physical Exam:
_____
_____
_____
_____
_____
_____

Action Taken:
_____
_____
_____

This Patient's condition requires Aeromedical transportation:

_____ M.D. (signature)

Lab Results- TIME_____	Flight Preparation-
_____ WBC _____ HGB _____ HCT	_____ C-Spine Immobilized
	_____ Airway (Type-_____)
_____ Na+ _____ K+ _____ C1−	_____ #1 IV guage _____ Site _____
	Solution _____ Total In _____
_____ C02 _____ ETOH _____ pH	_____ #2 IV guage _____ Site _____
	Solution _____ Total In _____
_____ PC02 _____ p02 _____ HC03	_____ MAST
	_____ NG
_____ FI02	_____ Foley U/O_____
	Urine heme (+) (−) circle one
Medications:	_____ X-Rays
_____	_____ Chart
_____	_____ Admission records
_____	_____ MD's orders & progress notes
_____	*(Please send with Patient)*
Tetanus Y or N	PLEASE WRITE ADDITIONAL NOTES ON BACK

Figure 7–4. Sample transfer sheet.

phase. Other procedures, such as placement of a Foley catheter, also may be done. A history of the injury or illness and the past medical history should be taken; current use of medications, immunization status, and drug allergies should be documented.

Documentation. Although documentation is a critical part of an ED admission, extensive laboratory and radiologic studies are not indicated for critically ill or injured children; indeed, they may prove detrimental. For example, a child presenting with fulminant meningitis should have antibiotic therapy and transport arrangements initiated immediately, even in the absence of a lumbar puncture, especially if the transferring staff feels uncomfortable performing a lumbar puncture. Some procedures and diagnostic studies can be delayed until the child arrives at the receiving center.

Documentation is often summarized on a transfer form (Figure 7–4). This form should include the child's name, demographic information, immunization and allergy status, chief complaint, vital signs, the therapeutic interventions initiated and the child's response, laboratory and radiologic findings, signed consent, and notes of communication with both the receiving facility and the transport team. This same information should be given in the oral nursing and medical report to the receiving facility.

On arrival of the transport team, an ideally prepared pediatric patient has a patent airway confirmed; the cervical spine immobilized; supplemental oxygen administered; two intravenous lines or an intraosseous line established; fluid resuscitation initiated if necessary; a nasogastric tube and Foley catheter in place if indicated; appropriate medications administered; and documentation ready.

Responsibilities of the Transport Team

Care of the child is generally assumed by the transport team after their arrival at the transferring hospital (Figure 7–5). The transport team should introduce themselves to the transferring staff to establish a collegial and cooperative relationship from the onset. The referring staff is a vital part of the transfer process. The team then re-assesses the child's condition and intervenes further if clearly indicated. The emphasis is on stabilization before the transport, because some procedures are difficult to perform in a noisy, moving vehicle. If the child's condition is stable and the child is well prepared, most interfacility transfers take 30 minutes or less.

One of the most difficult times for parents is witnessing their child sick or injured. Transferring a child miles away only contributes to this stress, and it may precipitate a family crisis. The transport team must be

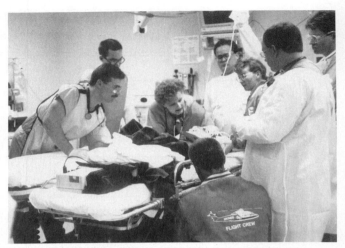

Figure 7–5. Roles and responsibilities of the referral facility and transport team must be clearly defined.

empathetic and supportive of both the child and the family. Whenever possible, the team should introduce themselves to the parents, explain the transportation process, and answer any questions. They should encourage the family to see the child before transport and, if possible, to stay with the child until the child leaves the referring facility. In some instances, the parents may accompany a child during transport, in which case they should receive a safety briefing. If parents do not accompany a child, the parents should receive directions and maps to the receiving facility and be advised to drive carefully.

En route, the transport team continues the care initiated by the transferring facility. Vital signs, a neurologic evaluation, and monitoring should be documented every 5–15 minutes, depending on the child's condition. All treatments and the child's response to them should be documented. Communication with the tertiary care center should also be documented. After the transport, evaluation of the transport and communication with the transferring hospital serve to strengthen the transport process.

CONCLUSION

Hippocrates stated many years ago that "healing is a matter of time, but sometimes also a matter of opportunity." For a critically ill or injured child, this opportunity begins even before the child reaches the referring hospital. Planning, adequate equipment, and specialized training are mandatory for the transferring staff (Figure 7–6). Add a well organized, responsive pediatric transport system, and one can be certain that optimal care is available for a critically ill or injured child requiring transport.

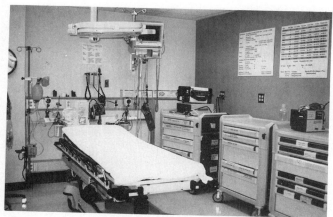

Figure 7–6. Planning and easy access to reference materials, such as wall charts with pediatric drug dosages and equipment, can greatly simplify the stabilization.

REFERENCES

American College of Emergency Physicians (1990). Principles of appropriate patient transfer: Position statement. *Annals of Emergency Medicine* 19:337–338

Aoki BY, McCloskey K (1992). *Evaluation, stabilization, and transport of the critically ill child.* St. Louis: Mosby Year Book, pp 329–341

Baxt WG, Moody P (1987). The impact of a physician as part of the aeromedical prehospital team in patients with blunt trauma. *Journal of the American Medical Association* 257:3246–3250

Bhende MAS, Thompson AE, Cook DR, et al (1992). Validity of disposable end-tidal CO_2 detector in verifying endotracheal tube placement in infants and children. *Annals of Emergency Medicine* 21:142–145

Black RE, Mayer T, Walker ML, et al (1982). Air transport of pediatric emergency cases (special report). *New England Journal of Medicine* 307:1465–1468

Brink LW, Neuman B, Wynn J (1993). Air transport. *Pediatric Clinics of North America* 40:439–456

Chou MM, MacDonald MG (1989). Landmarks in the development of patient transfer systems. In MacDonald MG, Miller MK (eds), *Emergency transport of the perinatal patient.* Boston: Little, Brown, pp 2–31

Continenza K, Hill JH (1990). Transport of the critically ill child. In Blumer JL (ed), *A practical guide to pediatric intensive care* (3rd ed). St. Louis: Mosby Year Book, pp 17–28

Day S, McCloskey K, Orr R, et al (1991). Pediatric interhospital critical care transport: Consensus of a national leadership conference. *Pediatrics* 88:696–704

Frew SA, Roush WR, LaGreca K (1988). COBRA: Implications for emergency medicine. *Annals of Emergency Medicine* 17:835–837

Ginzburg HM (1989). Legal issues in medical transport. In MacDonald MG, Miller MK (eds), *Emergency transport of the perinatal patient.* Boston: Little, Brown, pp 152–169

Haeger K (1988). *History of surgery.* New York: Bell, pp 159–161

Harris BH, Orr RE, Boles ET (1975). Aeromedical transportation for infants and children. *Journal of Pediatric Surgery* 10:719–724

Howell E (1988). Evolution of trauma care. In Howell E, Widra L, Hill MG (eds), *Comprehensive trauma nursing: Theory and practice.* Boston: Scott, Foresman, pp 5–33

Kissoon N (1992). Triage and transport of the critically ill child. *Progress in Pediatric Critical Care* 8:37–57

Luten RC, Wears RL, Broselow J, et al (1992). Length-based endotracheal tube and emergency equipment in pediatrics. *Annals of Emergency Medicine* 21:900–903

McCloskey KA, King WD, Byron L (1989). Pediatric critical care transport: Is a physician always needed on the team? *Annals of Emergency Medicine* 18:247–249

McCloskey KA, Orr RA (1992). Interhospital transport. In Barkin RM (ed), *Pediatric emergency medicine: Concepts in clinical practice.* St. Louis: Mosby Year Book, pp 41–43

Merrill M (1988). Timelines of emergency air-medical services. In American Society of Hospital Based Emergency Air Medical Services (ASHBEAMS), *Air medical crew national standards curriculum.* Pasadena, Calif, pp 1–5

Parsons CJ, Bobechko WP (1982). Airmedical transport: Its hidden problems. *Canadian Medical Association* 126:237–243

Pon S, Notterman DA (1993). The organization of a pediatric critical care transport program. *Pediatric Clinics of North America* 40:241–261

Rhee KJ, Burney RE (1990). Transfer and transport of patients. In Callahan ML (ed), *Current practice of emergency medicine* (2nd ed). Philadelphia: B.C. Decker, pp 75–79

Rhee KJ, Strozeski M, Burney RE, et al (1986). Is the flight physician needed for helicopter emergency medical services? *Annals of Emergency Medicine* 15:174–177

Smith DF, Hackel A (1983). Selection criteria for pediatric critical care transport teams. *Critical Care Medicine* 11:10–12

Southard PA (1989). COBRA legislation: Complying with ED provisions. *Journal of Emergency Nursing* 15:23–25

Todres D (1993). Pediatric airway control and ventilation. *Annals of Emergency Medicine* 22:440–444

PART 2

Psychosocial Emergencies

CHAPTER 8

Child Abuse and Neglect

SUSAN J. KELLEY

INTRODUCTION

Child maltreatment is one of the most serious health problems in the United States. Although child abuse has existed for centuries, its comprehensive identification and treatment is a relatively recent phenomenon. In 1962 Dr. C. Henry Kempe and colleagues (Kempe et al, 1962) introduced the concept of battered child syndrome. It was not until 1967, however, that all states had passed child abuse reporting laws.

Estimates of the actual scope of the problem of child maltreatment are difficult to ascertain for several reasons. Definitions of child maltreatment and investigative procedures vary among states. In addition, cases of child maltreatment that are reported to child protective services represent only the tip of the iceberg because many maltreated children remain unidentified and therefore unreported to officials.

Estimates of the numbers of children maltreated each year speak to the urgency of the problem and underscore the need for emergency nurses to keep an open mind to the fact that child abuse occurs on a frequent basis. In 1991 child protective services (CPS) agencies in the US received 2,694,000 reports of maltreatment (Daro and McCurdy, 1992). This reflects a 40% increase over the number of reports received in 1985, the first year in which the National Committee for the Prevention of Child Abuse (NCPCA) began their annual, 50-state survey (Daro and McCurdy, 1992). Factors to which this dramatic increase are attributed include increased reporting due to public awareness and an actual increase in maltreatment as a consequence of economic stress (Daro and McCurdy, 1992).

DEFINITIONS OF ABUSE AND NEGLECT

Child maltreatment is generally categorized into four major categories: (1) physical abuse; (2) sexual abuse; (3) emotional abuse; and (4) neglect. Each state's reporting law provides definitions of physical abuse, sexual abuse, and neglect, with definitions varying slightly from state to state (Myers, 1992). Some generally accepted definitions follow.

Physical abuse refers to intentionally inflicted physical injury to a child by a parent or caretaker.

Sexual abuse refers to any sexual contact between a child and adult (or considerably older child) whether by physical force, persuasion, or coercion. (Sexual abuse is addressed in Chapter 9).

Neglect refers to acts of omission and failure to meet a child's basic needs, including food, shelter, clothing, health care, education, and a safe environment.

Emotional abuse refers to parental behaviors that are cruel, degrading, terrorizing, isolating, or rejecting.

The American Association for the Protection of Children estimates that 26% of all child maltreatment reports involve charges of physical abuse, 16% involve charges of sexual abuse, 55% involve charges of child neglect, 8% involve charges of emotional maltreatment, and 8% involve other forms of abuse (American Association for Protecting Children, 1988).

ETIOLOGY OF CHILD ABUSE AND NEGLECT

Various theoretical frameworks have been used to explain the complex phenomenon of child abuse. Although most models have focused on parental and family dysfunction, other models incorporate environmental influences. One of the most comprehensive models applied to the phenomenon of child abuse is the ecology of human development (Belsky, 1980; Zuvarin, 1989). Within this framework child maltreatment is conceptualized as a social and psychological phenomenon that is determined by multiple forces at work in the individual, family, community, and culture. Cultural support for the use of physical force against children and the inadequate use of family support systems are identified as necessary conditions for child maltreatment.

Perpetrator Characteristics

Many factors contribute to the likelihood that a person will abuse a child, including a combination of individual, familial, and societal factors. Stress factors, such as economic difficulty, crowded or inadequate housing, and unemployment can contribute to a parent's abusive potential. Parenting factors that contribute to the potential for abuse include unrealistic expectations of children, lack of preparation for the parenting role, and poor parental role models. Psychological factors may include poor impulse control, substance abuse, and depression. Abusive parents are often socially isolated, without adequate support from extended family members and peers.

Physical abuse may be the result of excessive corporal punishment. Parents who overdiscipline their children often have good intentions. The abuse may take place while they are attempting to "teach the child a lesson" to change what they perceive as unacceptable or bad behavior. Unrealistic parental expectations of their children also can lead to abuse. This problem is related to a parent's lack of knowledge and understanding of normal or age-appropriate behavior. For example, some parents actually believe that their young infant cries only for attention or merely to annoy them.

Another major factor leading to child maltreatment is the type of parenting one received as a child; most people internalize, to some degree, the parenting they received during childhood. Many abusive parents were themselves abused as children and relate to their children as their parents related to them— through physical or emotional abuse. Abusive parents have unmet emotional needs of their own and are therefore unable to meet their child's basic emotional needs. To make matters worse, they look to the child to meet their own emotional needs and are often disappointed.

Table 8–1 summarizes characteristics of abusive parents (Milner and Chilamkurti, 1991). Clearly, every abusive parent does not possess each of these charac-

TABLE 8–1. CHARACTERISTICS OF ABUSIVE PARENTS

Low self-esteem
Social isolation
Negative perceptions of their children's behavior
Lack of knowledge of normal child development
Reliance on physical punishment techniques for discipline
Role reversal
Negative parent-child interactions
Childhood history of abuse
Substance abuse
Antisocial personality disorder
Neurologic and psychoneurologic problems
Physical health problems
Abnormal physiologic reactivity
Depression
External locus of control

(From Milner JS, Chilamkurti C (1991). Physical child abuse perpetrator characteristics. Journal of Interpersonal Violence *6:345–366)*

teristics; it remains unknown which combination of characteristics places parents at greatest risk for abusing or neglecting their children.

Child Risk Factors

Factors that are believed to place children at increased risk for maltreatment are outlined in Table 8–2. Needless to say, many children are maltreated who do not possess any of these characteristics and many children who possess these characteristics are not maltreated.

EFFECTS OF CHILD ABUSE AND NEGLECT

Many studies have attempted to identify the impact of abuse. Research on the developmental sequelae of child maltreatment indicates that various areas of a child's development are adversely affected. Research findings indicate that abuse and neglect negatively affect the intellectual, emotional, and social development of a child.

Numerous studies have documented the relationship between various types of child maltreatment and psychological harm to the child (Claussen and Crittenden, 1991; Famularo et al, 1990; Kelley, 1989; Kelley, 1992; Kolko et al, 1988). Child physical abuse and neglect are also associated with lower intelligence, devel-

TABLE 8–2. CHILD RISK FACTORS FOR MALTREATMENT

Premature birth
Congenital defect
Prenatal drug exposure
Product of multiple birth
Developmental disability
Physical disability
Chronic illness

opmental delays, and poor academic performance on the part of the child (Burke et al, 1989).

Results of a prospective study of 309 children indicated that physical abuse is a risk factor for development of chronic aggressive behavior patterns, even when other ecologic and biologic factors are known (Dodge et al, 1990). In addition, abused children were found to acquire deviant patterns of processing social information, which may later perpetuate the cycle of violence.

TYPES OF CHILD ABUSE AND NEGLECT

Neglect

Neglect is the most prevalent form of child maltreatment. Child neglect usually involves acts of omission, or failure to meet the basic needs of a child. These basic needs include food, shelter, clothing, medical care, and a safe environment. Neglect is often unintentional because of a lack of money, education, parenting skills, motivation, or appropriate judgment. Physical neglect, in contrast to physical abuse, tends to be more chronic than episodic. In addition to physical neglect, a child may be subjected to emotional, medical, or educational neglect.

Neglect is often not obvious, and many cases go undetected for long periods of time. Because neglect is sometimes difficult to distinguish from poverty, recognition of neglect often involves value judgments. Therefore, when neglect is suspected, it is important to consider what the family should be doing, as opposed to what they are economically capable of doing.

Physical indicators of neglect include malnourishment, poor hygiene, and inappropriate dress, such as light clothing in the winter or very soiled clothing. Bald patches on the scalp of an infant may be the result of an infant's lying in a crib in one position for extended periods of time. The child may have evidence of inadequate medical care, including unattended medical problems or lack of proper immunization. It is sometimes difficult to differentiate between medical neglect and lack of compliance. When harm to a child is the result, it is medical neglect. Neglected children often have extensive untreated dental caries and other dental problems. Neglected children may have a history of numerous accidental injuries due to inadequate supervision. There may be a history of truancy and school avoidance. Infants and young children may be brought to the ED because of abandonment.

Behavioral indicators of neglect include developmental delays, particularly in the area of language development. Malnourished children generally do poorly in school because they have a low energy level and an inability to concentrate. Neglected children of-

TABLE 8–3. INDICATORS OF NEGLECT

Malnutrition
Failure to thrive syndrome
Poor housing, such as unsanitary or unsafe conditions
Unattended medical problems
Lack of proper immunizations
Poor hygiene
Inappropriate dress or clothing
Bald spots on scalp
Extensive unattended dental caries
Developmental delays
Dull, inactive, and excessively passive and fatigued appearance
Abandonment
Lack of supervision
Educational neglect, such as frequent absences

ten fall asleep during class because they have inadequate sleep at night. Neglected infants and toddlers may appear dull, inactive, and excessively passive. Table 8–3 provides a summary of clinical indicators of neglect.

Failure to Thrive Syndrome

Failure to thrive (FTT) is a clinical diagnostic term used to describe a lack of growth according to expected norms (Ludwig, 1992). Non-organic FTT is a term often used to describe poor weight gain without apparent physical cause and is therefore believed to be related to environmental or psychosocial factors. Organic FTT refers to a failure to grow adequately as the result of an identified medical condition, which may include a cardiac, metabolic, endocrine, or neurologic disorder. The term *mixed FTT* refers to cases in which a child fails to grow normally in the presence of a minor health problem and an abnormal family environment.

Because most cases of FTT are of mixed etiology, the distinction between organic and non-organic FTT is often impossible to make. According to Alexander (1992), by the time a diagnosis of FTT is made, organic and non-organic causes are inevitably intertwined, making the question of which came first difficult and often pointless. Much more important is what can be done to remedy the situation. Failure to thrive is caused by one of three problems: not enough calories are going into the child; too many calories are being excreted by the child; too many calories are being lost internally (Alexander, 1992).

Failure to thrive usually occurs in the first 2 years of life. The criteria for the diagnosis of FTT are usually based on the infant's or child's falling below the third percentile for weight on an anthropometric chart. Appendix D contains anthropometric charts for height and weight that can be used by ED nurses to identify FTT.

Infants and young children with FTT who arrive

at the ED and are found to be below the third percentile in weight and height should be referred to their primary care provider for an evaluation. Some infants with FTT are admitted to the hospital for a comprehensive evaluation. Indications for hospitalization include the following: an infant is less than 6 months old; an infant below birth weight at 6 weeks; head circumference less than fifth percentile; signs of abuse or gross neglect; failure of outpatient treatment; medical problem suspected; an unsafe environment or an inadequate caretaker (Ludwig, 1992). Infants who are being neglected at home often gain weight while in the hospital.

Emotional Abuse

Emotional abuse is the result of parents failing to provide a nurturing environment. Although physical and sexual abuse are always accompanied by emotional abuse, emotional maltreatment can occur independently. Emotional abuse can be just as devastating to a child's well-being as other forms of abuse. Like neglect, emotional abuse is often a chronic impediment to normal development.

Emotional abuse includes constant criticism, beratement, belittlement, verbal abuse, threats, and exposure to domestic violence. Emotional maltreatment is more difficult to identify and document than physical maltreatment. There are rarely enough objective data to prove emotional abuse. Indicators of emotional abuse may include persistent vomiting, sleep disorders, enuresis, speech disorders, hyperactivity, or FTT syndrome. An emotionally abused child may demonstrate behavior that is excessively passive or aggressive. Emotional abuse in adolescents may be manifested by alcohol or drug abuse and runaway behavior. Table 8–4 summarizes indicators of emotional abuse.

Substance Abuse

It is estimated that 675,000 children are seriously mistreated annually by a substance abusing caretaker (National Committee for Prevention of Child Abuse, 1989). Research findings indicate that substance abusing mothers are at increased risk for maltreating their children (Kelley et al, 1991; Kelley, 1992; Famularo et al, 1989). Of particular concern is the dramatic increase

TABLE 8–4. INDICATORS OF EMOTIONAL ABUSE

Failure to thrive syndrome
Feeding disorders
Sleep disorders
Developmental delays
Speech disorders
Hyperactivity
Excessively passive or aggressive behavior
Depressed or suicidal behavior

TABLE 8–5. INDICATORS OF PARENTAL SUBSTANCE ABUSE

- INDICATORS OF PRENATAL DRUG EXPOSURE IN INFANTS
  Irritability
  Depressed interactive abilities
  Impaired organizational abilities
  Easy overstimulation
  Hypertonia
  Mottling
  Excessive yawning and sneezing

- INDICATORS OF PARENTAL SUBSTANCE ABUSE
  Erratic, unpredictable behavior
  Paranoid behavior
  Urgency to leave emergency department
  Neglect of child
  Criminal activity
  Prostitution
  Lack of prenatal care
  Premature delivery

in drug use among pregnant women. Table 8–5 contains a summary of indicators of prenatal drug exposure of infants and indicators of maternal substance abuse.

Fatal Child Maltreatment

One of the most tragic clinical situations encountered by emergency nurses is the death of a child caused by abuse or neglect. The actual number of child fatalities related to child abuse is difficult to determine with any degree of certainty. The National Committee on the Prevention of Child Abuse estimates that in 1991 almost 1400 children died from abuse or neglect. This means that almost four children die each day in the US as a result of maltreatment; half of these children are younger than 1 year of age (Daro and McCurdy, 1992). Of these children, 36% died from neglect and 64% died from abuse. Fifteen percent of deaths were linked to parental substance abuse. Between 1985 and 1991, the number of deaths related to child maltreatment rose 54% (Daro and McCurdy, 1992).

Homicide is the second cause of injury deaths among children. While almost two-thirds of these deaths are among 15–19 year olds, 23% occur among children younger than 5 years of age (Centers for Disease Control, 1990). The high rate of homicide among children younger than 5 years is primarily due to caretaker abuse and neglect (Christoffel, 1990). About half of all homicides among children aged 0 to 4 years are inflicted with blows, and about 10% of children in this age group are killed by firearms (Centers for Disease Control, 1990).

Children are at greatest risk of being killed during the first month of life; the rate of child homicide decreases as the child's age increases (Crittenden and Craig, 1990). The most likely explanations for the inverse relation between age and risk of fatal child abuse are: infants have greater biologic vulnerability to assault because of immaturity of the brain and other organs; younger children are less mobile; and more annoying child behaviors (Christoffel, 1992). Child abuse homicide victims are generally the youngest or second to youngest child in a family (Christoffel, 1992). After the first year of life boys are at greater risk than girls for fatal child maltreatment; for boys younger than 1 year, the incidences may be similar (Christoffel, 1992). Most cases of fatal child abuse among infants are committed by mothers (Crittenden and Craig, 1990). Mothers who begin childbearing at an early age are considered at increased risk for fatally maltreating their children.

Most children who die as a result of abuse or neglect have experienced maltreatment before the fatal incident. Korbin (1989) studied a sample of women incarcerated for killing their children and found that in each case the fatal incident was not the first time a parent or caretaker had become abusive with the murdered child, but rather was the culmination of a series of abusive incidents. In the annual national surveys conducted by the NCPCA between 1989 and 1991, 39% of the children who died of maltreatment had had current or prior contact with CPS agencies (Daro and McCurdy, 1992). These findings speak to the importance of early detection and reporting of maltreating families by emergency nurses before fatal incidents of maltreatment occur.

Unfortunately, no single health care, social service, law enforcement, or judicial system exists to track and comprehensively assess the circumstances of child death (Durfee et al, 1992). Currently, only 21 states have inter-agency multidisciplinary child death review teams at the local or state level for systematic evaluation and case management of suspicious child deaths (Durfee et al, 1992). Child death review teams are typically comprised of representatives of the medical examiner's office, law enforcement, prosecutors, CPS, pediatricians with child abuse expertise, and nurses (Durfee et al, 1992). The advantages of child death review teams include improved communication and cooperation among agencies, increased knowledge of risk factors for child homicide, systematic evaluation of agency actions and inactions, and identification of surviving siblings at risk for maltreatment (Durfee et al, 1992).

Münchhausen Syndrome by Proxy

Münchhausen syndrome by proxy (MSBP) is a form of child abuse in which a parent falsifies an illness in a child through fabrication or creation of symptoms and then seeks medical care. The syndrome was named after Baron Von Münchhausen, an 18th century story teller who entertained people with fabricated stories. The term *Münchhausen syndrome* was first used for adults who fabricated illnesses with false medical histories and altered laboratory and physical findings. Subsequently the term *Münchhausen syndrome by proxy* was used to describe cases in which a parent created or fabricated a medical problem in their child.

Victims of MSBP usually range in age from infancy to 6 years. Older children may aid in the parents' deceptions to protect them or because of an intense fear of retribution by the abusive parents. False histories given by parents often include seizures, apnea, cardiopulmonary arrest, hematuria, and hematemesis. Parents may induce physical findings in their children by suffocation, administration of drugs or toxic substances, or placing their own blood in the child's urine, vomitus, or stool specimens. Drugs often used in MSBP include laxatives to induce severe diarrhea; insulin to induce hypoglycemia and seizures; ipecac to induce vomiting; and drugs or alcohol to cause an alteration in level of consciousness. Salt may be added to an infant's formula to induce hypernatremia. Clinical indicators of Münchhausen syndrome by proxy are summarized in Table 8–6.

Most reported cases of MSBP involve the child's mother (Rosenberg, 1987). Often the mother has Munchausen syndrome with the same physical complaints as her child. In many reported cases the mother has had some nursing or allied health care education and is therefore quite adept at making falsified information appear credible. The mother often appears genuinely concerned over her child's illness. When the child is hospitalized, the mother rarely leaves the child's bedside.

Rosenberg (1987) reviewed 117 cases of MSBP and found the most common presentations of MSBP were bleeding, seizures, central nervous system depression, apnea, diarrhea, vomiting, fever, and a rash. In these cases, the mortality was 9%; the long-term morbidity rate, 8%; and the short-term morbidity rate, 100%. Failure to thrive was associated with MSBP in 14% of the children. All perpetrators were the victims' mothers.

Cases in which multiple children in a family are victimized, referred to as serial Münchhausen syn-

TABLE 8–6. INDICATORS OF MÜNCHHAUSEN SYNDROME BY PROXY

Recurrent illnesses for which no cause is identified
Unusual symptoms that do not make clinical sense
Symptoms that are only observed by the parent
Frequent visits to various hospitals with normal findings
Presence of drugs that induced the symptoms in a toxic screen
Discrepancies between history and physical findings
Numerous hospitalizations at many different hospitals

drome by proxy, have been reported in the literature by Alexander et al (1990b). These cases were found to be associated with a high mortality (31%) and a high incidence of maternal psychiatric illness.

PHYSICAL ABUSE

Nurses must be knowledgeable about all possible indicators of abuse and neglect, especially those that are manifested before a child suffers a serious injury, emotional impairment, or developmental delay. Early recognition and intervention are the keys to prevention of subsequent abuse and negative sequelae.

History

A meticulously taken history is invaluable in distinguishing between intentional and unintentional injuries. Table 8–7 summarizes the characteristics that should alert nurses to the possibility of child abuse.

Emergency nurses should elicit a careful, detailed history of all injuries and compare the explanation offered with the observed injury. Abusive parents may give an implausible explanation for the injury or a vague account of events surrounding the injury, or they may deny any knowledge of how the injury occurred. If a discrepancy exists between the account given for the cause of an injury and the physical findings, abuse should be suspected.

Whenever possible, the child and each caretaker present should be interviewed separately because discrepancies may exist between the parents' and the child's accounts. Also, when interviewed alone, the child is more likely to report accurately the cause of the injury and the identity of the abuser. If more than one caretaker has accompanied the child to the emergency department (ED), interviewing each separately may reveal discrepancies in explanations offered. Evoking as many details as possible helps reveal any inconsistencies.

The child's past medical history, including any previous injuries, should be carefully elicited. When

TABLE 8–7. CHARACTERISTICS IN HISTORIES OF CHILD ABUSE

History inconsistent with existing injury
Denial of any knowledge of cause or mechanism of injury
Parent reluctant to give information
Parent blames sibling for injury
Child developmentally incapable of specified self injury
Delay in seeking medical attention
Inconsistencies in history
History of repeated injuries or hospitalizations
Inappropriate response to severity of injury
Previous placement of a child in foster care
Previous involvement with child protective services agency

available, the child's medical record should be reviewed for previous suspicious injuries. Occasionally, caretakers may claim that a child bruises easily. Laboratory tests, including a platelet count, prothrombin time (PT), and partial thromboplastin time (PTT) readily determine if the child has a bleeding disorder. Previously undiagnosed hemophilia is a rare cause of bruising in older children (Johnson, 1990). Because hemophilia is a chronic and stressful disease, hemophiliac children may be at increased risk for abuse, and their increased tendency to bruise may mask intentional injury (Johnson, 1990). Therefore, because a child has hemophilia does not eliminate the possibility that the child is abused.

A delay in seeking medical attention for an injury should raise suspicion of abuse; some abusive parents ignore the seriousness of an injury in the hope that the injury will heal without medical attention, thereby avoiding detection and legal action.

Another important factor to consider is the distance the parent traveled to seek care. If they have traveled an unusual distance for medical attention, bypassing closer hospitals, the family may be trying to avoid detection by staff who have suspected them of abuse on previous occasions. Abusive parents often seek medical care at many different treatment facilities to prevent being identified.

Knowledge of normal child growth and development is essential when assessing for possible abuse (see Chapter 4). One must consider, "Is it developmentally possible for the child to have injured him or herself in such a manner?" For example, if the mother of a 1-month-old infant with a skull fracture states that the baby rolled over in the crib and fell out onto the floor, abuse should be suspected because infants are not capable of rolling over until 3–5 months of age. Likewise, noninflicted fractures of the limbs are unusual in infants who have not yet learned to walk.

Physical Assessment

A complete physical assessment should be conducted on all children of whom abuse or neglect is suspected. It is important to be cognizant of the fact that many cases of child abuse are identified while a child is being treated for a condition other than the inflicted injury. For example, inflicted rib fractures may be found during a chest x ray to rule out pneumonia in an infant who has presented with an upper respiratory tract infection. Old, previously undiagnosed fractures of an extremity may be detected on x rays while assessing a recent, unintentional injury. Table 8–8 summarizes indicators of physical abuse.

Cutaneous Lesions. Cutaneous lesions are the most common manifestation of physical abuse and are the

TABLE 8–8. INDICATORS OF PHYSICAL ABUSE

- CUTANEOUS INJURIES
  Bruises
  - In various states of healing
  - Bilateral, linear, or geometric injuries
  - In configuration of object
  - Pinch marks, pair of crescent bruises
  - Located on face, neck, thighs, genitals, back, inner upper arms, thorax
  - Grip marks on upper arms
  Human bite marks
  - Oval shape pattern of teeth marks
  Traction alopecia
  - Irregular areas of hair loss
  - Broken hair
  - Subgaleal hematoma
  Abrasions, lacerations
  - Circumferential abrasions or friction burns from ropes at neck, wrist, ankles, torso
  - Chain imprints
  - Linear puncture marks from fork

- BURNS
  Immersion burns
  - Uniform in depth, sharp lines of demarcation
  - Bilateral burns of feet, hands, and buttocks
  - Flexion creases spared because child flexes extremities
  Contact burns
  - Resemble configuration of object
  - In various stages of healing
  - Circular crater the diameter of a cigarette
  - Commonly located on face and dorsum of hands and feet

- HEAD TRAUMA AND CENTRAL NERVOUS SYSTEM INJURIES
  - Bilateral skull fractures
  - Multiple skull fractures
  - Skull fractures with widths greater than 5 mm
  - Subdural hematomas
  - Separation of sutures due to chronic subdural hematoma
  - Subgaleal hematoma
  - Decreased level of consciousness
  - Grip marks on upper arms
  - Spinal cord injury

- OPHTHALMIC INJURIES
  - Hyphema
  - Retinal detachment
  - Dislocated lens
  - Retinal hemorrhage
  - Subconjunctival bleeding
  - Periorbital ecchymosis

- NECK TRAUMA
  - Subluxation or dislocation

- SKELETAL INJURIES
  - Multiple fractures, especially bilateral
  - Fractures of various ages
  - Spiral fractures of humerus (forcible twisting)
  - Transverse fractures (blunt trauma)
  - Rib fractures, especially if multiple, bilateral, or posterior
  - Fractures of the sternum, spinous processes, scapula
  - Fractures of femur in children younger than 3 years
  - Fractures of the epiphyseal-metaphyseal junction
  - Digital fractures

- BLUNT ABDOMINAL TRAUMA
  - Abdominal distention, tenderness, bruising
  - Absent bowel sounds
  - Peritoneal or mesenteric bleeding
  - Persistent vomiting or abdominal pain
  - Bilious vomiting
  - Hypovolemic shock
  - Injury to liver, spleen, pancreas, duodenum, jejunum, kidneys
  - Signs of peritonitis

most easily recognized sign of abuse. Cutaneous lesions caused by maltreatment include contusions, abrasions, lacerations, burns, bite marks, and hair loss. The most important aspects of cutaneous lesions are location, configuration, and chronology (Reece, 1992). The size, shape, location, distribution, and color of all injuries should be carefully documented.

Bruises. Cutaneous lesions that are the result of unintentional injury are most commonly found on the skin over the bony prominences such as the chin, knees, elbows, iliac crests, and forehead. Bruises on the buttocks (Figure 8–1), genitals (Figure 8–2), perineum, trunk (Figure 8–3), upper legs (Figure 8–4), face (Figure 8–5) and neck (Figure 8–6) may be indicative of abuse. The depth of bruises varies by location. The loose, tender skin of the eyelids and genitalia bruises easily. Bruises on the buttocks (Figure 8–7) and thighs may not appear for hours or several days because of the thick muscular support of blood vessels and because of the initial extravasation of blood into deeper

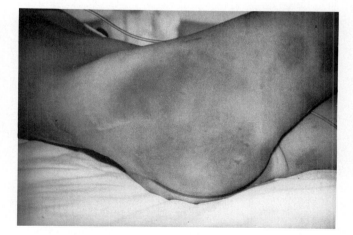

Figure 8–1. Extensive bruising of buttocks and thighs. (Courtesy of Dr. Seth Asser, University of California San Diego Medical Center)

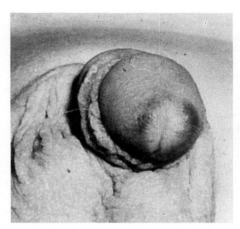

Figure 8–2. A pinch mark bruise on the end of the penis caused by fingernails. Note the two small crescent-shaped bruises that face each other. This injury was inflicted when the child was punished for touching his penis. (Courtesy of Barton Schmitt MD, The Children's Hospital, Denver)

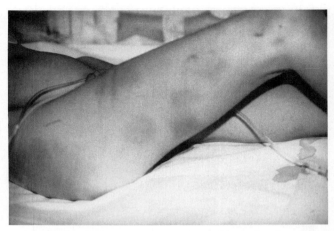

Figure 8–4. Multiple bruises of upper leg and buttocks. (Courtesy of Seth Asser MD, University of California San Diego Medical Center)

tissues. Careful inspection of these sites may reveal tenderness and swelling. Deep contusions may remain red or purple for days or weeks after an injury.

Bruises change color with time as blood is reabsorbed. It is, therefore, important to compare the reported date of injury with the color or age of the existing bruises to detect any discrepancies. Table 8–9 provides a guide for estimating the age of bruises. Multiple bruises in various stages of healing should raise concern.

The pattern of a bruise often reflects the method or instrument used to strike a child. Straight lines are uncommon in nature and in uninflicted injuries; thus injury from a manmade object should be considered when linear contusions or unusual configurations with sharp angles are present (Barnett, 1992). Configurations of objects frequently used to strike children include the characteristic loop mark from an extension cord; linear marks from a belt, strap, or stick; and imprints from a spoon, buckle, paddle (Figure 8–8); spatula, hair brush, or hand.

Linear marks 1–2 inches wide (Figure 8–9), often found over curved body surfaces, generally indicate beating with a belt or strap (Kessler and Hyden, 1991). In some cases, an imprint of the belt buckle is noted. If a hand is used to strike a child, characteristic parallel

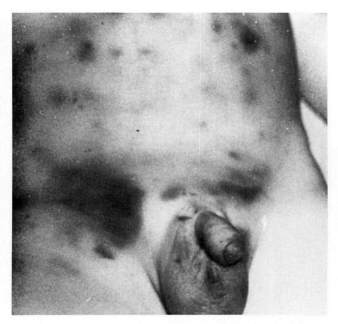

Figure 8–3. Multiple inflicted bruises on a child's lower abdomen, groin, and genitals in various stages of healing. (Courtesy of Barton Schmitt MD, The Children's Hospital, Denver)

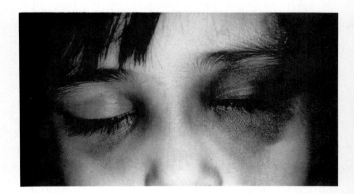

Figure 8–5. Blunt trauma to the face. (Courtesy of Seth Asser MD, University of California San Diego Medical Center)

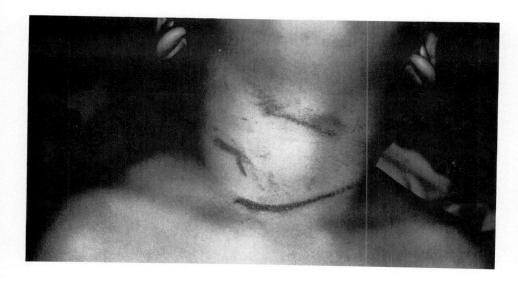

Figure 8–6. Strangulation marks on neck. (Courtesy of Seth Asser MD, University of California San Diego Medical Center)

linear marks (Figure 8–10) may be noted; these represent the spaces between the fingers (Kelley, 1988).

A doubled-over electrical extension cord or lamp cord leaves characteristic loop-shaped marks (Figure 8–11) that are typically found on the back, buttocks, upper arms, and thighs. In contrast, marks from a coat hanger leave a wider loop mark caused by the flat base of the coat hanger (Johnson, 1990).

Circular or oval marks on the upper arm may be the result of a caregiver's forcibly grasping a child and applying pressure to the site. Other cutaneous lesions that are indicative of abuse are rope marks on the

ankles, wrist, or torso indicating that a child has been bound. Cords or rope used to bind ankles and wrists leave thin, circumferential bruises; thicker marks may indicate friction burns from sheeting material used to tie a child (Kessler and Hyden, 1991). Infants and young children may be gagged or have clothes or objects stuffed in their mouths to stop their crying. Gag marks leave down-turned lesions at the corners of the mouth.

Burns. Inflicted burns are involved in approximately 10% of substantiated cases of child abuse and are the third leading cause of death related to child abuse. Ten to 25% of burns of children are deliberately inflicted by adults. Two-thirds of these cases involve children younger than 3 years.

Children who repeatedly come to the ED with burns should be carefully evaluated for abuse. Suspicion should be raised when treatment of a child's burns is delayed more than 24 hours or when the parent who was not home at the time of the burning brings the child to the ED.

Burns intentionally inflicted often leave identifiable patterns on the skin; they may involve hot liquids or objects. Purdue and Hunt (1992) found that al-

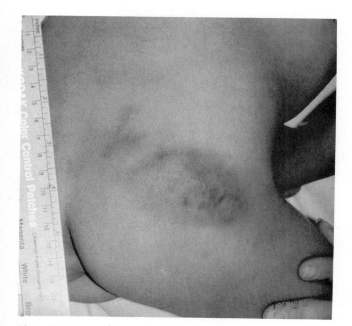

Figure 8–7. Severe bruising to buttocks. (Courtesy of Seth Asser MD, University of California San Diego Medical Center)

TABLE 8–9. GENERAL GUIDE TO ESTIMATION OF AGE OF BRUISES

Color	Age of Bruise
Red-blue	1–2 days
Blue-purple	2–4 days
Greenish yellow	5–7 days
Yellow-brown	7–14 days
Normal skin color	14–21 days

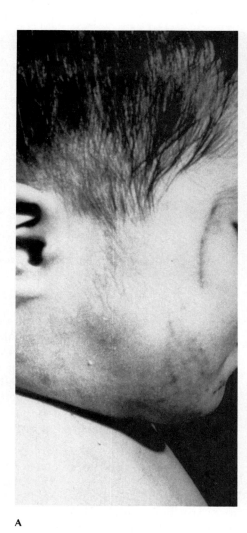

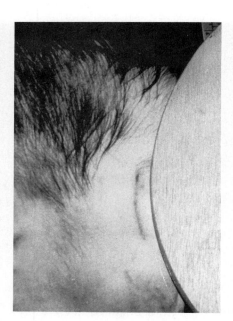

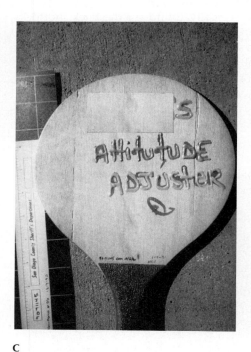

Figure 8–8. A. Contusion on face of a 1½-year-old, fatally maltreated boy with trisomy-21. Photographs taken postmortem. **B.** Matching of implement (paddle) with injury. **C.** Implement used to strike child (paddle). (Courtesy of Seth Asser MD, University of California San Diego Medical Center)

though burn injuries result from a wide variety of causes, most (82%) inflicted burns are caused by hot water. A large proportion (86%) of these scald injuries are caused by tap water; less than 16% of accidental injuries are caused by tap water.

IMMERSION BURNS. As noted, tap water scald burns are

often inflicted. Intentional scald burns are often the result of the child's being immersed in hot water. The resulting injury is typically uniform in depth and has sharp lines of demarcation. Immersion burns often involve bilateral burns of the feet, hands, and buttocks. Flexion creases are usually spared because the child flexes his or her extremities in the hot water. Inflicted

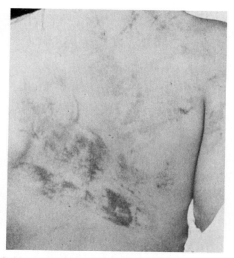

Figure 8–9. Numerous belt-mark bruises on the back and upper arms of an abused school-aged girl. (Courtesy of Barton Schmitt MD, The Children's Hospital, Denver)

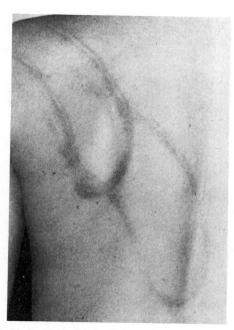

Figure 8–11. Bruises in this configuration are referred to as loop marks and are the result of being struck with a doubled over extension cord, lamp cord, or rope. (Courtesy of Barton Schmitt MD, The Children's Hospital, Denver)

immersion burns are typically symmetric, whereas accidental burns are usually asymmetric. Inflicted immersion burns often appear sock-like on the feet (Figure 8–12), glove-like on the hands, and doughnut-like (Figure 8–13) on the buttocks or genitalia. Immersion burns of the hands can be caused by the exploratory behavior of a child. However, when an immersion burn involves the buttocks and lower extremities of an infant, it is more likely to have been caused by the caretaker and to be associated with frustrated attempts to toilet train the child (Johnson, 1990).

Accidental burns display splash marks, varying depths of burn, indistinct borders between burned and unburned skin, and multiple areas of burn as the child struggles. The depth of an accidental burn tapers from deep to shallow as the body part is immersed, pain is felt by the child, and the limb is withdrawn (Purdue and Hunt, 1992).

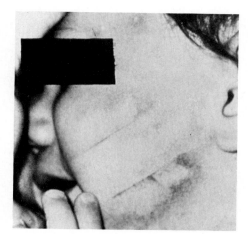

Figure 8–10. Fresh bruising on the cheek from a slap across the child's face. The configuration of the bruise indicates the child was struck from the front. (Courtesy of Barton Schmitt MD, The Children's Hospital, Denver)

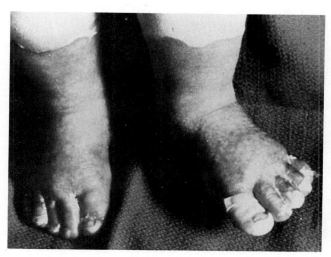

Figure 8–12. Forced immersion burns of both legs of a toddler. (Courtesy of Barton Schmitt MD, The Children's Hospital, Denver)

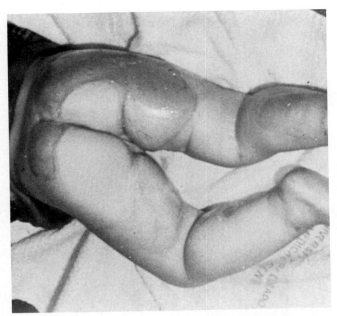

Figure 8–13. Child forced to sit in scalding water, resulting in a doughnut-shaped burn to the buttocks and legs. The unburned skin is the result of the child's being forcibly held down against the bottom of the tub and being spared prolonged contact in that area with the hot water. (Courtesy of Barton Schmitt MD, The Children's Hospital, Denver)

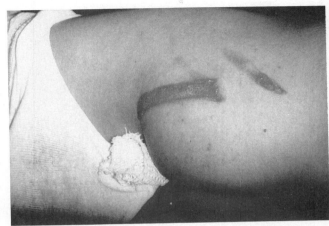

Figure 8–14. Burn to buttocks of a 7-year-old mentally retarded boy able to state that his mother heated a knife on the stove and burned him with it. (Courtesy of Seth Asser MD, University of California San Diego Medical Center)

The extent of an immersion burn depends on the temperature of the water, the duration of exposure, and the presence of clothing. Water with a temperature of 130°F (54° C) or higher can cause a full-thickness burn in less than 30 seconds. The presence of clothing tends to cause more severe burns because there is longer contact between the hot water with the skin. Accidental hot water burns are usually not as clearly demarcated on the edges as inflicted immersion burns. Inflicted burns tend to be full thickness, whereas the unintentional burns are often partial thickness.

PATTERNED BURNS

Cigarette Burns. Accidental cigarette burns, which may occur when sudden movement causes momentary contact with a lighted cigarette, typically occur about the face when a child walks into a lighted cigarette held by an adult at waist height (Purdue and Hunt, 1992). Cigarette burns found on the soles of the feet, palms of the hands, buttocks, or back are often inflicted. Inflicted cigarette burns are typically 8–10 mm in diameter and are indurated at the margins. Accidental cigarette burns are usually shallower, more irregular, and less circumscribed than deliberately inflicted ones. Multiple cigarette burns are pathognomonic of child abuse (Purdue and Hunt, 1992).

Contact Burns. Contact burns in the configuration of a heating object are often inflicted. Objects often involved in intentional contact burns include steam irons, electric stove burners, hot plates, forks, knives (Figure 8–14), curling irons (Figure 8–15), car cigarette lighters, cigarette lighters (Figure 8–16), radiators, hair dryers (Figure 8–17), and candles (Figure 8–18). Toddlers in the process of being toilet trained have been known to be placed on radiators to dry their wet diapers, resulting in burns to the buttocks.

Bite Mark Injuries. Human bite marks may resemble a double horseshoe or may appear to be an irregular doughnut-shaped mark (Sperber, 1989). Bite marks can be measured to determine if they were inflicted by an adult or a child. If the distance between the canines

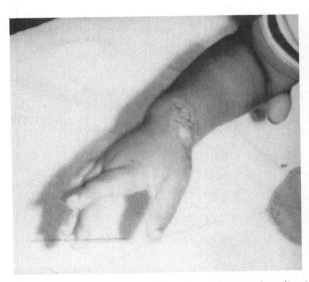

Figure 8–15. Isolated contact, nonaccidental injury with curling iron. Burn deep to back and side of wrist extending to palm. (Courtesy of Seth Asser, MD, University of California San Diego Medical Center)

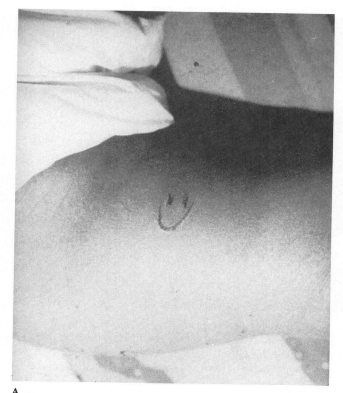

A

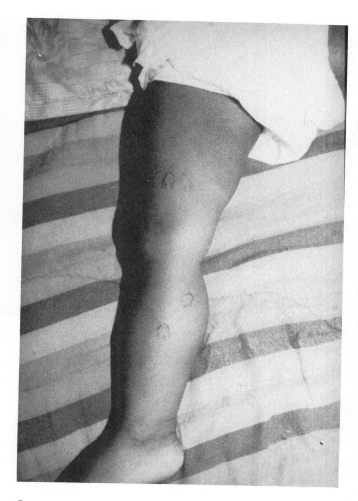

B

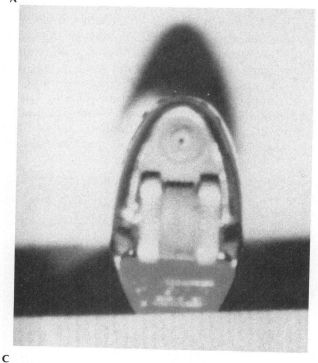

C

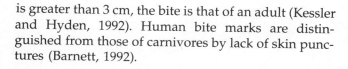

Figure 8–16. A. Nonaccidental burn of thigh with cigarette lighter. **B.** This infant had 19 of these burns. **C.** Cigarette lighter used to injure infant. (Courtesy of Seth Asser MD, University of California San Diego Medical Center)

is greater than 3 cm, the bite is that of an adult (Kessler and Hyden, 1992). Human bite marks are distinguished from those of carnivores by lack of skin punctures (Barnett, 1992).

Oral Trauma. Oral burns may occur from excessively hot food or fluids placed in the child's mouth. Injuries to the labial frenulum and lingual frenulum may be the result of a bottle's or a spoon's being forced into the child's mouth. Teeth may be loosened or knocked out from blunt trauma to the face. Oral lacerations also may occur from a direct blow to the face. Taking an

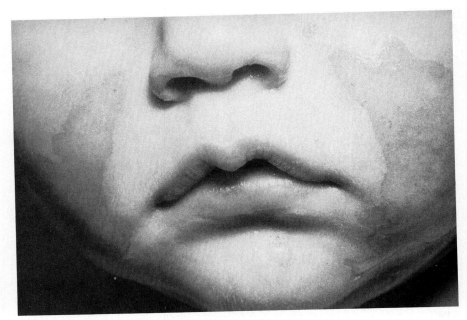

Figure 8–17. Burns to cheeks of 6-month-old infant from hair dryer. Burn inflicted by mother's boyfriend the first time he was left alone with the infant. (Courtesy of Seth Asser MD, University of California San Diego Medical Center)

accurate history is important as it may be the only way to determine if the trauma was accidentally or intentionally inflicted.

Traction Alopecia. Areas of baldness of the scalp may be the result of a child's being pulled by the hair, referred to as traction or traumatic alopecia. In such cases there are irregular areas of hair loss characterized by broken, uneven hair. Subgaleal hematomas also may result from the hair pulling.

Fractures. Although less common than other types of injuries related to abuse, fractures are present in 36% of abused children (Merten and Carpenter, 1990). Injuries to bones are more common in abused children

younger than 4 years, whereas accidental fractures occur more commonly among school-age children (Kessler and Hyden, 1991). Fractures and dislocations that are inconsistent with the history of the mechanism of the injury are highly suspect. In cases of inflicted injury, caretakers often delay seeking medical treatment; therefore, manifestations typically seen in the acute phase of skeletal injury, such as swelling and tenderness, may not be present.

Transverse fractures may occur as a result of inflicted, blunt trauma. Spiral fractures of long bones may be the result of an intentional twisting of the extremity; spiral fractures of the humerus are particularly suspicious. Fractures of the femur in children

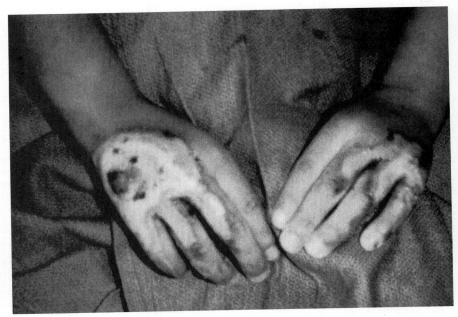

Figure 8–18. Old, scarred injury, after debridement. Note the bull's eye or target-like appearance from the child's hands being held over a candle. (Courtesy of Seth Asser MD, University of California San Diego Medical Center)

younger than 3 years are often a result of abuse (Barnett, 1992).

Rib fractures, common in abused children, are frequently multiple and bilateral, often reflecting a squeezing injury to the chest (Barnett, 1992). Multiple fractures in various stages of healing, especially involving the epiphyses and metaphyses, indicate repeated abuse. Fragmentation at the epiphysis may be the result of vigorous shaking of a young child. Fractures of the epiphyseal-metaphyseal junction are pathognomonic of abuse (Barnett, 1992). Fractures of the skull, nose, or facial structures are frequently the result of abuse.

The possibility that multiple fractures are related to an underlying disease, such as osteogenesis imperfecta, scurvy, syphilis, rickets, neoplasia, or osteomyelitis should be considered. The presence of these rare disorders can be ruled out by appropriate diagnostic procedures.

Head Injuries. Inflicted head injuries are the leading cause of deaths from child abuse. Inflicted head injuries may be the result of direct trauma, vigorous shaking, or a combination. Eighty percent of deaths from head trauma among children younger than 2 years are the result of nonaccidental trauma (Bruce and Zimmerman, 1989). The most common intracranial injuries are subdural and subarachnoid hemorrhage and retinal hemorrhage; skull fractures are present in about 50% of children with intracranial injuries resulting from abuse (Kessler and Hyden, 1991).

Subdural hematomas in children are often the result of abuse, such as direct trauma to the head from being struck, thrown, dropped, or shaken severely. Accidental falls from elevated surfaces usually result in single linear fractures of the skull, whereas nonaccidental trauma is more likely to cause multiple or complex fractures; depressed fractures; involvement of more than one cranial bone; nonparietal skull fractures; and associated intracranial injuries (Kessler and Hyden, 1991).

Shaken Baby Syndrome (Shaken Impact Syndrome). Some infants with intracranial injury have no external evidence of head trauma; these injuries are the result of acceleration-deceleration injuries from vigorous shaking, rather than of direct blows (Barnett, 1992). Such injuries are often termed shaken baby syndrome. The constellation of findings includes retinal hemorrhages; subdural or subarachnoid hemorrhages, or both; cerebral edema, contusion, and infarction; rib fractures; and multiple traction changes in the long bones of the limbs from violent shaking (Kessler and Hyden, 1991).

Controversy exists over whether shaking alone is sufficient to cause a serious head injury (Bruce and Zimmerman, 1989). Thus, the term *shaken impact syndrome* has been suggested as more accurate than *shaken*

baby syndrome. In one study of 24 infants initially receiving the diagnosis of shaken baby syndrome, half of the patients demonstrated signs of external head trauma (Alexander et al, 1990a). The mortality was not found to be statistically different between infants with evidence of direct trauma and those without such evidence. These findings suggest that shaking in and of itself is sufficient to cause serious intracranial injury or death. A substantial number of instances, however, represent a combination of shaking and impact injuries.

Presenting signs and symptoms of shaken baby and shaken impact syndrome include respiratory distress, irritability, lethargy, hypotonia, seizures, coma, vomiting, bradycardia, apnea, hypothermia, full or bulging fontanelle, and head circumference at or above the 90th percentile (Reece, 1992). Additional evidence of a shaking injury may be provided by grip marks on the upper arms (Figure 8–19) or shoulders. One study of 14 cases of shaken baby syndrome found a positive relationship between severity of retinal hemorrhage and acute neurologic findings (Wilkinson et al, 1989).

Ocular Injuries. Inflicted eye injuries may leave no external evidence of trauma. A funduscopic examination is, therefore, essential in suspected cases of child abuse. Eye injuries that can be the result of physical abuse include periorbital hematomas, fractures of the orbital or facial bones, subconjunctival hemorrhage, dislocated lens, retinal detachment, retinal hemorrhage, hyphema, corneal abrasion, and optic atrophy.

Ear Injuries. The external ear may show evidence of contusions. Ecchymoses on the internal surface of the pinna may be the result of boxing the ear and crushing it against the skull. A direct blow to the ear also may cause hemotympanum and perforation of the tympanic membrane. The presence of discoloration be-

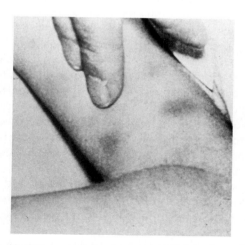

Figure 8–19. Grip marks on upper arm from infant's being held and shaken. (Courtesy of Barton Schmitt MD, The Children's Hospital, Denver)

hind the ear (Battle sign) may be a further indication of a basilar skull fracture.

Abdominal Trauma. Abdominal injuries related to child abuse, although infrequent, rank second only to head trauma as the leading cause of fatal child abuse. Blunt abdominal trauma, the most common type of inflicted abdominal trauma in children, is usually the result of a child's being punched or kicked in the abdomen. It may result in intra-abdominal hemorrhage with few external signs of trauma. The blow is usually to the midabdomen.

The child may present for treatment with persistent bilious vomiting, abdominal pain, or hypovolemic shock. Internal organs that may be injured by blunt trauma include the pancreas, duodenum, jejunum, mesentery, liver, spleen, and kidneys.

The high mortality resulting from these injuries may be due to exsanguinating intra-abdominal hemorrhage, a delay in seeking medical attention, or failure of emergency personnel to make the correct diagnosis when a life-saving operation is still possible. Severe internal injuries may not be immediately detected because of the parent's failure to give an accurate history of trauma and because there may be little or no external evidence of abdominal trauma at the time of examination.

Conditions that Mimic Child Abuse. Several conditions mimic child abuse. Mongolian spots—flat birth marks of varying sizes and shapes and are typically found on the lower back, buttocks, and shoulder—may be mistaken for inflicted contusions. Most Mongolian spots disappear by 3 years of age. They are present in 90% of black and Asian infants, 50% of Hispanic infants, and 10% of white infants (Kessler and Hyden, 1991).

Spontaneous bleeding into the skin and mucous membranes, resembling multiple bruises, can occur with idiopathic thrombocytopenic purpura, which often follows a viral illness (Kessler and Hyden, 1991). Bruising secondary to thrombocytopenia may be seen in children with neoplastic diseases such as leukemia or metastatic neuroblastoma and in adolescents with systemic lupus erythematosus or lymphoma (Kessler and Hyden, 1991).

Infected insect bites and impetigo often resemble cigarette burns. Impetigo is typically characterized by small, erythematous macules on the mouth, nose, and scalp that evolve into thin-walled, circular vesicular and pustular lesions that form honey-colored crusts when they rupture. Impetigo is highly contagious and spreads easily. Impetigo lesions, unlike cigarette burns, heal promptly without scarring when treated with antibiotics (Kessler and Hyden, 1991).

Several conditions that affect the skeletal system may be mistaken for intentional injury. These conditions include rickets, scurvy, osteomyelitis, congenital syphilis, infantile cortical hyperostosis, and osteogenesis imperfecta or brittle-bone disease (Kessler and Hyden, 1991).

Some folk medicine practices may be mistaken for child abuse. Cia Gao, or coin rubbing, is a folk remedy seen among Southeast Asians. It produces linear ecchymoses, usually on the back, when a coin heated in hot oil is rubbed over the body to treat fever, chills, and headaches (Kessler and Hyden, 1991). The Chinese practice of cupping, or applying a heated cup to the chest to treat congestion, may leave round burns.

Laboratory and Diagnostic Procedures
Radiologic Imaging. Computed tomography (CT) and magnetic resonance imaging (MRI) may be conducted in cases of suspected head injury. Body CT and ultrasonography may be performed in cases of suspected abdominal injury. X rays may reveal new and old fractures. Radionuclide skeletal scintigraphy (a bone scan) can reveal fractures and other skeletal injuries that are otherwise difficult to detect. A complete skeletal survey is usually indicated for all infants younger than 2 years who have clinical evidence of physical abuse and for infants younger than 1 year who are neglected (Merten and Carpenter, 1990).

Serologic Tests. Prothrombin time, PTT, and platelet counts can distinguish a child with a bleeding disorder who bruises easily from one who has been abused.

A toxicology screen should be obtained in all cases of suspected poisoning and MSBP.

Creatine phosphokinase (CPK) levels can identify muscle injuries. A complete blood count and amylase, lipase, serum glutamic-oxaloacetic transaminase (SGOT), and serum glutamic pyruvate transaminase (SGPT) levels should be obtained in cases of suspected inflicted abdominal trauma.

T R I A G E
Child Abuse and Neglect

Emergent
Any child with a life-threatening injury; decreased level of consciousness; unstable vital signs; impaired airway, breathing, or circulation.

Urgent
Child who has suspicious burns, bruises, skeletal injury; family in crisis; uncooperative or unreliable caretaker who might leave ED before discharge.

Non-urgent
Child with chronic neglect; reliable and cooperative caretaker.

Nursing Diagnosis
Altered Parenting

Defining Characteristics

- Inattentive to child's needs
- Negative identification with child's needs
- Evidence of physical and psychologic trauma to child
- Inappropriate discipline practices

Nursing Interventions

- Use empathetic approach
- Acknowledge the demands of parenting
- Discuss alternatives to use of corporal punishment

Expected Outcomes

- Parent verbalizes frustrations regarding parenting
- Parent verbalizes alternatives for discipline

Nursing Diagnosis
Ineffective Individual Coping (Parent)

Defining Characteristics

- Verbalization of inability to cope
- Anxiety, fear, anger, irritability

Nursing Interventions

- Assist parent in identifying social supports
- Refer parent to parenting group

Expected Outcomes

- Parent identifies social supports available to the family
- Parent verbalizes willingness to attend parent support group

Nursing Diagnosis
Altered Growth and Development

Defining Characteristics

- Delay in meeting developmental milestones
- Weight and height below normal

Nursing Interventions

- Refer child for early intervention program
- Discuss strategies for promoting growth and development

Expected Outcomes

- Parent agrees to seek services for child
- Parent verbalizes strategies for promoting child's growth and development

MANAGEMENT

It is common for health care professionals in encounters with an abused or neglected child to have feelings of sympathy for the child and anger toward the abusive caretaker. When encountering an abusive parent it is important to be understanding and empathetic. It is always counterproductive to display anger. Likewise, one should never act disapprovingly of a parent in front of an abused child.

Every effort must be made not to overidentify with a child. An abused child can be helped only through services for the entire family. It is unrealistic to believe that every child who comes from a suboptimal home environment should be removed from the parents. In many cases this would be a great disservice to the child, who usually loves the parent despite the maltreatment.

A multidisciplinary approach to child abuse involving nurses, physicians, and social workers is advantageous for several reasons. First, consultation with other health care professionals in the ED is helpful in validating suspicions of child abuse and neglect. Because intentional and unintentional injuries are difficult to differentiate, several clinical opinions are useful in collecting and interpreting data. It is important to have more than one professional interview the child and parents, so that each history obtained can be carefully compared for any inconsistencies. A child protection, multidisciplinary team approach is also useful so that members can share their thoughts and feelings and provide support to each other. It is important to establish an ED protocol that clearly outlines the management of child abuse and the responsibilities of each member of the child protection team. The demands of managing child abuse are lessened when the responsibilities· are shared with other health care professionals. Conferences that include all involved members of the ED staff should be held after difficult child abuse cases are seen. This serves as an opportunity for staff to express their feelings of anger and disbelief.

Documentation
Careful documentation in all cases of suspected abuse and neglect is of the utmost importance. It is not enough to write "multiple bruises in various stages of healing noted." Rather, each bruise, lesion, or burn needs to be described in detail according to size, location, color, and shape. Color photographs should be taken with a 35-mm camera and an instant camera whenever possible. In some jurisdictions parental permission to take a child's photograph is needed, whereas

in others photographs can be taken without parental consent.

Even the most severely abused children are often physically healed at the time of a court hearing. The photographs help the judge or jury understand the extent of injury. All significant statements by parents and children should be carefully recorded with as many direct quotes as possible. The behavior of the child and parents should be described carefully. Medical records, including the nurse's notes, are often subpoenaed and introduced as evidence. The nurse, therefore, has an important responsibility to carefully report all of the facts while never providing subjective opinion.

Disposition

The disposition of the child from the ED depends on many variables. One must look at the severity of the presenting injury and under what circumstances it occurred. The most important single factor to assess is whether the child is at immediate risk for further abuse if returned home from the ED. If it is perceived that the child will be at risk upon returning home, the child may be temporarily removed from the home through (1) admission to the hospital; (2) placement in the home of a relative such as a grandparent or aunt; or (3) placement in an emergency foster home. Often temporary removal from the home allows time for the parent to receive necessary support services.

All states provide a mechanism to protect children in emergencies (Myers, 1992). If a parent refuses to allow a child to be admitted to the hospital or to be placed with a relative or in foster care, an emergency care and protection order can be obtained from a judge over the telephone in most jurisdictions. This gives the hospital authority to temporarily remove the child from the home pending a further investigation into the child's safety; it also allows time for arrangement of support services for the family.

Reporting Suspected Child Abuse and Neglect

Child abuse legislation in each of the 50 states mandates the reporting of suspected child abuse and neglect by professionals who work with children. The list of mandated reporters includes educators, physicians, nurses, mental health professionals, social workers, and day care providers. In most states, mandated reporters have no discretion as to whether or not to report cases of suspected abuse or neglect (Myers, 1992).

The conditions for reporting, who the mandated reporters are, to which agency one reports, and protection for those who report in good faith are all defined by individual state statutes. In most states, nurses are identified as mandated reporters. It is important to be knowledgeable of child abuse laws in the jurisdiction

in which one practices. The statutes of many states include penalties for those who fail to report suspected abuse and neglect. Those who report in good faith are usually immune from criminal and civil liability.

It is important to understand that only a suspicion of abuse or neglect is necessary for reporting a case; actual proof or evidence is not required by law. According to Myers (1992), reporting is mandatory when a professional has evidence that would lead a competent professional to believe abuse or neglect is reasonably likely. A professional who postpones reporting until all doubt has been eliminated probably violates the reporting law (Myers, 1992). The ultimate decision about whether abuse or neglect occurred is the responsibility of investigating officials, not mandated reporters (Myers, 1992).

Reporting of suspected abuse should never be viewed as an accusation or punitive action but rather as a referral for further investigation into the child's environment and well-being and a referral for social services for the family. Reporting should never be used as a threat to force cooperation, nor should parents ever be told they will be given a second chance and that no report will be filed. If a report is not made immediately after suspicion has been raised, there may be subsequent injury to the child and a delay in services for the family. Also, if a health care professional had reason to suspect child abuse and failed to report it and the child was reinjured, the health care provider could be held liable for those injuries. (See Chapter 6 for further information on the legal responsibilities of nurses in cases of suspected abuse.)

Nurses should always inform the parents that a report is being made and should explain the purpose of the report. Parents need to know that the report is not a criminal complaint but rather a referral for services. They should also be told to expect a telephone call or home visit from a caseworker from the CPS agency as a follow-up to the report. Table 8–10 summarizes the ED nurse's responsibilities in cases of child abuse.

TABLE 8–10. RESPONSIBILITIES OF THE EMERGENCY NURSE IN CHILD ABUSE

Knowledge of indicators of child abuse and neglect
Case identification
Obtaining careful history and comparing it with existing injury
Observation of interactions between parent and child
Collaboration with other members of the health care team
Careful documentation of all objective data
Reporting of all suspected cases of abuse and neglect to child protective services
Assessment of immediate risk to child if returned home
Protection from subsequent abuse through hospitalization or foster placement
Referral to services for family
Emotional support to child and parents

REFERENCES

Alexander R (1992). Failure to thrive. *The Advisor* 5:11–13

Alexander R, Sato Y, Smith W, Bennett T (1990a). Incidence of impact trauma with cranial injuries ascribed to shaking. *American Journal of Diseases of Children* 144:724–726

Alexander R, Smith W, Stevenson R (1990b). Serial Münchhausen syndrome by proxy. *Pediatrics* 86:581–585

American Association for Protecting Children (AAPC) (1988). Highlights of official child neglect and abuse reporting. Denver: American Humane Association

Barnett TM (1992). Abuse and neglect. In Barkin RM (ed), *Pediatric emergency medicine.* St. Louis: Mosby, pp 537–555

Belsky J (1980). Child maltreatment: An ecological integration. *American Psychologist* 35:320–335

Bruce DE, Zimmerman RA (1989). Shaken impact syndrome. *Pediatric Annals* 18:482–494

Burke A, Crenshaw D, Green J, Schlosser M, Strocchia-Rivera L (1989). Influence of verbal ability on the expression of aggression in physically abused children. *Journal of the American Academy of Child and Adolescent Psychiatry* 28:215–218

Centers for Disease Control (1990). Childhood injuries in the United States. *American Journal of Diseases in Children* 144:627–646

Christoffel KK (1990). Violent death and injury in U.S. children and adolescents. *American Journal of Diseases in Children* 144:697–706

Christoffel KK (1992). Child abuse fatalities. In Ludwig S, Kornberg AE (eds), *Child abuse: A medical reference.* New York: Churchill Livingstone, pp 49–59

Claussen AH, Crittenden PM (1991). Physical and psychological maltreatment: Relations among types of maltreatment. *Child Abuse and Neglect: The International Journal* 15:5–18

Crittenden PM, Craig SE (1990). Developmental trends in the nature of child homicide. *Journal of Interpersonal Violence* 5:202–216

Daro D, McCurdy K (1992). Current trends in child abuse reporting and fatalities: The results of the 1991 annual fifty-state survey. Chicago: National Committee for Prevention of Child Abuse

Dodge KA, Bates JE, Pettit GS (1990). Mechanisms in the cycle of violence. *Science* 250:1678–1683

Durfee MJ, Gellert GA, Tilton-Durfee D (1992). Origins and clinical relevance of child death review teams. *Journal of American Medical Association* 267:3172–3175

Famularo R, Kinscherff R, Fenton T (1990). Symptom differences in acute and chronic presentation of childhood post-traumatic stress disorder. *Child Abuse and Neglect: The International Journal* 14:439–444

Johnson CF (1990). Inflicted injury versus accidental injury. *Pediatric Clinics of North America* 37:791–814

Kelley SJ (1989). Stress responses of children to sexual abuse and ritualistic abuse in day care centers. *Journal of Interpersonal Violence* 4:502–513

Kelley SJ (1988). Physical abuse of children: Recognition and reporting. *Journal of Emergency Nursing* 14:82–90

Kelley SJ (1992). Child maltreatment, stressful life events, and behavior problems in school-aged children in residential treatment. *Journal of Child and Adolescent Psychiatric and Mental Health Nursing* 5:5–13

Kelley SJ, Walsh JH, Thompson K (1991). Prenatal exposure to cocaine: Birth outcomes, health problems, and child neglect. *Pediatric Nursing* 17:130–135

Kempe CH, Silverman FN, Steel BF et al (1962). The battered child syndrome. *Journal of the American Medical Association.* 181:17–24

Kessler DB, Hyden P (1991). Physical, sexual, and emotional abuse of children. *Clinical Symposia* 43:2–32

Kolko D, Moser J, Weldy S (1988). Behavioral and emotional indicators of sexual abuse in child psychiatric in-patients: A controlled comparison with physical abuse. *Child Abuse and Neglect: The International Journal* 12:529–541

Korbin J (1989). Fatal maltreatment by mothers: A proposed framework. *Child Abuse and Neglect: The International Journal* 13:481–489

Ludwig S (1992). Failure-to-thrive/starvation. In Ludwig S, Kornberg AE (eds), *Child abuse: A medical reference.* New York: Churchill Livingstone, pp 303–319

Merten DF, Carpenter BL (1990). Radiologic imaging of inflicted injury in the child abuse syndrome. *Pediatric Clinics of North America* 37:815–837

Milner JS, Chilamkurti C (1991). Physical child abuse perpetrator characteristics. *Journal of Interpersonal Violence* 6:345–366

Myers JEB (1992). *Legal issues in child abuse and neglect practice.* Newbury Park, Calif: Sage, pp 100–105

Purdue GF, Hunt JL (1992). Burn injuries. In Ludwig S, Kornberg AE (eds), *Child abuse: A medical reference.* New York: Churchill Livingstone, pp 105–116

Reece RM (1992). Child abuse. In Reece RM (ed), *Manual of emergency pediatrics.* Philadelphia: Saunders, pp 129–134

Rosenberg DA (1987). Web of deceit: A literature review of Münchhausen syndrome by proxy. *Child Abuse and Neglect: The International Journal* 11:547–563

Sperber ND (1989). Bite marks, oral and facial injuries: Harbingers of severe child abuse? *Pediatrician* 16:207–211

Wilkinson WS, Han DP, Rappley MD, Owings CL (1989). Retinal hemorrhage predicts neurologic injury in the shaken baby syndrome. *Archives of Ophthalmology* 107:1472–1474

Zuravin SJ (1989). The ecology of child abuse and neglect: Review of the literature and presentation of data. *Violence and Victims* 4:101–120

CHAPTER 9

Sexual Abuse

SUSAN J. KELLEY

INTRODUCTION

Because of the high rate of sexual victimization of children in our society, emergency nurses frequently encounter sexually abused children. Few clinical encounters for emergency nurses carry the intense legal, social, and professional implications of contact with a sexually abused child. The physical, emotional, and behavioral stress placed on the child as the result of sexual abuse can be overwhelming. Despite the increased awareness that sexual abuse is a serious health problem, emergency care professionals often feel inadequately prepared to deal comfortably and effectively with a case of suspected sexual abuse. The psychological trauma a child suffers can be alleviated by informed, sensitive, and appropriate intervention on the part of the nurse involved. It is, therefore, essential that emergency nurses be adequately prepared to assess and intervene in cases of suspected sexual abuse.

DEFINITION

The legal definition of sexual abuse varies by state. In general, most state statutes define sexual abuse as any sexual contact or sexual activity between a child and an adult, whether by force or coercion, because children are legally and developmentally incapable of informed consent when it comes to sexual activity with an adult. Children are unaware of the moral, legal, emotional, and physical implications of sexual activity with an adult or considerably older child. Most children are bribed, threatened, coerced, or tricked into the sexual activity.

TYPES

Sexual abuse includes a wide range of behaviors, including exhibitionism; fondling or manipulation of the genitals; digital penetration; orogenital contact; vaginal or rectal penile penetration; insertion of foreign objects in the genitals, penis, or rectum; and use of children in pornography or prostitution. Sexual abuse also includes noncontact sexual activity such as sexually explicit language directed toward the child; obscene telephone calls; showing the child pornographic materials; and voyeurism. Most children who are sexually abused experience multiple types of several of these sexually abusive acts. Table 9–1 provides a summary of types of child sexual abuse.

The nature of the sexual activity is important to understand. Typically, sexual activity between the adult and child involves a steady progression or escalation in the severity of the sexual acts committed. Often, the sexual activity is initially presented to the child as a "game," "secret," or "something special."

TABLE 9–1. TYPES OF SEXUAL ABUSE OF CHILDREN

Exhibitionism
Voyeurism
Fondling of breasts, vagina, buttocks, penis
Digital penetration of vagina or rectum
Orogenital contact
Vaginal penile contact
Vaginal penile penetration
Rectal penile penetration
Insertion of foreign object into vagina, rectum, or urethra
Pornography
Prostitution

The sexual abuse may begin with the offender exposing him- or herself to the child or viewing the child naked. The activity may then involve masturbation by the offender in front of the child and then encouraging the child to imitate this behavior. Very often, the activity progresses to fondling, digital penetration of the vagina or rectum, and orogenital contact. Finally, the activity may involve vaginal or rectal intercourse. In some cases the offender does not attempt vaginal intercourse but instead simulates intercourse by rubbing his penis against the genitorectal region of the child.

OFFENDERS

Most adults who sexually abuse children are relatives, friends of the family, or other trusted adults who are well known to the child victims. According to Faller (1990), there are two prerequisites for sexual abuse—sexual arousal to children and the willingness to act on the arousal. Although most reported cases of childhood sexual abuse involve male offenders, women are perpetrators approximately 10% of the time. Many offenders commit their first offenses during adolescence.

PREVALENCE AND RISK FACTORS

Research findings indicate that sexual abuse of children occurs quite commonly in our society. In a large, nationally representative survey of 2,626 American adults, a childhood history of sexual abuse was disclosed by 27% of women and 16% of men (Finkelhor et al, 1990).

The following are considered risk factors for sexual abuse: presence of a stepfather; children who are living without one or both of their biologic parents; a mother who is disabled, ill, or extensively out of the home; poor parenting; and paternal violence (Finkelhor, 1993). It is important to note that race, social class, and ethnicity have not been found to be risk factors for child sexual abuse (Finkelhor, 1993).

IMPACT OF SEXUAL ABUSE

Although research has empirically validated the negative impact of child sexual abuse, the degree of impact varies. The initial and short-term sequelae of child sexual abuse include increased behavioral problems (Kelley, 1989; Kelley, 1992; Waterman, et al, 1993); anxiety and depression (Kelley, 1989; Kelley, 1992; Waterman et al, 1993); increased fears (Kelley, 1989; Waterman et al, 1993); and increased exhibition of sexualized behaviors (Friedrich, 1993; Friedrich et al, 1992; Kelley, 1989).

Factors associated with increased impact during childhood include frequency and duration of the abuse; use of physical force; sexual acts involving penetration; and abuse by a biologic father or a stepfather (Beitchman et al, 1991). Family belief of the child's disclosure and family support of the child mitigate the immediate negative impact of abuse (Berliner, 1991).

Sexual abuse is also associated with long-term sequelae. Adult women who report histories of child sexual abuse are at increased risk for sexual disturbances, homosexual experiences, anxiety and fear, depression, suicidal ideation and behavior, and revictimizing experiences (Beitchman et al, 1992). Male victims of childhood sexual abuse are at increased risk for disturbances in adult sexual functioning (Beitchman et al, 1992).

Factors associated with increased long-term impact include long duration of abuse; use of physical force or threat of force; abuse involving penetration; and abuse involving a father or stepfather (Beitchman et al, 1992).

ASSESSMENT

History

A sexually abused child may come to the emergency department (ED) for a variety of reasons. Some children have a chief complaint of sexual abuse or assault. These children have previously disclosed sexual abuse and may be accompanied by a parent, caretaker, police officer, or child protective worker. Another common type of presentation involves children with physical indicators of sexual abuse, such as trauma to the genitals or rectum or symptoms of a sexually transmitted disease, but who have not previously disclosed sexual abuse. Other sexually abused children may present with nonspecific complaints such as headache or abdominal pain, vaginal itching, or behavioral changes.

A careful, detailed history is critical in cases of suspected sexual abuse. Obtaining separate histories from the child and parents is preferable for several reasons. First, many children are hesitant to disclose abuse in the presence of a parent or other caregiver, especially if the offender is a family member or friend of the family. Some children are threatened by their parent or caretaker not to disclose the abuse or to identify the abuser. It is not uncommon for all involved to attempt to protect the identity of the offender. Some children are hesitant to disclose the abuse because they believe their parents will be angry at them and blame them for the abuse. This fear is often induced by the offender's telling the child that the child will be punished or not believed if he or she ever discloses the abuse. Other children are simply too embarrassed to disclose the abuse with a parent present.

Another reason for interviewing children and parents separately is that parents need an opportunity to express their feelings related to the suspected abuse, which may include shock, disbelief, and anger, as well as any other concerns they may have without the child present. The intense emotional reactions of parents at the time of disclosure can be frightening to the child. Unfortunately, children often view themselves as willing participants in the sexual abuse; they fear that their parents will be angry with them and hold them responsible. Often children misinterpret parental displays of anger and erroneously believe that the anger is directed toward them, which in turn compounds the fear and guilt children may already be experiencing. Even when children and parents are not trying to protect an offender, children are often embarrassed to describe the details of the sexual activity with parents present.

Interview of Parents and Caretakers

The information needed from parents or caretakers includes, when appropriate, why they believe their child has been abused and who they suspect abused their child. If the parent does not know who may have abused the child they should be asked who has access to the child, such as a babysitter, day care worker, teacher, or relatives. Parents may be hesitant to reveal their suspicions or to identify the offender, especially if the offender is a family member or friend. Parents should be carefully questioned regarding any previous family history of sexual victimization. It is not unusual for more than one child in a nuclear or extended family to be victimized by the same offender or for a child to be abused by multiple relatives. The possibility of multigenerational sexual abuse should be explored, especially if the offender is a grandparent.

Physical and behavioral indicators of child sexual abuse should be elicited in the history obtained from the parent or caretaker. Physical symptoms of possible sexual abuse of girls include vaginal discharge, bleeding, trauma or irritation; rectal lacerations or bleeding; foreign bodies in the vagina or rectum; and dysuria. Pregnancy in a young adolescent (10–14 years of age) should raise concern, especially if the adolescent attempts to conceal the pregnancy for an extended period of time. The issue of paternity should be pursued in such cases to determine if an adult or older adolescent had forced or coerced the adolescent into the sexual activity that resulted in the pregnancy.

Physical indicators of sexual abuse in boys include dysuria, penile discharge, foreign bodies in the urethra or rectum, rectal bleeding or laceration, or trauma to the penis or testicles. Table 9–2 summarizes physical indicators of sexual abuse.

TABLE 9–2. PHYSICAL INDICATORS OF CHILD SEXUAL ABUSE

Trauma to the genitals or rectum
Chafing, abrasions or bruising of the inner thighs
Scarring or tears of the hymen
Decreased amount of hymenal tissue
Vaginal or rectal bleeding
Vaginal, penile, or rectal lacerations
Vaginal or penile discharge
Foreign bodies in the urethra, vagina, or rectum
Pregnancy, especially in young adolescents
Complaint of vaginal or rectal pain
Presence of sexually transmitted disease
   Chlamydia
   Gonorrhea
   Syphilis
   Herpes genitalis
   Condyloma acuminata (anogenital warts)
   Trichomonas vaginalis

Behavioral changes are more common than physical complaints in child sexual abuse. Therefore, a careful history for behaviors that could be associated with sexual abuse should be elicited. Sexually abused children often act out sexually with peers, siblings, and adults. Sexual behaviors that are seen more often in sexually abused children than in nonsexually abused children include placing the mouth on another child's genitals; asking others to engage in sexual acts; masturbating with objects; inserting foreign objects in their vaginas or rectums; imitating intercourse; and making sexual sounds (Friedrich et al, 1992). Sexually abused children often make precocious remarks or ask questions that indicate their increased awareness of adult sexual behavior. There also may be a history of frequent and compulsive masturbation.

Any history of regressive behavior should be noted. Other behavior problems consistent with sexual abuse include extreme fears; becoming hysterical or uncooperative during physical examination of the genitals; refusing to sleep alone; and locking or barricading the bedroom door to prevent the offender from entering the bedroom. Sexually abused children may become obsessed with cleanliness, demonstrated by their taking excessive numbers of baths to conceal blood or secretions related to the abuse or to alleviate "feeling dirty." Table 9–3 summarizes behaviors often observed in sexually abused children. It is important to note that presence of one or more of these behaviors does not necessarily mean a child has been sexually abused, but they should be used in conjunction with other data.

Interview of Child

An interview of a sexually abused child has several important objectives. First, it is important to determine if there is reason to believe that the child has been

TABLE 9–3. BEHAVIORS SUGGESTIVE OF SEXUAL ABUSE

Sexual acting out with siblings, peers, or adults
Preoccupation with sexual matters
Precocious knowledge of adult sexual behavior
Excessive masturbation
Masturbation with objects
Aggressive or hostile behavior
Regressive behavior
Enuresis
Encopresis
Sleep disorders such as night terrors or nightmares
Refusal to sleep alone at night
Excessive fears, phobias
Eating disorders such as overeating or loss of appetite
Depression
Suicidal or self-destructive behavior
Substance abuse
Running away
Unusual behavior during examination of genitalia

sexually abused in order to provide appropriate nursing, medical, legal, and psychological intervention. The second objective is to protect the child from subsequent abuse by determining whether or not the child is at risk for further abuse or retaliation if returned home upon discharge from the ED.

Need for an Interview. Several circumstances determine if the child needs to be interviewed by the ED nurse. If the child is accompanied by child protective services (CPS) or law enforcement personnel, has already disclosed sexual abuse, and is being seen primarily for medical evaluation and evidence collection, a subsequent interview by an ED staff member may be unnecessary and detrimental to the child. It may also be unnecessary for an ED staff member to interview the child if sexual abuse specialists are available to come to the ED to conduct the interview. Some hospitals employ sexual assault nurse examiners (SANE), who are specially trained and on call to conduct interviews, examine victims, collect evidence, provide counseling, follow up on cases, and testify in court (Lenehan, 1991). Nurse examiners provide the much needed continuity and support that is often lacking as abused children and their families deal with the complexities of the health care, child protective, and legal systems.

Guidelines for the Interview. It is important to keep the number of people who interview the child to a minimum because child victims can be further traumatized by repeated interviews. The staff member with the most expertise should interview the child. That person can then share the information obtained during the interview with other ED staff as needed. Some hospitals have a sexual abuse team on call to interview children believed to be sexually abused.

Children should be interviewed before the physical examination when sexual abuse is suspected. The physical examination may be stressful for a child, and as a result the child becomes reluctant to disclose the abuse.

The importance of objectivity during the interview cannot be overemphasized. The interview should begin with general questions and proceed to more specific questions as details of the abuse are described. Open-ended questions are preferred to closed-ended questions. An open-ended question invites a child to discuss whatever the child wants to discuss about a subject (Myers, 1992). Examples of open-ended questions include "Did anything happen to you?" and "Do you know why you are here today?" It is crucial to avoid asking leading questions. A leading question is one that contains a suggestion of what the answer should be (Myers, 1992). An example of a leading question is "Your father hurt your private part, didn't he?" Faller (1990) identified five types of questions used in sexual abuse interviews: general questions; focused questions; multiple-choice questions; yes-or-no questions; and leading questions. Table 9–4 illustrates how these types of questions exist on a continuum and gives examples of each type of question.

A rapport with the child should be established before the child is separated from the parent. At first the child may be reluctant to separate from the parent or caretaker and needs reassurance. The child should then be brought to a quiet, private room for the interview.

Putting the Child at Ease. The first step in the interview is establishing a trusting relationship with the child by conveying interest, sincerity, and respect. This can be accomplished by explaining one's role as a nurse and initially discussing topics that are nonthreatening to the child such as school, friends, sports, and favorite television programs. Next, the child's understanding of why he or she is in the ED should be determined. This may provide insight into the child's perception of the situation. Often children do not understand that they are at the hospital because of the abuse.

Any fears the child is experiencing should be determined early on. The child may describe fear of retribution by the offender for disclosing the abuse; loss of offender's approval; disapproval from family members; and being placed in a foster home. Often the child believes that he or she is responsible for the abuse and fears being punished. Determining the child's fears and concerns early on in the interview provides the nurse an opportunity to reassure the child that he or she has done nothing wrong and will be supported.

The child should be asked if he or she has any requests. The child may ask the interviewer to prom-

TABLE 9–4. A CONTINUUM OF TYPES OF QUESTIONS USED IN INTERVIEWING CHILDREN ALLEGED TO HAVE BEEN SEXUALLY ABUSED AND CONFIDENCE IN RESPONSES (by Kathleen Coulborn Faller)

Question Type		Example	Child Response	
Open-ended	General	How are you?	Sad, 'cause my dad poked me in the pee-pee	More confidence
	Focused	How do you get along with your dad?	OK, except when he pokes me in the pee-pee	
	Multiple choice	Did anything happen to your pee-pee?	My daddy poked me there	
		What did he poke you with?	He poked me with his ding-dong	
		Did he poke you with his finger, his ding-dong, or something else?	He used his ding-dong	
		Did this happen in the daytime or nighttime?	In the day and night	
	Yes-or-no questions	Did he tell you not to tell?	No, he didn't say anything like that	
		Did you have your clothes off?	No, just my panties	
Closed-ended	Leading questions	He took your clothes, didn't he?	Yes	
		Didn't he make you suck his penis?	Yes	Less confidence

(Reprinted with permission from Faller KC. The Advisor, Vol. 3, No. 2 (Spring 1990). The Advisor is a quarterly publication of the American Professional Society on the Abuse of Children, Chicago, Illinois)

ise not to share the information obtained during the interview with parents and others. Such promises should never be made. Rather, the interviewer explains to the child that to help the child the interviewer needs to share information with others.

Type of Information Obtained. Once the child appears comfortable, the interviewer attempts to obtain general information regarding the abuse and then elicits specific details. It is important to avoid asking the child too many questions and to let the child tell the story at his or her own pace. The interviewer's vocabulary should be kept simple and concise. The child's limited vocabulary often interferes with the interviewer's ability to communicate and gather important information. For example, it is necessary to identify terms the child uses to describe the genitals and other private parts of the body, such as breasts, penis, rectum, and vagina. Children often have pet names for their genitals such as pee-pee, bum, hot cakes, and couchie. In most instances, parents can provide this information before the interview. If parents are not able to provide this information, anatomic drawings or anatomically detailed dolls can be used to obtain this information. (Use of anatomically detailed dolls and anatomic drawings is discussed in further detail in the section on age-appropriate media). Once the interviewer has determined the child's terms for the various body parts, the interviewer should use these terms; the time of crisis is not the appropriate time to teach a child the proper terms of anatomy.

Information obtained from the child should include the name of the offender; the types of sexual acts committed; the number of incidents; the time and location of the abuse; and the use of any violence, force, threats, or bribes. Children should be asked if they have any secrets or play any special games. Often the sexual abuse has been presented to the child as something fun or special. The use of threats should be noted. Typical threats made to child victims include "If you tell anyone, I won't love you any more" or "I'll kill your parents if you tell anyone about our secret." Such threats are very real to children and serve as a tremendous source of fear and pressure not to disclose the abuse. Threats and other pressures to keep the activity a secret are often as emotionally traumatizing as the sexual acts themselves.

Because of the extent of exploitation of children in pornography and sex rings, child victims should be asked if any photographs or videos were taken of the sexual activity. The child should also be asked if they were ever shown any adult or child pornography by the perpetrator. Offenders often show children sexually explicit material in an attempt to desensitize the child to sexual activity. The involvement of multiple victims or multiple offenders should be explored. Often, in intrafamilial abuse, the child knows of other siblings or cousins involved. In extrafamilial abuse, the child may know of other children or perpetrators involved in the sexual activity.

Careful documentation of the content of the interview is crucial; as many direct quotes from the child as possible should be used. All information obtained should be clarified with the child.

Sexual abuse cases are extremely stressful for all professionals involved. Although it is difficult, the interviewer must avoid indicating his or her own negative feelings during the interview because children incorporate the reactions of adults into their own thoughts and feelings. Because the disclosure of the sexual abuse is disturbing to the interviewer, the interviewer should be aware of any negative facial expressions, body language, or verbal responses. Remarks such as "you poor thing" or "what he did to you was terrible" only intensify the child's anxiety. At the same time, however, the interviewer should clearly communicate to the child that the sexual abuse is not acceptable through such statements as "What he did to you was wrong" or "Adults are not supposed to do that with children." Most important, children need constant reassurance that they have done nothing wrong and that the offender is totally responsible for the abuse.

Use of Age-Appropriate Media
Because of their lack of a sophisticated adult vocabulary, as well as fear and embarrassment, sexually abused children often have great difficulty describing the abuse. Questions can stimulate many emotions and trigger an inability to respond verbally, which can cause additional assessment and treatment problems. Sexually abused children, therefore, need age-appropriate ways to express their fears, anger, and other feelings surrounding the abuse (Burgess and Hartman, 1993; Kelley, 1984; Kelley, 1985). Communication can be facilitated through the use of anatomically detailed dolls, anatomic drawings, and drawings by the child.

Anatomically Detailed Dolls. Anatomically detailed dolls, such as those in Figure 9–1, are valuable tools for interviewing sexually abused children. In addition to the usual body parts of dolls, anatomically detailed dolls include genitals, rectal openings, and breasts. A complete set that includes a man, a woman, a girl, and a boy should be available.

In the ED, there are three major purposes for using anatomically detailed dolls: (1) to facilitate verbal communication; (2) to help the child identify body parts; and (3) to confirm the nurse's understanding of the child's verbal descriptions of events. It is important to understand that anatomically detailed dolls are not a test of whether abuse has occurred and that a decision about sexual abuse cannot be based solely on a child's interaction with the dolls (Myers, 1992). Rather the dolls are used to facilitate communication with the child.

Use of anatomically detailed dolls should be postponed until a child has had a full opportunity to describe the events. Myers (1992) recommends that if a child has provided a detailed verbal description of abuse, it may be wise for the interviewer to avoid using dolls, so that at a later time, a defense attorney cannot argue the use of the dolls influenced the child's disclosure.

Before the dolls are introduced, the interviewer should explain that "These are special dolls that have all of the body parts, just like real people." The dolls should be introduced fully dressed. The child is allowed to choose the dolls the child wants to use during the interview. The dolls may be used to assess the child's knowledge of body parts and functions. As the

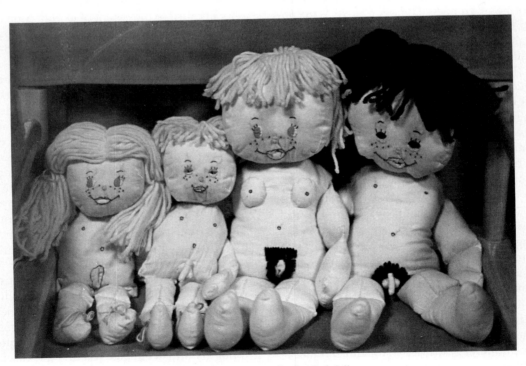

Figure 9–1. Anatomically detailed dolls.

interviewer points at first to nonsexual body parts followed by the genitals, breasts, and buttocks, the child is asked to name them. As stated earlier, this process helps identify which terms the child uses for the genitalia. Carefully observe how the child plays with the dolls and reacts to the genitals.

The interviewer should ask open-ended, non-leading questions. If the child demonstrates sexualized behaviors with the dolls, ask "What are the dolls doing?" and "Who are they?" If the child has previously verbalized sexual abuse, but the nurse wants to confirm his or her understanding of the child's statement, the child can be asked, "You already told me what happened to you. Now, do you think you can show me with the dolls what happened?" Sexually abused children are often quite graphic in demonstrating with the dolls the sexual acts performed. They often demonstrate intercourse, digital penetration, and orogenital activity with the dolls. All behaviors should be carefully observed and described in detail in the hospital record. This includes the child's positioning of the dolls and any verbal, nonverbal, or affective responses, such as crying, anxiety, fear, anger, or regression (Myers, 1992).

Anatomic Drawings. Anatomic drawings are another means of facilitating communication with sexually abused children. Anatomic drawings are simple line illustrations of male and female preschool, school-aged, adolescent, and adult figures. After they are explained to the child, the child is asked to name the body parts. If the child verbalizes sexual touching by an adult, the child can be asked to place an X on the areas where the child was touched by the offender. The adult illustrations can be used in a similar way for the child to indicate where he or she was made to touch or view the offender. Each anatomic drawing should be carefully labeled with the child's name, patient number, and interviewer and entered into the medical record. All statements made should be carefully recorded verbatim.

Drawings by the Child. Communicating through drawings is an effective and nonthreatening mode of communication for sexually abused children (Burgess and Hartman, 1993; Kelley, 1984; Kelley, 1985). Other advantages include the fact that most children enjoy drawing pictures and that the materials needed are inexpensive and easily accessible. In addition to whatever pictures the child may draw spontaneously, the child should be encouraged to draw a self-portrait, a portrait of the offender, a family portrait, and a picture of what happened in relation to the abuse. In addition to facilitating oral disclosure of abuse, the impact of the abuse is often reflected in the children's drawings.

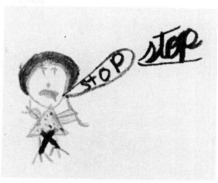

Figure 9–2. Self-portrait drawn by a 7-year-old girl who was being sexually abused by her stepfather. Of special significance is the sign she is holding that says "STOP" and the large "X" she has placed over her genital region. (Reproduced with permission from Kelley SJ [1985]. Interviewing the sexually abused child: Principles and techniques. *Journal of Emergency Nursing* 11:234–241)

Self-portraits drawn by sexually abused children often contain genitalia, reflecting their increased awareness of and concern and anxiety about these body parts. Sexually abused children may draw themselves with hands missing, reflecting feelings of helplessness. Self-portraits also may reflect low self-esteem, poor body image, and gender identity confusion (Kelley, 1984; Kelley, 1985). Figures 9–2, 9–3, and 9–4 are examples of self-portraits drawn by sexually abused children.

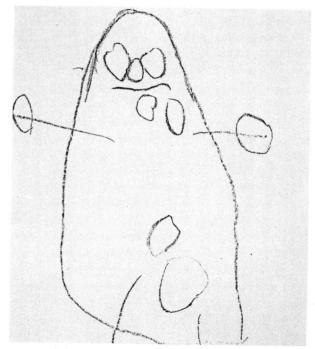

Figure 9–3. Self-portrait of a 4-year-old girl who was sexually abused by her uncle. She came to the emergency department with vaginal and rectal gonorrhea. Inclusion of prominent breasts, vagina, and rectum suggests anxiety and preoccupation with these parts of the body.

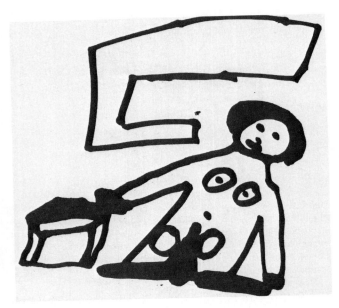

Figure 9–4. Self-portrait drawn by a 9-year-old boy who was sexually abused at overnight camp by his camp counselor. The prominent genitals indicate his increased awareness of the genitals after sexual victimization. The inclusion of breasts on a male figure is unusual; it reflects the boy's gender identity confusion after a sexual experience with another male. The boy's right hand holds a suitcase. (Reproduced with permission from Kelly SJ [1985]. Interviewing the sexually abused child: Principles and techniques. *Journal of Emergency Nursing* 11:234–241)

Children can be asked to draw a portrait of the offender. Doing so often helps a child verbalize thoughts and feelings related to the abuse. Often, both positive and negative feelings toward the offender are expressed. Figure 9–5 is an example of a picture of an offender drawn by a sexually abused child.

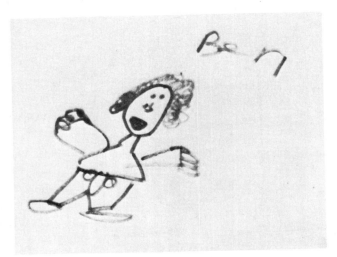

Figure 9–5. This portrait of the offender was drawn by the 9-year-old male victim whose self-portrait is shown in Figure 9–4. The prominent genitals and increased emphasis on the mouth are significant and are related to the type of abuse that occurred. (Reproduced with permission from Kelley SJ [1985]. Interviewing the sexually abused child: Principles and techniques. *Journal of Emergency Nursing* 11:234–241)

Sexually abused children should also be encouraged to draw pictures of what happened in relation to the abuse. Some sexually abused children are capable of graphically portraying the abuse or assault in their drawings. Drawing pictures of the event, or "what happened," enables children to organize their thoughts and feelings related to the abuse on paper before verbalizing them. Drawing pictures also assists a child in recalling some of the important details of the abuse. Figures 9–6, 9–7, and 9–8 are drawings done by sexually abused children showing "what happened." All drawings should be carefully marked with the child's name, patient number, date, and the name of the interviewer and should be entered into the medical record. Any relevant statements made by the child while drawing should be recorded verbatim.

Physical Assessment and Collection of Evidence

In some situations, such as when there is no recent history of sexual abuse, the physical examination can be deferred to a later date with the child's primary care nurse practitioner, pediatrician, or a sexual abuse specialist. Deferral of the examination is often in the child's best interest given that the child will be examined in a more relaxed atmosphere than the ED.

Normal physical findings are common in child sexual abuse. In a review of 21 studies of reported medical findings in children who were allegedly sexu-

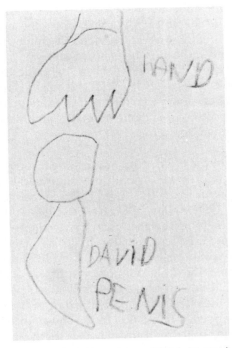

Figure 9–6. Picture drawn by a 6-year-old girl showing how she was forced to touch the penis of an adult male.

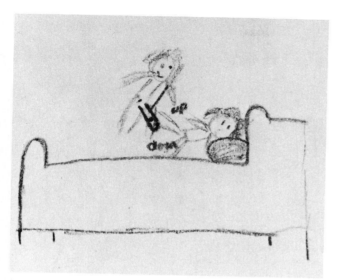

Figure 9–7. Drawing depicting rape scene of an 8-year-old female incest victim. Drawings such as this illustrate how the child has a clear mental image of the abuse. (Reproduced with the permission of Anthony J. Jannetti, Inc., Publisher, from Kelley SJ [1985]. Drawing: Critical communications for sexually abused children. *Pediatric Nursing* 11:421–426)

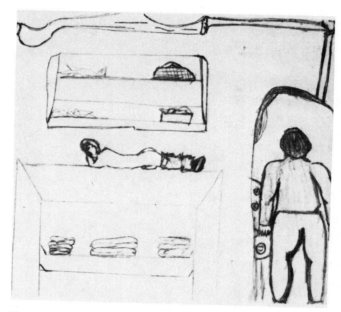

Figure 9–8. Drawing of "what happened" to a 9-year-old male rape victim. The victim (lying on the table) was tricked into believing that he was going to have a physical examination by an 18-year-old neighbor (standing on right) but instead was sodomized by the offender.

ally abused, Bays and Chadwick (1993) found that normal findings were reported in 26–73% of girls (mean of 50%) and 17–82% (mean of 53%) of boys. Findings diagnostic of sexual abuse, such as the presence of genital trauma, sexually transmitted diseases (STDs), or semen, were found in only 3–16% of victims (Bays and Chadwick, 1993). It is important to note that physical findings are more common in cases of recent, forced or violent sexual assaults.

Bays and Chadwick (1993) cite numerous reasons for lack of physical findings in sexually abused children: (1) delay in seeking medical attention; (2) semen and ejaculate are unlikely to be found, particularly if the child has washed, urinated, or defecated, or if more than 72 hours have elapsed since the assault; (3) when injuries do occur, healing can be rapid; (4) many types of sexual abuse such as fondling and oral sex typically do not leave physical evidence; (5) sexual abuse can occur without ejaculation or damage to the hymen; (6) offenders who victimize children may suffer from erectile or ejaculatory dysfunction; (7) the anal sphincter allows routine passage of stools larger than the diameter of a penis without damage; and (8) hymenal tissue is elastic, so full penetration by a finger or penis, particularly in an older child, may cause no visible trauma or may simply enlarge the hymenal opening.

Physical examination of a child typically is the last part of the assessment. Children younger than 12 years should be examined by a pediatrician or pediatric nurse practitioner; adolescents should be examined by a gynecologist or nurse practitioner. It is important to determine if this is the patient's first gynecologic examination. Reassurance from the nurse present during the examination may alleviate some of the child's anxiety. All procedures should be carefully explained to the child and parents. If the child desires, a parent or other caretaker should remain in the examining room to provide support. A hysterical or combative child should never be restrained during the examination because this causes further emotional trauma. In some instances, the medical examination can be deferred until the child has regained composure and is emotionally prepared for the examination. If necessary, the child should be sedated and then examined. If lacerations need to be sutured, or foreign objects removed from the vagina, rectum, or urethra, the child may be examined and treated under general anesthesia.

The genitals and anus should be examined within the context of a complete physical examination to avoid overemphasis on the genitals and to examine other areas for signs of abuse. Therefore, the examination is usually conducted in a head-to-toe manner. Common sites of nongenital trauma include the upper thighs, buttocks, and upper arms.

Several different positions are used for examination of a prepubertal child. The age and emotional state of the child help determine which type of position is used. The supine frog-leg position offers the child relative comfort and provides the examiner with a clear view of the genitalia and anus (Giardino et al,

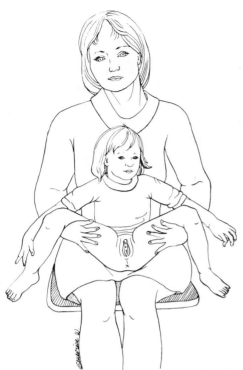

Figure 9–9. Supine frog-leg position in mother's lap.

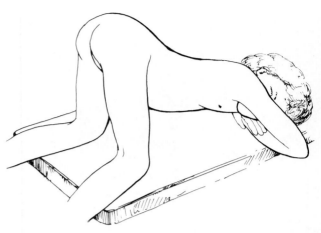

Figure 9–11. Girl in the knee-chest position with exaggerated lordosis and relaxed abdominal muscles. The examiner can inspect the interior wall of her vagina by gently separating her buttocks and labia using an otoscope without an attached speculum for illumination. (From Fleisher GR, Ludwig S [eds] [1993]. *Textbook of Pediatric Emergency Medicine.* [3rd ed]. Baltimore: Williams & Wilkins, p 915)

1992). This position may be assumed in the lap of a parent (Figure 9–9) or on the examining table (Figure 9–10). An older child can be examined in the supine frog-leg position with a parent or other support person sitting behind her or him on the examining table. A cooperative child should be allowed to hold her own labia majora apart during the examination of the genitalia. This gives the child a sense of control during the examination.

The prone knee-chest position (Figure 9–11) offers an excellent view of the anus and allows for another view of the hymenal membrane. The child is placed on the examining table and lies prone with her knees

tucked under her chest. This allows easy visualization of the perineum, labia majora and minora, introitus, and hymenal ring. As the child takes deep breaths, letting her abdomen sag forward, the vaginal orifice falls forward to allow easy visualization of the hymen. The standard lithotomy position is used for adolescents.

In prepubertal girls, only the external genitalia (Figure 9–12) need be examined, unless there is an indication of an intravaginal injury or the presence of a foreign body. A foreign body can often be removed by

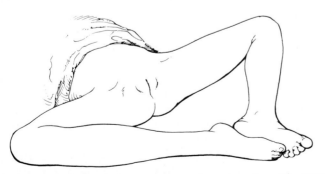

Figure 9–10. Girl in the frog-leg position for examination of the external genitalia. (From Fleisher GR, Ludwig S [eds] [1993]. *Textbook of Pediatric Emergency Medicine.* [3rd ed]. Baltimore: Williams & Wilkins, p 915)

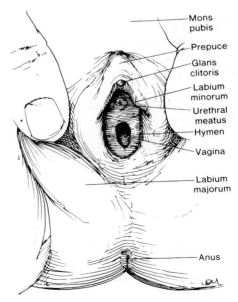

Mons pubis
Prepuce
Glans clitoris
Labium minorum
Urethral meatus
Hymen
Vagina
Labium majorum
Anus

Figure 9–12. External structure of the female genitalia. (From Fleisher GR, Ludwig S [eds] [1993]. *Textbook of Pediatric Emergency Medicine* [3rd ed]. Baltimore: Williams & Wilkins, p 914)

irrigation of the vagina using a feeding tube. The prepubertal vagina is quite short, and vaginal lacerations or foreign bodies are easily observed. If internal visualization of the vaginal canal is necessary, a small pediatric vaginal speculum, nasal speculum, or pediatric laryngoscope may be used. A colposcope, originally used to visualize the cervix in women, is used to assist in the visualization of the external genitalia of children (Giardino et al, 1992). It provides magnification and an excellent light source. When the colposcope is attached to a camera, the examination can be documented with either 35-mm photographs or a videotape (Giardino et al, 1992).

Any signs of trauma, including lacerations, ecchymosis, hematomas, abrasions, erythema, dried blood or secretions; signs of STDs; or foreign bodies should be noted. A description of the condition of hymen, including shape and contour, transverse diameter of the hymenal orifice; and signs of healed injury should be recorded. The size of the hymenal opening varies considerably, depending on the age of the child, the position in which the child is examined, the degree of relaxation, and the amount of traction on the labia used during the examination (Giardino et al, 1992). Therefore, the transverse diameter of the hymenal orifice alone is rarely sufficient to determine whether a child has or has not been sexually abused (Giardino et al, 1992).

Trauma to the penis, testicles, or urethra in male victims is usually easily observed. The urethra should be examined for presence of a discharge.

The anus and perianal area should be observed for signs of trauma, discharge, STDs, changes in pigmentation, and anal sphincter tone. The anal rugae are usually symmetric. A wide, gaping anal opening with poor-to-absent reflex tightening and no stool present in the ampulla is an abnormal finding (Giardino et al, 1992).

If there is a history of a recent assault, female and male victims should be examined with a Wood lamp for the presence of semen on the perineum, rectum, abdomen, or thigh and on clothing worn during the assault. Seminal fluid may be fluorescent.

Laboratory and Diagnostic Tests

Evidence Collection. Emergency departments should have a protocol for a standard sexual abuse laboratory evaluation and collection of specimens. The protocol should specify careful labeling of all specimens and documentation of the chain of evidence. Documentation each time evidence is transferred from one person to another is essential. The use of standardized collection kits should be used for orderly collection of all the necessary specimens. Table 9–5 contains a protocol for

TABLE 9–5. PROTOCOL FOR COLLECTING FORENSIC SPECIMENS IN CHILD SEXUAL ABUSE

Obtain two or three swabbed specimens from each area of body assaulted for sperm, acid phosphatase, P 30, mouse anti-human semen-5 (MHS-5), antigen, and blood group antigen determinations. Most laboratories require air-dried specimens.

Mouth—Swab under the tongue and at the buccal pouch next to the upper and lower molars.

Vagina—Use a dry or moistened swab or a 2-ml saline wash. Overdilution of secretions may produce false-negative results for acid phosphatase. Secretions also may be collected with a pipette or eyedropper.

Rectum—Insert swab at least 0.5–1 inch beyond the anus.

Specimens should be taken from any other suspicious site on the body or clothing.

Make a saline wet mount of specimens from all assaulted orifices and examine immediately for presence of sperm and whether it is motile or nonmotile.

Some forensic laboratories request that a dry smear be made of each secretion sample using clean glass microscope slides; others prepare their own slides from swab specimens.

Collect a saliva specimen to determine the victim's antigen secretion status. Saliva can be collected using three or four saline swabs or a 2 × 2-inch gauze pad.

Obtain a venous blood sample from the victim for antigen secretor status.

Save torn or bloody clothes or any clothing when semen staining is suspected. Semen may fluoresce with a blue or green color under the ultraviolet light of a Wood lamp.

If the victim was wearing a tampon, pad, or diaper during the assault, or if a fresh tampon, pad, or diaper was used after the assault, save it for analysis. Seminal fluid products may be found on these items. Do *not* pack these items or clothing in plastic bags. Paper bags may be used.

Save any foreign material found during removal of clothing.

Collect samples of combed pubic hair or scalp hair and fingernail scraping if required by local law.

Collect specimens to test for presence of STDs. This includes cultures from the vagina, urethra, rectum, and pharynx and blood samples for syphilis, human immunodeficiency virus and Hepatitis B infection.

(Adapted from DeJong AR, Finkel M [1990]. Sexual abuse of children. Current Problems in Pediatrics *20:495–567)*

collecting forensic specimens in cases of suspected child sexual abuse. These specimens should be collected if there has been a recent assault (within 72 hours before ED visit) and as indicated by the patient's history and physical findings.

Tests for Sexually Transmitted Diseases. Any child with an STD must be suspected of being a victim of sexual abuse. Table 9–6 categorizes the American Academy of Pediatrics' report on the probability that an STD in a child is acquired through sexual abuse. Table 9–7 summarizes the recommendations of the Centers for Disease Control (1993) for procedures and tests to be performed at the initial and follow-up evaluations of any prepubertal child suspected of being sexually abused. The decision to evaluate a child for an STD must be made on an individual basis.

TABLE 9–6. IMPLICATIONS OF COMMONLY ENCOUNTERED SEXUALLY TRANSMITTED DISEASES (STDs) FOR THE DIAGNOSIS AND REPORTING OF SEXUAL ABUSE OF PREPUBERTAL INFANTS AND CHILDREN

STD Confirmed	Sexual Abuse	Suggested Action
Gonorrhea[a]	Certain	Report[b]
Syphilis[a]	Certain	Report
Chlamydia[a]	Probable[c]	Report
Condylomata acuminata[a]	Probable	Report
Trichomonas vaginalis	Probable	Report
Herpes 1 (genital)	Possible	Report[d]
Herpes 2	Probable	Report
Bacterial vaginosis	Uncertain	Medical follow-up
Candida albicans	Unlikely	Medical follow-up

[a] If not perinatally acquired.
[b] To agency mandated in community to receive reports of suspected sexual abuse.
[c] Culture only reliable diagnostic method.
[d] Unless there is a clear history of autoinoculation.
(Reprinted with permission from Academy of Pediatrics Committee on Child Abuse and Neglect [1991]. Guidelines for the evaluation of sexual abuse of children. Pediatrics 87:257)

Gonococcal Cultures. Gonorrhea cultures should be obtained from the oropharynx, rectum, and vagina and urethra.

Chlamydia. Chlamydia cultures of the vagina and urethra (males) and the rectum should be obtained.

Syphilis. A serologic test for syphilis—rapid plasma reagin (RPR) or Venereal Disease Research Laboratory (VDRL)—should be obtained. If the abuse was a recent assault, the result serves as a baseline and the test should be repeated in 12 weeks.

Human Immunodeficiency Virus. Testing for the human immunodeficiency virus (HIV) in child victims of sexual abuse remains controversial. Several factors

TABLE 9–7. CENTERS FOR DISEASE CONTROL RECOMMENDATIONS FOR LABORATORY TESTS IN CASES OF SUSPECTED SEXUAL ABUSE

■ INITIAL EVALUATION
  Gram stain of any genital or anal discharge
  Culture for *Neisseria gonorrhea* (vagina and urethra, rectum, pharynx)
  Culture for *Chlamydia trachomatis* (vagina and urethra [if urethral discharge is present], rectum, pharynx)
  Culture and mount vaginal secretions for *Trichomonas vaginalis*
  Culture of lesions for Herpes simplex virus
  Serologic test for human immunodeficiency (HIV), *T. pallidum* and Hepatitis B virus
  Frozen serum sample

■ FOLLOW-UP EVALUATION
  Syphilis and HIV serology to be repeated in 12 weeks
  All other cultures to be repeated 2 weeks after initial examination in cases of recent assault

T. pallidum, Treponema pallidum.

need to be taken into consideration in making the decision whether or not to test. They include the type of sexual activity or abuse reported, the HIV status of the offender, offender risk factors (eg, is the offender a known user of intravenous drugs or homosexual?), and community risk factors (eg, does the perpetrator live in a community with known high rates of HIV infection?). The laboratory test used most often for screening of antibodies to HIV is the enzyme-linked immunoadsorbent assay (ELISA). The Western blot is used to confirm presence of the virus.

Other. If a vaginal, urethral, or anal discharge is present, collection of the following specimens is indicated: a specimen of discharge for Gram stain; wet preparation for *Trichomonas;* and a specimen of discharge for culture of other STDs (Giardino et al, 1992).

TRIAGE
Sexual Abuse

Emergent
Child or adolescent with history of sexual contact within the past 72 hours.

Urgent
Child with history of sexual abuse occurring more than 72 hours before ED visit; child with symptoms suggestive of sexual abuse.

Nursing Diagnosis
Rape Trauma Syndrome

Defining Characteristics
- Child discloses sexual abuse
- Child verbalizes anger, self-blame

Nursing Interventions
- Provide emotional support to child
- Alleviate feelings of self-blame
- Refer child for therapy
- Report suspected abuse to child protective services

Expected Outcomes
- Child remains calm and cooperative
- Child attends therapy
- Child is protected from subsequent sexual abuse

Nursing Diagnosis
Ineffective Family Coping: Compromised

Defining Characteristics

- Parent unable or unwilling to provide emotional support to child victim
- Nonoffending parent in denial of child's abuse

Nursing Interventions

- Provide support to nonoffending parent
- Assist parent in believing the child's disclosure

Expected Outcomes

- Parent demonstrates supportive actions toward child
- Parent verbalizes belief in child's disclosure

TABLE 9–8. EMERGENCY NURSE'S RESPONSIBILITIES IN CHILD SEXUAL ABUSE

Identify presenting condition as possible sexual abuse
Perform rapid triage; child receives priority
Conduct sensitive, non-leading interviews using age-appropriate media
Carefully document all statements made by child
Support child during physical assessment
Assist in evidence collection and preservation of evidence
Administer medication to prevent pregnancy
Administer antibiotics for sexually transmitted diseases
Report all suspected cases to child protective agency
Refer child and family for therapy and follow-up medical care
Participate on hospital- or community-based interdisciplinary child abuse teams
Provide community education
Become involved in professional organizations concerned with child abuse

TABLE 9–9. SEXUALLY TRANSMITTED DISEASES IN CHILDREN

Disease	Presentation	Laboratory Test	Treatment[a]
Gonorrhea	Penile discharge Vaginal discharge Rectal inflammation, discharge Pharyngitis Dysuria, frequency May be asymptomatic	Pharyngeal, rectal, vaginal, and urethral (male) cultures	Ceftriaxone: < 45 kg, 125 mg IM > 45 kg, 250 mg IM If allergic to ceftriaxone: spectinomycin: < 45 kg, 40 mg/kg IM > 45 mg, 2 gm IM
Syphilis	Primary syphilis: chancres may appear on penis, vulva, cervix, rectum, mouth Secondary syphilis: fever, pharyngitis; rash on trunk, upper extremities, palms, and soles of feet; lymphadenopathy; splenomegaly Late syphilis: Vasculitis; neurologic and cardiac involvement	VDRL or RPR serologic tests Microscopic exam of lesion scrapings reveals spirochete	Benzathine penicillin G 50,000 units/kg im (max dose 2.4 million units)
Chlamydia	May be asymptomatic Discharge Dysuria Pelvic pain	Culture is only reliable test for children	Younger than 8 years: erythromycin, 40 mg/kg/day PO for 7 days Older than 8 years: doxycycline, 100 mg bid PO for 7 days
Herpes genitalis	Dysuria Vulvar pruritis and burning Painful lesions on vulva, perianal area, vagina, cervix	Microscopic exam of cells from lesion Viral culture	Analgesics Antipruritics Acyclovir in adolescents Sitz baths
Condylomata acuminata	Nontender lesions (warts) on genitals or perirectal area	Biopsy	Liquid nitrogen Trichloroacetic acid Podophyllin for older children
Trichomoniasis	Vaginitis; discharge Asymptomatic in boys	Saline wet prep to identify the protozoa	Metronidazole: < 45 kg, 5 mg/kg PO tid × 7 days > 45 kg, 500 mg PO bid × 7 days

[a] Treatment may differ for adolescents.
VDRL, Venereal Disease Research Laboratory; RPR, rapid plasma reagin; IM, intramuscular; PO, by mouth.

MANAGEMENT

Table 9–8 provides a summary of the nurse's responsibilities in cases of child sexual abuse.

Treatment of STDs

Prophylaxis for STDs in sexually abused children is not indicated unless an infection is present in the perpetrator or the patient or parent requests it (Centers for Disease Control, 1993). The treatment of STDs is outlined in Table 9–9.

Pregnancy Prevention

The need for pregnancy prevention depends on the child's age, menstrual history, and type of sexual activity reported. If the patient is postmenarchal, has negative pregnancy tests, and coitus occurred within the past 72 hours, pregnancy prophylaxis with two oral contraceptive tablets containing 0.05 mg ethinyl estradiol and 0.5 mg norgestrel within 72 hours of the assault and two more tablets 12 hours later are effective in preventing pregnancy (Barnett, 1992). A repeat pregnancy test should be obtained 2 weeks after the ED visit.

Reporting Responsibilities

Sexual abuse of children is a crime in every state in the US, although specific laws pertaining to sexual abuse vary from one jurisdiction to another. Emergency department nurses need to be knowledgeable with the laws of their own jurisdiction pertaining to child sexual abuse.

The reporting of child sexual abuse is mandated in all 50 states. However, the official agency to which one reports varies with each jurisdiction. Nurses are mandated reporters of child abuse in almost every state and should take this obligation seriously. According to Myers (1992) the duty to report does not require the professional to "know for sure" that abuse occurred; rather it requires information that raises a reasonable suspicion of abuse. In most cases, the reporting is made to a CPS agency or the local police department. Table 9–10 contains the American Academy of Pediatrics' guidelines for deciding whether or not to report a case of suspected child sexual abuse.

Patient and Family Education and Support

As in all cases of child abuse, the ED staff must determine if a child victim is safe from further abuse or

TABLE 9–10. GUIDELINES FOR MAKING THE DECISION TO REPORT SEXUAL ABUSE OF CHILDREN

Data Available			Response	
History	Physical Findings	Laboratory Findings	Level of Concern About Sexual Abuse	Action
None	Normal	None	None	None
Behavioral changes	Normal	None	Low (worry)	Report or not[a]; follow closely (possible mental health referral)
None	Nonspecific	None	Low (worry)	Report or not[a]; follow closely
Nonspecific history by child or history given by parent only	Nonspecific	None	Possible (suspect)	Report or not[a]; follow closely
None	Specific	None	Probable	Report
Clear statement	Normal	None	Probable	Report
Clear statement	Specific	None	Probable	Report
None	Normal, nonspecific, or specific	Positive culture for gonorrhea; positive serologic test for syphilis; presence of semen, sperm, acid phosphatase	Definite	Report
Behavioral changes	Nonspecific changes	Other sexually transmitted diseases	Probable	Report

[a] A report may or may not be indicated. The decision to report should be based on discussion with local or regional experts and child protective services agencies.
(Reprinted with permission from Academy of Pediatrics Committee on Child Abuse and Neglect [1991]. Guidelines for the evaluation of sexual abuse of children. Pediatrics 87:257)

retribution if returned home. If the child appears to be at immediate risk for subsequent harm, an alternative disposition—such as discharge to a responsible relative's home or foster care placement—should be considered. All child and adolescent victims should be referred for therapy and medical follow-up care. When possible, the referral should be made within the same institution to provide continuity of care.

Nonoffending parents of victimized children experience acute and chronic psychological distress as a result of their child's abuse (Kelley, 1990) and therefore need an opportunity to express their thoughts and feelings about the victimization. Parents of female victims are often concerned with what they perceive to be loss of innocence or virginity, whereas parents of male victims are often concerned with what they perceive to be a threat to their child's masculinity. Although there is no evidence to support the belief that sexually abused boys will become homosexual later in life, many parents harbor this fear. In addition, many parents experience tremendous fear that their child may have contracted acquired immodeficiency syndrome (AIDS) during the sexual abuse.

Parents, therefore, need as much support as their children. They should be forewarned that the child may demonstrate regression in behavior, become fearful and clinging, refuse to be left alone, experience eating and sleeping disorders, and experience school phobias. Parents cope more effectively if they know in advance that these types of behaviors are typical reactions to sexual abuse. Parents need reassurance that their child should be able to adjust and integrate the experience over time with therapy and family support. Regardless of how well the child and family appear to be coping, they should be referred for therapy. When possible, this referral should be made directly from the ED to increase the likelihood the family will follow through with therapy.

Professional Involvement in the Field of Child Abuse

Nurses concerned with the problem of child abuse should become involved in the American Professional Society on the Abuse of Children (APSAC), 332 South Michigan Ave., Suite 1600, Chicago, IL 60604, 312-554-0166. This interdisciplinary society for professionals supports research, education, and advocacy that enhances efforts to respond to abused children, those who abuse them, and the conditions associated with child abuse.

REFERENCES

Academy of Pediatrics Committee on Child Abuse and Neglect (1991). Guidelines for the evaluation of sexual abuse of children. *Pediatrics* 87:254–260

Barnett TM (1992). Abuse and neglect. In Barkin RM (ed), *Pediatric emergency medicine*. St. Louis: Mosby, pp 537–555

Bays J, Chadwick D (1993). Medical diagnosis of the sexually abused child. *Child Abuse and Neglect* 16:91–110

Beitchman JH, Zucker KJ, Hood JE, DaCosta GA, Arkman D, Cassavia E (1992). A review of the long-term effects of child sexual abuse. *Child Abuse and Neglect* 16:101–118

Beitchman JH, Zucker KJ, Hood JE, DaCosta GA, Arkman D (1991). A review of the short-term effects of child sexual abuse. *Child Abuse and Neglect* 15:537–556

Berliner L (1991). Effects of sexual abuse on children. *Violence Update* 1:1, 8, 10–11

Burgess AW, Hartman CR (1993). Children's drawings. *Child Abuse and Neglect* 17:161–168

Centers for Disease Control and Prevention (1993). Sexually transmitted diseases treatment guidelines. MMWR;42 (No. RR-14): pp 1–102

DeJong AR, Finkel M (1990). Sexual abuse of children. *Current Problems in Pediatrics* 20:495–567

Faller KC (1990). *Understanding child sexual maltreatment.* Newbury Park, Calif: Sage, pp 38–67

Finkelhor D (1993). Epidemiological factors in the clinical identification of child sexual abuse. *Child Abuse and Neglect* 17:67–70

Finkelhor D, Hotaling G, Lewis IA, Smith S (1990). Sexual abuse in a national survey of adult men and women: Prevalence, characteristics, and risk factors. *Child Abuse and Neglect* 14:19–28

Friedrich WN (1993). Sexual victimization and sexual behavior in children: A review of recent literature. *Child Abuse and Neglect* 17:59–66

Friedrich WN, Grambsch P, Damon L, et al (1992). The sexual behavior inventory: Normative and clinical findings. *Psychological Assessment* 4:303–311

Giardino AP, Finkel MA, Giardino ER, Seidl T, Ludwig S (1992). *A practical guide to the evaluation of sexual abuse in the prepubertal child.* Newbury Park, Calif: Sage, pp 29–81

Kelley SJ (1984). The use of art therapy with sexually abused children. *Journal of Psychosocial Nursing* 22:12–18

Kelley SJ (1985). Drawings: Critical communications for sexually abused children. *Pediatric Nursing* 11:421–426

Kelley SJ (1989). Stress responses of children to sexual abuse and ritualistic abuse in day care centers. *Journal of Interpersonal Violence* 4:502–513

Kelley SJ (1990). Parental stress responses to sexual and ritualistic abuse of children in day care centers. *Nursing Research* 39:25–29

Kelley SJ (1992). Child maltreatment, stressful life events, and behavior problems in school-aged children in residential treatment. *Journal of Child and Adolescent Psychiatric and Mental Health Nursing* 5:5–13

Lenehan GP (1991). Sexual assault nurse examiners: A SANE way to care for rape victims. *Journal of Emergency Nursing* 17:1–2

Myers JEB (1992). Legal issues in child abuse and neglect. Newbury Park, Calif: Sage, pp 100–105

Waterman J, Kelly RJ, Oliveri MK, McCord J (1993). *Beyond the playground walls: Sexual abuse in preschools.* New York: Guilford, pp 79–165

CHAPTER 10

Psychiatric Emergencies

CATHERINE KNOX-FISCHER

INTRODUCTION

Pediatric emergency nurses are in a key position to assess and intervene when children and adolescents and their families experience emotional crises. Unfortunately, the number of psychiatric emergencies among children and adolescents is on the rise. Suicide is the third leading cause of death among teenagers and young adults; accidental death and homicide are the two most frequent causes of death (Kuperman et al, 1988). It is generally thought that the rate of suicide may be even higher than thought because some accidental deaths may mask an actual suicide attempt. Similarly, the number of young people using and being injured by guns is also rising. Violence among youth, including adolescent homicide, has been increasing across the United States (Srnec, 1991). It is critical that nurses who encounter children and adolescents undergoing a psychiatric emergency such as a suicide attempt develop skills to assess and intervene effectively; the goal is to stabilize the crisis.

This chapter focuses on a variety of psychiatric emergencies involving children and adolescents. They include depression and suicide, psychosis, and aggression and violence on the part of both children and their families. Common nursing diagnoses for each emergency are presented, and nursing management principles for each category are discussed.

Definition of a Crisis

Emotional crises occur when a person cannot resolve a problem utilizing coping mechanisms that proved effective in the past (Aguilera and Messick, 1986). Tension and anxiety increase, the possibility of finding solutions decreases, and feelings of helplessness and distress occur, resulting in the array of psychiatric crises treated in emergency departments (EDs) today.

Aguilera and Messick (1986) wrote that a crisis may be thought of as a danger in that it may overwhelm the child and family. Likewise, it can be viewed as an opportunity for change; during crises, the child and family may be more open to intervention. The nursing goal is to assist the child and family to restore their previous level of functioning by collecting relevant data and intervening with the immediate problem (Aguilera and Messick, 1986).

Reactions of Caregivers

Psychiatric symptoms generate many reactions in caregivers; they range from avoidance, irritation, anger, and fear to sympathy and understanding. Psychiatric disorders are not as clear cut as medical disorders, which usually have a clearly delineated etiology. Psychiatric disorders can be understood according to an array of theoretical frameworks. Intervention strategies are usually based on principles and therapeutic use of self as opposed to specific protocols. Because the symptoms of a psychiatric disorder may be unusual and because the symptoms vary from child to child and family to family, professionals may feel anxious and unsure about how to best deal with people experiencing psychiatric problems. When caring for children experiencing a psychiatric emergency, the nurse must clearly identify her or his personal reactions to these situations. A mental health nurse specialist or clinical nurse specialist can provide a safe outlet for staff to sort out and address their reactions. Doing so increases a nurse's ability to intervene in objective and therapeutic ways and to help stabilize the condition of the child and the family.

Underlying a caregiver's ability to intervene effectively in any type of psychiatric emergency is the ability to contain one's own anxiety and reactivity to the situation and to remain calm. Families experiencing emotional crises are sensitive to the reactions of others. Just as anxiety is contagious, so is calmness. The process of remaining calm during the crisis is as important as what the nurse says and does. Calmness and reassurance on the part of the staff communicate to the child and family that the nurse is not fearful of what is occurring and that the situation will be under control. A calm approach better enables the nurse to make a connection with the child and family in an effort to establish the helping relationship that serves as the foundation for all nursing interventions.

Limit-Setting

Limit-setting is a strategy used in most psychiatric emergencies; it assists the child and family in feeling safe and in control. Limit-setting is the process by which someone determines temporary ego boundaries for another person. Defining boundaries protects the child and others, provides security, and decreases anxiety (Lyon, 1970). Acting-out behavior on the part of children and adolescents may be in part a request for assistance in regaining control. Specifics of limit-setting are addressed in categories of emergencies.

Assessment

Nurses are instrumental in collecting relevant data from children and families, not only during specific emergencies but also for early identification of families at risk. Facilitative communication skills and exploratory interviewing are useful in assessing the family's perspective of the problem. Strategies used in assessment incorporate nonverbal and verbal techniques. Nonverbal strategies include active listening, respect, provision of privacy, and awareness of body posture. Verbal strategies include the use of open-ended questions, focusing, communicating in a nonjudgmental way, clarifying information, and providing support (Haber, 1987). Because younger children may not respond to classic interviewing techniques, the use of nondirective approaches such as drawings and observation of play may be helpful in revealing a child's perceptions (Pfeffer, 1985). Using behaviors observed in the clinical setting to explore a child's experience can generate more information. For example, the nurse may ask, "I notice you are having trouble concentrating. What are you thinking about?" Acknowledging a patient's current situation may enable the child to feel

listened to. The nurse asks, for example, "It sounds like it has been tough at school. Any ideas about what's been going on?" The more strongly a child denies a problem, the more likely it is that there is one. It is important not to force the issue but to stay connected with the child and the family.

It is important to acknowledge that a child's symptoms do not occur in isolation but in the context of a family's interaction with the environment. Family systems theorists say that psychiatric symptoms in children and adolescents reflect disturbances in the larger family system. Collecting data from the child and family to ascertain the context in which the child's symptoms are occurring may help to decrease the child's anxiety. General areas to assess include the following.

Areas of Assessment in Psychiatric Emergencies

- Family perception of the problem
- Child's perception of the problem
- Precipitating event for the ED visit
- Baseline level of functioning (cognitive, behavioral, peer relations, and any changes)
- Current stresses or changes (possible losses)
- Family structure and nature of relationships
- Family coping and baseline family health

DEPRESSION

Depression and suicide among children and adolescents are receiving much attention by health care providers. Studies demonstrate that youth who have completed suicide, attempted suicide, or expressed suicidal ideation have shown symptoms of depression (Pfeffer, 1987). Depression in children and adolescents manifests itself differently than in adults. Whereas adults can usually verbalize feelings of depression, young people often exhibit mood or behavioral changes that are indicative of depression. Although it can be seen in young children, childhood depression occurs more commonly among 9–12-year-olds and even more frequently among adolescents (Poster, 1987). Nursing assessments need to incorporate screening for overt or covert symptoms of depression in any age group to provide preventive care to children and families.

Etiology

A variety of theoretic frameworks exist to explain the cause of depression in youth. Psychodynamic theory focuses on a child's response to separation and loss as the grounds for depression. Losses may include a significant person in the child's life, or life experiences or developmental tasks. It is hypothesized that a child experiences anger that becomes directed toward self, resulting in depression and possibly suicide (Poster, 1987). Much of today's research focuses on the biochemical theory of depression. Biologic theory hypothesizes that depression results from a deficiency in the amount or transmission of the following neurohormones: norepinephrine, serotonin, dopamine, and acetylcholine (Krupnick and Wade, 1993). A third theory, family systems theory, proposes that symptoms of depression and suicide in youth usually reflect larger family problems or family dysfunction. Many of the problems with depression and suicide in youth are associated with families that have difficulty adjusting to life-cycle changes. These changes are experienced as losses rather than as opportunities for gain or growth. Symptoms in a child or adolescent reflect a disturbance in the balance of relationships in the family so that the family unit becomes the focus of care and the child's symptoms are considered in the context in which they occur. In addition, social factors, such as living in a highly mobile society, the increased divorce rate, pressures to succeed, fear of failure, and pressures to grow up, may also contribute to the development of depression.

Assessment

Like other clinical skills, the ability to recognize covert and overt symptoms of depression in young people develops with knowledge and experience. Early recognition of these symptoms in youth may promote earlier treatment and referral. Table 10–1 contains some of the more common behavioral manifestations of depression in children and adolescents (Muse, 1990; Patros and Shamoo, 1989; Poster, 1987). Table 10–2 lists risk factors and aspects of the history related to depression (Muse, 1990; Patros and Shamoo, 1989; Poster, 1987).

The presence of symptoms and family risk factors, as outlined in Table 10–2, assists to identify a child who may be depressed or at risk for depression. The nurse uses direct observation and an interview to assess the child and family. Direct and clear questioning is an efficient approach to gathering data about depression. The child should be asked about how well he or she sleeps, whether or not he or she likes school, and what he or she likes to do. The child is asked to tell the nurse about friends, what they do together, and how often they see each other. The nurse attempts to get a sense of the child's hopes for the future to determine the degree of hopelessness because hopelessness has been linked to adolescent depression and suicide (Rotheram-Borus and Trautman, 1988).

TABLE 10–1. BEHAVIORAL MANIFESTATIONS OF DEPRESSION IN CHILDREN AND ADOLESCENTS

- DEPRESSED MOOD
  Presence of sadness
  Mood changes, irritability
  Hypersensitivity
  Anxiety

- BEHAVIORAL CHANGES, AS IN SCHOOL PERFORMANCE
  Difficulties concentrating
  Memory problems, forgetfulness
  Changed attitude or performance in school

- WITHDRAWN BEHAVIORS
  Decreased interest in friends and activities
  Lack of friends

- POOR SELF ESTEEM
  Negative comments about self
  Difficulty receiving compliments

- INCREASED OR DECREASED ENERGY
  Boundless energy
  Decreased pleasure in activities
  Fatigue

- AGGRESSIVE BEHAVIOR
  Hostility or agitation, which may mask an underlying depression by serving as a defense against sadness or hopelessness

- SLEEP DISTURBANCES
  Difficulty arising
  Insomnia or hypersomnia
  Restless sleep, awakening during night

- THOUGHTS OF DEATH AND DYING

- PHYSICAL FINDINGS
  Loss or gain in weight
  Increase or decrease in appetite
  Gastrointestinal symptoms
  Unexplained somatic complaints

TABLE 10–2. RISK FACTORS FOR DEPRESSION IN CHILDREN AND ADOLESCENTS

- FAMILY HISTORY AND ASSESSMENT
  History of depression or suicide
  History of drug and alcohol usage
  Significant losses—moves, deaths, divorce, loss of body part or other function, loss of pet
  Current stresses or changes—illness, unemployment, remarriage
  Family disorganization—abuse, incest, violence, lack of parenting skills
  Lack of identified resources or supports

TRIAGE
Depression

Emergent
Child or adolescent with five or more of the following symptoms present during a 2-week period that represent a change in previous functioning (American Psychiatric Association, 1987): depressed or irritable mood all the time; decreased interest in activities all the time; weight loss or gain; insomnia or hypersomnia; psychomotor agitation or retardation every day; fatigue or loss of energy every day; feelings of worthlessness every day; decreased ability to think or concentrate every day; recurrent thoughts of death, suicidal ideation.

Urgent
Child or adolescent exhibiting depressed or irritable mood, the quality of which is milder than in an emergent situation. At least two of the following symptoms are present (American Psychiatric Association, 1987): poor appetite or overeating; insomnia or hypersomnia; low energy or fatigue; low self esteem; poor concentration or indecisiveness; sense of hopelessness.

Non-urgent
Child or adolescent with mild mood disturbance occurring within 3 months of a clearly identified precipitating event (American Psychiatric Association, 1987). Patient has support systems in place.

Nursing Diagnosis
Self Esteem Disturbance

Defining Characteristics

- Critical of self or others
- Difficulty accepting compliments
- Decreased responsibility for self care
- Lack of eye contact
- Self-destructive behavior

Nursing Interventions

- Convey acceptance, respect, and empathy. Provide support and do not try to talk patient out of what he or she is feeling
- Assist patient to identify positive aspects of self, strengths, and accomplishments
- Assess for suicide risk

Expected Outcomes

- Patient verbalizes current strengths
- Patient is safe and controls impulses for self harm

Nursing Diagnosis
Ineffective Individual Coping

Defining Characteristics

- Low self esteem
- Chronic depression
- Inability to meet basic needs

Nursing Interventions

- Establish rapport and trusting relationship
- Assess for presence of depressive symptoms
- Assist patient to identify current stresses
- Assess previous coping strategies
- Assess for drug and alcohol use
- Encourage patient to verbalize feelings, fears, anxieties, and concerns using age-appropriate medium

Expected Outcomes

- Patient identifies current fears and concerns
- Patient identifies current stresses

Nursing Diagnosis
Ineffective Family Coping: Compromised

Defining Characteristics

- Unresolved anger, depression, hostility, and aggression
- Denial of patient's health problem
- Helplessness

Nursing Interventions

- Assist family to identify stresses affecting child and family
- Ask family to describe behavioral changes
- Assess family coping strategies
- Assess family support network
- Collaborate with family and team to determine disposition

Expected Outcomes

- Family verbalizes stress and its impact
- Family identifies supports
- Family identifies one way it has managed a crisis successfully
- Family verbalizes understanding of disposition

Management

Initial stabilization of a depressed child involves the accurate identification of the symptoms, collection of relevant data, provision of support and safety to the child, and appropriate referral. Children experiencing severe depressive symptoms should be evaluated by a child psychologist, psychiatrist, or a child mental health nurse clinician to evaluate the need for in-patient psychiatric care. The triage guidelines can serve as a framework for referral and disposition in collaboration with the medical and psychiatric teams. Disposition may include discharge to home, discharge with psychiatric outpatient referral, or transfer to a psychiatric facility or other alternative care setting. Because safety and support are the priorities, it is also important to assist the family in defining the resources they have or need if the child is to be discharged. Collaboration with social services is helpful in this area.

Antidepressant medication including tricyclic agents and monoamine oxidase (MAO) inhibitors may be prescribed by a child psychiatrist after extensive evaluation. Although physicians are unlikely to prescribe antidepressants in the ED, the patient may be using these drugs before the ED visit. Because they may have life-threatening side effects, MAO inhibitors are not recommended for children younger than 16 years (Keltner, 1991). Adverse reactions to tricyclic antidepressants include dry mouth, constipation, dizziness, tremors, sedation, blurred vision, confusion, mouth sores, difficulty urinating, and fever (Keltner, 1991). The child and family should be taught to report any of these symptoms to the physician.

Patient and Family Teaching and Psychosocial Support

Families with a depressed or suicidal child require a great deal of support, information, and acknowledgment. Family teaching should include

Components of Family Teaching on Depression

- A discussion of the prevalence of depression and suicide in our culture coupled with information regarding normal development and situational crisis
- Early identification and review of common symptoms
- Counseling referrals including suicide hotline numbers
- A discussion of the importance of open communication among family members in regard to stresses and feelings
- A reminder about the importance of openly discussing the risk for suicide

SUICIDE

Suicide among youth is a tragedy that is on the rise. It consists of any self-destructive behavior that has the intent to damage or result in death (Castiglia, 1990). As previously mentioned, suicide is the third leading cause of death among people 15–24 years of age, and the rate increases each year through a person's early twenties.

Most teenagers who kill themselves do so with a firearm. Hanging is the second most common method among boys and jumping from a great height among girls. Drug overdoses are another frequent method (Castiglia, 1990). The incidence of suicidal behavior among children younger than 12 years has not been firmly established; suicide is not classified by the National Center for Health Statistics as a cause of death among children younger than 10 years (Gemma, 1989). Several authors and clinicians, however, describe the presence of suicidal thinking, preoccupations with death, and suicidal behavior in children younger than 12 years (Pfeffer, 1985; Valente, 1987). Because attempts may be underreported or masked as other injuries, statistics may not reflect actual rates. As rates increase, emergency nurses are key in the assessment of suicidal risk in addition to providing immediate care to patients after a suicide attempt.

Etiology

As for depression, a variety of theories exist to provide a framework for understanding suicidal behavior among children. Theories outlined for depression are also used to explain suicidal behavior. In addition, the expendable child concept described by Sabbath (1970) proposes that a suicidal youth perceives his or her family to want covertly or overtly the child gone. The child responds to this perceived death wish in the family and acts accordingly by attempting suicide. Other stresses of adolescence that may contribute to suicide are peer pressure, crisis, change, and impulsiveness. Current research findings have linked the presence of hopelessness with adolescent suicide (Rotherman-Borus and Trautman, 1988).

Assessment

Distinctions between children and adolescents in regard to their concepts of death and other cognitive functions are useful to the assessment process. How children present to the ED relates to their level of development. Although it is clearly documented that younger children are capable of understanding the concept of death, many children may not view death as final because their capability for abstract thinking is incomplete (Valente, 1987). Suicidal behavior in a child

TABLE 10–3. RISK FACTORS FOR SUICIDE IN CHILDREN AND ADOLESCENTS

Presence of depressive symptoms
Past attempts by child or within family
Aggressive behavior
Use of drugs or alcohol
Poor impulse control
Altered mental status
Conduct problems
Current crises, such as loss, death, separation, change
Recent conflicts with parents
Break-up with significant other
Anniversary of a loss
Recent perceived personal or school failure or public humiliation
Family disorganization
Preoccupation with death themes
Pattern of recurrent accidental injuries
Statements indicating a wish to be gone
Statements about the future indicating the child or adolescent does not expect to be a part of it
Giving away possessions, saying goodbye
Quick affective shifts from depressed to elated affect

may represent an escape from unpleasant parts of life rather than permanent death; teenagers generally have a better sense of permanence. Children use less cognition to explain suicidal behavior; they may view suicide as an opportunity to join a lost loved one, make a significant other love them, or punish those who have hurt them. Adolescents are capable of using rationalization and cognition to explain suicidal behavior. Suicide by younger children is less peer driven than that of teenagers. Adolescence as a developmental stage is more vulnerable to external variables and involves more risk-taking, which may lead to impulsive behavior. Gould and Shaffer (1986) addressed the susceptibility of adolescents to imitation and cluster suicide. They found an increase in the rate of attempted suicide in a group of adolescents after the adolescents viewed films about suicide on television. Table 10–3 contains factors that increase the risk of suicide among youth (Castiglia, 1990; Gemma, 1989; Muse, 1990; and Valente, 1987).

Once risk is identified, it is critical to raise the subject of suicide directly to assess current risk for self injury. Many caregivers feel awkward discussing suicide; they fear they may introduce the idea. By discussing suicide directly, caregivers provide an opportunity to address a serious problem. Often people are relieved when their suicidal cues are heard and the patient receives a response.

Assessment for suicide risk should include direct questioning about intent, current plan, lethality and availability of means, and presence of resources (Valente, 1992). Intent addresses the patient's desire to die. Questions to ask might include, "When kids feel bad it's not unusual to have thoughts about wanting to be dead. Have you ever had thoughts like that?" and "What did you want to happen when you took the pills?" Because younger children may not respond to an interview, the nurse should assess the child's play for destructive themes and ask the child to describe what is happening. If a child indicates intent, the nurse assesses for the presence of a specific plan and past history. Questions to ask include "Have you ever tried to hurt yourself in the past?" and "Have you thought about how you might harm yourself?" Ascertain when the child was thinking of doing something and when they last had thoughts of self harm. The more lethal the method and more available the means, the higher is the risk for suicide. A child who expresses intent, who has a clear plan with high lethality, and who has few or no resources or support is at high risk (Patros and Shamoo, 1989; Valente, 1987).

TRIAGE
Suicidal Behavior

Emergent

Child or adolescent with clear desire to harm self with intent to die. Presence of specific plan, means, intense family stress, anxiety, poor impulse control and minimal perceived support. Patient entering the emergency room after a suicide attempt.

Urgent

Child or adolescent with self-destructive thoughts but has no plan or means and identifies support network. Total breakdown in coping has not occurred.

Non-urgent

Child or adolescent with depressive symptoms, with no clear intent or plan, and with evidence of family coping.

Nursing Diagnosis

High Risk for Violence: Self-directed or directed at others

Defining Characteristics

- Presence of self-destructive behavior
- Suicidal ideation
- Vulnerable self esteem

Nursing Interventions

- Assess for presence of intent, plan, lethality, and availability and presence of support
- Provide safe environment
- Contract with patients that they will not harm self during specific times
- Obtain specimens for drug screen
- Review disposition plans

Expected Outcome

- Patient does not injure self

Management

Suicidal behavior can occur in the ED as ideation, gesture, or an actual attempt. Regardless, all suicidal behavior is taken seriously by clinicians. During assessment it is crucial to convey support, acknowledgment, and a nonjudgmental attitude. The following are the goals of crisis intervention in the care of a suicidal child: (1) provision of safety; (2) communication of a sense of hope that the current situation can change; and (3) mobilization of resources (Aguilera and Messick, 1987).

Initial stabilization of a child who enters the ED after a suicide attempt involves the medical treatment of the complications of the attempt according to the injury presented. Safety precautions should be taken, and one-to-one supervision should be provided until further psychiatric evaluation occurs. Young people may become more agitated or aggressive as they become more aware of what occurred; one-to-one supervision may decrease further harm to self or others. Initial stabilization for patients who are assessed to be suicidal also involves provision for safety and staff supervision. To provide a safe environment, sharp objects such as scalpels, needles, and glass should be removed from the reach of the patient. Youth with suicidal ideation and no plan should remain within staff vision and have a family member present. The nurse acknowledges the stressful situation and encourages the family to participate in the care of the child. The child psychiatry and social services departments should be consulted for evaluation in all triage categories for collaboration in risk assessment and disposition. Children who require medical care after a suicide attempt are admitted to the hospital; children assessed to be at high risk but in a stable medical condition may require admission to a child psychiatric inpatient facility. Children assessed to be at lower risk may be discharged home with referral. For families who are given outpatient referrals, compliance may increase if the caregiver makes the appointment in the ED rather than giving the family a telephone number to call (Castiglia, 1990).

Patient and Family Teaching and Psychosocial Support

In providing support, the nurse assists the child and family in verbalizing their feelings, fears and frustrations and assists in identifying support. The nurse can acknowledge potential ambivalent feelings between the child and family during the initial contact after a suicide attempt. Acknowledging feelings such as anger and relief legitimizes the family's experience. Teaching includes an explanation of the rationale and the process of safety precautions emphasizing that all attempts are taken seriously. A review of behavioral clues, triggers for suicide, and suicide hotline numbers can enable parents to identify risk early on and to gain access to the mental health system as needed.

PSYCHOSIS

Psychosis involves the disintegration of ego functioning resulting in altered and distorted perceptions, thoughts, behavior, and feelings (Bernstein, 1987). Massive amounts of anxiety that cannot be adequately managed by the child or family are a major factor in psychotic behavior.

In general, psychosis indicates a substantial loss of contact with reality; it includes hallucinations, delusions, and disordered thinking. Common psychiatric disorders in youth that result in psychotic behavior include schizophrenia, bipolar affective disorder, brief reactive psychoses, and acute psychiatric episode (Bair, 1990). Disorders that occur in the first year of development include the pervasive developmental disorders such as autism. Schizophrenia and other psychotic disorders usually manifest themselves in middle to late adolescence (Pearson, 1992).

Although pure thought disorders are rare in children and adolescents, they do occur (Pearson, 1992). Emergency nurses play an important role in assessment and intervention. In addition, psychotic behavior from a youth may be caused by other than pure psychiatric disorders, so nursing interventions are used broadly.

Psychotic behavior can be anxiety provoking for staff. Behavior is often unpredictable, and it may be difficult to establish a connection with the child. Effective emergency care depends on increased knowledge of the principles of managing psychosis.

Etiology

Several theories exist to explain the causes of psychotic disorders. Current research findings suggest a connection between genetic predisposition and the development of schizophrenia. Additional biologic findings suggests that alterations in the biochemical, metabolic, and electrical functioning of the brain may play a part as well (Krupnick and Wade, 1993). Psychosocial theories, such as family systems, view psychotic symptoms in children as reflective of dysfunctional family relationships characterized by increased anxiety and over-involvement between parents and children, resulting in an inability to trust and distortions of reality (Krupnick and Wade, 1993). Children in these families may receive conflicting and ambivalent messages that affect self image and self concept.

Initial theories that underlie the present understanding of autism focused on a specific parenting style. It was thought that a cold, detached, non-nurturing parenting style contributed to autism (Zoltak, 1986). At present, autism is more commonly identified as a reflection of an underlying abnormality in brain functioning. Biologic theories include genetic transmission, perinatal factors, hemispheric specialization, and alteration in neurotransmitters, including dopamine, serotonin, and opioid neuroregulators (Dalton and Howell, 1989).

Assessment

Assessment of psychoses in children and adolescents involves observation of overt behavior and observation for the presence of age-appropriate norms and a history of identified patterns. The initial symptoms of psychoses in children may manifest as deviations from age-appropriate norms. Younger children may present as odd, shy, withdrawn, and isolated whereas adolescents may present with psychotic symptoms similar to those of adults (Pearson, 1992). Table 10–4 contains

TABLE 10–4. SYMPTOMS OF PSYCHOSIS IN CHILDREN AND ADOLESCENTS

Auditory or visual hallucinations
Delusional thinking
Strange movements or posturing
Lack of connectedness with environment
Fragmented, unfocused play
Impulsitivity
Aggressiveness
Disorientation
Inappropriate affect (laughs at sad situations)
Speech alterations
   Mutism
   Echolalia
   Difficult to understand speech
   Unusual flow or rhythm
Concrete thinking
Lack of interest in self care
Unusually great focus on child by family members to the neglect of their own needs
Increased family anxiety
Changes in peer relationships (note nature and level of relatedness with others)

symptoms of psychosis in children and adolescents (Dalton and Howell, 1989; Keltner, 1991; Pearson, 1992).

Autism as a syndrome was identified and described by Kanner in 1943. It usually manifests before 2½ years of age, although symptoms may occur later. Kanner (1943) identified the first five specific behaviors of autistic children given in the following list. The other behavioral characteristics of autism were described by Dalton and Howell (1989), Zoltak (1986), and the American Psychiatric Association (APA) (1987). These behaviors occur variably in autistic children.

Behaviors of Autistic Children

- A pervasive inability to develop social relationships
- A desire to maintain environmental sameness
- A preoccupation with objects
- Mutism
- A normal physical appearance
- Self-stimulating behavior that may be ritualistic (ie, finger sucking, rocking, head banging)
- Attachment to and inappropriate use of objects
- Repetitive play
- Difficulties with change in routine
- Withdrawn behavior (prefers to be alone and is unaware of others)
- Limited number of activities
- Destructive behavior or tantrums
- Inconsistency in development and motor activity (hyperactivity and hypoactivity)
- Impaired verbal and nonverbal communication
- Impaired social interactions—unaffectionate and unresponsive to nurturing; emotionally distant; poor to no eye contact; poor response to social activities.

It is important to obtain a brief developmental history to place symptoms in a larger context. For a child with a pre-existing diagnosis of autism, current patterns can be identified by the family because they have an impact on how the ED nurse approaches the child.

TRIAGE
Psychosis

Emergent

Child or adolescent with active hallucinations, delusions, disorganized thinking, disorientation, and agitation. Presence of aggressive or other destructive behaviors indicating child may hurt self or others in response to psychotic thinking. Unable to focus or respond to verbal interventions by nurse.

> ### Urgent
> Child or adolescent preoccupied with hallucinations, delusions, or other internal stimuli. Possible increased motor activity and agitation but responds to calming verbal interventions.
>
> ### Non-urgent
> Child or adolescent mildly withdrawn and preoccupied, able to engage with nurse.

Nursing Diagnosis
Altered Thought Processes

Defining Characteristics

- Distractibility or preoccupation
- Inaccurate interpretations of environment
- Inappropriate affect

Nursing Interventions

- Convey acceptance and caring
- Reinforce and focus on reality
- Avoid challenging disturbed thoughts
- Communicate clearly and concisely
- Promote safety
- Assist child in verbalizing fears
- Administer medications as ordered

Expected Outcome

- Patient is calmer, safe, able to focus on reality, and able to communicate in ways that are understood by others

Nursing Diagnosis
High Risk for Violence: Self-directed or directed at others

Defining Characteristics

- Self mutilation
- Overt aggressive acts
- Pacing and increased motor activity
- Rigid, tight body posture
- Hostile verbalizations

Nursing Interventions

- Protect child from self mutilation
- Identify possible precipitating event
- Decrease stimuli and observe frequently
- Remove dangerous objects
- Redirect behavior to physical outlets
- Give medications as ordered
- Use mechanical restraints as a last resort

Expected Outcomes

- Patient does not mutilate self or act aggressively
- Patient does not sustain injury

Nursing Diagnosis
Impaired Verbal Communication

Defining Characteristics

- Echolalia
- Mutism
- Inability to communicate in ways that are understood by others

Nursing Interventions

- Have same staff member care for child throughout visit
- Use good eye contact, simple words, and sentence structure in interacting with patient

Expected Outcome

- Patient has needs understood and addressed

Nursing Diagnosis
Anxiety

Defining Characteristics

- Increased tension, apprehension, and fear
- Helplessness
- Restlessness, increased motor activity
- Poor eye contact

Nursing Interventions

- Decrease stimuli
- Communicate calmly
- Remain with patient and reassure safety
- Administer medication as ordered

Expected Outcome

- Patient's anxiety is reduced by the decrease or absence of symptoms

Nursing Diagnosis
Impaired Social Interaction

Defining Characteristics

- Observed inability to relate
- Lack of responsiveness or interest in others
- Observed use of unsuccessful social skills

Nursing Interventions

- Promote trusting relationship

- Remain with patient
- Use favorite activities or familiar objects to join with patient

Expected Outcomes

- Patient uses eye contact and other forms of non-verbal communication
- Patient uses verbal contact with others
- Patient does not withdraw from attempts to relate

Management

Management of psychoses is complicated and involves a multidisciplinary approach. The goal in the pediatric ED is stabilization of the psychotic crisis, provision of safety, and involvement of psychiatric resources to provide evaluation and referral. Children with pre-existing psychotic disorders may come to the ED for treatment of a physical disorder, or they may arrive for treatment of an emotional crisis. Attempts are made to differentiate between an organic and a functional cause of the psychosis. A comprehensive approach to treatment includes therapy, parental involvement, therapeutic communication, in-patient or outpatient management and medication management.

Antipsychotic medication as one component of treatment may be initiated in the ED for the management of psychosis. Antipsychotic drugs are used to decrease thought disorganization and to allow a return to baseline functioning. Antipsychotic drugs also are used to manage assaultive, aggressive, and self-destructive behavior. These medications have a neuroleptic effect, which acts to sedate, and an antipsychotic effect, which acts to normalize thoughts and behavior. Antipsychotic agents can be used for autistic and psychotic children. The neuroleptic effect calms the agitation and aggression of an autistic or psychotic child and the antipsychotic effect calms the thought disorganization of a psychotic child (Keltner, 1991). Table 10–5 presents common medications.

Campbell and Spencer (1988) suggest that the drugs of choice for children and adolescents be high potency drugs such as haloperidol and thiothixone because these drugs have a less sedative effect at recommended dosages. In administering these medications, the nurse must be alert for two categories of side effects. Anticholinergic effects include dry mouth, blurred vision, constipation, urinary hesitation or retention, tachycardia, and nasal congestion. Extrapyramidal effects include muscle rigidity, dystonia, muscle spasms, motor restlessness, and oculogyric crisis, which is a medical emergency because the patient's airway can become blocked (Keltner, 1991). Benztropine mesylate, trihexyphenidyl, and diphenhydramine are medications that can be given to counteract extrapyramidal

TABLE 10–5. COMMONLY USED ANTIPSYCHOTIC MEDICATION FOR PSYCHOSES IN CHILDREN AND ADOLESCENTS

Name	Dosage and Route	Side Effects
Chlorpromazine	0.55 mg/kg q 6–8 hours po For acute crises 0.55 mg/kg q 6–8 hours im.	Anticholinergic and extrapyramidal effects
Thioridazine	0.5–3.0 mg/kg/day PO or 10 mg bid or tid for mild symptoms 25 mg bid or tid for severe symptoms	Same
Trifluoperazine	1 mg once a day or bid For rapid control 1 mg IM	Same
Fluphenazine	0.025–0.05 mg/kg up to 0.03 mg/kg per day	Same
Thiothixene	0.15–0.3 mg/kg day	Same
Haloperidol	0.05–0.15 mg/kg day	Same

side effects. Anticholinergic effects are managed by comfort measures such as the use of lozenges.

Interventions with psychotic children are geared primarily toward decreasing anxiety. The nurse approaches the child and family calmly and explains what is occurring in simple terms. Attempts are made to decrease environmental stimuli by having the patient and family wait in a separate room or alcove as opposed to a busy waiting area. A staff member who stays with the family can establish trust, provide support, and monitor for escalation of symptoms. Reassurance, support, and an emphasis on keeping the child safe and secure can decrease confusion and fear in both the child and family. Listening to their concerns and offering choices about aspects of care about which they can decide may enable a family to feel more empowered during a crisis. Assisting the child and family to focus on what is happening currently and what decisions need to be made serves to keep discussions focused on reality. While acknowledging the child's fear and anxiety, the nurse should keep interactions focused on the child's behavior rather than challenge the content of the disturbed thinking.

It may become necessary to physically restrain a psychotic child if less restrictive interventions are unsuccessful and the child's safety is compromised because of violent or aggressive behavior. Specific strategies for restraint are covered in the section on violence.

Establishing trust is also key in providing care to autistic children. Although a challenge in the ED, it may be helpful to slowly introduce an autistic child to a procedure in the presence of an adult the child trusts and with objects familiar to the child at hand. Zoltak (1986) suggests demonstrating procedures on parents first. Keeping directions concrete and using one-to-three word sentences may promote communication with an autistic child (Zoltak, 1986). Such strategies may help to prevent self mutilation, which sometimes occurs in response to anxiety. The nurse can utilize protective devices such as helmets or hand mitts to protect the child during episodes of self mutilation.

During psychotic episodes in children it is necessary to involve social workers and child psychiatrists in evaluation and referral. It is likely that a child with an acute functional psychosis will be admitted to an in-patient child psychiatric facility for safety and further treatment. Support to the family in making the decision to hospitalize a child is important; many families are ambivalent and uncertain as to whether or not they are doing the right thing. Children whose psychosis is not acute or who have a history of psychiatric illness may receive treatment and consultation in the ED and be discharged home with a specific plan, such as parental observation, medication and follow-up care at an outpatient facility or with their regular therapist. A social worker helps manage these linkages.

Patient and Family Teaching and Psychosocial Support

In addition to previously outlined support measures, successful management of a child's psychosis involves teaching on several different levels. Teaching should include assessment of parental use of resources and support groups, such as the National Society for Autistic Children and the National Alliance for the Mentally Ill, which are advocacy groups. There are many local chapters throughout the US. These support groups can enable families to increase their knowledge about psychiatric disorders and provide information about specific techniques in parenting, such as behavior management. Families are empowered through knowledge and sharing with others in similar situations.

Teaching also includes information about the uses, actions, and effects of prescribed medications. Parents are advised that drug therapy is but one aspect of a multifaceted approach so that their expectations of the medications are realistic. The nurse considers and integrates the child's developmental stage when teaching.

The parents are taught how to recognize a relapse of symptoms and what to do about them. Discharge and referral plans are reviewed. It may be helpful to provide the family with an appointment card.

VIOLENCE

Violent and aggressive behavior on the part of patients, their parents, and visitors is becoming common in pediatric EDs. Because the focus is on children, it is often easy to minimize the potential for violent behavior. The ways in which families cope with stress, frus-

tration, and grief seem to be escalating as families become easily angered, upset, aggressive, and violent. The trend parallels the rise in violence across the US as murder rates have doubled in the last 20 years (American College of Emergency Physicians, 1988). An increase in drug and alcohol use has been associated with increased homicidal behavior among teenagers (Muscari, 1992). Violence is being recognized as a major social problem.

Violence in a pediatric ED is complicated in that both children and families can exhibit violent behavior under stress. Caring for potentially violent children and family members presents a challenge to an emergency nurse. Given current trends, it is critical that preventive and acute approaches to the management of violence in the ED focus on the development of skills in staff to manage potentially violent situations and on institutional strategies to promote a safe and secure environment for the staff. The goal of crisis intervention with a violent child or family member is stabilization and safety for the child, family, and staff.

Etiology

The potential for violence is a state in which an individual is or may be assaultive toward others or the environment (Kim, 1984). The central theme in violent behavior is helplessness and powerlessness. Aggressive and assaultive behavior often is a defense against overwhelming feelings of helplessness. It can be understood as an attempt to regain some power and control in a situation. Violence usually is not random; it occurs in response to specific stresses and goes through phases related to goal obstruction and frustration (Kurlowicz, 1990; Maynard and Chitty, 1979). Many potentially violent people are fearful of losing control and want assistance in maintaining control. Mahoney (1991) identified four factors in EDs that contribute to violent behavior: (1) 24-hour-a-day accessibility; (2) an overstimulating physical environment that promotes tension and agitation; (3) the impact of illness and injury on the coping skills of families, resulting in aggressive behavior; and (4) staff frustration in regard to the nature of emergency nursing.

Violent behavior by pediatric patients may occur as a result of physical conditions masked by behavioral symptoms (eg, meningitis); emotional crisis (eg, underlying psychiatric disorders); or drug and alcohol consumption (Johnston, 1987). In addition, violent behavior on the part of family members may occur as a result of long waits, inadequate resources, domestic tensions, overstimulation, grief and loss, and drug or alcohol use.

Assessment

The prevention of violence involves recognizing which patients and families are at high risk. Specific behaviors that may indicate the potential for violence are as follows (Bjorn, 1991; Johnston, 1987; Kurlowicz, 1990; Nickens, 1984).

Indicators of a High Risk for Violence

- *History of aggression or violence*—one of the best predictors of violent behavior
- *Current Use of Drugs or Alcohol*—The use of substances decreases inhibitions and increases the risk for violent behavior. Laboratory testing includes a toxicology screen.
- Nonverbal and physical cues
    Increased psychomotor activity, such as pacing and restlessness
    Clenching of fists
    Intense facial expressions
    Rigid posture and increased muscle tension
    Quick, extreme changes in behavior and mood
    Confusion or difficulty cooperating
    Hostile body language and gesturing
    Overt aggressive acts

- Verbal cues
    Hallucinations and delusions, especially those of a persecutory nature
    Verbal threats of violence
    Angry, hostile statements
    Fear and expressed fear of losing control
    Suspiciousness
    Loud, intense, threatening speech

- Staff perception that a child or family member might lose control

The emergency nurse should assess for a history of assaultiveness or loss of control. She or he also should ascertain the circumstances of the violent act: "What was happening when the episode occurred?" The nurse should also find out if the child is exhibiting a typical reaction to stress and if the behavior is related to a physical condition.

As part of the assessment process, emergency nurses should evaluate all patients and families for the presence of indicators in addition to obtaining historical data.

Some physical conditions are masked by violent behavior. These include seizure disorders, meningitis, diabetes, head trauma, and hypoxia.

TRIAGE
Violence

Emergent ———————————————
Child, adolescent, parent, or visitor with minimal to no ability to focus on interview, listen to inter- viewer, or accept external direction. Person exhibiting assaultive behavior toward others or objects or is under the influence of drugs or alcohol.

Urgent ———————————————
Child, adolescent, parent, or visitor with decreasing ability to focus on interview. Person exhibiting argumentative behaviors as manifested by increased voice tone with threatening content and other nonverbal cues. Person making verbal or physical threats to others. Person who is receptive to calming efforts by staff, including external direction and limit-setting.

Non-urgent ———————————————
Child, adolescent, parent, or visitor who is mildly anxious.

Nursing Diagnosis
High Risk for Violence: Directed at Self or Others

Defining Characteristics

- Threatening body language, increased motor activity
- Overt aggressive acts
- Hostile, threatening verbalizations

Nursing Interventions

- Promote safe environment for child, family, and staff
- Reduce stimuli
- Maintain and convey a calm attitude and good eye contact
- Listen to concerns and assist in solving problems
- Convey clear, concise limits and expectations
- Have other staff available for back-up
- Administer medications as ordered
- Use mechanical restraints as last resort

Expected Outcomes

- Patient decreases violent behavior
- Patient, family, and staff are free from injury

Nursing Diagnosis
Ineffective Individual Coping

Defining Characteristics

- Inability to solve problems
- Chronic anxiety
- Poor self esteem

Nursing Interventions

- Establish trust through honesty and acceptance of the person
- Acknowledge patient's and family's response to stressful environment and loss of control
- Provide choices to promote sense of control
- Assist violent person in using alternative ways to handle frustration

Expected Outcome

- Patient and family are able to express anger or frustration in nondestructive ways

Management

Many clinicians agree that the most effective intervention in violent behavior is prevention (Johnston, 1987; Kurlowicz, 1990). Prevention occurs on two levels: (1) institutional systems that promote a safe environment, and (2) development of staff skills to recognize and intervene in violent situations. Institutional strategies to promote a safe and secure environment are outlined in Table 10–6 (Emergency room violence, 1989).

Treatment of a potentially violent patient or family member involves verbal communication strategies, pharmacologic agents, external controls to protect others from harm, and an evaluation of the underlying causes of the violence (Kurlowicz, 1990; Johnston, 1987) (Table 10–7). Talking is most effective when a person is in the beginning phases of escalation and has not yet demonstrated overt violence. Bjorn (1991) emphasizes the importance of communicating in a calm, confident, and nonjudgmental manner when dealing with aggression. Provision of information regarding procedures and what the child and family can expect along with reassurance that the child is in a safe place can have a calming effect. Listening, taking concerns seriously, and acknowledging the truth in what people are angry about also act to defuse aggressive behavior. Additional defusion techniques include offering sim-

TABLE 10–6. INSTITUTIONAL STRATEGIES TO PROMOTE SAFETY IN EMERGENCY DEPARTMENT

Visibility and control of ED entrances
Use of metal detectors
Use of silent alarm system
Provision of comfort (strategies to make waiting less stressful, such as snacks, drinks, magazines)
Separate space for seclusion and treatment of potentially violent people
Use of debriefing principles with staff
Facilities to separate patients with acute illness from those less seriously ill

Information from Emergency room violence: Dealing with a frightening and still growing problem. Hospital Security and Safety Management. 1989:10(4);5–12.

TABLE 10–7. PRINCIPLES IN THE MANAGEMENT OF POTENTIALLY VIOLENT PATIENTS AND FAMILY MEMBERS

- **VERBAL COMMUNICATION STRATEGIES**
  Use calm, confident voice tone
  Have nonjudgmental attitude
  Provide information
  Reassure the person of his or her safety
  Listen
  Take concerns seriously
  Offer choices
  Reduce stimuli
  Use the same caregivers throughout the visit
  Set limits

- **PHARMACOLOGIC AGENTS**
  Use antipsychotic medications as outlined in Table 10–5

- **EXTERNAL CONTROLS**
  Use physical restraints
  Have four staff members present; each one holds a limb
  Assess circulation
  Provide fluids and bathroom breaks
  Allow range of motion

- **EVALUATION OF THE UNDERLYING CAUSES OF VIOLENCE**
  Assess source of anger
  Perform toxicology screens
  Determine if there are underlying medical reasons for the violence

ple choices, reducing environmental stimuli, reorienting the person to the surroundings, and allowing the patient to interact with the same staff members throughout the visit (Bjorn, 1991; Kurlowicz, 1990).

Nurses attempt to identify the source of aggression as early as possible. It is important to allow the angry person to describe their experience rather than interpreting his or her actions. Observable behaviors are used as cues, for example, "I noticed you pacing the hallway. Would you sit down and tell me what's happening?" Multiple people interacting with the potentially aggressive person may promote impulsive behavior. Therefore, it is critical that one staff member intervene. As aggression continues to escalate, the nurse may need to set limits on maladaptive behavior. Limit-setting provides boundaries and promotes a safe environment. Limits placed on counterproductive behaviors should be simple and enforceable. Limits are not placed on feelings but on how the feelings are enacted (Lyon, 1970). For example, "I know you are upset about the long wait. I would like things to move along more quickly, but we cannot allow you to scream at the other families. Let's find some ways to make the time more bearable for you."

The nurse also monitors their own communication for undertones of frustration and anger. Aggressive behavior in children and families can escalate in response to perceived frustration in the caregiver, so a calm manner cannot be overemphasized. Common sense safety principles for staff in dealing with aggression include: (1) ready access to an exit; (2) maintenance of a safe distance from the aggressor; (3) keeping the person within view; and (4) mobilization of other staff.

Physical Restraints. If preventive measures and defusion techniques are ineffective or when the staff is confronted with overt violence by a child or adolescent, it may become necessary to restrain the violent patient with physical restraints. The priority is always the safety of others and the patient. Restraints are used in conjunction with crisis intervention measures and possibly with medication. Mechanical restraints are viewed as a temporary external means of assisting a patient to regain control when he or she is unable to do so. Just as code teams exist for medical emergencies, a restraint team of four or five staff members should be assembled for psychiatric emergencies. One person is in charge and each staff member is assigned a limb. The extra staff member can restrain limbs while the patient is being contained. During the restraint procedure, one staff member explains what is happening (Splawn, 1991). While a child is restrained, a staff member remains with him or her to observe the response to restraint and to provide reassurance. Other interventions for a child or adolescent in restraints include: (1) assessment of circulation at the restraint site; (2) provision of fluids and bathroom breaks; (3) periodic range of motion exercises for limbs; and (4) periodic release of the restraints (Splawn, 1991). Once the child has regained control, two restraints, such as the opposite arm and leg, are removed for 15 minutes; then the other two limbs are released. This process assists the child in making the transition from total external control toward gradual self control.

Medications. Chemical restraints in the form of medication may be used in addition to physical restraints to calm an agitated and violent patient. Although it is critical to treat the underlying medical reasons for assaultive behavior, as in acute meningitis, antipsychotic medication may be used as an adjunct. Antipsychotic medication also may be given for violence associated with an emotional crisis. Haloperidol is commonly given to calm violent behavior (Table 10–5). A minor tranquilizer such as lorazepam may be used in the earlier stages of agitation and aggression. If the patient's behavior has not escalated to the point of loss of physical control, oral medication may be offered with an emphasis on the patients' safety and security. If violence has escalated to the point that physical restraint becomes necessary, medication should be given quickly and efficiently, usually by intramuscular injec-

tion. This procedure should be explained to the patient as it is occurring. For example, "I am giving you some medicine to help you be calmer and in better control."

Children who exhibit violent behavior as a result of an emotional crisis are evaluated by a child psychiatrist for possible in-patient psychiatric treatment. Children who experience aggression with an organic cause have treatment initiated in the ED and may be admitted to the pediatric or intensive care unit for further treatment of the underlying medical disorder. A psychiatric consultation may be used to assist in managing aggressive behavior, both in the ED and once the child is admitted. Outpatient referral and counseling may be recommended for children who are mildly aggressive.

Unique to pediatric nursing is the issue of parental or visitor violence. The stress of having an acutely ill child can tax an already stressed family to the point of violence. Emergency department staff can use many of the principles used to manage violence on the part of a patient to treat aggressive family members. Protocols that stage aggressive behavior can be developed to guide nursing practice (Green, 1989).

Patient and Family Teaching and Psychosocial Support

Families with an aggressive and violent child often feel anxious and out of control themselves. Teaching should include the following.

Points to Include in Patient and Family Teaching on Violence

- Rationale for aggressive behavior (eg, underlying medical disorders, fear)
- Information and updates regarding care
- Rationale for use of chemical and or mechanical restraints, emphasizing patient safety
- Identification of triggers indicating potential for aggression
- Referral information

REFERENCES

Aguilera D, Messick J (1986). *Crisis intervention: Theory and methodology.* St. Louis: Mosby, pp 17–28

American College of Emergency Physicians (1988). *Emergency department violence: Prevention and management.* Dallas, TX: American College of Emergency Physicians

American Psychiatric Association (1987). *Diagnostic and statistical manual of mental disorders-R* (Revised). Washington DC: American Psychiatric Association

Bair S (1990). Acute psychiatric disorders. In Grossman M, Dieckmann R (eds), *Pediatric emergency medicine.* Philadelphia: Lippincott, pp 593–597

Bernstein L (1987). Patterns of dysfunctional reality orientation. In Haber J, et al (eds), *Comprehensive psychiatric nursing*. New York: McGraw-Hill, pp 719–769

Bjorn P (1991). Nurse educator: An approach to the potentially violent patient. *Journal of Emergency Nursing*, 17:336–339

Campbell M, Spencer EK (1988). Psychopharmacology in child and adolescent psychiatry: A review of the past five years. *Journal of the American Academy of Child and Adolescent Psychiatry* 27:269–279

Castiglia P (1990). Suicide in adolescents. *Journal of Pediatric Health Care* 4:149–151

Dalton S, Howell C (1989). Autism: psychobiological perspectives. *Journal of Child and Adolescent Psychiatric and Mental Health Nursing* 2:92–96

Emergency room violence: Dealing with a frightening and still growing problem (1989). *Hospital Security Safety Management* 10:5–12

Gemma P (1989). Coping with suicidal behavior. *Maternal Child Nursing Journal* 14:101–103

Gould MS, Shaffer D (1986). The impact of suicide in television movies. *New England Journal of Medicine* 315:690–694

Green E (1989). Patient care guidelines: Management of violent behavior. *Journal of Emergency Nursing* 15:523–528

Haber J (1987). Communication theories and application. In Haber J, et al (eds), *Comprehensive psychiatric nursing*. New York: McGraw-Hill, pp 225–254

Kanner L (1943). Autistic disturbances of affective contact. *Nervous child* 2:217–250

Johnston J (1987). Violence in the emergency department. *Emergency Nursing Reports* 1(12):1–7

Keltner N (1991). Psychopharmacology. In Clunn P (ed), *Child psychiatric nursing*. St Louis: Mosby, pp 380–395

Kim M, McFarland G, McLane A (1984). *Pocket guide to nursing diagnoses*. St Louis: Mosby, p 61

Krupnick S, Wade A (1993). *Psychiatric care planning*. Springhouse, PA: Springhouse Corp, pp 83–102

Kuperman S, Black DW, Burns TL (1988). Excess suicide among formerly hospitalized child psychiatry patients. *Journal of Clinical Psychiatry* 49:88

Kurlowicz L (1990). Violence in the emergency department. *American Journal of Nursing* 90(9):35–40

Lyon GL (1970). Limit setting as a therapeutic tool. *Journal of Psychiatric Nursing and Mental Health Services* Nov/Dec: 8(6);17–24

Mahoney B (1991). The extent, nature and response to victimization of emergency nurses in PA. *Journal of Emergency Nursing* 17:282–292

Maynard C, Chitty K (1979). Dealing with anger: Guidelines for nursing intervention. *Journal of Psychiatric Nursing and Mental Health Services* 17:36–41

Muscari M (1992). The acting out adolescent: Identification and management. *Pediatric Nursing* 18:362–366

Muse N (1990). *Depression and suicide in children and adolescents*. Austin, Texas: Pro ed, pp 7–41

Myers K, McCauley E, Calderon R, Mitchell J, Burke P, Schloredt K (1991). Risks for suicidality in major depressive disorder. *Journal of American Academy of Child and Adolescent Psychiatry* 30:86–94

Nickens HW (1984). Assessment and management of the violent patient. In Dubin WR (ed), *Psychiatric emergencies*. New York: Churchill Livingstone, pp 101–109

Patros P, Shamoo T (1989). *Depression and suicide in children & adolescents*. Boston: Allyn & Bacon, pp 81–104

Pearson G (1992). Nursing interventions with children and adolescents experiencing thought disorders. In West P, Evans C (eds), *Psychiatric and mental health nursing with children and adolescents*. Gaithersburg, Maryland: Aspen, pp 329–342

Pfeffer C (1985). Death preoccupations and suicidal behavior in children. *Issues in Comprehensive Pediatric Nursing* 8:261–277

Pfeffer C (1987). *The suicidal child*. New York: Guilford, pp 60, 173–192

Poster E (1987). Behavioral problems. In Smith M, Goodman J, Ramsey N. *Child and family: Concepts of nursing practice* New York: McGraw-Hill, pp 1263–1293

Rotheram-Borus M, Trautman P (1988). Hopelessness, depression and suicidal intent among adolescent suicide attempters. *Journal of the American Academy of Child and Adolescent Psychiatry* 27:700–704

Sabbath JC (1970). The suicidal adolescent: The expendable child. *Journal of American Academy of Child Psychiatry* 8:272–289

Splawn G (1991). Restraining potentially violent patients. *Journal of Emergency Nursing* 17:316–317

Srnec P (1991). Children, violence and intentional injuries. *Critical Care Nursing Clinics of North America* 3:471–478

Valente S (1987). Assessing suicide risk in the school age child. *Journal of Pediatric Health Care* 1:14–20

Valente S (1992). Nursing interventions with children and adolescents experiencing self-destructive tendencies. In West P, Evans C (eds), *Psychiatric and mental health nursing with children & adolescents*. Gaithersburg, Maryland: Aspen, pp 315–328

Zoltak B (1986). Autism: Recognition and management. *Pediatric Nursing* 12:90–94

SUGGESTED READING

Barlow D (1989). Therapeutic holding: Effective intervention with the aggressive child. *Journal of Psychosocial Nursing* 27:10–14

Fremouw W, Perczel M, Ellis T (1990). *Suicide risk: Assessment and response guidelines*. New York: Pergamon

Hogarty S, Rodaitis C (1987). A suicide precautions policy for the general hospital. *Journal of Nursing Administration* 17:36–40

Martin L, Francisco E, Nicol C, Schweiger J (1991). A hospital wide approach to crisis control: One inner city hospital's experience. *Journal of Emergency Nursing* 17:395–401

Newell-Withrow C (1987). Observations of children, youth & violence. *Journal of Pediatric Health Care* 1:77–83

Pfeffer C (1989). *Suicide among youth: Perspectives on risk and prevention*. Washington, DC: American Psychiatric Press

Saunders D (1991). Family violence. *Emergency Care Quarterly* 7:51–56

Walker M, Moreau D, Weissman M (1990). Parents awareness of children's suicide attempts. *American Journal of Psychiatry* 147:1364–1366

CHAPTER 11

Sudden Infant Death Syndrome

MARY E. McCLAIN

INTRODUCTION

Sudden infant death syndrome (SIDS) is the sudden death of an infant younger than 1 year of age that remains unexplained after the performance of a complete postmortem investigation, including an autopsy, an examination of the scene of death, and a review of the case history (National Sudden Infant Death Syndrome Clearing House, 1990b). Families whose babies die of SIDS face an extraordinary crisis. There is no preparation and no warning for the infant's death. The shock of finding an unresponsive infant leaves family members in disbelief and in a state of disorganization. The entire family system is changed (Mandell and McClain, 1988). According to the National Center for Health Statistics, SIDS is the leading cause of post-neonatal deaths (deaths occurring 28 days–1 year after birth) in the United States. The worldwide incidence of SIDS is 2 deaths per 1000 live births; the incidence in the US is 1.37 deaths per 1000 live births. Five to seven thousand infants in the US die of SIDS each year. In 1986, SIDS accounted for an estimated 336,884 years of potential life lost (YPLL) and was ranked as the eighth leading cause of YPLL (National Sudden Infant Death Syndrome Clearing House, 1990).

Sudden infant death syndrome occurs in families from all racial, cultural and socioeconomic backgrounds. In 1987 the National Center for Health Statistics reported 5230 deaths of SIDS in the United States. Racial and cultural differences accounted for different rates of occurrence. The incidence of SIDS in the US in 1987 was reported by the National SIDS Clearinghouse as 1.37 deaths per 1000 live births for all infants; for whites it was 1.20 deaths per 1000 and for African

Americans it was 2.26 deaths per 1000. The incidence of SIDS among the Northern Plains Indians is reported to be 5.7 deaths per 1000 births (Oyen et al, 1990) and among Asian American babies in California to be 1.1 deaths per 1000 live births (Grether et al, 1990). Sixty percent of infants who die of SIDS are boys. Infants who die of SIDS are usually 2–4 months of age. Infants usually die in their sleep. Death occurs within a matter of seconds and is silent. For these reasons, it is believed that the death does not cause pain or suffering to the baby.

ETIOLOGY AND PATHOPHYSIOLOGY

Many theories related to the cause of SIDS have been proposed, yet the cause remains unknown. The National Institute of Child Health and Human Development (NICHD) SIDS Cooperative Epidemiological Study identified statistically significant risk factors for SIDS, but identifying the factors has not resulted in the prevention of SIDS in vulnerable infants (Hoffman et al, 1988). Fifty to seventy percent of infants who die of SIDS have a slight cold when they die, but the cold is not considered to be the cause of or a risk factor for SIDS. The risk of recurrence of SIDS in a family is low (Guntheroth et al, 1990; Irgens et al, 1984; Peterson et al, 1986). Additional maternal and infant risk factors (Hoffman et al, 1988) are listed in Table 11–1.

Sudden infant death syndrome is not caused by external suffocation, vomiting, or choking. It is not contagious, and it cannot be predicted or prevented, even by a physician. No increased risk for SIDS is associated with diphtheria-pertussis-tetanus (DPT)

TABLE 11–1. RISK FACTORS FOR SIDS

- MATERNAL RISK FACTORS
  Maternal age < 20 years at first pregnancy
  Maternal education < 12 years
  Inadequate prenatal care
  Weight gain less than 20 lbs
  Cigarette smoking
  Urinary tract infection
  Anemia
  Illicit drug use

- NEWBORN RISK FACTORS
  Cyanosis
  Tachycardia
  Fever
  Irritability
  Respiratory distress
  Hypothermia
  Poor feeding
  Tachypnea

- INFANT RISK FACTORS
  Male sex
  Parity > 2
  Prematurity
  Low birthweight
  Multiple gestation
  Diarrhea and vomiting during last 2 weeks before death
  Listless or droopy appearance in last 2 weeks before death

immunization or newborn apnea. An autopsy reveals no identifiable cause of death. Typical autopsy findings are summarized in Table 11–2. The American Academy of Pediatrics (AAP) in 1992 issued a statement indicating a possible relation between the prone sleeping position and SIDS. The AAP recommended that a healthy infant be positioned on its side or back when being put in its bed (American Academy of Pediatrics Task Force on Infant Positioning and SIDS, 1992). Other reports (Hunt and Shannon, 1992; Mit-

TABLE 11–2. AUTOPSY FINDINGS FOR SIDS

- AUTOPSY
  No identifiable cause of death found

- FINDINGS INCLUDE
  Pulmonary congestion and edema
  Inflammatory changes in trachea
  Intrathoracic petechial hemorrhages (85% of cases)

- AUTOPSY RULES OUT
  Infection—sepsis, meningitis, encephalitis, pneumonia, botulism
  Cardiac disease—myocarditis, congenital heart disease, sudden arrhythmia
  Aspiration or airway obstruction
  Trauma
  Congenital anomalies
  Genetic disorders

chell and Mandell, 1992), however, called for scientific research to investigate the relation between sleeping position and SIDS before recommending a major change in infant sleeping practices in the US.

The NICHD in its 5-year research plan for SIDS seeks to study the occurrence of SIDS and the biologic, medical and physical aspects of the syndrome (National Sudden Infant Death Syndrome Clearing House, 1990). Research projects include studies of infants at high risk, investigation of cardiorespiratory and sleep factors, infant behavior, and infectious diseases; and immunologic, metabolic, neurologic, and pathologic studies. The NICHD research plan flows from the hypothesis "that infants who die of SIDS are more vulnerable than average infants to internal or external stress factors due to some developmental abnormalities that occur in fetal development" (National Sudden Infant Death Syndrome Clearing House, 1991, p 3). Future research to prevent SIDS will explore how internal and external factors interact to cause infants to die.

When an unresponsive infant is brought to a hospital emergency department (ED), nurses provide care to both the infant and the family. The use of a form in the ED (Figure 11–1) is helpful in obtaining the information needed in cases of SIDS.

THE INFANT

Assessment

History. Typically, a parent or caretaker states that their apparently well infant was put down for sleep and was found unresponsive seconds, minutes, or hours later. The infant is often found face down on a crib mattress, occasionally covered with a blanket. The infant also may be found unresponsive in a parent's bed, carriage, car seat, infant carrier, or a parent's arms. The infant may be in a supine position or on its side. No outcry or apparent sign of struggle is noted by the parent. The infant may have had recent symptoms of a slight cold, ie, sniffles, a runny nose, a cough, or a stuffy nose. Cardiopulmonary resuscitation (CPR) may be initiated by a parent or caretaker, a police officer, or an emergency medical technician and continued during transport to the hospital.

In general, the infant is apparently well, often was seen recently by a pediatrician, is taking no medication, and has no history of allergies. The infant seldom is a subsequent sibling of an infant who has died of SIDS, seldom has a history of infantile apnea, and seldom has a history of illness within the previous 2 weeks.

Massachusetts Center for SIDS
Emergency Room Form

Patient Information

Name: _____   Age: _____   Sex: M _____   F _____

Birthdate: _____

Last seen alive: Date _____   Time _____

Found dead: Date _____   Time _____

By whom: _____

Place: Crib, parent's bed, other _____

Position: _____

Appearance of Infant: Body temperature _____

Color of skin _____

Nasopharyngeal discharge: Yes _____   No _____

Resuscitative Efforts

CPR: Yes _____   No _____

Intracardiac medication: Yes _____   No _____

Other medication (Please specify) _____

_____

Birth and Medical History

Birthweight: _____   Gestational age: _____   Birthplace: _____

Source of medical care: _____

Well baby visits: Yes _____   No _____   Unknown _____

Most recent visit _____

Most recent weight _____

Immunizations: Yes _____   No _____   Date _____

Type of feeding: Breast _____   Bottle _____   Both _____

Illness in last two weeks: Yes _____   No _____

Cold, sniffles, stuffy nose _____

Figure 11–1. An emergency department information form. (From McClain M, Project Coordinator (1992). *SIDS: A guide for emergency department personnel*. Boston: Massachusetts Center for Sudden Infant Death Syndrome)

(*continued*)

GI symptoms _____

Other minor/major _____

Describe _____

Medical Examiner

Name: _____

Autopsy: Yes _____   No _____   By whom: _____

Parental Data:

Mother: _____   Age: _____   Father: _____   Age: _____

Address: _____

Telephone: _____   Emergency phone: _____

Pregnancy complications: _____

_____

Type of delivery: _____   Anesthesia: _____

Complications during labor, delivery or neonatal period: _____

_____

_____

Previous infant deaths: Yes _____   No _____   Cause _____

Number of siblings: _____

Report filed by: _____

Date: _____

Figure 11–1. (*Continued*)

Physical Assessment and Findings. There are no signs that vital organ systems are functioning. The infant on arrival to the ED is unresponsive, pale, and cyanotic and has a cool body temperature. There may be a blood-tinged frothy discharge from mouth or nose and vomitus on the face. The diaper is usually wet and full of stool. Lividity and rigor mortis (purple mottled markings on the head and face) may be present. The infant appears to be well nourished and well developed.

Laboratory and Diagnostic Tests. The medical team evaluates the appropriateness of continuing or terminating resuscitative measures. Full body x rays and a blood culture may be ordered by the attending physician. The infant's body is examined for obvious signs of abuse, injury, or neglect, such as broken bones, bruises, burns, cuts, head trauma, scars, welts, wounds, and malnutrition. Any diagnosis made in the ED is tentative pending an autopsy unless there is a documented disease or obvious severe injury. When the infant's history is compatible with SIDS, a presumptive diagnosis of SIDS can be made.

T R I A G E
Sudden Infant Death Syndrome

Emergent ——————————————
Any infant in cardiopulmonary arrest.

Nursing Diagnosis
Inability to Sustain Spontaneous Ventilation

Defining Characteristics

- Vital signs absent
- Cool body temperature
- Blood tinged frothy fluid from mouth or nose
- Vomitus on face
- Diaper wet and full of stool
- Lividity
- Rigor mortis

Nursing Interventions

- Initiate or continue cardiopulmonary resuscitation
- Administer oxygen
- Administer medication as ordered
- Administer intravenous fluids as ordered
- Monitor vital signs

Expected Outcome

- The infant cannot be successfully resuscitated if SIDS has occurred

THE FAMILY

Assessment

History. Family members have a variety of reactions. The parents are in a state of shock precipitated by finding an unresponsive infant with physical changes associated with SIDS. Parents whose child dies in the care of someone else may not have seen the infant before arriving at the hospital and may have little information about what happened to the baby.

Physical Assessment. Parents respond to crisis in several ways. Their emotional state is influenced by cultural background, the severity of the grief reaction, and previous coping in response to other losses. Assessment should determine if the parent is using medication, especially tranquilizers or mood altering drugs; is using alcohol or other drugs; has a history of depression or suicide attempts; or has had another infant, child, or family member die or has had another serious loss. The special circumstances of grieving single parents, adolescent parents, childcare providers, siblings, families with multiple problems, and parents newly arrived in the US require assessment. The family's religious, folk, or spiritual beliefs and language barriers may require special intervention.

T R I A G E
Sudden Infant Death Syndrome

Emergent ——————————————
Family with infant in cardiopulmonary arrest.

Nursing Diagnosis
Functional Grieving

Defining Characteristics

- Shock
- Agitation
- Anxiety
- Hysteria
- Crying, screaming
- Collapse

- Physical shaking
- Immobilization
- Flat affect
- Sadness
- Anger
- Striking out
- Injurious behavior toward oneself

Nursing Interventions

- Provide private space for parents
- Assign staff member to remain with parents
- Inform parents of status of resuscitation
- Gather family support system—family members, clergy
- Inform parents in a sensitive and caring manner that resuscitation has been unsuccessful and that infant has died
- Discuss need for autopsy and explain the autopsy procedure to parents or family
- Allow free expression of grief
- Validate what parents are expressing
- Refer to the baby by name and encourage parents to talk about the baby
- Assure parents they are in no way responsible for the baby's death
- Encourage parents to see and hold the baby's body (accompany them if necessary)
- Be emotionally available
- Assist parents in relinquishing the baby's body
- Help parents with decision-making and guide them toward healthy grieving
- Give parents permission to leave hospital
- Encourage parents to participate in local SIDS program support services (National Sudden Infant Death Syndrome Clearing House, 1991a)
- Provide anticipatory guidance that it is normal to experience sleep and appetite disturbances, dreams, hearing and seeing the baby, especially the sight of the baby's body when found
- Inform parents of 24-hour availability of professional support services through local SIDS program, hospital counselors, or other mental health counselors

Expected Outcomes

- Parents express grief
- Parents are aware baby has died
- Parents acknowledge autopsy will be performed
- Parents recognize SIDS as one possible cause of infant's death
- Family members have seen or held infant
- Social supports are available to parents in emergency setting
- Parents relinquish baby's body

Nursing Diagnosis
Ineffective Family Coping: Compromised

Defining Characteristics

- Severe expressions of grief continue or increase in severity, ie, hysteria, undirected screaming, striking out at others, injurious behavior to oneself
- Parents refuse to see or hold baby's body
- Parents deny baby is dead
- Parents unable to relinquish baby's body

Nursing Interventions

- Continue interventions
- Continue assessment of severity of grief reactions
- Provide medication if necessary
- Enlist psychiatric nursing or social service support
- Continue assurance to parents they did not cause the baby's death
- Admit parents with extreme or psychotic episode to hospital if necessary
- Provide anticipatory guidance regarding grieving process

Expected Outcomes

- Severe grief reaction decreases
- Parents verbalize awareness they did not cause baby's death
- Parents acknowledge wide range of feelings and reactions are normal for the trauma they have experienced

Nursing Diagnosis
Knowledge Deficit (Sudden Unexpected Death of Infant)

Defining Characteristics

- Parents indicate infant suffocated or choked
- Parents indicate lack of knowledge of what happened to the baby
- Parents express guilt that the baby's death was their fault

Nursing Interventions

- Provide information about SIDS if medical differential diagnosis indicates SIDS as presumptive cause of death
- Assure parents the death was not their fault
- Explain the necessity for an autopsy, the autopsy procedure, where the infant will go for the autopsy, when the parents will be notified of results
- Refer family to local SIDS support program

Expected Outcomes

- Parents are able to recognize SIDS as one possible cause of their infant's death
- Parents are aware an autopsy will be performed
- Parents are aware they will receive preliminary autopsy findings within 24–48 hours
- Parents and extended family are aware of local SIDS support services and how to contact SIDS 24-hour hotline or other psychiatric emergency services

Management

When an infant is found unresponsive by a parent or caretaker, the emergency response system is called. The police and emergency medical technicians who arrive at the scene assess the status of the infant, initiate or continue resuscitative measures, and transport the infant to the nearest ED. Occasionally an infant may not be transported if she or he has been dead for a long period of time. Parents sometimes transport the infant to the hospital themselves.

Figure 11–2 provides a summary of interventions in the form of a checklist that can be used by ED personnel to assure that each intervention is completed in cases of SIDS. In the ED the infant is evaluated and emergency resuscitative measures instituted or continued. A nurse should remain with the parents and inform them of what is happening to their baby. Parents need to be assured that everything possible is being done for the child.

When resuscitative efforts are ineffective, the infant is pronounced dead by the attending physician. The medical examiner who has jurisdiction in the case is notified, investigates the circumstances of death, makes the final decision concerning the performance of the autopsy, and releases the infant's body for transportation for autopsy.

Informing the Parents. It is desirable that the physician in charge of the resuscitative effort or the primary care physician and the emergency team member assigned to the family be present when the family is informed of the baby's death. Before speaking with the family, attending personnel should review the circumstances of death and the infant's medical history. If the findings are compatible with SIDS, that is, an apparently well infant who may have had a mild upper respiratory infection and is younger than 1 year died in its sleep, a *presumptive* diagnosis of SIDS may be made. Any presumptive diagnosis in the emergency setting is tentative pending an autopsy unless there is documented disease or obvious severe injury. Case review assists the team in discussing the child's death with the family. Through a sensitive approach, ED staff can assist family members as they grieve. The first contacts at the time of the infant's death are extremely important, and parents long remember what is said to them.

The family can be told that an autopsy will confirm the cause of death. Often parents are reluctant or resistant to an autopsy because of cultural and religious beliefs or fear that the baby's body will be mutilated. It is helpful for the physician or nurse to explain that an autopsy is a medical procedure similar to an operation. The parents are told the autopsy is performed by a pathologist in a respectful manner and that they will be able to see the baby after the autopsy. The autopsy eliminates any unsuspected illness, congenital anomaly, inherited disorder, injury, and aspiration as the cause of death. Often when autopsies are not performed, parents regret the decision because of lingering doubts about the cause of death (McClain, 1992).

It may be difficult for parents in a state of shock to assimilate what has happened. It is important to provide adequate information to families, especially to assure grieving parents that they were in no way responsible for their baby's death.

Psychosocial Support. Each person reacts differently to the sudden unexpected death of a baby. It is important for ED personnel to respond to the needs of family members keeping in mind individual differences and cultural beliefs and practices. A member of the emergency team should stay with the parents as much as possible to provide support and to answer questions. In the event of complicated grief reactions, a social worker, psychiatric nurse, or member of the clergy may be contacted for immediate crisis intervention.

The nurse should be prepared for difficult situations, including extremes in behavior, such as screaming, collapsing, or even expressing no emotion. Parents should be encouraged to talk about the baby using the baby's name. Permission is given for the family to grieve as they must. Professional intervention at this time, soon after the death, may set the tone for the entire process of grieving. A caring, sensitive approach facilitates healthy grieving.

Parents should be encouraged to see and hold their baby after the baby has died to enable them to focus on the reality of the death and to provide an opportunity to say good-bye. The baby should be bathed and wrapped in a blanket before the parents see the body. Resuscitative equipment (tubes, catheters) should be removed. If it is not possible to remove equipment because of legal requirements, the equipment should be covered or made as inobtrusive as possible. The member of the emergency staff who has

EMERGENCY DEPARTMENT CHECKLIST
FOR SUDDEN INFANT DEATH

☐ Resuscitation

☐ Staff person assigned to family members

☐ Primary care physician notified

☐ Medical examiner notified

☐ Clergy called (hospital chaplain and/or family clergy) if parents desire

☐ Family notification of death and tentative cause (essential family members present
   in emergency department)

☐ Family permitted to see baby

☐ Family given keepsakes such as lock of hair, footprint and Polaroid picture of infant

☐ Family allowed to express grief; staff responds to individual needs

☐ Family understands how they may receive autopsy report

☐ If tentative SIDS diagnosis—SIDS facts pamphlet given to family

☐ Family informed of follow-up services by the Massachusetts SIDS Center

☐ ED chart completed

☐ ED staff conference

Patient's name: ─────────────────────────────

Staff member: ──────────────────   Date: ──────────────

Figure 11–2. An emergency department checklist for SIDS. (From McClain M, Project Coordinator (1992). *SIDS: A guide for emergency department personnel.* Boston: Massachusetts Center for Sudden Infant Death Syndrome)

been with the family should accompany the parents to view the baby's body and reassure them as they touch and hold their child. Support should be given to the parents during and after the time they see their infant.

Efforts should be made to contact absent family members or any individual whose presence and support is important to the family. The presence of a member of the clergy or the performance of rituals such as baptism should be discussed. Because many parents are unfamiliar with procedures concerning funeral arrangements, it may be helpful to inform the family of the necessity of contacting a funeral director and a member of the clergy for assistance. The funeral director assumes the responsibility for the infant's body after it is released from the medical examiner or hospital.

Follow-up Care
The parents are referred to the local SIDS support program. If necessary they are referred to the mental health crisis team in the hospital or the community.

Emergency Team Conference
It may be helpful for the ED staff to meet for support and to discuss feelings and concerns regarding the unsuccessful resuscitation and the family's anguish. The emotional drain on the ED staff needs to be taken into account and addressed. It is helpful to evaluate intervention strategies with families to gain a sense of competency. Was the family supported at the time of crisis and was provision made for follow-up care? Appropriate intervention in the emergency setting sets the tone for how parents begin to cope with the impact of an infant's death. Supportive care in the immediate crisis period in conjunction with long-term follow-up care promotes mental health and reduces the incidence of psychiatric morbidity.

PATIENT OUTCOME

If a nurse has been successful caring for parents whose child has died suddenly the parents' intense reactions have decreased. That is, hysteria has been allayed, and undirected screaming, striking out at others, and injurious behavior toward themselves have stopped. The parents are aware the baby has died and they understand an autopsy will be performed. The parents have seen and held the infant after resuscitative efforts have been discontinued. The parents recognize feelings of guilt about the infant's death even if they are unable to control these feelings. The parents recognize SIDS as one possible cause of the infant's death. The parents and extended family are aware of the local SIDS support services and know how to contact them. The parents are aware they will be notified of the preliminary autopsy results within 24 hours. Before the family leaves the ED they should be told when and by whom they will be informed of the autopsy results. The nurse should find out where the family can be reached; frequently parents do not return to their own homes. The nurse should contact the SIDS program in the area (Table 11–3) to facilitate family follow-up counseling (National Sudden Infant Death Syndrome Clearing House, 1991a). If appropriate, the family is given a SIDS fact sheet and the local SIDS program telephone number.

TABLE 11–3. NATIONAL SIDS ORGANIZATIONS

Association of SIDS Program Professionals
C/O Massachusetts Center for SIDS
Boston City Hospital
818 Harrison Avenue
Boston, MA 02118
617-534-7437

Sudden Infant Death Syndrome Alliance
10500 Little Patuxent Parkway
Suite 420
Columbia, MD 21044
800-221-7437

National SIDS Resource Center
8201 Greensboro Drive
Suite 600
McLean, VA 22102
703-821-8955

REFERENCES

American Academy of Pediatrics Task Force on Infant Positioning and SIDS (1990). Positioning and SIDS. *Pediatrics* 89:1120–1126

Grether JK, et al (1990). Sudden infant death syndrome among Asians in California. *Journal of Pediatrics* 4:525–528

Guntheroth W, Lohrmann R, Spiers P (1990). Risk of sudden infant death syndrome in subsequent siblings. *Journal of Pediatrics* 4:520–524

Hoffman H, Damus K, Hillman L, Krongrad E (1988). Risk factors for SIDS: Results of the National Institute of Child Health and Human Development SIDS cooperative epidemiological study. *Annals New York Academy of Sciences* 533:13–30

Hunt C, Shannon D (1992). Sudden infant death syndrome and sleeping position. *Pediatrics* 90:115–118

Irgens LM, Skjaerven R, Peterson DR (1984). Prospective assessment of recurrence risk in sudden infant death syndrome. *Journal of Pediatrics* 104:349–351

Mandell F, McClain M (1988). Supporting the SIDS family. *Pediatrician* 15:180

McClain M (1992). *Sudden infant death syndrome: A guide for emergency department personnel.* Boston, Mass: Massachusetts Center for SIDS, 1992 (Revised)

Mitchell A, Mandell F (1992). Critical review: Does the prone sleep position cause SIDS? *Pediatric Alert* 17:3–6.

National Sudden Infant Death Syndrome Clearinghouse (1990). Sudden infant death syndrome statistical review. *Information Exchange* January: 1–3

National Sudden Infant Death Syndrome Clearinghouse (1991a). *Directory of State Title V. Maternal and Child Health Directors, and SIDS Program Coordinators.* McLean, Va: National Sudden Infant Death Syndrome Clearinghouse, pp 1–21

National Sudden Infant Death Syndrome Clearinghouse (1991b). SIDS research. Part II. Current and future directions. *Information Exchange* November: 1–8

Oyen N, Bulterys M, Welty TK, Kraus JF (1990). Sudden unexplained infant deaths among American Indians and whites in North and South Dakota. *Pediatric and Perinatal Epidemiology*, 4 (1990): 175–182

Peterson DR, Sabotta EE, Daling JR (1986). Infant mortality among subsequent siblings of infants who died of sudden infant death syndrome. *Journal of Pediatrics* 108:911–914

SUGGESTED READING

Corr CA, Fuller H, Barnickol CA, et al (eds) (1991). *Sudden infant death syndrome: Who can help and how?* New York: Springer.

DeFrain J, Ernst L, Jacub D, Taylor J (1991). *Sudden infant death: Enduring the loss.* Lexington, Mass: Lexington Books

Guist C (1986). Responding to an unexpected infant death. *Emergency Update* 4:1–4

Mandell F (ed) (1988). *Pediatrician,* Volume 15. (Entire issue on SIDS)

Willinger M (1989). SIDS: A challenge. *Journal of NIH Research* 1:73–80

PART 3

Cardiorespiratory Emergencies

CHAPTER 12

Newborn Care and Resuscitation

VIRGINIA L. DODD

INTRODUCTION

Delivery of a baby, or admission of a newborn baby, does not occur frequently in the emergency department (ED). Most emergency personnel are unfamiliar or unpracticed in handling perinatal emergencies. In one study, one of every 160 deliveries occurred before the mother arrived at the hospital or in the ED (Brunette, 1989). Of these, one-third of the children were born at home and almost one-half were born in the ED. The mortality for unplanned home deliveries is 10–20 times the mortality of in-hospital deliveries (Burnett et al, 1980; Schramm et al, 1987; Tyson, 1991). The morbidity is also considerably higher than for hospital deliveries. Harper et al (1990) reported that many of the mothers who had these deliveries had some prenatal care. Most mothers were multiparous, since the duration of labor is shorter after the first baby, though some were primiparous. Many of the deliveries are associated with unusual bleeding.

This chapter discusses management when delivery is imminent, care of a healthy newborn, and resuscitation of a compromised infant. Care of a premature infant, and of possible congenital defects, especially congenital heart problems also is presented. Preparation for transport and support of the family are described.

IMMINENT DELIVERY

If at all possible, delivery of a baby should not occur in the ED. Delivery should occur under sterile conditions; facilities should be available for emergency cesarean section, and personnel should be skilled, not only in the delivery process but also in newborn resuscitation. Although EDs usually are considered the appropriate location for emergency care, in the case of delivery of a baby, every effort should be made to transport the mother to a delivery room.

Etiology and Physiology

A woman may come into the ED for delivery for many reasons. She may have experienced trauma, acute hypertension induced by pregnancy, abrupt separation of the placenta, profuse bleeding, or very rapid onset and progression of labor. Other reasons for women to come to the ED in labor may be denial of pregnancy, acute abdominal pain, and recent ingestion of cocaine. Delivery may have occurred before arrival in the ED because of complications of a planned home delivery or labor progressing too rapidly for the woman to get to the ED before delivery.

Stages of Labor. The first stage of labor involves the thinning and dilation of the cervix. In first pregnancies it generally takes 11 hours (2.3–19.7 hours) for the cervix to dilate completely (Friedman, 1978). In multiparous pregnancies dilation usually lasts 7.2 hours (0.1–14.3 hours). The second stage of labor is the passage of the infant down the birth canal and delivery. The second stage lasts 1.1 hours (0.3–1.9 hours) in first pregnancies and 0.39 hours (0.09–.69 hours) in subsequent pregnancies. It is still unknown what triggers the onset of labor.

Assessment

History. The most urgent aspects of the history to ascertain are the expected due date, any prenatal problems, whether membranes are ruptured, whether there is any bleeding or meconium staining, if there have been changes in fetal movement, and if there are multiple fetuses (Boychuk, 1991; Higgins, 1987). Additional quickly ascertained factors include whether there are allergies or chronic illnesses, whether any medications or street drugs have been taken and the time of the last dose, and information on past pregnancies and outcomes (Lamb and Rosner, 1987). If time permits, and to make the history more complete, information about other risk factors (Table 12–1) should be elicited.

Physical Assessment. Assessment should begin as soon as health care personnel come in contact with the mother. The stage of labor should be assessed first along with maternal vital signs, including blood pressure. Assessment of the stage of labor includes timing contractions and examination for visualization of fetal parts. Imminent delivery is characterized by an uncontrollable urge to push, which may be exhibited by involuntary holding of breath and subtle or obvious pushing or the mother's statement that something's pushing; perineal bulging; rectal bulging; the sensation of an impending bowel movement or involuntary emptying of the rectum; and crowning of the fetus's head or presentation of another fetal part (Doan-Wiggins, 1991; Higgins, 1987). Fetal heart tones should be auscultated. The fetal heart beat should vary beat to beat; it slows with the onset of a contraction. The heart rate should increase as the contraction ends and should never go below 100 beats per minute. When decelerations are prolonged after a contraction ends, the fetus is in distress, experiencing hypoxia, and intervention is needed. Fetal vital signs indicating fetal distress are presented in Table 12–2.

TRIAGE
Delivery

Emergent

Infant delivered before arrival at the hospital or in the emergency department.

Management

If delivery is imminent, preparations should be made to deliver the infant on the spot instead of trying to reach a delivery facility. Preparations should be made

TABLE 12–1. NEONATAL HIGH-RISK FACTORS

Prenatal	Perinatal	Postnatal
■ MATERNAL	■ MATERNAL	■ FETAL
Older than 35 years	Hypotension	Respiratory distress
Younger than 16 years	Prolonged labor	Asphyxia
Diabetes	Placenta previa	Hypotension
Hypertension	Abruptio placenta	Meconium staining
Third-trimester bleeding	Drug use	Prematurity
Infection	Cesarean section	Small for dates
Premature rupture of membranes	■ FETAL	
Drug ingestion or therapy	Abnormal presentation	
Drug abuse	Prolapsed cord	
Anemia	Abnormal heart rate	
Rh sensitization	Meconium-stained fluid	
Cardiac, hepatic, or renal disease	Poly- or oligohydramnios	
Toxemia	Forceps delivery	
Preeclampsia, eclampsia	Asphyxia	
No prenatal care		
■ FETAL		
Fetal distress on monitor		
Meconium-stained amniotic fluid		
Premature labor		
Postmature labor		
Intrauterine growth retardation		

(Reproduced with permission from Schafermeyer R (1993). Neonatal Resuscitation. In Fleisher G, Ludwig S [eds.], Textbook of pediatric emergency medicine [3rd ed]. Baltimore: Williams & Wilkins, p 33)

calmly but expeditiously, and every effort should be made to avoid upsetting the mother. Trying to delay delivery or attempting to push the baby back is contraindicated. Higgins (1987) provides a review of ED delivery and includes a section related to emergency cesarean section during resuscitation of the mother to increase the chance of survival of both the mother and the infant.

TABLE 12–2. SIGNS OF FETAL DISTRESS

Loss of beat-to-beat variability
Heart rate >160 beats per minute for >10 minutes
Heart rate <120 beats per minute for >10 minutes
Fetal scalp pH <7.20
Short-term variability, variable decelerations to <80 beats per minute or if unrelenting and not corrected by maternal repositioning
Long-term variability, late decelerations

(By permission from Lamb FS, Rosner MS [1987]. Neonatal resuscitation. Emergency Medicine Clinics of North America 5:541–557).

Family Support

Having a baby is supposed to be a joyful occasion. Having an emergency delivery causes great anxiety regarding the outcome of both the mother and the infant. Proceeding in a calm manner provides some reassurance. A significant other should be allowed to stay with the mother during labor and delivery to provide reassurance; this person usually has a stabilizing effect.

DELIVERY OF A HEALTHY INFANT

Whether in the ED or before the mother arrives at the hospital, delivery of even a healthy-appearing infant should be considered an emergency until assessment confirms a healthy status. Before and during delivery, the outcome remains unknown. Even a healthy-appearing infant is exposed to risks that can result in precipitous changes in physiologic status.

Etiology and Physiology

Fetal Circulation and Transition to Extrauterine Life. In utero the fetus exists in a dependent symbiosis with the mother. The uterine artery carries oxygenated blood and nutrients to the placenta. The oxygen and nutrients diffuse across the placental membrane based on concentration gradients. Likewise, carbon dioxide and wastes diffuse from the fetus into the mother's circulation. The umbilical vein carries the oxygenated blood (pO_2, 35 mmHg; pCO_2, 40 mmHg) (Phibbs, 1987) to the fetus. This blood is diluted with unoxygenated blood from the fetal circulation before it reaches the right atrium of the fetus. Most of the blood streams across the foramen ovale to the left atrium, where a small amount of unoxygenated blood from the fetal lungs is added. Blood leaving the left ventricle initially has a pO_2 of approximately 30 mmHg; this blood perfuses the brain and coronary arteries of the fetus. In the descending aorta, unoxygenated blood from the right ventricle, which has been diverted from the fetus's lungs because of high pulmonary pressure through the ductus arteriosus, joins the systemic circulation of the fetus at a lower pO_2.

Because the fetal lungs are not inflated, the pulmonary arterioles are constricted. The systemic circulation is a large low-pressure pool produced because of the presence of the placenta. Thus, in the fetus the pulmonary system is at a higher pressure than the systemic circulation. It is this relationship that keeps the foramen ovale open, shunting blood from right to left and allowing the direction of flow in the ductus arteriosus to be toward the aorta.

During labor and delivery multiple events occur that result in appropriate transition to air breathing and normal circulation. With vaginal delivery, the infant's chest is compressed and then re-expands as the baby exits the vaginal canal. The infant may cry on exposure to noise, light, and cold (Nelson, 1987), inflating the lungs with air, stretching and expanding the pulmonary circulation and decreasing pulmonary vascular resistance. It also allows intake of oxygen, enriching the oxygen concentration in the blood, stimulating pulmonary vasodilatation and closure of the ductus arteriosus.

Clamping the umbilical cord cuts off the large systemic vascular pool, effectively raising the systemic pressure. The combination of decreasing pulmonary vascular resistance and increasing systemic vascular resistance results in the closure of the foramen ovale, halting the right-to-left shunt within the heart. The pCO_2 and pO_2 rise quickly with the exchange of gases in the lungs. The pH rises over the first few hours (Table 12–3).

Thermoregulation. A healthy-appearing newborn who breathes immediately after delivery and appears to have good color, perfusion, and respiratory effort is still exposed to potential problems. The most common is temperature instability. Before birth a fetus is in an environment that is close to body temperature. After birth the environmental temperature is at least 20°F cooler, and the infant is wet with amniotic fluid. The infant has minimal insulation, has a large surface-to-mass ratio, and is already compromised with transitional oxygenation and acid balance.

Neonates have a limited ability to respond to thermal stress. They do not shiver because of neurologic immaturity and can only generate heat by an increase in metabolism. They do this by metabolizing brown fat, a richly vascularized supply of fat found around the kidneys, adrenal glands, scapulae, neck, and axillae (Dodman, 1987). Burning this brown fat requires high amounts of oxygen and calories, which a newborn in transition can ill afford. Healthy infants are known to drop core temperatures to 96°F within minutes of delivery. This results in peripheral vasoconstriction, promoting lactic acid production and pulmonary vasoconstriction, leading to ventilation perfusion mismatches and evidence of respiratory distress in the form of grunting. In some infants this phenomenon can produce a downward spiral to pulmonary hypertension and severe hypoxia.

Infection. Healthy-appearing infants may have been exposed to infection during the labor process. As soon as the amniotic membrane ruptures, the fetus becomes exposed to microbes resident in the vaginal canal. This exposure is augmented by manual examinations and

TABLE 12–3. NORMAL BLOOD GAS VALUES AFTER BIRTH

	Immediately after birth					
	Value	SD	Range	5 minutes	10 minutes	1 hour
pH						
Umbilical artery	7.28	± .05	7.20–7.43			7.3
High altitude	7.32	± .05	7.20–7.42			
Umbilical vein	7.35	± .05	7.26–7.48			
pCO$_2$ (mmHg)						
Umbilical artery	47.5	± 7	30–40			38.8
High altitude	44.7	± 7	23–65			
Umbilical vein	38	± 5.6	25–50			
pO$_2$ (mmHg)						
Umbilical artery	17.5	± 6.4	4–37			85
High altitude	18.1	± 5.4	6.8–33			
Umbilical vein	29	± 6.2	15–47			
HCO$_3$ (mEq/L)						
Umbilical artery	22	± 2.5	15–27			
High altitude	22.9	± 2.3	16.7–28			
Umbilical vein	20.4	± 2.3	16–25			
O$_2$ sat (%)						
Umbilical artery	26.3	± 16	2.2–71			
High altitude	27	± 12.6	3.6–68.6			
Umbilical vein	54	± 14	18.5–83.5			
Right hand	72	± 6.5		83.3	90.7	
Right foot	63	± 4.3		76.6	87.1	

Data from Carlo and Waldemar, 1991; Dimich et al, 1991; Yancey et al, 1992; Yeomans et al, 1985.

any instrumentation. A full-term fetus has limited immune capabilities and can be easily overwhelmed by infection. Although immunoglobulin-G has been transmitted across the placenta, immunoglobulin M, the initial responder to infection and the early trigger of the immune response, is essentially not present. Therefore it may take hours before an immune response is mounted. Infants who appear healthy may already be ill from bacterial invasion.

Most infections of a newborn are not a danger to healthy caregiving personnel. Sexually transmitted or blood-borne diseases may be present, however, and universal precautions are required. Because newborns are covered with vernix and the mother's body fluids, wearing gloves is required when handling an infant. During the delivery, goggles and gowns protect against splatters.

Assessment

Immediate. Assessment of a newly born infant must be divided by priorities. First is assessment of the infant as he or she is born and his or her response to immediate care. Does the infant begin respiration without assistance? Is the heart rate adequate? Does the infant's color improve with the onset of respiration? Does the baby have good muscle tone? This assessment occurs simultaneously with care activities. If

there are negative findings, resuscitation must be begun immediately.

Apgar Score. The 1-minute Apgar score is the first formal assessment (Apgar et al, 1958). The Apgar score assesses five physical signs—heart rate, respiratory effort, reflex irritability, muscle tone, and color—as 0, 1, or 2 (Table 12–4). The total score ranges from 0 (none of these signs present) to 10 (a completely healthy infant). The 1-minute score should be assessed beginning 55 seconds after complete emergence of the infant (Jepson et al, 1991). A timer is necessary. Infants rarely score 10 at 1 minute. With a score of 5 or less the infant should already be receiving resuscitation. A 1-minute score of 7 or more indicates an infant making a good transition.

If an infant is making a good transition, physical assessment can be carried out during the 5-minute period before the next Apgar score is taken. The 5-minute Apgar score has been used to predict mortality and developmental outcome. It lacks sensitivity for prediction because it fails to account for congenital defects, low birth weight, and other factors. A 5-minute Apgar score of 0–3 (in spite of resuscitative efforts) for a full-term, normal-weight infant is associated with an increased incidence of cerebral palsy (Committee on Fetus and Newborn, 1986).

If resuscitation is continuing at this point, Apgar

TABLE 12–4. APGAR SCORING

Sign	Score		
	0	1	2
Heart rate	Absent	Slow (<100 beats/min)	≥100 beats/min
Respirations	Absent	Slow, irregular	Good, crying
Muscle tone	Limp	Some flexion	Active motion
Reflex irritability (catheter in nares, tactile stimulation)	No response	Grimace	Cough, sneeze, cry
Color	Blue or pale	Pink body with blue extremities	Completely pink

(Reproduced with permission from Emergency Care Committee and Subcommittees [1992]. Guidelines for cardiopulmonary resuscitation and emergency cardiac care. Journal of the American Medical Association 268(16):2277)

scoring is done every 5 minutes until the infant's vital signs are stabilized or resuscitative efforts are discontinued.

Gestational Age Assessment. Along with a gross assessment for visible defects, assessment of gestational age should be performed as soon as possible (Kraybill, 1987). An infant could be full-term but have growth retardation or be premature but weigh as much as a term infant and be at risk for respiratory distress syndrome (RDS). Estimating gestational age and making weight comparisons provides an estimation of risk for mortality and guidance as to which complications the neonate may be most at risk.

Gestational age is assessed using the Ballard method (Ballard et al, 1987). The skin, breast and ear tissue, genitalia, and foot creases are assessed. According to Constantine et al (1987), doubling the physical maturity score provides a valid estimation of gestational age at birth, whereas using the neuromuscular maturity section of the Ballard method is not optimal until the child is 30–42 hours of age (Ballard et al, 1987).

Physical Examination. General assessment of a newborn should be done in the following manner. Infants are unable to cooperate with an examination, and portions of the examination may be enough to arouse crying, thereby making other parts difficult if not impossible to carry out.

Observation of the infant when he or she is quiet allows assessment of breathing effort, muscle tone, color, spontaneous movement, and alertness. Full-term newborns hold their extremities in a flexed position and exhibit spontaneous movements. Prematurity or illness is responsible for decreased muscle tone and flexion. The infant should be pink, either robust or pale, with good perfusion as evidenced by capillary

refill in less than 3 seconds. Many infants have acrocyanosis (dusky hands and feet) and sometimes circumoral cyanosis. This coloring is normal and is caused by immature circulatory control. Respiratory effort should be easy, with no retractions of the chest muscles. An awake, non-crying infant should be looking at the environment and be responsive to sounds and visual stimuli.

Because of the small area of the chest, breath sounds are primarily bronchovesicular, with no rales or rhonchi. The normal respiratory rate of a newborn ranges from 40 to 60 breaths per minute. A newborn's heart is situated centrally, and it is common to hear heart sounds on the right sternal border. A murmur may be heard in the first hours after birth because the ductus arteriosus may not yet be functionally closed. This murmur is heard over the right or left upper sternal border. If there is a murmur, pulses in all four extremities, color, perfusion, and respiratory effort should be assessed for the possibility of a congenital heart defect. The normal heart rate after birth may range from 110 to 160 beats per minute and may slow several hours after birth.

The abdomen should be soft and slightly rounded, with some scattered bowel sounds. The umbilical cord is about the size of an adult finger and should be gelatinous, not already drying. It contains three vessels—a large vein and two small arteries. The genitalia should be examined for any abnormalities, and the rectum should be examined for patency. This examination should be done visually. Use of a rectal thermometer or other insertions into the rectum should be avoided because of risk of rectal tear or vagal stimulation. The liver may be palpated up to 1 cm below the costal border.

The spine and extremities should be examined carefully for myelomeningocele, club foot, extra or absent digits, and any other abnormalities.

A newborn's head may be elongated because of molding during delivery. The sutures are not fused and the parts of the skull may actually override each other. The anterior fontanelle should be open, soft, and flat. The posterior fontanelle may be tiny. The ears should appear normal; the upper insertion of the ear falls along or above an imaginary line drawn from the inner and outer canthus of the eyes to the occipital prominence. If the ear insertion falls below this line, it may be retroverted or low-set, a configuration associated with Down syndrome. The eyes should appear normal with no defects in the pupil or lids. The nasal septum should appear straight. Each naris can be occluded separately to determine that air passes easily. The examiner should be certain that the mouth is closed during this maneuver. The mouth should appear normal and the infant should open his or her mouth when the lips are touched and suck on a finger or nipple when one is inserted. The high arched hard palate should be palpated for a cleft.

The clavicles should be palpated for fractures. A more complete physical examination should be performed in the nursery.

Laboratory and Diagnostic Tests. Even if there appear to be no problems, a blood glucose screening and a hematocrit should be done by heelstick. If the blood glucose level is below 40 mg/dl, a serum glucose level should be obtained, and early feedings should be initiated or intravenous administration of glucose (10% dextrose in water, $D_{10}W$) should be started. The hematocrit level should be 50–65%. If the hematocrit level is lower, and the infant has any respiratory distress or oxygen needs, a blood transfusion may be needed. If the hematocrit level is higher than 65%, a central hematocrit should be done, because there are risks associated with plethora.

T R I A G E
Delivery

Emergent ————————————————————
Infant delivered before arrival at the hospital or in the emergency department.

Nursing Diagnosis
High Risk for Altered Body Temperature

Defining Characteristics

- Fluctuations in body temperature above or below normal

- Increased radiant and evaporative cooling

Nursing Interventions

- Provide radiant heat source
- Dry quickly and remove wet blankets

Expected Outcome

- Temperature stays within normal range (97°F–99°F axillary)

Nursing Diagnosis
High Risk for Infection

Defining Characteristic

- Prolonged or premature rupture of membranes

Nursing Interventions

- Identify risk factors for exposure
- Provide clean environment to prevent infection
- Assign one nurse to care for infant

Expected Outcome

- Infant remains free of infection

Nursing Diagnosis
Ineffective Airway Clearance

Defining Characteristics

- Cyanosis
- Dyspnea
- Apnea

Nursing Intervention

- Clear airway using bulb syringe

Expected Outcomes

- Even pink color
- Improved tone
- Respiratory rate of 40–60 breaths per minute

Nursing Diagnosis
Ineffective Breathing Pattern

Defining Characteristics

- Dyspnea
- Retractions
- Altered chest excursions

Nursing Interventions

- Dry infant vigorously to stimulate deep breath
- Stimulate cry

Expected Outcomes

- Pink color
- Easy respirations at a rate of 40–60 breaths per minute

Nursing Diagnosis
Ineffective Family Coping: Compromised

Defining Characteristics

- Protective behavior disproportionate to baby's needs
- Fear, anxiety, anticipatory grief

Nursing Interventions

- Provide ongoing information about baby's condition
- Allow holding as soon as possible

Expected Outcomes

- Parent expresses relief that baby's condition is satisfactory
- Parent exhibits bonding behaviors

Management
The focus in providing adequate resuscitation and care for a newborn in the ED is to *be prepared*. Two areas require preparation—training and equipment.

Training. Sufficient ED staff should be certified in the Neonatal Resuscitation Program (NRP) to have a trained person available anytime a newly born infant enters the ED for care. Just as caregivers are certified in advanced life support (ALS) for adults and pediatric ALS (PALS) for children, personnel need to be trained and to have regular practice in newborn resuscitation. The NRP was designed by the American Heart Association (AHA) and the American Academy of Pediatrics (AAP). It includes equipment and preparation, the ABCs (airway-breathing-circulation) of cardiopulmonary resuscitation (CPR), CPR techniques, the special procedure for endotracheal intubation of a newborn, and emergency medications (American Heart Association and American Academy of Pediatrics, 1990).

Equipment. Adequate and regularly checked equipment suited to newborn resuscitation should be available in the ED (Table 12–5). This includes a radiant heat source for the resuscitation table, endotracheal tubes (ET), suction catheters, feeding tubes, and masks in the appropriate sizes for full-term and premature infants. Resuscitation bags should not exceed 750 ml (American Heart Association and American Academy of Pediatrics, 1990) and should have a pressure release

TABLE 12–5. RESUSCITATION EQUIPMENT IN THE DELIVERY ROOM

Radiant warmer
Stethoscope
Cardiotachometer with electrocardiogram (oscilloscope desirable)
Suction with manometer
Bulb syringe
Meconium aspirator
Wall oxygen with flowmeter and tubing
Suction catheters, 5F or 6F, 8F, and 10F
Neonatal resuscitation bag (manometer optional)
Face masks, newborn and premature sizes
Oral airways, newborn and premature sizes
Endotracheal tubes, 2.5, 3.0, 3.5, and 4.0 mm
Endotracheal tube stylets
Laryngoscope
Laryngoscope blades, straight no. 0 and 1
Umbilical catheters, 3.5F and 5F
Three-way stopcocks
Sterile umbilical vessel catheterization tray
20-mL syringe and 8F feeding tube for gastric suction
Needles, syringes
Medications
   Epinephrine (1:10 000)
   Naloxone hydrochloride (1mg/mL or 0.4 mg/mL)
   Volume expander
   Sodium bicarbonate (0.5 mEq/mL)

(Reproduced with permission from Emergency Care Committee and Subcommittees [1992]. Guidelines for cardiopulmonary resuscitation and emergency care. Journal of the American Medical Association 268(16):2277)

valve or pressure gauge. Some of the drug concentrations and fluids required are different than for other patients. Umbilical catheters also should be included with the other equipment and supplies standard for any resuscitation.

As soon as it is known that a newborn will be in the ED, the radiant heat should be turned on to warm the bedding on which the infant will receive care, and the rest of the equipment should be checked and prepared.

Care of a Newborn at Birth. When an infant's head emerges, the mouth and nose should be suctioned with a bulb syringe. When the infant is completely expelled, he or she is dried vigorously (this should initiate breathing), wrapped in warm sterile blankets, and placed on the mother's abdomen. The cord should be double-clamped several inches from the baby and cut between the clamps. This need not be done immediately but should be completed before the cord stops pulsating.

After cord clamping, the infant should be placed under a radiant heat source and drying continued. The wet towels should be removed quickly and replaced with dry ones. The infant should be placed with the neck slightly extended to open the airway, and gentle suction of the mouth and nares should be done. The infant should have begun breathing by this point. Vigorous suctioning of the mouth and nose should be avoided because this can stimulate a reflex that results in bradycardia and apnea. If the infant is not breathing, gentle stimulation by rubbing the back or tapping the soles of the feet should start the breathing. If the infant does not respond, the infant's heart rate, color, and respiratory effort should be evaluated. Further steps should be taken to initiate resuscitation.

After breathing begins, Apgar scores are assigned. Identification bands are prepared and placed on the infant, preferably in the presence of the mother. A complete physical assessment also can be performed in the presence of the mother. This alleviates anxieties she may have about the infant's welfare in the face of the emergency delivery.

In most states or hospitals, it is routine to provide vitamin K and prophylaxis against ocular gonorrhea and chlamydia. These procedures can be deferred until after transfer to the nursery, but clear communication regarding the status of these treatments is important. Eye prophylaxis consists of a ribbon of erythromycin ophthalmic ointment in each eye. Silver nitrate solution can be used, but it may cause chemical conjunctivitis. Tetracycline ophthalmic ointment is also effective.

Vitamin K should be given within several hours of birth to prevent hemorrhagic disease of the newborn (Kraybill, 1987). The dose is 1 mg intramuscularly into the thigh.

Blood glucose levels and hematocrit by heelstick should be done ½ to 1 hour after delivery. Blood glucose levels should be repeated every hour until the baby is under nursery care.

If an infant is born before arrival at the ED, he or she should be placed on a radiant warmer, and resuscitation should be carried out as necessary. If resuscitation is not necessary, an Apgar assignment, temperature reading, hematocrit, and blood glucose screening should be done immediately. Additional assessment of labor and delivery circumstances, timing of delivery, infant responses to delivery and transport, and pregnancy history for neonatal risk factors should be made.

Family Support

To assist in preventing ineffective family coping, and to promote bonding, the infant should be wrapped and presented to the mother to hold and even breast feed as soon as the infant's condition is stable and the mother is available. The mother may want to unwrap the infant. This should only be done if a radiant heat source can be supplied to prevent hypothermia. The father or significant other should continue to be present and may also be allowed to hold the infant.

RESUSCITATION OF A DISTRESSED INFANT: ASPHYXIA

A fetus is particularly vulnerable to hypoxia during labor and delivery. Transient hypoxemia occurs during uterine contractions, and a healthy fetus tolerates this fairly well. Circumstances that complicate and augment hypoxia, however, can quickly produce asphyxia.

Conditions that Produce Asphyxia

- Compression of the umbilical cord between the descending fetus and the wall of the birth canal, interrupting flow of oxygenated blood to the fetus
- Interruption of placental exchange, if the placenta separates prematurely
- Maternal hypotension and poor uterine arterial blood flow to the placenta. This can occur as a result of compression on the uterine artery by the extremely gravid uterus; it may be relieved by repositioning the mother on her side
- Infant compromise due to severe anemia, growth retardation, or postmaturity
- Mechanisms that prevent adequate lung inflation and aeration after birth (Phibbs, 1987)

Physiology of Asphyxia and Apnea

Fetuses and newborns respond in a well-described sequence of events when experiencing hypoxia. First, there is a period of rapid breathing, followed by apnea. This is called primary apnea. In primary apnea, stimulation and administration of oxygen are usually adequate to induce respiration and reverse the condition. During primary apnea the heart rate and blood pressure rise, initially blood flow is shunted to vital organs, and the heart rate then falls to a rate of 80–100 beats per minute. As asphyxia continues, the infant begins gasping respirations; the heart rate then begins to fall further; and blood pressure begins to fall. The gasping is irregular until a last gasp is made. Secondary apnea follows with final decreases in heart rate and blood pressure. In secondary apnea, full resuscitation is needed. As resuscitation is successful, the vital functions return in reverse order to their failure.

The problem is knowing in which stage of apnea a newly born infant is presenting when he or she does not take a breath after delivery. The infant may have completed both stages of apnea in utero, and the stages are indistinguishable at birth when the heart rate is less than 100 beats per minute and there is no respiratory effort. Therefore, one must proceed as if the apnea were secondary and begin resuscitation without hesitation.

Assessment

If time allows before delivery, the prenatal and perinatal history should be assessed for factors that put the infant at risk for asphyxia (Table 12–1). A newly emerging infant should be assessed for distress as initial care is given. The initial assessment is based on respirations, heart rate, and color. If an infant does not respond to being dried by exhibiting spontaneous movement and respirations, or if the heart rate is less than 100 beats per minute, the nurse should not wait for 1-minute Apgar scores to be assigned before beginning resuscitation.

TRIAGE
Asphyxia

Emergent —————————————————
Infant experiencing a hypoxic episode.

Nursing Diagnosis
Decreased Cardiac Output

Defining Characteristics

- Variations in blood pressure
- Decreased peripheral pulses
- Color changes in skin, mucous membranes
- Dyspnea
- Weakness, decreased tone

Nursing Interventions

- Administer oxygen
- Assess vital signs frequently
- Administer volume expanders and vasopressors as ordered

Expected Outcomes

- Pink color
- Pulses and perfusion return to normal
- Vitals signs are normal

Nursing Diagnosis
Impaired Gas Exchange

Defining Characteristics

- Hypercapnia
- Hypoxia
- Restlessness, irritability

Nursing Intervention

- Perform oxygen and bag ventilation

Expected Outcomes

- Pink color
- Normal breathing
- Normal vital signs

Nursing Diagnosis
Ineffective Airway Clearance

Defining Characteristics

- Abnormal breath sounds
- Dyspnea
- Cyanosis

Nursing Interventions

- Perform suction
- Assist with intubation

Expected Outcomes

- Adequate airway established
- Infant is able to ventilate

Nursing Diagnosis
Ineffective Breathing Pattern

Defining Characteristics

- Dyspnea, apnea
- Cyanosis
- Decreased breath sounds

Nursing Interventions

- Perform bag ventilation
- Administer oxygen
- Assist with ventilation

Expected Outcomes

- Pink color
- Normal respiration

Nursing Diagnosis
Altered Cardiopulmonary Tissue Perfusion

Defining Characteristics

- Pale, cyanotic, or mottled skin color
- Cold extremities
- Decreased muscle tone

Nursing Interventions

- Administer oxygen
- Administer medications as ordered

Expected Outcomes

- Even pink color
- Improved tone

Nursing Diagnosis

Anticipatory Grieving

Defining Characteristics

- Potential loss of baby (real or perceived)
- Expressed distress or denial of potential loss

Nursing Interventions

- Keep parents informed of baby's condition
- Facilitate verbalization of feelings

Expected Outcomes

- Parents remain rational
- Parents are able to participate in care
- Parents can make decisions regarding care of baby

Management

Resuscitation of newborns is delineated by the American Heart Association and the American Academy of Pediatrics (1990). The guidelines are based on the premise that neonatal asphyxia occurs because of two basic problems—the lungs are not properly inflated and cleared of lung fluid, and blood flow to the alveoli has not been adequately increased.

Airway. Regardless of an infant's appearance at birth, which is initially cyanotic because of the low pO_2 in utero, the infant should be placed under a radiant heat source, dried, and positioned for an adequate airway (Figure 12–1). Suctioning the mouth first and then the nose should be adequate stimulation to initiate respiration, unless the infant's condition is compromised. Tactile stimulation such as slapping or flicking the sole of the foot or rubbing the infant's back should be tried briefly. No one should slap the infant's back or hold him or her upside down.

Breathing. If stimulation is not effective in initiating respiration, bag and mask ventilation with 100% oxygen should be started. There should be no hesitation or indecision in proceeding with resuscitation because there is no way of knowing how long the infant's condition has been compromised. The infant's heart rate should be assessed after ventilation is initiated. If the heart rate is greater than 100 beats per minute, the nurse evaluates the infant's color and watches for resumption of spontaneous respirations. If spontaneous

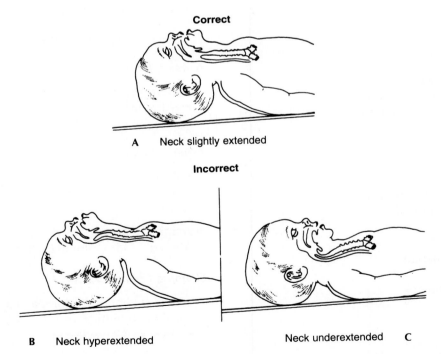

Figure 12–1. A. The neonate should be placed on his or her back or side in a slight Trendelenburg position with the neck slightly extended. Care should be taken to prevent hyperextension (**B**) or underextension (**C**) of the neck because either may decrease air entry. (Reproduced with permission from the American Heart Association and the American Academy of Pediatrics [1990]. *Textbook of neonatal resuscitation.* Elk Grove Village, Ill: American Academy of Pediatrics, p 2)

respirations begin, continue to ventilate briefly while assessing breathing. Gasping respirations require on-going ventilation. If regular respirations are sustained, ventilation may be stopped while administration of free-flow oxygen is continued; the free-flow oxygen is gradually withdrawn as the infant's condition stabilizes. If respirations and heart rate are acceptable, but color is poor, administration of oxygen is continued. If the heart rate is less than 100 beats per minute, positive pressure ventilation should continue, regardless of respiration.

Bag and mask ventilation of a newborn requires special knowledge and equipment. The bag can be self-inflating with a pressure pop-off valve and an oxygen reservoir, or it can be an anesthesia bag with a pressure manometer. The bag should not exceed a capacity of 750 mL (some self-inflating bags are as small as 250 mL). Full-term infants require only 6–8 mL/kg or 20–30 ml of oxygen in each ventilation. The mask should fit over the infant's mouth and nose without causing overriding eye pressure or damage (Figure 12–2). The person providing resuscitation should be trained in using the bag properly on a newborn. After an adequate seal is obtained, ventilating breaths should be delivered for 15–30 seconds at a rate of 40–60 breaths per minute. Pressures may be very high for the first 1 or 2 breaths (40 cm H_2O or more) to inflate an unused lung, and then 15–20 cm H_2O. Details can be found in the AHA NRP (American Heart Association and American Academy of Pediatrics, 1990).

If ventilation continues for more than 2 minutes, a nasogastric tube may be inserted to decompress the stomach, relieving pressure on the diaphragm and improving lung expansion.

An oral airway is not necessary unless the infant has a chin or lower jaw malformation that might keep the tongue in a posterior position. Neonates are obligate nose breathers because their posterior soft palate and epiglottis are in approximation, except when the child is crying.

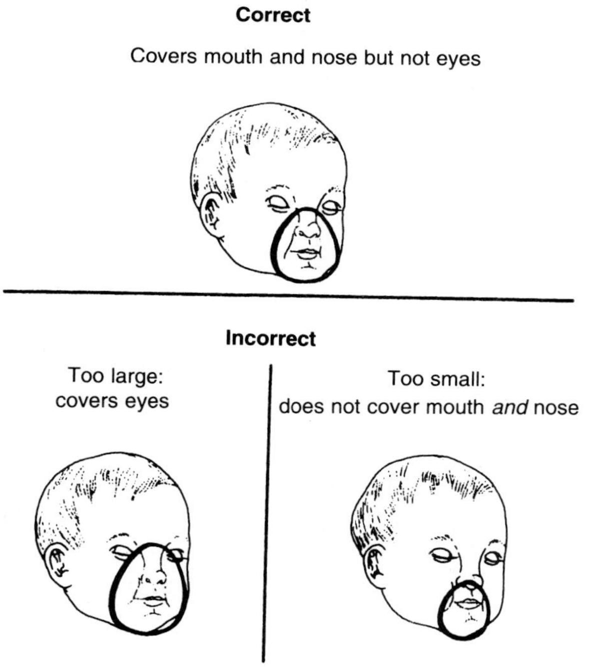

Circulation. Heart rate can be assessed apically with a stethoscope or by feeling the umbilical pulse at the base of the cord. If the heart rate is 60–100 beats per minute and increasing, ventilation is continued. If the heart rate is not increasing and is below 80 beats per minute, chest compressions are begun. Again, there is a special technique for neonatal chest compressions; either two fingers or both thumbs are used (Figure 12–3). The chest should be depressed ½–¾ inch at a rate of 120 compressions per minute. The effectiveness of chest compressions can be evaluated by palpating the brachial, carotid, or femoral pulses.

Color. Most infants have some degree of cyanosis initially. If their color does not become pink by 60–90 seconds with regular respirations and good heart rate, free-flow oxygen should be given. The reasons for persistent cyanosis may be inadequate respiration or congenital defects. Free-flow oxygen can be provided by face mask or by oxygen tube held to the nose. At 5 liters/minute flow of 100% oxygen you can deliver 80% oxygen when the tube is ½ inch, 60% oxygen when it is 1 inch, and 40% oxygen when the tube is 2 inches from the nose (American Heart Association and American Academy of Pediatrics, 1990). As color improves, oxygen should be gradually withdrawn, and the infant's color should be assessed continually. Neonates have a left shift in their ability to release oxygen from their hemoglobin; as a result cyanosis appears at low levels of oxygen saturation. Therefore, efforts should be directed to keeping the infant pink. If possible, a pulse oximeter should be used to keep the oxygen saturation at 95–100% in full-term infants.

Wall oxygen is cold and dry. It should be warmed and humidified to prevent heat loss and drying of the mucosa if it must be given for more than a few minutes. Cold oxygen should never be directed to the infant's forehead; this stimulates the trigeminal nerve, and profound heat loss can occur.

Correct

Covers mouth and nose but not eyes

Incorrect

Too large: covers eyes

Too small: does not cover mouth *and* nose

Figure 12–2. Correct and incorrect positioning of air masks on infants. (Reproduced with permission from the American Heart Association and the American Academy of Pediatrics [1990]. *Textbook of neonatal resuscitation.* Elk Grove Village, Ill: American Academy of Pediatrics, p 3)

A

B

Figure 12–3. A. Two-finger method. The tips of the middle and index or ring finger are used for compression. **B.** The balls of the thumbs are used for compression. (Reproduced with permission from the American Heart Association and the American Academy of Pediatrics [1990]. *Textbook of neonatal resuscitation.* Elk Grove Village, Ill: American Academy of Pediatrics, pp 11–13)

Intubation. During chest compressions, ventilation can be done after every third compression. However, ventilation during chest compressions is difficult at these rates. Therefore, it is more effective through an ET. Indications for intubation are prolonged ventilation, ineffective bag and mask ventilation, the need for tracheal suctioning (as in meconium aspiration), or a diaphragmatic hernia. Intubation should be done only by a skilled practitioner; it is not required for most resuscitations. A no. 0 or 1 laryngoscope blade, straight, not curved, is used. Oral intubation is preferred in an emergency, and forceps are not used because of lack of space and the potential for injury. A stylet is used to stiffen the tube for insertion, and it is removed immediately. Endotracheal tubes are uncuffed for infants and children.

The laryngoscope blade is inserted into the vallecula at the base of the tongue (Figure 12–4), the vocal cords visualized; and the tube is inserted so that the black mark is at the cords. The process should not take longer than 20 seconds, and free-flow 100% oxygen should be provided during the process. After 20 seconds, some ventilation is done before the intubation attempt is repeated. Once the tube is inserted and ventilation resumed, placement of the tube should be evaluated immediately by auscultation of the lungs and stomach. Care should be taken to evaluate more than upper lobe aeration because esophageal sounds may seem to be lung inflation since the lungs and esophagus are so close to one another. Proper placement produces bilaterally equal breath sounds; an observer can see the chest rise with each breath, and there is no gastric distention. Once proper placement is established, the ET should be cut so that no more than 4 cm protrudes from the lips, to reduce dead space.

Medications. If the heart rate remains below 80 beats per minute after 30 seconds of chest compressions and positive pressure ventilation with 100% oxygen, or if the heart rate is zero, medications might be used to stimulate the heart, to increase tissue perfusion, and to restore acid-base balance. The drugs can be administered through the umbilical vein (the preferred route), through peripheral veins, or by endotracheal instilla-

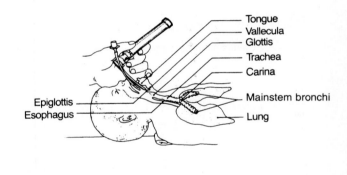

Tongue
Vallecula
Glottis
Trachea
Carina
Mainstem bronchi
Lung
Epiglottis
Esophagus

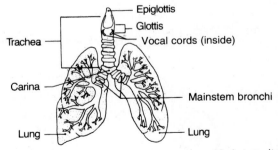

Epiglottis
Glottis
Vocal cords (inside)
Trachea
Carina
Mainstem bronchi
Lung
Lung

Figure 12–4. The goal in inserting the laryngoscope blade is to slide it over the tongue with the tip of the blade resting on the vallecula (the area between the base of the tongue and the epiglottis). (Reproduced with permission from the American Heart Association and the American Academy of Pediatrics [1990]. *Textbook of neonatal resuscitation.* Elk Grove Village, Ill: American Academy of Pediatrics, p 5)

TABLE 12-6. MEDICATIONS FOR NEONATAL RESUSCITATION

Medication	Concentration to Administer	Preparation	Dosage/ Route	Total Dose			Rate and Precautions
Epinephrine	1:10,000	1 mL	0.1–0.3 mL/kg IV or ET	weight (kg) 1 2 3 4		total (mL) 0.1–0.3 0.2–0.6 0.3–0.9 0.4–1.2	Give rapidly
Volume expanders	Whole blood 5% albumin Normal saline solution Ringer lactate	40 mL	10 mL/kg IV	weight (kg) 1 2 3 4		total (mL) 10 20 30 40	Give over 5–10 min
Sodium bicarbonate	0.5mEq/mL (4.2% solution)	20 mL or two 10-mL pre-filled syringes	2 mEq/kg IV	weight (kg) 1 2 3 4	total dose (mEq) 2 4 6 8	total (mL) 4 8 12 16	Give *slowly*, over at least 2 min Give only if infant is being effectively ventilated
Naloxone	0.4 mg/mL	1 mL	0.1 mg/kg (0.25 mL/kg) IV, ET, IM, SC	weight (kg) 1 2 3 4	total dose (mg) 0.1 0.2 0.3 0.4	total (mL) 0.25 0.50 0.75 1.00	Give rapidly IV, ET preferred IM, SC acceptable
	1.0 mg/mL	1 mL	0.1 mg/kg (0.1 mL/kg) IV, ET, IM, SC	1 2 3 4	0.1 0.2 0.3 0.4	0.1 0.2 0.3 0.4	
Dopamine	$\dfrac{6 \times \text{weight (kg)} \times \text{desired dose (mcg/kg/min)}}{\text{desired fluid (mL/hr)}} = \text{mg of dopamine per 100 mL of solution}$		Begin at 5 mcg/kg/ min (may increase to 20 mcg/kg/ min if necessary) IV	weight (kg) 1 2 3 4	total (mcg/min) 5–20 10–40 15–60 20–80		Give as a continuous infusion using an infusion pump Monitor HR and BP closely Seek consultation

IM, intramuscular; ET, endotracheal; IV, intravenous; SC, subcutaneous; HR, heart rate; BP, blood pressure.
(*From Textbook of Neonatal Resuscitation © 1987, 1990 American Heart Association*)

tion. Epinephrine is the first drug chosen to stimulate heart rate. If there is an inadequate response, or if acute volume loss occurs during delivery, a volume expander such as 5% albumin is used. If there is documented acidosis or prolonged hypoxia, sodium bicarbonate is given. If the infant continues to show evidence of shock, a dopamine infusion might be started. Naloxone is given when the infant's condition is depressed from maternal analgesia. Naloxone should not be given when the mother has been abusing narcotics, because it could precipitate severe withdrawal. Table 12-6 provides dosages and administration of medications for neonatal resuscitation.

Resolution. If the heart rate is 80 beats per minute and rising, chest compressions are discontinued, but ventilation with 100% oxygen is continued. If the heart rate is greater than 100 beats per minute with spontaneous respirations, bag ventilation may be stopped but oxygen is withdrawn gradually.

If the baby is not responding to resuscitation, mechanical factors should be assessed. When mechanical factors have been ruled out, assessment for medical factors should be continued (Table 12-7).

If an infant's heart rate was initially zero, compressions and ventilation should be continued until a medical decision is made to discontinue resuscitation. Figure 12-5 provides an overview of newborn resuscitation.

Family Support

During resuscitation the mother is usually nearby undergoing the last stage of labor, and is exposed to the activities of neonatal resuscitation. The anxiety of emergency admission is aggravated by the baby's

TABLE 12–7. REASONS FOR LACK OF RESPONSE TO BASIC CARDIOPULMONARY RESUSCITATION

- INADEQUATE VENTILATION
  Misplaced endotracheal tube
  Inadequate pressure
  Air leak

- SHOCK
  Asphyxial
  Hypovolemic
  Septic

- CONGENITAL ANOMALIES
  Airway
  Pulmonary hypoplasia
  Severe cardiac disease

(By permission Edwards M [1988]. Delivery room resuscitation of the neonate. Pediatric Annals 17:464)

need for resuscitation. If possible, the infant resuscitation should be carried out in another room or away from the area of the mother. At the least, activities around the baby should be shielded from the mother's sight. Reassurances are needed that everything possible is being done by skilled professionals; regular up-

dates of the status of the baby should be given to the mother. Honest but sensitive reports prepare the mother and any other family members present for an unfortunate outcome and provide reassurance when the outcome is good. Even if an infant remains ill, the mother should be allowed to see and touch the baby before either of them is transferred out of the ED. If at all possible the mother should hold the baby, even briefly.

Infants who have needed resuscitation usually are admitted to an intensive care nursery, at least for a period of observation if not for ongoing support. The family needs a great deal of support; intensive care symbolizes a life-threatening situation. Although some infants may be in such a condition, others need only observation, and their condition is not critical. The family needs information about visiting, who the physician will be, and about what their role will be. Anticipatory grieving occurs, even if the baby is not likely to die. The parents are experiencing grief over the loss of the happy delivery experience they were expecting and over the seemingly lost joy of having a new baby.

If resuscitation fails, or if the infant was stillborn, the family should be given every opportunity to hold,

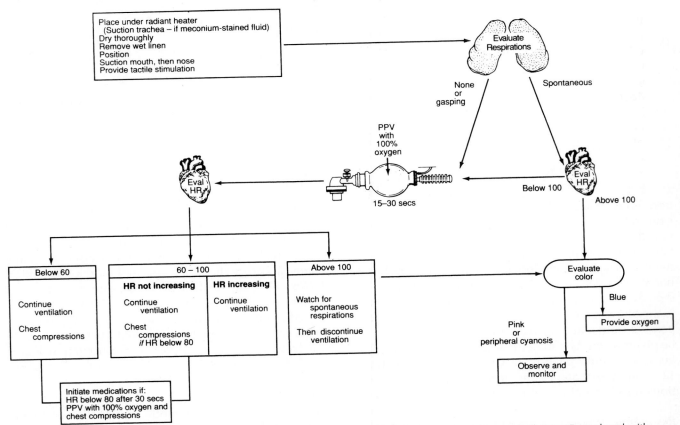

Figure 12–5. Overview of resuscitation in the delivery room. HR, heart rate; PPV, positive pressure ventilation. (Reproduced with permission from the American Heart Association and the American Academy of Pediatrics [1990]. *Textbook of neonatal resuscitation.* Elk Grove Village, Ill: American Academy of Pediatrics, p 1)

bathe, and dress the infant if desired. Photographs should be taken and saved for the parents. A lock of hair, the identification band, and any clothing also should be kept. It has been shown that mothers experience incomplete grieving if not given opportunities to see or hold their infants. Any tokens of memorabilia serve to provide for healthy grieving. These tokens and photographs may be requested later, even if they are rejected initially.

MECONIUM ASPIRATION AND PULMONARY HYPERTENSION

Meconium staining occurs in up to 22% of all live births (Katz and Bowes, 1992). Meconium is found in the lungs of 35% of these infants, and respiratory distress occurs in 10%. The presence of meconium is associated with fetal hypoxia and fetal distress.

Etiology and Physiology

Meconium is a blackish green tarry substance that is the product of intrauterine digestion. When sufficient hypoxia occurs, the rectal sphincter relaxes, releasing meconium into the amniotic fluid. At first the meconium occurs in small blobs. If inhaled in this form it lodges in the large and small airways. As respiration occurs, some airways become completely blocked and some allow inhalation but block exhalation, resulting in atelectasis and air trapping and producing a pneumothorax.

Meconium becomes dissolved in the amniotic fluid in a relatively short time and resembles pea soup. As time progresses this fluid turns yellow. If this fluid is inhaled, an aspiration pneumonia is produced that irritates the alveolar membranes and provides an excellent substrate for infection before it is eventually absorbed.

Along with these effects, it must also be remembered that it was severe hypoxia at some point that caused the release of meconium, placing the baby at high risk while he or she sustains the rigors of delivery. Indeed, meconium is often the marker for intrauterine hypoxia, which can produce the increased smooth muscularization of the arterioles that is responsible for persistent pulmonary hypertension (Cunningham et al, 1989).

Pulmonary hypertension with persistence of fetal shunting is the most critical disease seen in neonatal intensive care nurseries. Newborns have thick smooth muscle lining the pulmonary arteries, possibly because of the low oxygenation levels experienced in utero. If there is any additional hypoxia, additional smooth muscle is grown. The pulmonary vasculature is highly susceptible to hypoxia and acidosis as vaso-constrictors. When these conditions are experienced during labor and delivery or during resuscitation, a viscous circle of pulmonary vasoconstriction and deepening hypoxia can occur. Because of the high pulmonary vascular resistance sustained after birth, the foramen ovale remains open, and because of hypoxia, the ductus arteriosus remains dilated. That is, the fetal shunts persist.

The babies most at risk for meconium or pulmonary hypertension are those who experience hypoxia and asphyxia before delivery, and those who have experienced chronic stress in utero, ie, infants who are postmature or infants with growth retardation.

Assessment

If the amniotic fluid is stained with meconium but is thin and watery, no special management is needed. If the amniotic fluid is like pea soup or has particulate meconium, steps should be taken to prevent aspiration before the first breath is taken. After resuscitation is complete, assessment of breath sounds, respiratory effort, and oxygenation help determine if there are effects of meconium aspiration. If there is unequal aeration of lung fields, a barrel chest, or tachypnea, aspiration of meconium may have occurred. Babies who seem to have good aeration and heart rate, but do not have good color and have decreased perfusion, may have a cyanotic congenital heart defect or may have persistent pulmonary hypertension.

TRIAGE
Meconium Aspiration and Pulmonary Hypertension

Emergent
Newborn with suspected meconium aspiration syndrome or pulmonary hypertension.

Nursing Diagnosis
High Risk for Aspiration

Defining Characteristics
- Reduced reflexes
- Reduced level of consciousness
- Presence of meconium in oropharynx
- Unequal breath sounds

Nursing Interventions
- Assist with intubation
- Perform suction by endotracheal tube

Expected Outcomes

- Removal of meconium
- Adequate respirations

Nursing Diagnosis
Impaired Gas Exchange

Defining Characteristics

- Hypercapnia
- Hypoxia

Nursing Interventions

- Administer oxygen
- Assist with intubation

Expected Outcomes

- Color and perfusion return to normal
- Blood gasses at acceptable levels
- Normal vital signs

Nursing Diagnosis
Alteration in Cardiac Output: Decreased

Defining Characteristics

- Variations in blood pressure
- Decreased peripheral pulses and perfusion
- Color changes in skin, mucous membranes
- Dyspnea
- Weakness, decreased muscle tone

Nursing Interventions

- Administer medications as ordered
- Administer oxygen
- Assess vital signs frequently

Expected Outcomes

- Pulses, perfusion return to normal
- Pink color
- Vital signs are normal

Management
When meconium stains the amniotic fluid, specific measures should be taken to prevent aspiration of this fluid after delivery. As soon as the head is delivered (before the shoulders emerge), the nose, mouth and oropharynx should be suctioned with a 10 F or larger catheter. As soon as the infant is placed under the radiant warmer, before drying, residual fluid should be removed from the hypopharynx, and the trachea should be suctioned through an ET. This is done by intubating and using the ET as a suction catheter, applying continuous suction. Meconium particles are too large to suction through a suction catheter that is threaded through an ET. During intubation the trachea can be visualized for the presence of meconium. Linder et al (1988) suggest that intubated suctioning may not be necessary for vigorous infants who have already initiated respiration. The AHA recommends using clinical judgment in this situation.

Whenever there are indications of hypoxia, such as low Apgar scores, or need for oxygen or any resuscitation, or there has been meconium staining, it is wiser to give a full-term infant oxygen to keep him or her pink than it is to withhold oxygen when the color is equivocal. Adequate oxygenation helps prevent the spiral of pulmonary vasoconstriction, hypoxia, pulmonary hypertension, and persistence of fetal shunting. However, when an infant is vigorous and has good color, oxygen is not needed.

Family Support
Family support is the same as for any infant who needs resuscitation. The mother needs reassurance that the meconium aspiration was not something she could have prevented.

PREMATURE DELIVERY

Prematurity covers a relatively wide range of weights and risk groups. The smaller and more premature the baby, the greater are the risks. A 36-week infant (1 month premature) may weigh 6 or 7 pounds, be healthy, and have no apparent problems. A 32-week infant (2 months premature) may weigh 3 pounds, need some initial support, and then be fine. A 28-week infant (3 months premature) may weigh 2 pounds or less, need some ventilator support for a week or more, and have several risks for complications. A 24–25-week infant may survive, but only if expert care is given from the beginning, including delivery in a center with a perinatal program and a neonatal intensive care unit (Hack and Fanaroff, 1989).

The best option for a premature delivery is to provide therapies that delay delivery and to transfer the mother to a center for high-risk deliveries. If that is not possible, special precautions for the premature infant promote an optimum outcome.

Etiology and Pathophysiology

Reasons for Premature Labor and Delivery. Premature labor occurs for many reasons. Often there is a rupture of membranes before labor has begun. Or chorioamnionitis stimulates uterine contractions. Other reasons for premature delivery are an incompetent cervix, inability of the uterus to hold the pregnancy to term, and ingestion of cocaine. Teenage pregnancy, malnutrition, smoking, alcohol and narcotic abuse, and chronic illness are also associated with a high incidence of premature delivery.

Respiratory Distress Syndrome. The primary problem of premature infants is that their organ systems are not mature enough for function in the extrauterine world. The most well-known and the most imminently threatening problem at delivery is the immaturity of the pulmonary surfactant system. Though the fetus begins making surfactant as early as 20 weeks of gestation, the surfactant is not available until about 24 weeks of gestation and is weak and sparse until about 34 weeks. Between 34 and 36 weeks the production of surfactant increases, preventing the development of idiopathic respiratory distress syndrome (IRDS), previously known as hyaline membrane disease. Babies born before 34–36 weeks of gestation may have minimally adequate surfactant, and IRDS may not develop as long as the pulmonary system is not stressed by hypoxia or acidosis, which can inhibit the production of surfactant or break down whatever surfactant is present.

Infection. If infection is the stimulus for premature labor, the infant is exposed and is ill-equipped to resist. The minimal immunity a newborn has develops during the last trimester of pregnancy. The more premature an infant, the weaker is the immune response he or she can mount. Therefore, quite frequently, a premature infant must be treated for sepsis until cultures prove none is present.

Intraventricular Hemorrhage. Premature babies are at risk for intraventricular hemorrhage (IVH). The hemorrhaging occurs because a premature infant has almost no cerebral autoregulation. Any changes in systemic blood pressure are expressed directly in changes in intracranial pressure. At the same time vessels in the subependymal area of the lateral ventricles are very fragile and have little supporting tissue. Stresses that can increase pressures and cause rupture of these vessels are hypoxia, acidosis, and general handling. Labor and delivery are a substantial stress for these infants, as are the resuscitation and admission activities that follow. Although large infants are at reduced risk for IVH, smaller, immature infants are at high risk. Intraventricular hemorrhage is most likely to occur around labor and delivery and within the first 24 hours after delivery (Hack and Fanaroff, 1987). There are four grades of IVH. Recovery from grade 1 IVH is almost always complete. Severe developmental handicaps and death are associated with grade 4 IVH.

Other Problems of Prematurity. Premature infants have less fat and less ability to generate heat. So they are at high risk for hypothermia and have minimal ability to recover from it. Hypothermia is also a trigger for surfactant breakdown. Premature infants also have few glycogen stores and are at greater risk for hypoglycemia.

Assessment

A premature infant is smaller, has less fat, and less muscle tone than a full-term infant. Premature infants should be active and alert like full-term infants, moving around in response to stimuli and giving focused attention to a caregiver. However, the premature infant's attention is easily overwhelmed. A premature infant should have the same response to birth and resuscitation as a full-term infant, although such an infant is at greater risk for hypothermia, hypoxia, and acidosis. A premature infant is at higher risk for asphyxia than is a full-term infant.

A premature infant's most difficult transition is making an adequate effort to expand his or her lungs and keep them expanded. This primary atelectasis plus the atelectasis associated with surfactant deficiency puts the infant at risk for IRDS.

Idiopathic respiratory distress syndrome is characterized by grunting respirations and retractions of the chest wall. Retractions occur because mineralization of the bones is not complete, and the chest wall is not rigid enough to resist the negative pressure needed to inhale. Grunting occurs when the infant tries to compensate for ineffective lung expansion by partially closing the glottis, thereby keeping air trapped in the lungs. On auscultation breath sounds are diminished and have very shortened excursion. Cyanosis may or may not be present. These findings also are present for other respiratory diseases, such as pneumonia.

Physical assessment and assessment of gestational age proceed as for full-term infants. A blood sugar screening and hematocrit also should be done. Careful plotting of weight and height against gestational age on premature growth curves should be done—many low-birth-weight infants actually are not premature but have growth retardation, which carries different risks.

T R I A G E
Premature Infant

Emergent ———————————————
A newborn of less than 37 weeks' gestational age.

Nursing Diagnosis
Ineffective Breathing Pattern

Defining Characteristics

- Nasal flaring and grunting
- Cyanosis
- Retracting

Nursing Interventions

- Administer oxygen
- Assist with intubation

Expected Outcomes

- Color returns to normal
- Normal chest excursion

Nursing Diagnosis
Impaired Gas Exchange

Defining Characteristics

- Hypoxia
- Hypercapnia
- Diminished breath sounds

Nursing Interventions

- Administer oxygen
- Provide continuous positive airway pressure
- Assist with intubation if necessary
- Administer surfactant as ordered

Expected Outcomes

- Blood gases are adequate
- Color returns to normal
- Breath sounds are normal

Nursing Diagnosis
Ineffective Thermoregulation

Defining Characteristics

- Immature thermoregulatory center
- Exposure to radiant and evaporative cooling

Nursing Interventions

- Place infant on radiant warmer
- Wrap infant in warmed blankets
- Dry infant quickly
- Remove wet blankets

Expected Outcome

- Axillary temperature remains normal

Nursing Diagnosis
Altered Nutrition: Less than body requirements

Defining Characteristics

- Inadequate glycogen stores
- Blood sugar less than 30 mg/dl
- Apnea
- Decreased muscle tone

Nursing Interventions

- Administer intravenous glucose as ordered
- Monitor blood glucose levels

Expected Outcome

- Blood glucose levels remain higher than 40 mg/dl

Nursing Diagnosis
Anticipatory Grieving

Defining Characteristics

- Potential loss of baby
- Expressed distress of potential loss

Nursing Interventions

- Keep mother informed of baby's condition
- Facilitate verbalization of feelings

Expected Outcomes

- Parent is able to understand information
- Parent can make decisions regarding care of the baby

Management
Resuscitation of a premature infant proceeds in the manner previously described. It is necessary, however, to take extra precautions to reduce the risks of IVH and the increased utilization of oxygen associated with stress. In addition, a premature infant must be assessed for adequate initial inflation of the lungs. If respiratory distress is exhibited by retraction and grunting, intubation with pressure-limited ventilation that results in moderate chest excursion and positive end expiratory pressure (4–6 mmHg) should be provided. The level of oxygen provided should be adequate to keep the baby pink but just so. If pulse oximetry is available, saturations should be kept at or about 95%. Excess oxygenation should be avoided to prevent oxygen toxicity damage to the immature retinas. Oxygen given by endotracheal intubation or hood should be warmed to near body temperature and humidified.

Surfactant replacement therapy can be given, but it has been shown that for infants of more than 26 weeks' gestational age, no difference in outcome occurs if therapy is held until there is a need for it (Kendig et al, 1991). It is also recognized that when surfactant is given, experts in managing premature infant ventilation must be present to adjust ventilator settings appropriately as pulmonary dynamics change rapidly. For infants of less than 27 weeks' gestational age, the preferred approach is to intubate and give a prophylactic dose of surfactant. Again, the surfactant should be administered only by someone who has experience in managing very-low-birth-weight infants; administration can be postponed until the infant is under the care of the neonatal team.

Keeping the infant warm and assuring glucose balance is as important as resuscitation of the premature infant.

Family Support

Parents are aware that premature births are risky; they are anxious about the outcome of a premature delivery, more so if the infant is more than 1 month premature. They experience anticipatory grief and a lack of knowledge of the specific risks relative to the level of prematurity and the specific problems of a premature infant. Because the infant is in an intensive care unit separated from the mother, perhaps even in a different hospital, anxiety is intensified. In addition, mothers may believe the baby is incompletely formed because he or she was born early.

It is very important that mothers see and touch the baby before it is taken to the neonatal intensive care unit, even if the infant is being taken to another facility. An instant photograph helps the mother to adjust to the separation. Mothers should also have accurate information regarding the status of the infant. This information is best supplied by the neonatal team who transports the infant.

OTHER PROBLEMS OF NEWBORNS

Congenital Heart Defects

There are a variety of congenital heart defects, only some of which may be symptomatic at birth. Transposition of the great vessels has blood circulating in parallel circuits, the oxygenated blood returning back to the lungs and the unoxygenated blood recirculating through the body. The pO_2 may be in the teens, and oxygen therapy has no effect. These infants are often not acidotic initially, yet resuscitation efforts seem unsuccessful. If 100% oxygen has little effect, and the infant is breathing spontaneously with good breath sounds and pulses appear to be normal, further resuscitation is not required. One hundred percent oxygen may be given to improve oxygenation of blood cross-ing into the systemic circulation through persistent fetal shunts.

Several congenital heart defects require the ductus arteriosus to remain open for adequate circulation to either the lungs or the heart. In coarctation of the aorta, one of the more common defects, a narrowing or even blockage of the aorta occurs. Pulses and perfusion in the lower extremities may be decreased. Systemic circulation depends on the ductus arteriosus remaining open. Because the ductus tends to remain open on the first day of life anyway, these defects do not usually present as problems in the emergency room.

Assessment of a newborn should always include pulses in all four extremities, perfusion, color, and auscultation for murmurs to determine cardiac function. Ductal murmurs are heard frequently on the first day of life. A ductal murmur is heard loudest at the upper right or left sternal border. If pulses do not appear to be equal or are weak, blood pressures should be taken on all four extremities; there should not be more than a 10-mmHg difference. If giving 100% oxygen is ineffective after an open airway and adequate lung inflation are assured, there may be a cardiac anomaly. Neonatal and cardiac experts should determine this, however, and 100% oxygen should be continued until pulmonary hypertension has been ruled out.

Other Congenital Anomalies

There are two conditions in which the abdominal contents protrude from the abdomen. In *omphalocele* the intestines protrude encased in a membrane continuous with the umbilical cord. The membrane should be protected from injury or rupture by wrapping it in a warm saline-soaked dressing and then with plastic to prevent cooling by evaporation. Additional efforts should be taken to prevent hypothermia. In *gastroschisis*, the intestines and possibly other abdominal organs are loose outside the abdominal cavity. They should be carefully protected in sterile, warm saline-soaked dressings. Transport to a pediatric surgical facility should be arranged.

Myelomeningocele is a protrusion of the spinal cord, usually in the lumbar area and sometimes encased in a membrane through the back. If the defect is open, the exposed tissue is spinal cord and the fluid draining is spinal fluid. A warm, sterile saline-soaked dressing should be applied. Usually the defect is covered with a membranous sac. If there is any drainage, a sterile dressing should be applied. The infant should be kept prone to keep pressure off the defect and to protect the sac from rupture. Usually the infant is in no other distress. Assessment can include observation of movement in the lower extremities and urine stream.

There are many *defects that can occur in the limbs*

and face that require no immediate treatment and do not distress the infant. Examples are cleft lip and palate, webbed fingers or toes, and clubbed foot. Congenital anomalies often occur together, and whenever one anomaly appears in a newborn infant, a thorough examination should be done to rule out other, perhaps more serious defects.

STABILIZATION AND PREPARATION FOR TRANSPORT

After resuscitation has stabilized the infant's condition, the newborn should be transported in a heated transport incubator as quickly as possible to an appropriate level of nursery care. Only a completely healthy infant who has had no distress should go to a well-baby nursery. If any risks have occurred, or if the infant has had any difficulties, he or she should be transported to a level II or III nursery for further evaluation and observation. Most nurseries have a transport team or can provide personnel for transport who are experienced in care of newborns at high risk.

While awaiting the arrival of the transport team, the ED nurse monitors vital signs, including blood pressure and oxygenation. Blood sugar screening can be done by a heelstick every 30 minutes. An intravenous line of $D_{10}W$ either peripherally or through the umbilical vein should be established if the blood sugar level falls below 40 mg/dL or if any respiratory distress is present. A chest x ray can be done to evaluate placement of the ET and to evaluate cardiopulmonary status. A copy should be sent with the transport team if the baby is going to another hospital. Immediately after delivery a large sample of blood from the umbilical cord and placenta should have been drawn to accompany the baby. A complete copy of the mother's and baby's charts should be made to go with the baby.

CONCLUSION

Delivery and resuscitation of an infant are highly specialized tasks. Every effort should be made for the mother to be taken to a delivery suite before delivery occurs to assure an optimum outcome for both. If delivery is imminent, emergency personnel should proceed calmly and quickly to facilitate delivery and provide adequate care of the newborn. Emergency personnel should be certified in neonatal resuscitation and should always have ready equipment needed for resuscitation. As soon as delivery is anticipated, a neonatal transport team should be requested; transport to a neonatal facility should proceed when the infant's

condition is stabilized. A significant other should be with the mother during delivery, and the mother should see and touch the infant before transport. If the baby is well enough, he or she can be held and nursed.

REFERENCES

American Heart Association and the American Academy of Pediatrics (1990). *Textbook of Neonatal Resuscitation.* Elk Grove Village, Ill: American Heart Association

Apgar V, Holaday D, James L, Weisbrot I, Berrin C (1958). Evaluation of the newborn infant: Second report. *JAMA* 168:1985–1988

Ballard JL, Novak KK, Driver M (1987). A simplified score for assessment of fetal maturation of newly born infants. *Journal of Pediatrics* 110:921–928

Boychuk RB (1991). The critically ill neonate in the emergency department. *Emergency Medicine Clinics of North America* 9:507–522

Brunette DD (1989). Prehospital and emergency department delivery: A review of eight years' experience. *Annals of Emergency Medicine* 18:1116–1117

Burnett CA, Jones JA, Rooks J, et al (1980). Home delivery and neonatal mortality in North Carolina. *JAMA* 244:2741–2745

Carlo W (1992). Assessment of pulmonary function. In Fanaroff AA, Martin RJ (eds), *Neonatal Perinatal Medicine.* St. Louis: Mosby Year Book

Committee on Fetus and Newborn, American Academy of Pediatrics (1986). Use and abuse of the Apgar score. *Pediatrics* 78:1148–1149

Constantine NA, Kraemer HC, Kendall-Tackett KA, Bennett FC, Tyson JE, Gross RT (1987). Use of physical and neurological observations in assessment of gestational age in low-birth-weight infants. *Journal of Pediatrics* 110:921–928

Cunningham AS, Lawson EE, Martin RJ, Pildes RS (1989). Tracheal suction and meconium: A proposed standard of care. *Journal of Pediatrics* 116:153–154

Dimich I, Singh PP, Adell A, Hendler M, Sonnenklar N, Jhaveri M (1991). Evaluation of oxygen saturation monitoring by pulse oximetry in neonates in the delivery system. *Canadian Journal of Anaesthesia* 38:985–988

Doan-Wiggins L (1991). Emergency delivery. In Harwood-Nuss A (ed), MD. *The Clinical Practice of Emergency Medicine.* Philadelphia: Lippincott

Dodman N (1987). Newborn temperature control. *Neonatal Network* 5(6):19–23

Edwards MC (1988). Delivery room resuscitation of the neonate. *Pediatric Annals* 17:458–466

Friedman EA (1978). *Labor: Clinical Evaluation and Management* (2nd ed). New York: Appleton-Century-Crofts

Hack M, Fanaroff AA (1986). Changes in the delivery room care of the extremely small infant. *New England Journal of Medicine* 314:660–664

Hack M, Fanaroff AA (1989). Outcomes of extremely low-birth-weight infants between 1982 and 1988. *New England Journal of Medicine* 321:1642–1647

Harper RA, Seaton E, Spinazzola R, Schlessel JS (1990). Unexpected, unattended deliveries. *New York State Journal of Medicine* 90(6):330–331

Higgins SD (1987). Emergency delivery: Prehospital care, emergency department delivery, perimortem salvage. *Emergency Medicine Clinics of North America* 5:529–540

Jepson HA, Talashek ML, Tichy AM (1991). The Apgar score: Evolution, limitations, and scoring guidelines. *Birth* 18:83–91

Katz VL, Bowes WA (1992). Meconium aspiration syndrome: Reflections on a murky subject. *American Journal of Obstetrics and Gynecology* 166:171–183

Kendig JW, Notter RH, Cox C, et al (1991). A comparison of surfactant as immediate prophylaxis and as rescue therapy in newborns of less than 30 weeks' gestation. *New England Journal of Medicine* 324:865–872

Kraybill EN (1987). Needs of the Term Infant. In Avery GB (ed), *Neonatology: Pathophysiology and Management of the Newborn.* Philadelphia: Lippincott pp 258–263

Lamb FS, Rosner MS (1987). Neonatal Resuscitation. *Emergency Medicine Clinics of North America* 5:541–557

Linder N, Aranda JV, Tsur M, et al (1988). Need for endo-
tracheal intubation and suction in meconium-stained neonates. *Journal of Pediatrics* 112:613–615

Nelson NM (1987). The Onset of Respiration. In Avery GB (ed), *Neonatology: Pathophysiology and Management of the Newborn.* Philadelphia: Lippincott pp 176–200

Phibbs RH (1987). Delivery Room Management of the Newborn. In Avery GB (ed), *Neonatology: Pathophysiology and Management of the Newborn.* Philadelphia: Lippincott pp 212–234

Schramm WF, Barnes DE, Bakewell JM (1987). Neonatal mortality in Missouri home births. *American Journal of Public Health* 77:930–935

Tyson H (1991). Outcomes of 1001 midwife-attended home births in Toronto. *Birth* 18:14–19

Yancey MK, Moore J, Brady K, Milligan D, Strampel W (1992). The effect of altitude on umbilical cord blood gases. *Obstetrics and Gynecology* 79:571–574

Yeomans ER, Hauth JC, Gilstrap LC, Strickland DM (1985). Umbilical cord pH, PCO_2, and bicarbonate following uncomplicated term vaginal deliveries. *American Journal of Obstetrics and Gynecology* 151:798–800

CHAPTER 13

Resuscitation of Infants, Children, and Adolescents

ANN POWERS

INTRODUCTION

Cardiopulmonary arrest in infants and children is often an unexpected, emotionally charged, and tragic event. In many cases, it is also preventable. Most emergency nurses see few pediatric cardiac arrests unless they work in a large children's hospital. Successful resuscitation of a pediatric patient requires knowledge of the etiology and pathophysiology of pediatric cardiopulmonary arrest; knowledge of the anatomic and physiologic differences between infants, children, and adults; and competent assessment, intervention, organization, and priority-setting skills.

ETIOLOGY AND PATHOPHYSIOLOGY

Cardiopulmonary arrest in a pediatric patient usually occurs as a result of progressive hypoxia and acidosis secondary to an underlying respiratory or circulatory disorder. Without appropriate intervention, the hypoxia and acidosis lead to respiratory failure or shock, which immediately precede the arrest. The condition of a patient in this situation is severely compromised at the time of the arrest. Pediatric cardiopulmonary arrest is usually preceded by a compensated state, which has specific signs and symptoms. If these warning signs go unrecognized and untreated, rapid deterioration occurs, leading to arrest. This process is in sharp contrast to the etiology of adult cardiopulmonary arrests, which usually occur as a primary cardiac event with loss of perfusion at a time of relative homeostasis.

Most pediatric arrests occur secondary to a respiratory disorder characterized by progressive and prolonged hypoxia. Because of this, the outcomes are poor, the mortality exceeding 90% in some studies. Among children who do survive, many suffer permanent neurologic sequelae (Gillis et al, 1986; Torphy et al, 1984; Zaritsky, 1987). Respiratory arrest alone carries a much better prognosis, the survival rates being 40–50% (Friesen et al, 1982; Gillis, 1986). It is therefore critical to recognize that a child is in respiratory failure and to initiate appropriate intervention before circulatory failure and arrest follow.

Sudden, primary cardiac arrest in infants and children is rare, occurring most often in children with complex congenital heart disease. The incidence of lethal ventricular dysrhythmias increases after cardiac surgery in proportion to the child's age at the time of the operation, after a right ventriculotomy is done, or when residual cardiac defects are present (Krongrad, 1984). Although rare, these dysrhythmias are usually sudden, unanticipated events that can occur at any time. Ventricular fibrillation has been reported in less than 10% of children in pulseless arrest (Eisenberg et al, 1983).

Pediatric cardiopulmonary arrests occur most frequently during either the first year of life or in the teen years. More than one-half of arrests happen during infancy, most of these in infants younger than 4 months. The most common causes of infant arrests are sudden infant death syndrome (SIDS), airway obstruction, drowning, sepsis, and neurologic diseases. Beyond the first year of life, common causes include motor vehicle accidents, drownings, burns, gunshot wounds, and ingestions (American Heart Association, 1992a).

Anatomic and physiologic features in infants and

small children predispose them to respiratory and cardiac failure, which can result in cardiopulmonary arrest. Features in the upper and lower airways include the following. The nasal passages in infants are very narrow and can easily be obstructed by secretions or foreign bodies. Infants breathe through their noses for the first few months of life, which places them at high risk for respiratory distress and failure because of obstructed nasal passages. The respiratory tract is short, narrow, and compact. Because of this, pathogens have a shorter distance to travel to reach the terminal airways and pulmonary vasculature, which may result in respiratory or systemic infection. Because the pediatric airway is narrow, obstruction can easily occur from a foreign body, mucus, or edema. A 1-mm decrease in the diameter of an infant's airway produces a 75% decrease in the cross-sectional area and a 16-fold increase in airway resistance (Chameides, 1988). Infants and small children also have large tongues, which can easily obstruct the airway with improper positioning. The epiglottis is large, U-shaped, and lies cephalad; it can obstruct the airway with even a small amount of edema (ie, epiglottitis). The glottic opening is anterior and high in relation to the esophagus, predisposing infants and small children to aspiration. The cricoid ring is the narrowest portion of the airway until the middle of childhood. Because of this, small foreign bodies can be aspirated deeper into the trachea before they obstruct the airway; thus they are difficult to remove. The cartilage supporting both the upper and lower airways is poorly developed in early childhood. As a result, airways can be easily obstructed by mucus, blood, edema, or active constriction. Extrinsic factors, such as vascular rings, tumors, and congenital anomalies, also can compress the airway, thereby causing obstruction. Hyperextension or flexion of the neck can compress and obstruct the airway. Infants are especially susceptible to hyperextension and hyperflexion because they have poor head control during the first few months of life. It is important to remember that any disorder that contributes to airway obstruction increases airway resistance, and therefore increases the work of breathing. Without appropriate and timely intervention, this process can lead to respiratory failure and arrest. Only a small proportion of alveoli are present at birth, which limits gas exchange at the alveolar level. Alveoli increase in size and number from birth through the middle of childhood. Alveolar and bronchiolar pathways for collateral ventilation are incomplete during infancy and early childhood; therefore the ability to ventilate alveoli below the level of bronchiolar obstruction is decreased, compromising respiratory function.

Anatomic features of the thoracic cage also predispose infants and small children to respiratory dysfunction. The chest wall and sternum are soft and have a greater proportion of cartilage to hard bone. This configuration causes the chest wall to collapse inward when airway resistance and work of breathing increase. This phenomenon in turn decreases tidal volume, which further compromises effective ventilation. The ribs are more horizontal in infancy and early childhood than later in life and are not well supported by the intercostal muscles. Both the intercostal and accessory muscles are poorly developed and are unable to contribute to respiratory excursion when distress develops. Because of these factors, infants and small children are very dependent on effective diaphragmatic functioning to maintain adequate ventilation. Any problem that impedes this functioning, such as abdominal distention, a spica cast, or diaphragmatic paralysis, can contribute to the development of respiratory distress and failure. Premature infants are at particularly high risk for respiratory compromise. They have a poor medullary response to changes in pCO_2, which may result in apnea or periodic breathing. Surfactant insufficiency, which causes decreased lung compliance, can predispose premature infants to respiratory distress. Hypoglycemia and cold stress, with or without respiratory disease, can lead to respiratory arrest.

Another factor that predisposes infants and children to both respiratory and circulatory compromise is immaturity of the immune system, which increases susceptibility to infection. The metabolic rate also is higher, which increases oxygen demand and consumption and therefore results in faster development of hypoxemia and acidosis with any cardiopulmonary disorder. A child's brain has a particularly high oxygen demand and is very sensitive to hypoxemia, which can cause hypoxic-ischemic injury. Other problems that can contribute to cardiopulmonary arrest in the pediatric population include seizures, increased intracranial pressure, metabolic disturbances, neuromuscular diseases, gastroesophageal reflux, and administration of narcotics.

The physiologic compensatory response to hypoxia in pediatric patients includes an increase in respiratory rate, heart rate, and work of breathing. If this response is ineffective and hypoxia is prolonged, the body shifts from aerobic to anaerobic metabolism, which leads to metabolic acidosis through the production of lactic acid. The compensatory response to shock in a pediatric patient includes tachycardia, tachypnea, increased cardiac contractility, and peripheral vasoconstriction, which attempts to maintain blood flow to vital organs. Severe vasoconstriction leads to inadequate tissue perfusion, which causes metabolic acidosis. Because of these cardiovascular responses, oxygen consumption and demand increase, which can lead to hypoxemia and hypoxia. Without timely and effective intervention during the compensatory phases of respiratory failure and shock, decompensation rapidly follows. Both hypoxia and acidosis depress cardiac conduction and contractility, resulting in ineffective myocardial contraction, dysrhythmias, bradycardia, and, finally, asystole.

HISTORY

A designated emergency department (ED) staff member should immediately obtain a rapid and thorough history from the family member or witness to the arrest. The history should include events or circumstances before the arrest, the length of time the child had no breathing or pulse before the initiation of cardiopulmonary resuscitation (CPR), who administered CPR, and for how long CPR was given before arrival in the ED. If prehospital care providers responded to the arrest, a detailed report of treatments and procedures initiated in the field should be obtained. Other important facts to obtain are the circumstances surrounding the child's illness or injury, the child's activities and behavior in the previous 24 hours, past medical history, allergies, and immunization status.

PHYSICAL ASSESSMENT

As soon as the child arrives in the ED, the nurse must quickly perform an assessment for level of responsiveness, airway, breathing, circulation, and extent of injuries. Responsiveness is determined by tapping the child and speaking loudly, and assessing the level of the child's response. If head or neck trauma is suspected, the cervical spine should be immobilized until a spinal cord injury has been ruled out. When the patient is moved, the head and body must be supported and turned as a unit so that the head does not roll or twist.

Respiratory assessment includes evaluation of the patient's airway for patency, respiratory rate, air exchange, work of breathing, and color. Tachypnea is usually the first sign of respiratory distress in infants and children. Bradypnea is an ominous sign; it usually precedes respiratory arrest. A slow respiratory rate can be caused by hypothermia, fatigue, or central nervous system depression from a variety of causes. It is important for the nurse to know that a decreasing respiratory rate is not necessarily a sign of improvement and that it may actually indicate decompensation. Increased work of breathing in a pediatric patient presents as nasal flaring, use of accessory muscles, and intercostal, subcostal, and suprasternal retractions.

Head bobbing with each breath frequently signals impending respiratory arrest. Evaluation of air exchange includes assessment of chest wall movement and breath sounds. Stridor occurs with upper airway obstruction; prolonged expiration accompanied by wheezing occurs with lower airway obstruction.

Expiratory grunting is another sign of respiratory distress in infants and small children; it occurs in disorders in which interstitial or alveolar fluid accumulates. It is important to note that accurate assessment of breath sounds in a pediatric patient requires practice and skill. Breath sounds are easily transmitted from one area of the lungs to another because the chest wall is thin and compact. A change in pitch may be the only evidence of areas of compromise. Diminished breath sounds may or may not be heard on auscultation.

The child's color is assessed by checking the mucus membranes of the mouth and nailbeds. Cyanosis is a late sign of respiratory failure. Cyanosis of the extremities is more often due to vasoconstriction associated with shock or hypothermia than to respiratory failure. Arterial oxygen saturation should always be assessed by pulse oximetry if available to accurately determine oxygenation status.

Cardiovascular assessment includes evaluation of the patient's heart rate, perfusion status, and blood pressure. An increased heart rate is the normal compensatory response to many types of stress. Cardiac output is equal to heart rate times stroke volume. Infants depend on heart rate to maintain cardiac output, because they have limited ability to increase stroke volume with any compromise in cardiovascular function. The primary response of the neonatal myocardium to hypoxemia is bradycardia; in older children, tachycardia occurs first. When tachycardia fails to compensate adequately, tissue hypoxia and acidosis develop, resulting in bradycardia. Bradycardia in a distressed infant may be a sign of hypoxemia, which could lead to cardiac arrest. In a child bradycardia is usually a sign of impending cardiac arrest. Perfusion is assessed by evaluating peripheral pulses and blood flow to the skin, brain, and kidneys.

A decrease in the strength and volume of peripheral pulses is noted with vasoconstriction associated with hypothermia or early shock. As shock progresses, peripheral pulses become thready and, finally, impalpable. Loss of a central pulse is a sign of impending cardiac arrest. Decreased perfusion to the skin is also an early sign of shock. Mottling, pallor, coolness, a capillary refill time greater than 3 seconds, and peripheral cyanosis indicate poor perfusion to the skin.

Level of consciousness is the best indicator of cerebral perfusion. This is assessed in infants and toddlers by noting whether or not they recognize their parents; older children should be able to respond by speaking. In early shock, restlessness, agitation, confusion, and anxiety can occur. As shock progresses, the child becomes less responsive. It is important to identify other factors from the patient's history, such as head trauma or ingestion of narcotics, that may alter consciousness.

Urine output is an accurate reflection of renal perfusion, although it is not often helpful in the initial assessment because information regarding recent urine output is often vague or nonspecific. An indwelling urinary catheter should be placed as soon as possible to facilitate assessment of renal perfusion. The minimal acceptable urine output is 0.5 mL/kg/hr for a child and 1 mL/kg/hr for an infant.

Blood pressure is a less reliable indicator of adequate cardiac output in infants and children. Normal blood pressure can be maintained during shock as long as the patient compensates with tachycardia, vasoconstriction, and increased cardiac contractility. Hypotension is usually a late and sudden sign of cardiovascular decompensation; it signals imminent cardiac arrest in the pediatric population.

The patient should be undressed to facilitate quick and accurate assessment. It is important to provide external warming measures (lights or heat) because infants and children have a large body surface area relative to weight, and they quickly lose heat to the environment through convection and evaporation. Energy used to maintain body temperature increases oxygen consumption, which can further compromise the patient's status if either hypoxia or acidosis is present. Hypothermia also causes vasoconstriction and bradycardia, which can mimic shock or hinder successful resuscitation.

As soon as airway, breathing, and circulation are evaluated and appropriate basic life support is initiated, a quick head-to-toe assessment is performed to identify other problems. The head is inspected and palpated for signs of deformity, fracture, laceration, or other trauma. The pupils should be assessed for size and reactivity. Pupils become fixed and dilated with hypoxia and ischemia. Unilateral pupil dilation may indicate a localized lesion. Extraocular movements are assessed; these are asymmetric with structural coma. The anterior fontanelle is assessed in infants, preferably with the infant in a sitting position and when quiet and not crying. A tense, full, or bulging fontanelle occurs with increased intracranial pressure, whereas a depressed fontanelle may indicate hypovolemia. The neck is inspected and palpated for signs of deformity, trauma, subcutaneous air, and the position of the trachea. The chest wall is assessed for spontaneous and equal movement and trauma. The abdomen is evaluated for distention, rigidity, and trauma. Finally, the extremities are assessed for fractures and other signs of trauma.

LABORATORY AND DIAGNOSTIC TESTS

Blood tests should be done as soon as possible to assess for abnormalities that may be contributing to the child's status or that may hinder successful resuscitation efforts. These tests should include arterial blood gas determinations, measurement of electrolytes, calcium, glucose, urea nitrogen, hemoglobin levels, and a hematocrit. Resuscitation is not to be delayed while blood tests are performed.

TRIAGE
Cardiopulmonary Arrest

Emergent

Any child experiencing respiratory arrest; cardiac arrest; bradycardia with low cardiac output; respiratory failure; shock.

Nursing Diagnosis

Ineffective Airway Clearance

Defining Characteristics

- Obstruction by tongue
- Obstruction by secretion
- Inability to cough effectively

Nursing Interventions

- Open airway with chin lift maneuver
- Remove foreign object if visible
- Maintain head in a neutral position
- Insert oropharyngeal airway if unconscious
- Insert nasopharyngeal airway if conscious
- Suction oropharynx and nasopharynx to remove mucus or blood as needed

Expected Outcome

- Patency of airway is maintained

Nursing Diagnosis

Ineffective Breathing Pattern

Defining Characteristics

- Absence of spontaneous respiration
- Cyanosis

Nursing Interventions

- Determine presence of breathing: look, listen and feel for exhaled air
- Provide assisted ventilation mouth to mouth or with a bag-valve-mask device
- Assess breath sounds and chest wall movement during ventilation
- Assist with endotracheal intubation
- Administer 100% humidified oxygen

Expected Outcome

- Adequate ventilation maintains gas exchange

Nursing Diagnosis
Impaired Gas Exchange

Defining Characteristic

- Abnormal blood gases

Nursing Interventions

- Provide assisted ventilation mouth to mouth or with a bag-valve-mask device
- Assist with endotracheal intubation
- Assess breath sounds and chest wall movement during ventilation
- Initiate cardiopulmonary resuscitation

Expected Outcome

- Arterial blood gasses are maintained within normal limits

Nursing Diagnosis
High Risk for Aspiration

Defining Characteristics

- Presence of endotracheal tube
- Depressed gas reflex

Nursing Interventions

- Provide long inspiratory times with low pressure during assisted ventilation
- Assess for gastric distention
- Decompress stomach by inserting a nasogastric tube to remove air and stomach contents

Expected Outcome

- Aspiration is prevented

Nursing Diagnosis
Decreased Cardiac Output

Defining Characteristics

- Cardiopulmonary arrest
- Absence of palpable pulse

Nursing Interventions

- For a child, palpate the carotid or femoral pulse to assess presence of cardiac output
- For an infant, palpate the brachial or femoral pulse to assess presence of cardiac output
- Place child supine on a firm surface
- Initiate CPR if there is no pulse
- Monitor heart rate and rhythm continuously
- Administer drugs to support heart rate, rhythm, and cardiac output
- Monitor perfusion status and blood pressure continuously

Expected Outcomes

- Cardiac output is restored and maintained
- Tissue perfusion is adequate

Nursing Diagnosis
Fluid Volume Deficit

Defining Characteristics

- Bleeding
- Abnormal fluid losses

Nursing Interventions

- Administer appropriate intravenous fluids (crystalloid, colloid, or blood products) at desired rate (depending on volume status)
- Monitor vital signs and respiratory and perfusion status to assess response to fluids
- Measure intake and output

Expected Outcomes

- Expansion of circulation volume is achieved and maintained
- Tissue perfusion is adequate
- Vital signs are within normal limits for age and clinical condition

Nursing Diagnosis
Altered Tissue Perfusion

Defining Characteristics

- Weak or absent palpable pulses
- Cool skin, mottling
- Cyanosis
- Decreased urine output

Nursing Interventions

- Initiate basic or advanced life support
- Monitor arterial blood gases
- Assess strength of pulses, skin color and temperature, capillary refill time, level of responsiveness, and neurologic status continuously
- Hyperventilate the patient if there is evidence of increased intracranial pressure
- Place Foley catheter and monitor urine output

Expected Outcomes

- Adequate tissue perfusion is maintained as evidenced by presence of pulses
- Skin tissue is pink and warm
- Appropriate level of responsiveness is present.
- Urine output is adequate

Nursing Diagnosis
Hypothermia

Defining Characteristics

- Cool skin
- Slow capillary refill

Nursing Interventions

- Monitor rectal or tympanic temperature continually
- Use overhead radiant warmer or heat lamps
- Maintain warm ambient room temperature
- Use warming blankets
- Place hat on infants and small children
- Warm intravenous fluids, blood products, and gastric lavage fluids before administering them

Expected Outcomes

- Body temperature is stabilized and maintained within normal limits
- Peripheral perfusion is adequate

Nursing Diagnosis
Anticipatory Grieving

Defining Characteristic

- Potential loss of loved one

Nursing Interventions

- Provide a staff member for continuous communication and support to parents regarding their child's status
- Provide a private area for parents and family to grieve

- Provide emotional support using crisis intervention skills
- Contact family or clergy member to be with the parents
- Allow parents to see their child either during or as soon as possible after the resuscitation

Expected Outcomes

- Parents are informed about their child's condition
- Parents feel supported by the staff
- The grieving process begins
- Short-term goals are established

Nursing Diagnosis
Knowledge Deficit Related to Child's Condition and Resuscitation Process

Defining Characteristic

- Inadequate understanding of emergency procedures

Nursing Intervention

- Continually inform the parents of the child's status, resuscitation efforts, and the child's response to treatments

Expected Outcome

- Parents demonstrate an understanding of the child's condition and the treatments performed

BASIC LIFE SUPPORT

Basic life support is initiated to maintain or restore oxygenated blood flow to the brain and other vital organs when cardiopulmonary failure or arrest occurs. The steps taken to initiate basic life support are outlined in Table 13–1.

Establishing Unresponsiveness
Infants and children normally respond to tactile stimulation by moving, crying, or speaking. To establish unresponsiveness, loudly call to, and gently shake the patient. If head or neck trauma is suspected, care should be taken to avoid injury to the spinal cord. Any child who is conscious and experiencing respiratory distress should be allowed to assume the position of their choice; children usually position themselves to maximize airway opening.

Call for Help
If the patient is unresponsive, limp, not breathing, or is experiencing respiratory difficulty, the nurse should

TABLE 13–1. THE SEQUENCE OF CPR

Maneuver	Infant (<1 year)	Child (1 to 8 years)
Airway	Head tilt–chin lift (unless trauma occurred) Jaw thrust	Head tilt–chin lift (unless trauma occurred) Jaw thrust
Breathing		
Initial	2 breaths at 1 to 1½ seconds/breath	2 breaths at 1 to 1½ seconds/breath
Subsequent	20 breaths/min	20 breaths/min
Circulation		
Pulse check	Brachial/femoral	Carotid
Compression area	Lower third of sternum	Lower third of sternum
Compression with Depth	2 or 3 fingers Approximately ½ to 1 in	Heel of 1 hand Approximately 1 to 1½ in
Rate	At least 100 compressions/min	100 compressions/min
Compression-to-ventilation ratio	5 : 1 (pause for ventilation)	5 : 1 (pause for ventilation)
Foreign-body airway obstruction	Back blows, chest thrusts	Heimlich maneuver

(From American Heart Association [1992]. Guidelines for cardiopulmonary resuscitation and emergency cardiac care: Pediatric basic life support. JAMA 28:2257)

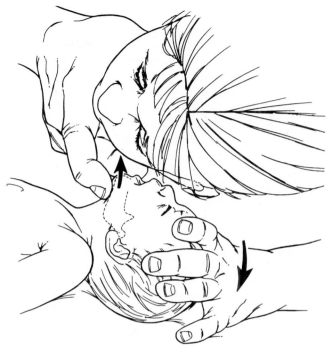

Figure 13–1. Opening the airway with the head tilt–chin lift maneuver. One hand is used to tilt the head, extending the neck. The index finger of the rescuer's other hand lifts the mandible outward by lifting on the chin. Head tilt should not be performed if cervical spine injury is suspected. (Reproduced with permission from the American Heart Association [1992]. Guidelines for cardiopulmonary resuscitation and emergency cardiac care: Pediatric basic life support. *JAMA* 268:2253)

call for help. If the nurse is alone and the child is not breathing and is pulseless, CPR should be performed for 1 minute before the nurse calls for help.

Position the Victim
The infant or child should be positioned supine on a firm, flat surface for CPR to be effective. If head or neck trauma is suspected, the patient must be supported and turned as a unit so that the head does not roll, turn, or twist in any direction during movement.

Open and Clear the Airway
Because of the anatomy of the pediatric airway, it easily obstructs during unconsciousness secondary to muscle relaxation and passive posterior displacement of the tongue. The airway should be immediately opened by the head tilt–chin lift method. To accomplish this maneuver, the nurse places one hand on the patient's forehead and tilts the head back gently into a neutral or slightly extended position for an infant (Figure 13–1) and slightly farther back for an older child. Hyperextension of the airway is avoided because this can obstruct the soft, pliable, and narrow airway of an infant or small child. The fingers, not the thumb, of the other hand are placed under the bony part of the lower jaw at the chin, and the chin is lifted. Special attention must be taken not to close the mouth or push on the soft tissues under the chin; doing so can cause further airway obstruction.

If a neck injury is suspected, the head tilt should

be avoided and the airway opened using a jaw thrust maneuver. To accomplish this maneuver the nurse rests her or his elbows on the surface where the patient is lying and places two or three fingers under the angle of the jaw and lifts it (Figure 13–2). If the jaw thrust

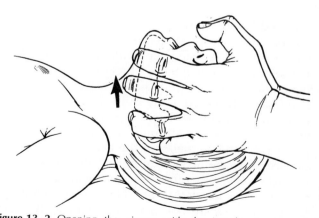

Figure 13–2. Opening the airway with the jaw-thrust maneuver. The airway is opened by lifting the angle of the mandible. The rescuer uses two or three fingers of each hand to lift the jaw while other fingers guide the jaw upward and outward. (Reproduced with permission from the American Heart Association [1992]. Guidelines for cardiopulmonary resuscitation and emergency cardiac care: Pediatric basic life support. *JAMA* 268:2254)

alone does not open the airway, a slight head tilt can be used with the jaw thrust as long as there is no evidence of an injury to the cervical spine. The patient's cervical spine should be immobilized by a second person as soon as possible.

The airway must be cleared to allow for effective ventilation. This is done with a finger swipe of the oropharynx only if an obstruction can be seen. This maneuver is especially important and often overlooked in toddlers; because they are inquisitive and unafraid, they frequently put objects in their mouths. Suctioning of the nasopharynx and oropharynx also may clear the airway. The appropriate amount of suction pressure to use varies with age. In general, 60–90 mmHg of suction pressure is used in infants, 90–110 mmHg in children, and 110–150 mmHg in adolescents (Zander and Hazinski, 1992).

Assessment of Respiration

Once patency of the airway is established, the nurse next determines whether or not the patient is breathing. This task is accomplished by observing the chest and abdomen for respiratory movement while listening and feeling for exhaled air from the patient's mouth. Because the diaphragm is the main muscle of respiration in infants and toddlers, symmetric chest wall movement is best observed at the lower chest and upper abdominal area as an indicator of adequate ventilation. Older children and adolescents use intercostal and accessory muscles for respiration; therefore, symmetric chest wall expansion is best observed at the upper chest as an indicator of effective ventilation. Auscultation of the neck and chest wall facilitates assessment of air exchange in the upper and lower airways. This part of the assessment can be done while observing chest wall movement during respiration if present.

Assisted Ventilation

If spontaneous respiration does not occur after the airway is opened, assisted ventilation must be provided. For infants, the nurse takes a breath and places his or her mouth over the infant's nose and mouth, forming a seal (Figure 13–3). For older children, the nurse makes a mouth-to-mouth seal while pinching the patient's nose closed with the thumb and forefingers while using the hand to maintain the head tilt. Emergency departments should be equipped with masks with a one-way valve, other infection control barriers, or self-inflating bags for staff to provide assisted ventilation. If such devices are not available, ventilation should not be delayed, and mouth-to-mouth breathing should be initiated (American Heart Association, 1992a). If mouth-to-mouth breathing is needed, the nurse should give two initial slow breaths, pausing after the first breath to take a breath, thereby maximizing oxygen and minimizing carbon dioxide content in the

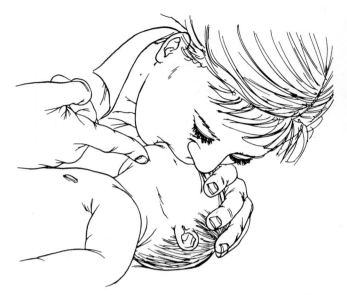

Figure 13–3. Rescue breathing in an infant. The rescuer's mouth covers the infant's nose and mouth, creating a seal. One hand performs head tilt while the other hand lifts the infant's jaw. Avoid head tilt if the infant has sustained head or neck trauma. (Reproduced with permission from the American Heart Association [1992]. Guidelines for cardiopulmonary resuscitation and emergency cardiac care: Pediatric basic life support. *JAMA* 268:2254)

breaths delivered (Terndrup et al, 1989). Regardless of how assisted breaths are delivered, adequate volume for each breath is the volume that causes the chest to rise. Breaths should be delivered slowly at a low inspiratory pressure. If breaths are delivered too rapidly, esophageal opening pressure (approximately 20 cm H_2O) is exceeded, and gastric distention may result. Gastric distention elevates the diaphragm and restricts lung capacity, which can hinder resuscitation efforts.

If air enters the lungs easily and the chest rises, the airway is clear. If this does not occur, then more breath volume or pressure may be needed, or the head and neck may be repositioned to open the airway. If these maneuvers fail and ventilation continues to be unsuccessful, a foreign body may be obstructing the airway. Assisted breaths should be delivered at a rate of 20 breaths per minute, or one breath every 3 seconds. Adjuncts to assisted ventilation are discussed in the section on advanced life support.

Circulation

Assessment of the pulse is done to check for ineffective or absent cardiac contractions. In children older than 1 year, the carotid artery is palpated. Because infants have short, stubby necks, it is difficult to locate the carotid artery quickly. Therefore, the brachial artery is palpated in infants younger than 1 year. The femoral artery also may be used to assess for cardiac contraction because it is easily located in all children and is accessible once the child is undressed. It is unac-

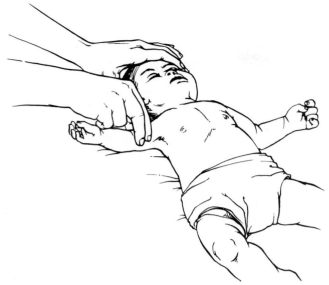

Figure 13–4. Palpating the brachial artery pulse. (Reproduced with permission from the American Heart Association [1992]. Guidelines for cardiopulmonary resuscitation and emergency cardiac care: Pediatric basic life support. *JAMA* 268:2255)

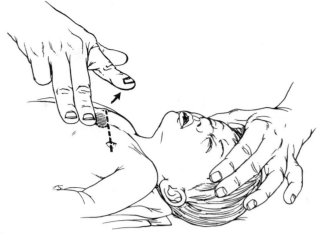

Figure 13–5. Locating proper finger position for chest compressions in infant. Note that the rescuer's other hand is used to maintain head position to facilitate ventilation. (Reproduced with permission from the American Heart Association [1992]. Guidelines for cardiopulmonary resuscitation and emergency cardiac care: Pediatric basic life support. *JAMA* 268:2253)

ceptable to use the apical pulse because a pulsation in this area actually may be an electrical impulse, not the mechanical pulsation of blood.

The carotid artery is located by sliding two or three fingers from the child's trachea toward the sternocleidomastoid muscle on the side where the nurse is standing while gently palpating for a pulse. The brachial artery is located by placing the thumb on the outer aspect of the infant's upper arm while palpating the inside of the upper arm with the index and middle fingers (Figure 13-4). If a pulse is present and the patient is not breathing, assisted ventilation alone may be sufficient, depending on the pulse rate and quality. If the pulse is absent, chest compressions are initiated and must be coordinated with assisted breathing. Continuous electrocardiographic monitoring should be initiated as soon as possible, as should blood pressure monitoring. It is important to note that the presence of cardiac electrical activity on the monitor screen does not necessarily indicate effective cardiac contraction. The pulse must be assessed to determine this.

Chest Compressions

The infant or child must be supine on a firm, flat surface for chest compressions to be effective. The purpose of providing compressions is to circulate oxygenated blood to the heart, lungs, and brain. The compressions, therefore, must always be accompanied by ventilation. Effective cardiac compressions generate only about 25–30% of normal cardiac output (Paradis et al, 1990). The American Heart Association (1992a) recommends the following technique for pediatric patients.

Infants

Compressions in infants are done over the lower third of the sternum (Figure 13–5). This area is located by drawing an imaginary line between the nipples over the sternum. The index finger on the hand farther away from the infant's head is then placed on the sternum just below this line. The middle and ring fingers are then placed on the sternum adjacent to the index finger. The sternum is compressed one finger breadth below the nipple line with the middle and ring fingers at a rate of 100 compressions per minute to a depth of ½–1 inch.

Children

Compressions in children between the ages of 1 and 8 years also are done over the lower third of the sternum (Figure 13–6). The correct spot is located by tracing the lower margin of the rib cage with the middle finger of the hand closest to the child's feet on the side of the chest where the nurse is standing. When the middle finger reaches the sternal notch, the index finger is placed adjacent to the middle finger. The heel of the same hand is then placed next to the point where the index finger was located. Compressions are done with the heel of the hand, care being taken to hold the fingers up off the ribs, at a rate 80–100 compressions per minute to a depth of 1–1½ inches.

Compressions for children older than 8 years and for adolescents are done in approximately the same location. The heel of one hand is placed on the lower half of the sternum, and the other hand is placed on top of the hand on the sternum. The fingers may be extended or interlocked, as long as they are kept off the ribs. The sternum is depressed to 1½–2 inches,

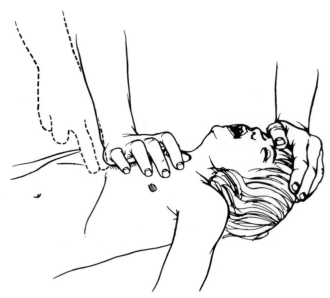

Figure 13–6. Locating hand position for chest compressions in child. Note that the rescuer's other hand is used to maintain head position to facilitate ventilation. (Reproduced with permission from the American Heart Association [1992]. Guidelines for cardiopulmonary resuscitation and emergency cardiac care: Pediatric basic life support. *JAMA* 268:2253)

depending on the size of the child at a rate of 80 to 100 compressions per minute.

Chest compressions should be smooth and rhythmic. The chest is allowed to return to its normal position between compressions, but the nurse's fingers or hands remain on the sternum. It is important to check for a pulse during CPR because adequate chest compressions should be strong enough to generate a central pulse. The ratio of compressions to assisted ventilation is 5:1; two people should provide CPR if at all possible. (If mouth-to-mouth breathing and compressions are performed on an infant, one-person CPR is appropriate). Table 13–1 gives a summary of the sequence of steps for basic life support.

ADVANCED CARDIAC LIFE SUPPORT

Adjuncts for Airway and Ventilation

Oxygen Delivery Systems. If an infant or child is breathing but is in acute respiratory distress, humidified oxygen should be administered at the highest possible concentration. Heated humidification systems are preferred over cool systems because cool mist may contribute to hypothermia in infants and small children. Oxygen can be delivered by face mask, hood, tent, or nasal cannula, depending on the size of the patient. Oxygen tents are avoided in acute situations because it is difficult to assess and observe a child in a

tent. An infant or unconscious child should be positioned (with a slightly elevated head and chest) to maximize airway opening and respiratory excursion. If the child is conscious, he or she is allowed to assume the position most comfortable to him or her. It is important to consider that administration of high concentrations of oxygen to infants and children with chronic respiratory disease may eliminate respiratory drive, resulting in bradypnea or apnea. These children must be closely monitored during the administration of oxygen.

Airways. Oropharyngeal airways can be used to maintain a patent airway in an unconscious infant or child. The use of such airways is contraindicated in conscious patients because placement can induce gagging, vomiting, and aspiration. Sizes range from 000 to 5 (4 to 10 cm long) to accommodate children of all sizes. Proper size is determined by placing the airway along the side of the face with the flange at the level of the central incisors, the bite block segment parallel to the hard palate, and the tip extending to the angle of the jaw. Appropriate size and placement are critical—an airway that is too small or too large or placed incorrectly can obstruct the airway.

Because they are better tolerated than oral airways, nasopharyngeal airways can be used to maintain a patent airway in a conscious infant or child. Sizes range from 12F to 36F. The smallest size, 12F, normally fits a full-term newborn. Because they can easily become obstructed with mucus or other debris, small airways require frequent suctioning and assessment of airway patency. The appropriate length is estimated by measuring the distance from the tip of the nose to the tragus of the ear. Careful insertion is necessary to avoid laceration of adenoidal tissue and subsequent bleeding, which could obstruct the airway and complicate management.

Bag-Valve-Mask Devices. Ventilation with a bag-valve-mask device with supplemental oxygen should replace mouth-to-mouth or mask-to-mouth breathing as soon as possible. An appropriately sized self-inflating bag with an oxygen reservoir and no pop-off valve is the ideal choice for resuscitation. Bags come in a variety of neonatal, pediatric, and adult sizes. It is important to know that tidal volume for pediatric patients ranges from 10 to 15 mL/kg of body weight. Pediatric size bags deliver approximately 500 mL per breath; they can be used for full-term newborns through to children of school age. Neonatal-sized bags deliver approximately 250 mL per breath and may be inadequate to ventilate infants effectively. Adult-sized bags deliver 750 to 1600 mL per breath, which may easily overinflate the compliant lungs of infants and small children, resulting in barotrauma, such as tension pneumothorax.

Bags without oxygen reservoirs deliver 30–80% oxygen, whereas bags with oxygen reservoirs deliver 60–95% oxygen. Pediatric-sized bags require at least 10–15 L/min of oxygen flow, whereas adult-sized bags require 15 L/min of oxygen flow to maintain high concentrations of oxygen (Finer, 1986).

Most self-inflating bags contain a pressure limited pop-off valve set at 35–45 cm H_2O to prevent over-inflation of the lungs and subsequent barotrauma. It is frequently necessary to utilize inspiratory pressures exceeding these limits to effectively ventilate a patient during CPR. Therefore, a bag without a pop-off valve, or one with a valve that can easily be occluded, should be used for resuscitation. Ventilation pressure can be measured with an inline manometer to determine the amount of pressure needed to effectively ventilate the patient, as evidenced by chest rise.

Cricoid pressure (the Sellick maneuver) can be used in conjunction with slow inspirations at low peak pressures to prevent gastric distention when ventilating an unconscious patient. Cricoid pressure also may prevent regurgitation and aspiration of gastric contents. Caution must be used to avoid excessive pressure because such pressure may cause tracheal compression and airway obstruction.

Face masks are available in a variety of sizes to accommodate infants, children, and adolescents. An appropriately sized mask covers the nose and mouth from the bridge of the nose to the cleft of the chin. The mask should provide a tight seal on the child's face to maximize inspired oxygen concentration during ventilation. Transparent masks should be used so that the child's lip color can be observed and vomiting can be promptly recognized. During bag-valve-mask ventilation, it may be necessary to reposition the patient's head to optimize airway opening for ventilation. The nurse uses one hand to maintain proper head position and a secure mask seal on the child's face while the other hand squeezes the bag. It is important to note that prolonged bag-valve-mask ventilation can cause gastric distention. This may cause vomiting, with possible aspiration, or elevation of the diaphragm, which decreases ventilation tidal volume. Therefore, placement of a nasogastric tube is recommended to decompress and empty the stomach when prolonged bag-valve-mask ventilation is anticipated.

Endotracheal Intubation. The indications for endotracheal intubation in the pediatric population include central nervous system dysfunction that results in inadequate ventilation; inability to protect the airway; respiratory failure; functional or anatomic airway obstruction; respiratory and cardiac arrest; and the requirement for prolonged mechanical ventilation, high peak inspiratory pressure, and positive end expiratory pressure (PEEP) to maintain adequate gas exchange.

Providing assisted ventilation through an endotracheal tube (ET) is the safest and most effective method to use during an arrest situation. Effective ventilation, delivery of oxygen, and continuous chest compressions can be maintained. The airway is isolated and can be suctioned to remove mucus or blood; it also can be used to deliver emergency medications. Gastric distention is minimized, which facilitates delivery of appropriate tidal volumes and reduces the risk of vomiting and pulmonary aspiration.

The recommended sizes of ETs and suction catheters for different ages are listed in Table 13–2. It has recently become evident that body length is a more reliable indicator of appropriate ET size than the patient's age. Use of the Broselow resuscitation tape (Figure 13–7) facilitates selection of the proper size ET (Hinkle, 1988). All EDs that care for infants and children should have such a tape. The tape lists appropriate equipment sizes and drug doses in color-coded sections that correspond to the patient's length. Use of the Broselow resuscitation tape has allowed more accurate selection of appropriate-sized equipment and medication dosages than other methods (Lubitz, 1988). The following formula can be used if necessary to calculate the appropriate size of ET to use for children older than 1 year

$$\text{size of ET in mm} = \frac{\text{age in years}}{4} + 4$$

Another method that can be used to estimate ET size is to choose the size equivalent to the diameter of the infant or child's little finger. Accurate estimation by this method is difficult. An ET 0.5 mm smaller and 0.5 mm larger than the estimated size by any of these methods should be available. Because the narrowest portion of an infant or small child's airway is at the cricoid cartilage, a natural cuff is formed around the ET in the trachea. Uncuffed ETs are therefore used in children younger than 8 years. Cuffed ETs are used in older children and adolescents. Laryngoscopic blades come in a variety of sizes to accommodate the pediatric population. A no. 1 straight blade is usually used for infants because it provides greater displacement of the tongue into the floor of the mouth and better visualization of the glottis. A curved blade provides better displacement of the tongue in older children because of its broader base and flange. A no. 2 straight blade is used for children up to the age of 7 or 8 years, and a no. 3 curved blade is preferred for older children and adolescents.

Intubation should be performed by a skilled health care provider. The technique used for infants and small children differs from that for older children and adolescents because of the anatomic differences in the airway previously discussed. The nurse should gather all equipment necessary for intubation, including an ET, laryngoscope with an appropriate-sized

TABLE 13–2. NORMAL PEDIATRIC RANGES

Age	Average Wt (kg)	Normal BP[a] Syst/diast (mmHg)	Heart Rate (Beats per minute)	ET Size (F)	Size of Suction Catheter (F)	Resp Rate (Breaths per minute)	IV Maintenance (mL/hour)
■ BIRTH							
1 month	4	60/90–120/60	120–160	3.5	6–8	30–60	17
3 months	5	74/100–50/70	120–160	3.5	6–8	30–60	21
6 months	7	74/100–50/70	120–160	3.5–4.0	8	30–60	29
9 months	9	74/100–50/70	120–160	3.5–4.0	8	30–60	38
12 months	10	80/112–50/80	90–140	3.5–4.0	8	24–40	42
15 months	10.5	80/112–50/80	90–140	3.5–4.0	8	24–40	43
18 months	11.5	80/112–50/80	90–140	4.0–4.5	8–10	24–40	45
21 months	12	80/112–50/80	90–140	4.0–4.5	8–10	24–40	46
24 months	12.5	80/112–50/80	90–140	5.0–5.5	10	24–40	47
30 months	13.5	80/112–50/80	90–140	5.0–5.5	10	24–40	49
3 years	14.5	82/110–50/78	80–110	5.5–6.0	10–12	22–34	51
4 years	16.5	82/110–50/78	80–110	5.5–6.0	10–12	22–34	55
5 years	18	82/110–50/78	80–110	5.5–6.0	10–12	22–34	58
6 years	21	84/120–54/80	75–100	6.0–6.5	12	18–30	64
8 years	27	84/120–54/80	75–100	6.0–6.5	12	18–30	70
10 years	32	84/120–54/80	60–90	6.5–7.0	12–14	18–30	75
12 years	39	94/140–62/88	60–90	7.0–7.5	14	12–16	82
14 years	49	94/140–62/88	60–90	7.0–7.5	14	12–16	93
16 years	56	94/140–62/88	60–90	7.0–7.5	14	12–16	100

[a]Blood pressure ranges include those in the 10th to 90th percentile.
(*From Curley MA, Vaughan SM* [1987]. *Assessment and resuscitation of the pediatric patient.* Critical Care Nurse *1:30*)

blade, suction catheters (a large size catheter to suction the oropharynx and a smaller size to suction the ET), Magill forceps, and a stylet. Smaller ET tubes are softer and more pliable than large tubes; therefore a stylet is used to facilitate proper placement. The tip of the stylet should be a few centimeters inside the ET and not extend beyond the length of the tube to prevent tracheal laceration or injury.

Bag-valve-mask ventilation with the maximum available concentration of oxygen should always precede intubation. Attempts should last no longer than 30 seconds, and the heart rate and rhythm should be closely monitored. If bradycardia develops (heart rate less than 80 beats per minute in infants and less than 60 beats per minute in children) or the patient's color or perfusion worsens, the procedure should be stopped and the patient should be ventilated and oxygenated by the bag-valve-mask method. Atropine should be used cautiously to prevent vagally induced bradycardia during intubation; this drug can mask hypoxia-induced bradycardia, particularly in infants. Morbidity can occur from hypoxia related to prolonged efforts at intubation and from improperly placed ET tubes.

After intubation, positive pressure ventilation is delivered with a bag; the chest wall is observed closely for symmetric movement; and breath sounds are auscultated over both lung fields and in the axillary areas. If breath sounds are decreased or of different quality on the right, the ET may have been placed in the right mainstem bronchus, and it should be pulled back slightly. This maneuver is followed by reassessment of breath sounds. Intubation of the right mainstem bronchus is a frequent occurrence in infants and small children because the trachea is short, and the angle of the right mainstem bronchus is less acute, providing a natural pathway for the ET. Breath sounds may be transmitted to the lung fields with esophageal intubation, therefore chest wall movement is an important indicator of proper placement of the ET. The nurse should not hear breath sounds when auscultating over the upper abdomen; this may indicate esophageal intubation. The presence of water vapor in the ET is not a reliable indicator of proper tube placement because this can occur with esophageal intubation (Andersen and Hald, 1989). A chest x ray should be obtained as soon as possible to confirm proper placement of the ET.

Once the position of the ET has been confirmed, the tube must be taped to prevent accidental extubation. A variety of creative methods are used to secure ETs in pediatric patients. One popular method is the cloth tape–suture method. The skin between the nose and upper lip is cleaned, dried, and painted with tincture of benzoin. After the benzoin is dry, a thin strip of

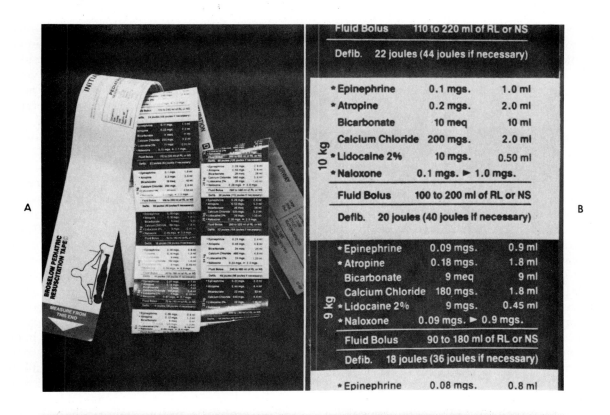

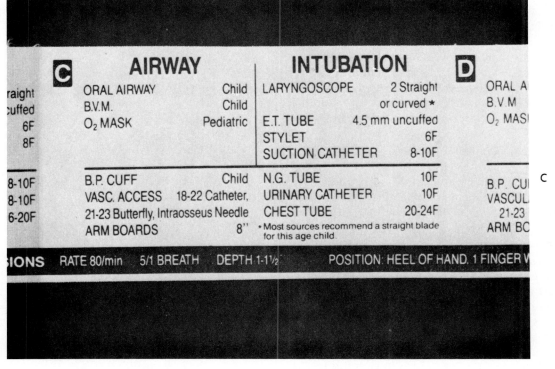

Figure 13–7. Broselow resuscitation tape. **A.** The two-sided tape measure displays proper dosages of emergency drugs and provides color-coded sections for rapid selection of pediatric equipment based on child's body length. **B.** Front side of tape displays appropriate dosages and administration volumes of resuscitation drugs (estimated weight and drug dosages determined from child's length). **C.** Second (color-coded) side of tape indicates appropriate sizes of emergency equipment based on child's length. Equipment sizes were determined by a panel of experts. (Photographs courtesy of Vital Signs, Inc., Totowa, NJ) (From Hazinski MF [1991]. *Nursing care of the critically ill child* [2nd ed] St Louis: Mosby, p 9)

cloth tape with one pleat in the middle is placed between the nose and upper lip. Suture of 00 silk on a cutting needle is tied around the tube, and then sewn to the pleat on the cloth tape (not the skin). Other methods involve various ways of applying cloth tape to anchor the tube. Cloth tape with benzoin is preferred over adhesive tape because it provides better hold in the presence of oral and nasal secretions. The patient's head must be kept in a neutral position to maintain the position of the ET. Flexion of the neck displaces the tube farther into the airway; extension of the neck pulls the tube farther out of the airway. It is frequently necessary to restrain infants and children to prevent movement of the ET and accidental extubation. If a child is biting down on the tube and obstructing the airway, an oral airway is placed.

Noninvasive Respiratory Monitoring. Pulse oximetry is a widely used and reliable noninvasive method for continuous monitoring of arterial oxygen saturation. The usefulness of pulse oximetry is limited if peripheral perfusion is inadequate because the method relies on the presence of pulsatile blood flow for accurate readings. Once perfusion is established, pulse oximetry provides an early warning of respiratory decompensation and hypoxemia. All EDs should have pulse oximetry available to facilitate patient assessment.

End tidal carbon dioxide monitors can be useful in confirming placement of the ET and displacement in infants larger than 2 kg who have spontaneous circulation (Bhende et al, 1992). These monitors are not reliable in asystolic arrest because they may give falsely low readings when esophageal intubation is used or a low cardiac output state is present.

Vascular Access. Establishing vascular access during cardiopulmonary arrest is essential for the administration of fluids and medications; it is often very difficult and challenging in the pediatric population. Infants and children have smaller veins than adolescents and adults, and these veins are usually extremely vasoconstricted when cardiac arrest occurs. The ideal site for vascular access is the largest and most accessible vein that does not require interruption of CPR. Peripheral venous access can provide adequate access if it can be obtained within a few minutes. Preferred peripheral sites in infants and children include the veins of the scalp, arm, hand, leg, or foot. Close observation of the site is necessary because medications used in resuscitation can cause local tissue injury if infiltrated. It is important to follow peripheral injections of medication with a fluid flush to facilitate moving the drug into the central circulation (3–5 ml, depending on the patient's size and distance of the site from the central circulation).

Central venous access can be attempted if a skilled provider is present. The femoral, internal or external jugular, or, in older children, the subclavian vein may be used. In general, the femoral vein is the safest and easiest site to access and can be cannulated without interfering with CPR. If the femoral vein is used, the tip of the catheter should be placed above the level of the diaphragm to assure delivery of medications to the central circulation and heart.

Intraosseous Access. Emergency departments should establish protocols for establishing vascular access during pediatric resuscitations. If vascular access cannot be obtained in three attempts, or within 90 seconds, whichever comes first, intraosseous access should be obtained in children 6 years of age and younger. Intraosseous vascular access provides a quick, safe, and dependable route for administering medications, fluids, and blood products during resuscitation. Access is accomplished by inserting a rigid intraosseous or bone marrow needle into the anterior tibial bone marrow (Figure 13–8). If these are not available, a 16 or 18 gauge hypodermic needle or a spinal needle with a stylet may be used. If rapid fluid administration is required, it may be necessary to use an infusion pump or pressure bag because resistance in the emissary veins can slow fluid flow rates (Orlowski et al, 1989). Few complications have been reported using the intra-

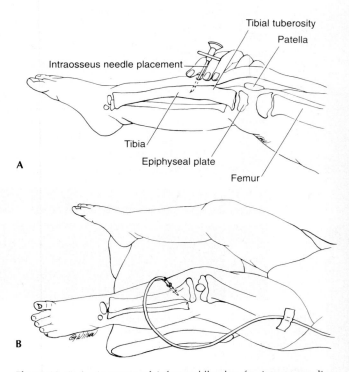

Figure 13–8. A. Anatomy of infant-toddler leg for intraosseus line placement. **B.** Site of choice for intraosseus needle placement.

osseous route. These include tibial fracture, lower extremity compartment syndrome, and osteomyelitis (La Fleche et al, 1989; Moscati and Moore, 1990). Observation of the extremity for infiltration is necessary. If blanching of the extremity occurs during administration of medication, dilution of the medication is recommended.

Endotracheal Drug Administration. Endotracheal administration of lipid-soluble medications is indicated if vascular access has not been established within 3–5 minutes, although any vascular access route is preferred over administration of medication through an ET (American Heart Association, 1992b). Drugs that can be given by the endotracheal route include epinephrine, atropine, lidocaine, and naloxone. Non-lipid-soluble drugs such as sodium bicarbonate and calcium cannot be given by this route. Recent studies have demonstrated wide variation in drug absorption by the endotracheal route in animal and adult models (Quinton et al, 1987; Ralston et al, 1985). A standard dose of epinephrine was found to produce serum levels of about one-tenth or less of those produced by equivalent intravenous doses of epinephrine. On the basis of this finding, the American Heart Association (1992b) now recommends the dose of endotracheally administered epinephrine to be ten times the recommended intravenous or intraosseus dose. Other doses of resuscitation medication also should probably be increased when given by the endotracheal route, but no specific dosage recommendations have been made. Dilution of drugs with normal or 0.45 normal saline solution and instilling them through a catheter or feeding tube beyond the tip of the ET may facilitate delivery into the peripheral airways, where the drugs gain access to the pulmonary circulation (Ralston et al, 1984).

Intravenous Fluid Therapy. Volume expansion is a crucial component of pediatric resuscitation, and one that is overlooked at times. Volume expansion is best achieved with crystalloid solutions, such as Ringer lactate or normal saline solution, or with colloid solutions, such as 5% albumin. Blood transfusions are indicated for hypovolemic states associated with acute hemorrhage. Solutions containing dextrose, such as 5% dextrose in water (D_5W) or 5% dextrose in normal saline solution (D_5NS), should not be used for children during resuscitation because the large volumes of fluid frequently required cause hyperglycemia. Hyperglycemia can cause neurologic sequelae such as decreased level of consciousness and cerebral edema. It also may induce an osmotic diuresis, which may contribute to hypovolemia or cause electrolyte imbalances, resulting in seizures. Because hypoglycemia occurs commonly, particularly in infants who are in

cardiopulmonary failure, bedside glucose testing should be done, followed by intravenous administration of glucose as indicated (see the section on Drug Therapy). During resuscitation, it is usually necessary to administer intravenous or intraosseous fluids as quickly as possible. Although it is crucial to carefully monitor the amount of fluid given to avoid pulmonary or cerebral edema, which can result from fluid overload, a successful resuscitation can occur only if the circulating volume is adequate. In many situations, the size of the intravenous catheter in pediatric patients and the use of the minidrip intravenous line sets hinder rapid volume administration. Attaching a three-way stopcock with a large syringe to the intravenous fluid line close to the patient allows boluses to be pushed at the desired rate and facilitates rapid and precise fluid administration.

Drugs Used for Resuscitation After Cardiac Arrest

Sympathetic Nervous System Review. Many of the drugs used for resuscitation act on the heart through stimulation of the sympathetic nervous system (Table 13–3). The sympathetic fibers originate in the adrenal medulla and thoracic nerves of the spinal cord and terminate in beta receptors in the atria and ventricles and in alpha receptors throughout the peripheral vasculature. Sympathetic nervous system stimulation occurs through alpha or beta adrenergic receptors. Beta-1 stimulation produces an increase in heart rate, an increase in cardiac contractility, and an increase in the speed of conduction of the electrical impulse. Beta-2 stimulation produces peripheral vasodilatation and bronchodilatation; alpha stimulation causes peripheral vasoconstriction.

Epinephrine. Epinephrine is the most commonly used drug in pediatric resuscitations. Epinephrine is an endogenous catecholamine with alpha- and beta-stimulating properties. It increases heart rate, stimulates spontaneous contraction and increases the force of myocardial contraction, and increases the vigor of ventricular fibrillation, thus making the heart more responsive to electrical defibrillation. During cardiac arrest, the most important pharmacologic action of epinephrine is vasoconstriction with subsequent elevation of aortic diastolic pressure and increased perfusion pressure, which facilitates oxygen delivery to the heart (Zaritsky and Chernow, 1984). Along with these desired effects, epinephrine increases myocardial oxygen demand and consumption. Catecholamines are ineffective in the presence of hypoxemia and acidosis. Therefore it is critical to provide effective ventilation, oxygenation, and circulation during cardiopulmonary arrests.

TABLE 13–3. DRUGS USED IN PEDIATRIC ADVANCED LIFE SUPPORT

Drug	Dose	Remarks
Adenosine	0.1 to 0.2 mg/kg Maximum single dose: 12 mg	Rapid IV bolus
Atropine sulfate	0.02 mg/kg per dose	Minimum dose: 0.1 mg Maximum single dose: 0.5 mg in child, 1.0 mg in adolescent
Bretylium	5 mg/kg; may be increased to 10 mg/kg	Rapid IV
Calcium chloride 10%	20 mg/kg per dose	Give slowly
Dopamine hydrochloride	2–20 μg/kg per minute	α-Adrenergic action dominates at ≥15– 20 μg/kg per minute
Dobutamine hydrochloride	2–20 μg/kg per minute	Titrate to desired effect
Epinephrine For bradycardia	IV/IO: 0.01 mg/kg (1:10 000) ET: 0.1 mg/kg (1:1000)	Be aware of effective dose of preserva- tives administered (if preservatives are present in epinephrine preparation) when high doses are used
For asystolic or pulseless arrest	First dose: IV/IO 0.01 mg/kg (1:10 000) ET: 0.1 mg/kg (1:1000) Doses as high as 0.2 mg/kg may be effective Subsequent doses: IV/IO/ET 0.1 mg/kg (1:1000) Doses as high as 0.2 mg/kg may be effective	Be aware of effective dose of preserva- tive administered (if preservatives pres- ent in epinephrine preparation) when high doses are used
Epinephrine infusion	Initial at 0.1 μg/kg per minute Higher infusion dose used if asystole present	Titrate to desired effect (0.1-1.0 μg/kg per minute)
Lidocaine	1 mg/kg per dose	
Lidocaine infusion	20–50 μg/kg per minute	
Sodium bicarbonate	1 mEq/kg per dose or 0.3 × kg × base deficit	Infuse slowly and only if ventilation is adequate

IV, intravenous route; IO, intraosseous route; ET, endotracheal route.
(*From American Heart Association* [1992]. *Guidelines for cardiopulmonary resuscitation and emergency cardiac care: Pediatric advanced life support.* JAMA *268:2268*)

The most common rhythm disturbances in infants and children with cardiopulmonary failure are brady-dysrhythmias and asystole. Epinephrine can generate a perfusing rhythm in such situations. The recommended dose of epinephrine for bradycardic states is 0.01 mg/kg (0.1 mL/kg of 1:10,000 solution) for the intravenous or intraosseous route, or 0.1 mg/kg (0.1 mL/kg of the 1:1000 solution) for the endotracheal route.

The results of animal and limited clinical studies (Brown and Werman, 1990; Goetting and Paradis, 1991) have suggested that high doses of epinephrine may improve neurologic outcome for children with no heart rate and no palpable pulse. The American Heart Association (AHA) therefore changed recommended dosages of epinephrine for pediatric patients in asystolic arrest. The initial dose remains 0.01 mg/kg for the intravenous or intraosseous route. If the initial dose is ineffective, subsequent doses of epinephrine should be increased to 0.1 mg/kg and should be ad-

ministered within 3–5 minutes of the initial dose. Doses as high as 0.2 mg/kg may be effective in generating cardiac rhythm and contraction. Higher doses should be administered every 3–5 minutes during the resuscitation. If asystolic arrest is prolonged, a continuous infusion of epinephrine at 20 μg/kg/min may be given until cardiac activity is restored. It should then be titrated down to more conventional doses. Because both the 1:1000 and 1:10,000 epinephrine concentrations may be necessary if these new dosing guidelines are followed, the nurse must be careful to select the appropriate concentration to avoid errors in dosing. The nurse also must be aware if the epinephrine solution contains preservatives, because of the risk of administering excessive preservatives and their subsequent side effects.

Calcium. Calcium is essential for effective myocardial electromechanical coupling. It has not been proved to improve outcomes of cardiac arrest; in fact it may worsen outcomes by contributing to cell death. Calcium is indicated for the treatment of documented hypocalcemia, hyperkalemia, hypermagnesemia, and overdose with calcium channel blockers. Calcium chloride 10% is the solution of choice because it provides greater bioavailability of calcium than calcium gluconate does. A dose of 20 mg/kg is given slowly by the intravenous or intraosseous route while observing for bradycardia. A second dose may be repeated in 10 minutes if needed. Subsequent doses should be based on documented deficits.

Glucose. Because infants have high glucose needs and low glycogen stores, hypoglycemia can develop quickly during periods of stress. Hypoglycemia can mimic shock and cause seizures, which can complicate resuscitation efforts. It is therefore necessary to monitor glucose concentrations closely by bedside and laboratory analysis in any compromised infant. Documented hypoglycemia is treated with 2–4 mL/kg of 25% dextrose solution. It is preferable to give a lower-dose continuous glucose infusion if possible to avoid a sudden increase in serum glucose level and subsequent osmotic diuresis, which may contribute to poor neurologic outcome and which has been associated with hypertonic glucose bolus therapy.

Sodium Bicarbonate. Sodium bicarbonate has long been used to treat metabolic acidosis. There is, however, no evidence that it improves outcome in cardiac arrests. Respiratory failure with respiratory acidosis is the major cause of cardiac arrest in children. Therefore, intubation, ventilation, and re-establishment of systemic perfusion are priorities in management. Administration of sodium bicarbonate may temporarily elevate carbon dioxide levels, which may worsen respiratory acidosis, and hinder resuscitation efforts. This drug should be administered to patients with prolonged arrest who are unresponsive to ventilation, compressions, and epinephrine therapy or when shock is associated with documented metabolic acidosis. No specific recommendation has been made regarding the degree of acidosis that requires treatment. The initial dose of sodium bicarbonate is 1 mEq/kg for infants and children and 0.5 mEq/kg for newborn infants by the intravenous or intraosseous route. The concentration of sodium bicarbonate should be 0.5 mEq/mL for neonates because the hyperosmolar 1 mEq/mL solution may cause intraventricular hemorrhage in this population. Subsequent doses of bicarbonate are based on blood gas results, although it is important to note that arterial blood gas analysis may not accurately reflect tissue and venous pH. Excessive administration of sodium bicarbonate may cause metabolic alkalosis with im-

paired oxygen delivery to the tissues, hyperkalemia, hypocalcemia, decreased fibrillation threshold, and impaired cardiac function. It is also important for the nurse to be aware that sodium bicarbonate inactivates catecholamines and precipitates with calcium salts. It is therefore extremely important to flush lines clear between administrations of these medications.

Drugs Used to Control Heart Rate and Rhythm

Atropine Sulfate. Atropine sulfate has parasympatholytic action and both peripheral and central effects. It is used to treat symptomatic bradycardia, which is accompanied by poor perfusion, hypotension, or atrioventricular (AV) block and vagally induced episodes of bradycardia during intubation attempts. Because hypoxia is a common cause of bradycardia, particularly in infants, atropine should be used to treat bradycardia that persists despite adequate oxygenation and ventilation. Caution must be used when atropine is given to prevent vagally induced bradycardia during attempts at intubation because it may also mask hypoxia-induced bradycardia. It is therefore important for the nurse to monitor oxygen saturation with pulse oximetry and to avoid prolonged intubation attempts. Atropine must be given in a vagolytic dosage to avoid the paradoxic bradycardia that may occur with smaller doses. Atropine is administered in a dose of 0.02 mg/kg, with a minimum dose of 0.1 mg and a maximum single dose of 0.5 mg in a child and 1.0 mg in an adolescent. The dose may be repeated in 5 minutes if the initial dose is ineffective. The maximum for subsequent doses is 1.0 mg in a child and 2.0 mg in an adolescent. Atropine may be administered endotracheally in the same dose. Tachycardia frequently occurs after the administration of atropine, but it is usually well tolerated by infants and children. Adverse effects include tachydysrhythmias and subsequent myocardial ischemia.

Isoproterenol. Isoproterenol is a pure beta-adrenergic receptor stimulator that increases heart rate, conduction velocity, and myocardial contractility. These actions, in conjunction with the peripheral vasodilatory effects of isoproterenol, usually result in improved peripheral perfusion. Isoproterenol is administered as a continuous infusion at a rate of 0.1–0.5 µg/kg/minute to treat bradydysrhythmias that are not responsive to atropine sulfate. Adverse effects include tachydysrhythmias and subsequent myocardial ischemia. It should be administered cautiously to children receiving digitalis; these children may be at increased risk for the development of dysrhythmias.

Lidocaine. Lidocaine is administered to treat ventricular ectopy, ventricular tachycardia, and ventricular fibrillation. Lidocaine suppresses the automaticity of ventricular pacemaker cells, which subsequently increases the threshold for ventricular fibrillation. This makes the myocardium more susceptible to electrical defibrillation. Lidocaine should be given in a dose of 1.0 mg/kg before attempts at defibrillation or cardioversion if it is readily available. Attempts should not be delayed if lidocaine or intravenous access is unavailable. If ongoing lidocaine therapy is needed, a continuous infusion of 20–50 μg/kg/minute may be given. The adverse effects of lidocaine include drowsiness, disorientation, muscle twitching, and seizures. Symptoms of central nervous system toxicity usually precede cardiac symptoms, which include decreased myocardial contractility, heart block, and asystole.

Bretylium Tosylate. Bretylium has been effective in treating adult ventricular fibrillation that is unresponsive to electrical defibrillation. No studies have been published on the usefulness of bretylium in pediatric patients. The recommended dosage of bretylium in pediatric patients is 5.0 mg/kg by rapid intravenous infusion if defibrillation and lidocaine fail to correct ventricular defibrillation. Administration of bretylium should be followed by a defibrillation attempt. If the attempt fails, an additional dose of 10 mg/kg may be given.

Adenosine. Adenosine is an endogenous nucleoside that temporarily blocks conduction through the AV node, thereby interrupting the re-entry circuits frequently associated with supraventricular tachycardia (SVT) in infants and children. Symptomatic SVT should be treated by synchronized electric cardioversion. If IV access is available, however, adenosine may be administered before cardioversion. Adenosine is the treatment of choice for children with nonsymptomatic SVT who are in a stable condition. After continuous cardiac monitoring is initiated, adenosine is given in a dose of 0.1 mg/kg as a rapid intravenous bolus. If this therapy is ineffective, the dose may be doubled and repeated. The maximum single dose is 12 mg. Adenosine is very effective and has minimal side effects because its half-life is only 10 seconds. It may be necessary to give a higher dose if the drug is administered through a peripheral rather than a central line because adenosine is metabolized so rapidly.

Drugs Used to Improve and Maintain Cardiac Output

Epinephrine. Epinephrine infusion is given to treat any type of shock with poor perfusion that is unresponsive to volume therapy (Table 13–4). It may be preferred to dopamine in infants and other pediatric

TABLE 13–4. PREPARATION OF DRUGS FOR CONTINUOUS INFUSION

Drug	Preparation[a]	Dose
Epinephrine	0.6 × body weight (kg) equals milligrams added to diluent[b] to make 100 mL	Then 1 mL/h delivers 0.1 μg/kg per minute; titrate to effect
Dopamine, dobutamine	6 × body weight (kg) equals milligrams added to diluent to make 100 mL	Then 1mL/h delivers 1.0 μg/kg per minute; titrate to effect
Lidocaine	120 mg of 40-mg/mL solution added to 97 mL of 5% dextrose in water, yielding 1200 μg/mL solution	Then 1 mL/kg per hour delivers 20 μg/kg per minute

[a]Standard concentration may be used to provide more dilute or more concentrated drug solution, but then individual dose must be calculated for each patient and each infusion rate:

$$\text{Infusion Rate (mL/h)} = \frac{\text{Weight (kg)} \times \text{Dose (μg/kg/min)} \times 60 \text{ min/h}}{\text{Concentration (μg/mL)}}$$

[b]Diluent may be 5% dextrose in water, 5% dextrose in half-normal saline solution, normal saline or Ringer lactate.
(*From American Heart Association* [1992]. *Guidelines for cardiopulmonary resuscitation and emergency cardiac care: Pediatric advanced life support. JAMA 268:2270*)

patients who may have low endogenous stores of catecholamines (see Dopamine). The initial dose is 0.1 μg/kg/minute and is titrated up to 1.0 μg/kg/minute in accordance with its hemodynamic effects. The goal of therapy is to improve systemic perfusion without excessive tachycardia, which can cause tachydysrhythmias, impaired coronary artery perfusion, and decreased cardiac output. Higher infusions may be used in asystole, as previously discussed. Epinephrine should be administered into a reliable and secure intravenous site because infiltration can cause local tissue ischemia and ulceration.

Dopamine. Dopamine is an endogenous catecholamine with alpha, beta, and dopaminergic effects that are dose related. Dopamine is indicated for the treatment of shock that is unresponsive to fluid replacement or after cardiopulmonary resuscitation. Dopamine is used to improve perfusion, urine output, and blood pressure. At low doses of 0.5 to 2 μg/kg/minute, dopaminergic effects cause an increase in renal and splanchnic blood flow. At doses of 5–15 μg/kg/minute, beta effects dominate and cause an increase in heart rate, AV conduction velocity, and myocardial contractility. It should be noted that dopamine acts both directly through stimulation of cardiac beta receptors and indirectly by stimulating the release of norepinephrine stored in cardiac sympathetic nerves. Norepinephrine stores may be limited in infants because sympathetic nervous system innervation of the myocardium is incomplete during the first few months of life. Norepinephrine stores also may be depleted in children with congestive heart failure. Because of this effect, the inotropic action of dopamine may vary and be diminished in such situations. At doses greater than 20 μg/kg/minute, the alpha effects of dopamine predominate, resulting in peripheral vasoconstriction. It is preferable to add either an epinephrine or dobutamine infusion if the desired inotropic effects are not achieved with a dopamine infusion of less than 20 μg/kg/minute. The side effects of dopamine include tachycardia, ventricular ectopy, and vasoconstriction. Infiltration can cause local tissue necrosis. It is important for the nurse to note that dopamine is deactivated by alkaline solutions such as sodium bicarbonate and should not be infused through the same intravenous line as sodium bicarbonate.

Dobutamine Hydrochloride. Dobutamine is a synthetic catecholamine with selective beta actions; it causes increased myocardial contractility and decreased peripheral vascular tone. Dobutamine is indicated for the treatment of low cardiac output and poor myocardial function. The clinical response to dobutamine varies in pediatric patients, the dose range is titrated from 2.0 up to 20 μg/kg/minute until the desired response is achieved. Side effects can occur at the higher doses; they include tachycardia and ventricular dysrhythmias.

Defibrillation, Cardioversion, and External Pacing

Defibrillation. Ventricular fibrillation is uncommon in the pediatric population, therefore defibrillation is indicated only after ventricular fibrillation is documented by an electrocardiogram (ECG) using more than one lead. Defibrillation works by producing a simultaneous depolarization of myocardial cells, which may then facilitate spontaneous depolarization if the myocardium is oxygenated, perfused, and not excessively acidotic.

A paddle 4–5 cm in diameter is recommended for infants who weigh less than 10 kg; the standard adult paddles 8–10 cm in diameter are recommended for children who weigh more than 10 kg or who are about 1 year of age. Proper paddle size reduces transthoracic impedance and maximizes current flow (Atkins et al, 1988). The nurse should be skilled at changing from the small to the large paddles so that valuable time is not wasted. Electrode cream or paste or adhesive monitoring defibrillation pads can be used to interface between the paddle or electrode and the chest wall. Any facility that has a defibrillator should have cream, paste, or adhesive pads available for use; but saline-soaked gauze may be used if these materials are not available. Bare paddles produce a very high impedance and therefore should never be used. Alcohol-soaked pads are also contraindicated because they can cause serious burns. Because electrical current follows the path of least resistance, it is imperative that the cream, paste, or saline gauze from one paddle not touch the other. If this happens, bridging occurs, causing a short circuit, and insufficient electrical current crosses the heart.

The paddles are placed on the chest wall using firm pressure. One paddle is placed over the right upper chest, and the other one is placed over the apex of the heart, to the left of the nipple. Health care workers should be cleared from contact with the patient and the bed during defibrillation. The recommended dosage for pediatric defibrillation is 2 watt-seconds or joules (J)/kg. If this dose is ineffective, the dose is doubled and repeated twice. The first three defibrillation attempts are done in rapid succession. If these are unsuccessful, then acidosis, hypoxemia, and hypothermia should be treated aggressively; epinephrine and lidocaine should be administered; and defibrillation should be attempted again at 4 J/kg. Adverse effects that can occur with defibrillation include myocardial injury from excessive current or multiple attempts in rapid succession. Skin and tissue injury may result if the interface between the electrode or paddle and the skin is inadequate.

Synchronized Cardioversion. Synchronized cardioversion is the timed depolarization of myocardial cells. It is used to convert symptomatic supraventricular or ventricular tachycardia accompanied by poor perfusion, hypotension, or heart failure. The synchronizer circuit must be activated on the defibrillator before each cardioversion attempt. The dose is 0.5–1.0 J/kg. Initially the lowest dose should be used; subsequent doses can be increased if necessary. Hypoxemia, acidosis, hypoglycemia, and hypothermia must be corrected, if present, to facilitate successful cardioversion.

Transcutaneous Pacing. Noninvasive transcutaneous pacing has been used for several years to treat adults with bradycardia or asystole. It has recently been used to a limited degree in children (Beland, 1987). Because it is extremely uncomfortable, this procedure is used only for children with prolonged symptomatic bradycardia unresponsive to basic and advanced life support.

Transcutaneous pacing uses two adhesive-backed

electrodes attached to an external pacing unit. Three sizes of electrodes are available. For neonates and infants, the infant-sized electrodes are used. For children weighing less than 15 kg, pediatric-sized electrodes are used; adult-sized electrodes are used for children weighing more than 15 kg. The negative electrode is applied over the heart on the anterior chest wall, and the positive electrode is placed behind the heart on the back. Ventricular fixed rate or inhibited pacing may be used. Adjustment of pacemaker output usually is necessary to assure that every pacer impulse results in ventricular capture and subsequent depolarization. Generally, a lower pacer output is required with smaller electrodes. If ventricular inhibited pacing is used, the sensitivity of the pacer must be adjusted to sense intrinsic ventricular electric activity.

Secondary Interventions

Treatment of Hypothermia. As previously discussed, infants and young children have a large body surface area relative to their weight. This results in rapid heat loss when the skin surface is exposed. Therefore, measures must be taken to maintain or restore normothermia during resuscitation efforts. Such measures include the use of radiant heat warmers, warmed intravenous fluids, and warmed fluid for peritoneal lavage if indicated. Because infants' heads are large in proportion to the rest of their body, covering an infant's head can be an important measure to decrease heat loss, which occurs through convection and evaporation. This is especially important during transport, when the patient may be exposed to extreme fluctuations in environmental temperature. It is important for the nurse to closely monitor the infant or child's temperature throughout resuscitation efforts because hypothermia may both mimic shock and hinder successful resuscitation.

Nasogastric Tube. A nasogastric tube should be placed as soon as possible during resuscitation to decompress the stomach and facilitate lung expansion with assisted ventilation, and to prevent vomiting and aspiration of stomach contents. It may be necessary to remove the nasogastric tube during intubation, but it should be replaced as soon as intubation is achieved. An orogastric tube should be placed if head trauma is suspected.

Foley Catheterization. A Foley catheter should be inserted as soon as possible during pediatric resuscitation. Urine output is an important indicator of vital organ perfusion because the kidneys are less affected than the brain or skin by extraneous factors. Large volumes of fluid are often given during resuscitation,

which makes accurate measurement of intake and output critical for planning appropriate interventions for fluid management, inotropic support, and diuretic therapy. Urine output should be at least 1 mL/kg/hour for an infant and 0.5 mL/kg/hour for a child.

Other Diagnostic Studies. Laboratory studies, including measurement of arterial blood gases, electrolytes, calcium, glucose, blood urea nitrogen (BUN), and creatinine, a complete blood count (CBC), and blood cultures, should be performed to identify abnormalities that may have contributed to the arrest or that may have been caused by resuscitation efforts. Appropriate intervention can then be initiated to correct disorders and to stabilize the patient's condition. A chest x ray should be obtained to verify the position of the ET and to evaluate lung status and heart size. Other radiologic studies should be based on the patient's history and current status.

Postresuscitation Assessment. Table 13–5 lists conditions that the patient should be assessed for after successful resuscitation.

Termination of Resuscitation in the Emergency Department

The decision to terminate resuscitation in the ED is the decision of the senior physician. Termination of resus-

TABLE 13–5. POSTRESUSCITATION ASSESSMENT

■ NEUROLOGIC Cerebral edema Cerebral acidosis Seizures	■ HEMATOLOGIC Disseminated intravascular coagulation
■ CARDIOVASCULAR Alterations in circulating blood volume Alterations in CO secondary to hypoxia, acidosis and fluid overload Cardiac tamponade from intracardiac injections	■ METABOLIC Acidosis/alkalosis Electrolyte imbalance Hyperkalemia: renal shutdown and cell destruction, blood- glucose disturbances, calcium imbalance
■ PULMONARY ARDS Right mainstem intubation Barotrauma pneumothorax pneumomediastinum pneumopericardium Aspiration pneumonia Pulmonary contusions	■ GASTROINTESTINAL Hepatic dysfunction Pancreatic ischemia Gastrointestinal bleeding ■ IATROGENIC TRAUMA Chest wall Liver Gastric distention/ perforation Skin trauma from IV Drug toxicity
■ RENAL Acute tubular necrosis	

(From Curley MA, Vaughan SM [1987]. Assessment and resuscitation of the pediatric patient. Critical Care Nurse 7:41)

citation should be considered after approximately 15 minutes for the normothermic child in cardiac arrest who does not respond to two doses of epinephrine and skilled CPR (Gillis et al, 1986; Nichols, 1986; Zaritsky, 1987). Because the heart tolerates hypoxia better than the brain does, normal heart function may return even though neurologic function is profoundly impaired. This may result in the infant or child's existing in a persistent vegetative state, requiring chronic nursing care. Meaningful neurologic recovery or long-term survival is unlikely. Unfortunately, it is impossible to determine the extent of neurologic injury in the ED once heart function has been restored. Absence of cranial nerve function, flaccid motor tone, unresponsiveness, and a long lapse of time between the arrest and resuscitation may suggest devastating brain damage or brain death. There are many factors, however, that can alter the neurologic findings after an arrest, such as acid base and electrolyte imbalances, hypothermia, and medications.

Patient and Family Education and Psychosocial Support

Psychosocial Issues. The child and family are inseparable. When an infant or child is critically ill or injured, the parents often experience as much fear and anxiety as the child. The parental response to cardiopulmonary arrest is very individual and may vary depending on the circumstances surrounding the arrest. For example, a parent whose child is chronically ill at home may react differently from one whose healthy child is hit by a car. Parents frequently blame themselves or the person who was caring for the child at the time of the illness or injury. Parents may experience feelings of disbelief, anger, outrage, despair, and hysteria on arrival in the ED. Although their feelings may be directed at the staff, it is important to realize that these feelings are more likely related to the family's shock and helplessness over the situation.

A nurse, social worker, or other appropriate member of the health care team should be assigned to remain with the family throughout the resuscitation. Ideally, this person can serve as a liaison between the resuscitation team and the family to provide continuous communication. Parents and other family members should be brought to a private location away from the resuscitation area. It is important to be aware that parents may not be able to support each other during this time, because each is dealing with her or his own feelings about what is happening. A staff member should offer to call other family members or clergy if the parents wish.

Parents need to be assured that everything possible is being done for the child. Information shared should be accurate and realistic and should not offer false hope to the parents. A calm, nonjudgmental approach should be used by all health care workers to alleviate any guilt the parents may be experiencing about the circumstances that led to the cardiac arrest. It is appropriate to ask parents if their child has been baptized, and if not, if they would like this to be done. It is also important to note that parents may not know what to do or be able to make their needs known to staff at this time. Therefore, direction and choices should be offered to them when indicated. It may be appropriate for some parents to be allowed to see and be with their child during resuscitation efforts. Although this is a foreign concept to many ED staff, it may facilitate the parents' grieving process and acceptance of their child's death, if that is the outcome. Some families have actually identified being removed from the patient's bedside during resuscitation as the least supportive action by the health care team (Hampe, 1975). Allowing parents to be present gives them the opportunity to see how much effort went into saving their child's life and that their child was not in pain during the resuscitation. It may also alleviate feelings of helplessness if they view their presence as supportive to their child. It may also facilitate closure for parents if the resuscitation is unsuccessful (Doyle et al, 1987). A knowledgeable and supportive member of the health care team should escort parents to the resuscitation area to provide explanations and prevent misunderstandings regarding what is going on.

Nurses and other members of the health care eam may be reluctant to allow parents to be present during resuscitation. This may be related to their fear that parents will be disruptive or interfere with resuscitation efforts, or that a grieving family may make it difficult for staff to maintain their own emotional composure during resuscitation. Some staff may fear that they will do or say something that may offend or upset the family. One study found that families were not disruptive during resuscitation, rather they were in awe of the activity in the room. Nurses were less able to remain emotionally distant during the resuscitation, because they saw the patient as a loved family member and not a clinical "case." The staff was able, however, to focus on clinical priorities and function appropriately (Hanson and Strawser, 1992). Regardless of whether parents or family are allowed to be present during the resuscitation, ED staff should have a forum to discuss their feelings and emotional response to these situations and to get whatever support they may need. This is especially important for staff who deal with infants and children, because tragedy and death among this age group can be more difficult for staff to deal with. This can be related to the sense of unfairness that someone so young should die before experiencing many of life's promises or the sense of identification with the parents if they are of similar age or if the child is close in age to any of the staff's children.

If the resuscitation is unsuccessful, the parents should be informed of the child's death as soon as possible. Information regarding the child's condition during the resuscitation and what treatment was done should be given. The parents should be given an opportunity to ask questions and to express their anger, disbelief, and sorrow. Parents should be given the opportunity to see, touch, and hold their child if they choose. This is an individual decision, which may allow parents to begin the grieving process and get closure with their child. If siblings are present, it may be appropriate for them to accompany the parents, if the children and the parents wish. An ED staff member should offer to remain with the parents during this time. Before the parents view the deceased child, the child and resuscitation area should be made as presentable as possible. Parents and other family members should be prepared ahead of time for the child's appearance. The amount of time the family may wish to be with their deceased child varies. Although it is important to allow enough time for the family to achieve closure, it may be necessary to direct them toward closure if they are having difficulty.

Most parents express strong feelings about whether or not they wish an autopsy to be done. The autopsy request should be explained by the physician in order for the parents to make an informed decision. Depending on the circumstances surrounding the child's death, an autopsy may be legally required. In these cases, parents should be so informed. A nurse should be present during any discussions with the parents during this time. This facilitates clarifying issues and answering questions that may come up at a later time.

It is important for the nurse to be aware that parents are frequently in a state of shock or numbness at the time of their child's death and may be unable to ask questions, retain information, or make their wishes and needs known. It is therefore critical to identify the name and telephone number of a nurse or physician the parents can contact for information or follow-up counseling. Some EDs have established programs for follow-up phone calls or meetings with families after an ED death. This can provide support and closure for both the family and the staff.

Emergency staff should inform the parents where their child's body will be sent from the ED, such as to the hospital, city, or county morgue. The nurse may offer to contact a funeral director for the family. If the parents desire, a clergy member may be called to pray with and comfort the grieving family.

The attitudes of health care workers in interacting with parents both during and after resuscitation are a very important determinant of how parents remember and cope with the experience. Staff members need to demonstrate care and concern and a willingness to be involved with parents during this time. After the high level of stress and activity involved in a resuscitation effort, it can be difficult for the nurse to slow down and be with the parents when there is nothing left to do for the child. Nurses may feel at a loss or helpless in such situations.

It may be beneficial for the nurse to prepare some keepsakes for the parents to take home with them. If appropriate, and the parents wish, the child's picture may be taken with an instant camera, a lock of the child's hair may be cut and placed in a plastic bag, or the child's hand and footprint can be imprinted on a card for the parents to take home. The staff involved in the resuscitation also may wish to send the family a sympathy card. A "bereavement packet" (Phelps, 1990) may be put together to be used after the death of an infant or child in the ED. It can include a bibliography, literature on death and grieving for parents and siblings, a list of area support groups, and materials for the collection of keepsakes. Nurses should be familiar with parent support groups in their geographic area so they can direct parents appropriately. This can be helpful in facilitating closure for both the parents and the staff in the ED. A parent should never be sent home from the hospital alone. The nurse can offer to contact a relative or friend to come and take the parent home. The child's primary care provider also should be contacted as soon as possible.

After the resuscitation, the health care team members involved should have the opportunity to discuss the resuscitation, both as a quality assurance measure and to provide support for each other. A psychiatric liaison nurse, social worker, or other appropriate resource should be available to provide an opportunity for staff to express feelings and be supported either individually or as a group.

Parent Education. Because most pediatric cardiopulmonary arrests are preventable, the major responsibility of nurses is to provide ongoing education whenever they interact with parents about the health of their children. Parents need to be taught childhood safety and to recognize when to seek medical attention for acute illness. Nurses have a unique opportunity to teach parents about the importance of such things as car seats, seat belts, providing for age-appropriate play in a safe environment, and health maintenance activities.

Nurse Education. Any nurses working in areas where infants and children are cared for should be certified in pediatric basic and advanced life support. Because pediatric resuscitations require special knowledge and skills, and occur infrequently in most EDs, resuscitation drills should be scheduled on a regular basis. These sessions can be used to identify learning needs, to maintain skills, and to give staff confidence in handling a pediatric arrest situation. Postresuscitation conferences or critiques should occur after each resuscitation to discuss any problems identified, to address concerns, and to provide constructive feedback regarding the performance of team members during the resuscitation. The findings can be used to make needed improvements in practice, with the goal of improving the outcome of pediatric cardiopulmonary arrests.

REFERENCES

American Heart Association (1992a). Guidelines for cardiopulmonary resuscitation and emergency cardiac care: Pediatric basic life support. *JAMA* 268:2251–2261

American Heart Association (1992b). Guidelines for cardiopulmonary resuscitation and emergency cardiac care: Pediatric advanced life support. *JAMA* 268:2262–2275

Andersen KH, Hald A (1989). Assessing the position of the tracheal tube: The reliability of different methods. *Anesthesia* 44:984–985

Atkins DL, Sirna S, Kiesko R, Charbonnier F, Kerber R (1988). Pediatric defibrillation: Importance of paddle size in determining transthoracic impedance. *Pediatrics* 82:914–918

Beland MJ (1987). Noninvasive transcutaneous cardiac pacing in children. *PACE: Pacing Clinics of Electrophysiology* 10:1262–1270

Bhende MS, Thompson A, Cook D, Saville A (1992). Validity of a disposable end-tidal CO_2 detector in verifying endotracheal tube placement in infants and children. *Annals of Emergency Medicine* 21:142–145

Brown CG, Werman HA (1990). Adrenergic agonist during cardiopulmonary resuscitation. *Resuscitation* 19:1–16

Chameides L (ed) (1988). *Textbook of Pediatric Advanced Life Support*. Dallas: American Heart Association, p 21

Doyle CJ, Post H, Burney R, Maino J, Keefe M, Rhee K (1987). Family participation during resuscitation: An option. *Annals of Emergency Medicine* 16:673–675

Eisenberg M, Berger K, Hallstrom A (1983). Epidemiology of cardiac arrest and resuscitation in children. *Annals of Emergency Medicine* 12:672–674

Finer N, Barrington K, Al-Fadley F, Peters K (1986). Limitations of self-inflating resuscitators. *Pediatrics* 77:417–420

Friesen RM, Duncan P, Tweed W, Bristow G (1982). Appraisal of cardiopulmonary resuscitation. *Canadian Medical Association Journal* 126:1055–1058

Gillis J, Dickson D, Rieder M, Steward D, Edmonds J (1986). Results of inpatient pediatric resuscitation. *Critical Care Medicine* 14:469–471

Goetting MG, Paradis NA (1991). High-dose epinephrine improves outcome from pediatric cardiac arrest. *Annals of Emergency Medicine* 20:22–26

Hampe S (1975). Needs of the grieving spouse in the hospital setting. *Nursing Research* 24:113–119

Hanson C, Strawser D (1992). Family presence during cardiopulmonary resuscitation: Foote Hospital emergency department's nine-year perspective. *Journal of Emergency Nursing* 18:104–106

Hinkle AJ (1988). A rapid and reliable method of selecting endotracheal tube sizes in children. *Anesthesia and Analgesia* 67:S92

Krongrad E (1984). Postoperative arrhythmias in patients with congenital heart disease. *Chest* 85:107–113

La Fleche FR, Slepin M, Vargas J, Milzman D (1989). Iatrogenic bilateral tibial fractures after intraosseous infusion attempts in a 3-month-old infant. *Annals of Emergency Medicine* 18:1099–1101

Lubitz DS (1988). A rapid method for estimating weight and resuscitation drug dosages from length in the pediatric age group. *Annals of Emergency Medicine* 17:576–581

Moscati R, Moore GP (1990). Compartment syndrome with resultant amputation following intraosseous infusion. *Annals of Emergency Medicine* 8:470–471

Nichols DG (1986). Factors influencing outcome of cardiopulmonary resuscitation in children. *Pediatric Emergency Care* 2:1–5

Orlowski JP, Julius C, Petras R, Porembka D, Gallagher J (1989). The safety of intraosseous infusions: Risks of fat and bone marrow emboli to the lungs. *Annals of Emergency Medicine* 18:1062–1067

Paradis NA, Martin G, et al (1990). Coronary perfusion and the return of spontaneous circulation in human cardiopulmonary resuscitation. *JAMA* 263:1106–1113

Phelps J (1990). *Bereavement Packet for PICU Families*. Hartford: Hartford Hospital

Quinton DN, O'Byrne G, Aitkenhead AR (1987). Comparison of endotracheal and peripheral intravenous adrenaline in cardiac arrest. *Lancet* 1:828–829

Ralston SH, Tacker W, Showen L, Carter A, Babbs C, Lafayette W (1985). Endotracheal versus intravenous epinephrine during electromechanical dissociation with CPR in dogs. *Annals of Emergency Medicine* 14:1044–1048

Ralston SH, Voorhees WD, Babbs CF (1984). Intrapulmonary epinephrine during prolonged cardiopulmonary resuscitation: Improved regional blood flow and resuscitation in dogs. *Annals of Emergency Medicine* 13:79–86

Terndrup TE, Kanter RK, Cherry RA (1989). A comparison of infant ventilation methods performed by prehospital personnel. *Annals of Emergency Medicine* 18:607–611

Torphy DE, Minter MG, Thompson BM (1984). Cardiorespiratory arrest and resuscitation of children. *American Journal of Diseases of Children* 138:1099–1102

Zander J, Hazinski MF (1992). Pulmonary disorders. In Hazinski MF (ed), *Nursing care of the critically ill child* (2nd ed). St. Louis: Mosby Year Book, pp 395–497

Zaritsky A (1987). CPR in children. *Annals of Emergency Medicine* 16:1107–1111

Zaritsky A, Chernow B (1984). Use of catecholamines in pediatrics. *Journal of Pediatrics* 105:341–349

SUGGESTED READING

American Heart Association (1992). Guidelines for cardiopulmonary resuscitation and emergency cardiac care: Adult basic life support. *JAMA* 268:2184–2198

Andropoulos DB, Soifer SJ, Schreiber MD (1990). Plasma epinephrine concentrations after intraosseous and central venous injection during cardiopulmonary resuscitation in the lamb. *Journal of Pediatrics* 116:312–315

Curley MA, Vaughan SM (1987). Assessment and resuscitation of the pediatric patient. *Critical Care Nurse* 7:26–42

Finholt DA, Kettrick R, Wagner H, Swedlow D (1986). The heart is under the lower third of the sternum: Implications for external cardiac massage. *American Journal of Diseases of Children* 140:646–649

Fredrickson JM (1988). Basic pediatric cardiopulmonary resuscitation (CPR) update. *Journal of Emergency Nursing* 14:76–81

Glaeser PW, Losek JD (1986). Emergency intraosseous infusions in children. *American Journal of Emergency Medicine* 4:34–36

Gray WA, Capone RJ, Most AS (1991). Unsuccessful emergency medical resuscitation: Are continued efforts in the emergency department justified? *New England Journal of Medicine* 325:1393–1398

Hasegawa EA (1986). The endotracheal use of emergency drugs. *Heart and Lung* 15:60–63

Hazinski MF (1992). Advances and controversies in cardiopulmonary resuscitation in the young. *Journal of Cardiovascular Nursing* 6:74–85

Horimoto Y, Yoshizawa M, Okazaki A, Hasumi K (1985). Five years' experience of cardiopulmonary resuscitation in a children's hospital. *Resuscitation* 13:47–55

Jost KE, Haase JE (1989). At the time of death: Help for the child's parents. *Children's Health Care* 18:140–146

Kanter RK, Zimmerman J, Strauss R, Stoeckel K (1986). Pediatric emergency intravenous access: Evaluation of a protocol. *American Journal of Diseases of Children* 140:132–134

Krischer JP, Fine E, Weissfeldt M, Guerci A, Nagel E, Chandra N (1989). Comparison of prehospital conventional and simultaneous compression-ventilation cardiopulmonary resuscitation. *Critical Care Medicine* 17:1263–1269

Lee CJ (1991). Determining the pulse for infant CPR: Time for a change? *Military Medicine* 156:190–193

Lewis JK, Minter M, Eshelman S, White M (1983). Outcome of pediatric resuscitation. *Annals of Emergency Medicine* 12:297–299

Ludwig S, Kettrick RG, Parker M (1984). Pediatric cardiopulmonary resuscitation: A review of 130 cases. *Clinical Pediatrics* 23:71–75

Miccolo MA (1990). Intraosseous infusion. *Critical Care Nurse* 10:35–47

O'Rourke PP (1986). Outcome of children who are apneic and pulseless in the emergency room. *Critical Care Medicine* 14:466–468

Orlowski JP (1986). Optimal position for external cardiac compressions in infants and young children. *Annals of Emergency Medicine* 15:667–673

Phillips GW, Zideman DA (1986). Relation of infant heart to sternum: Its significance in cardiopulmonary resuscitation. *Lancet* 1:1024–1025

Rice V (1987). Acid-base derangements in the patient with cardiac arrest. *Focus on Critical Care* 14:53–61

Sapien R, Stein H, Padbury J, Thio S, Hodge S (1992). Intraosseous versus intravenous epinephrine infusions in lambs: Pharmacokinetics and pharmacodynamics. *Pediatric Emergency Care* 8:179–183

Soud T (1992). Airway, breathing, circulation, and disability: What is different about kids? *Journal of Emergency Nursing* 18:107–116

Spivey W (1987). Intraosseous infusions. *Journal of Pediatrics* 111:639–642

Weatherly KS, McCallum AW, Young S (1991). Cost-effective resuscitation education. *Journal of Staff Development* 7:165–170

Zaritsky A (1988). Selected concepts and controversies in pediatric cardiopulmonary resuscitation. *Critical Care Clinics* 4:735–754

CHAPTER 14

Cardiac Emergencies

SANDRA MOTT

INTRODUCTION

Although cardiac emergencies are not frequent statistically, the level of acuity of these conditions is high. Cardiovascular conditions are one of the two top causes of sudden death among children older than 1 year (Denfield and Garson, 1990). The other condition is infectious diseases. The cardiovascular conditions most often responsible for these deaths are myocarditis (viral), hypertrophic cardiomyopathy, and congenital coronary artery anomalies. Myocarditis and cardiomyopathy are discussed more fully later in this chapter. Congenital anomalous origin of the left coronary artery is rare and is often asymptomatic before death. In this anomaly, the left coronary artery may be between the aorta and the pulmonary artery, putting it at risk for being compressed, or it originates from the pulmonary artery so desaturated blood flows through it to the left myocardium. Compression of the artery causes ischemia to the left ventricle and potential sudden death. Unfortunately, death occurs within the first year of life among 65% of infants with this diagnosis (Park, 1988). The more fortunate few demonstrate signs and symptoms of congestive heart failure (CHF) and myocardial infarction at 2–3 months of age, so surgical correction can be attempted. Rarely, children with artery compression experience exercise-induced syncope, which may be the only hint of their life-threatening anomaly.

Most infants and children who present with either undiagnosed cardiac disease or a worsening status of a previously diagnosed cardiac disease are either emergently or urgently ill. Their condition necessitates prompt recognition and skilled management by the emergency department (ED) staff. Although they vary, the presenting signs and symptoms all relate to an alteration in cardiac function that keeps the heart from pumping efficiently. Of critical importance is the realization that any clinical presentation of cyanosis, shock, or CHF has a potential cardiac cause, and immediate, competent intervention is required.

The initial nursing assessment, including a history and a physical examination, provides defining data that identify children with life-threatening, high-risk conditions from those with less emergent demands. The amount and type of data gathered vary with the physical presentation of the child and whether the onset is sudden with rapid deterioration or gradual with progressive worsening of signs and symptoms. Data gathered in the nursing history of an acutely ill child include all or some modification of the following.

Nursing History of an Acutely Ill Child

- Age of child
- Chief concern or complaint
- Definition of concern or complaint
    Onset—sudden or gradual, previous episodes
    Location of complaint—anatomically precise
    Quality—dull, sharp, aching, burning, itching
    Quantity—intensity and degree of discomfort
    Chronology—previous health, onset of problem, duration, frequency, change over time
    Setting—home or school
- Alleviating or aggravating factors
    Associated symptoms
    Actions taken to relieve problem

Epidemiologic information—exposure, contacts, travel
- Relevant medical and surgical history

Often the nurse is gathering health history data while performing the physical examination. These data help to focus the examination, making it more efficient and expediting the analysis of findings. Thorough assessment of the child's cardiac output is the critical aspect of the examination. This is especially true during the first couple of weeks of infancy when the possibility of an undiagnosed congenital anomaly exists, if the child is cyanotic, or if the child has a history of syncopal episodes, cardiac disease, or cardiac surgery.

Cardiac output is defined as the volume of blood ejected by the heart in 1 minute. When adequate, this volume is sufficient to maintain oxygenation and substrate delivery to the body tissues. Cardiac output is calculated by multiplying stroke volume by the heart rate. In infants and children, stroke volume is relatively fixed because of the immaturity of the sympathetic innervation to the ventricles. The child responds to increased cardiac output demands with tachycardia. Although tachycardia may initially compensate during periods of distress, prolonged rapid rates (more than 200 beats per minute for infants and 170 beats per minute for children) cause a shorter ventricular diastolic filling time and inadequate perfusion of the left coronary artery, resulting in diminished stroke volume and decreased cardiac output plus varying degrees of ischemia of the heart muscle. Physical assessment of cardiac output includes the following.

Physical Assessment of Cardiac Output

- Observing the child's color—pink, blue, gray, mottled. For children of color, check mucous membranes (tongue and conjunctivae) for adequacy of perfusion
- Checking capillary refill (should be brisk and less than 2 seconds)
- Noting the core as opposed to the skin temperature gradient—Are extremities warm, cool, or cold? How do they compare to core body temperature?
- Palpating the quality and character of distal pulses—bounding, strong, weak, thready, absent
- Describing level of consciousness, degree of irritability, interest in environment, and activity tolerance
- Noting variations in vital signs from developmental norms—heart rate and regularity, blood pressure, respiratory rate and effort

INFANT CYANOSIS

One of the more terrifying situations for both parents and health care providers is profound cyanosis in a previously healthy infant. When a cyanotic infant is brought to the ED, the highest priority is to determine whether the cyanosis is peripheral or central and if central, whether it has a pulmonary or a cardiac cause. Once this differentiation is made, a treatment plan can be implemented.

Etiology and Pathophysiology

Peripheral cyanosis usually has a vascular cause manifested by poor perfusion of the skin during times of environmental cold, sepsis, or shock. It is the result of pathophysiologic changes secondary to hemorrhage, trauma, infection, or metabolic abnormalities.

Central cyanosis, on the other hand, is caused by poor oxygenation of circulating blood related to either a pulmonary or a cardiac disorder. Pulmonary causes include an interference with gas exchange leading to retention of carbon dioxide and the inability of the respiratory system to breathe in sufficient oxygen. Ductal-dependent lesions are usually the cardiac cause of sudden onset neonatal cyanosis. Various congenital anomalies depend on a patent ductus arteriosus for blood flow either to the pulmonary artery through the left-to-right shunt or to the systemic circulation from a right-to-left shunt that occurs as long as the ductus remains patent. Generally, the ductus begins to close sometime during the first week of life. As it closes, pulmonary blood flow is compromised (either increased or decreased), and the infant's condition rapidly deteriorates.

Not all cardiac lesions that present with cyanosis during the first week of life are totally ductal dependent. With some lesions, a patent ductus masks the presence of a right-to-left shunt that only becomes apparent as the ductus arteriosus closes. With other lesions, the infant experiences a gradual increase in cyanosis or is cyanotic only when stressed. Still other infants have extensive collateral circulation or additional defects that allow sufficient mixing and avoid the sudden onset of deterioration that would otherwise occur with closure of the ductus arteriosus. Their symptoms appear gradually and may be more difficult to identify. In addition, a few neonates are discharged with cyanosis related to a cardiac anomaly; it must be determined if the current cyanosis is the same as or worse than the infant's baseline.

Assessment

History. Except for the small percentage of neonates with known cyanotic cardiac disease, the prenatal and birth histories are often unremarkable. The age of the infant and the suddenness of onset, however, are the two key factors that suggest the differential diagnosis of either septic or some other cause of shock or a ductus-dependent cardiac lesion.

Physical Assessment. The first objective of physical assessment is to ascertain whether the infant is experiencing peripheral or central cyanosis (Figure 14–1). Data supporting peripheral cyanosis include pink mucous membranes (tongue and conjunctivae), cool extremities, and slow capillary refill. Transcutaneous oximetry is unreliable. It should be within normal limits, but it may be low because of poor peripheral perfusion. Although the infant may have tachycardia, no murmur is heard during auscultation.

Data supporting central cyanosis include an infant who is warm and well perfused and whose cyanosis includes the tongue and conjunctivae. Transcutaneous oximetry is low (65–85%), indicating inadequate oxygen saturation of the red blood cells. A cue that helps differentiate between pulmonary and cardiac causes is the respiratory status of the infant at rest and when agitated. If dyspnea and increased work of breathing are present at rest, but decreased cyanosis occurs with crying, the cause probably is pulmonary. An infant with cardiac disease may show evidence of tachypnea but breathes comfortably until upset; then cyanosis deepens and dyspnea appears. Tachycardia is present and peripheral pulses may be decreased if there is an increased pulmonary flow lesion. Another cue, although not always as helpful, is auscultation of a cardiac murmur. Its presence indicates cardiac disease, but its absence does not eliminate it. If the cardiac lesion is very large or essentially closed, there is not enough turbulence of blood for a murmur to be heard.

Laboratory and Diagnostic Tests. Two tests are helpful in separating pulmonary and cardiac causes of central cyanosis. Arterial blood gases reveal a low PaO_2 for both, but the $PaCO_2$ is elevated, indicating retention of carbon dioxide, with pulmonary conditions and is normal with cardiac disease. Administration of oxygen lessens the cyanosis and improves transcutaneous oxygen saturation if the cause is pulmonary, but has little, if any, effect on either one if the cause is cardiac. Additional diagnostic tests, which may be done before but are often delayed until after initial treatment and which aid in the definitive diagnosis, are a chest x ray and electrocardiogram (ECG).

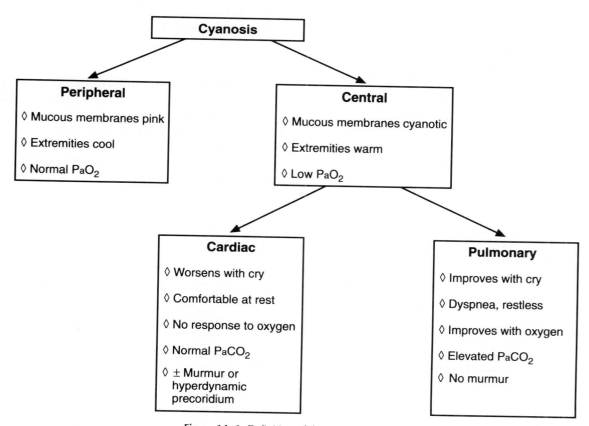

Figure 14–1. Definition of the cause of cyanosis.

TRIAGE
Cyanosis

Emergent

An infant 2 weeks of age or less with sudden onset of cyanosis and rapidly worsening of cardiorespiratory status and little or no response to 100% oxygen.

Urgent

Infant with gradual onset of cyanosis that increases with crying or straining, increased heart rate and respiratory rate, and who has little, if any, improvement in color with 100% oxygen.

Nursing Diagnosis
Decreased Cardiac Output

Defining Characteristics

- Variations in blood pressure readings
- Decreased peripheral pulses
- Color changes in skin and mucous membranes
- Dyspnea

Nursing Interventions

- Monitor cardiorespiratory status
- Administer medication as ordered
- Anticipate needs to decrease stress of crying
- Provide uninterrupted rest periods

Expected Outcomes

- Infant's color improves
- Cardiorespiratory status stabilizes
- Oxygen saturation improves

Nursing Diagnosis
Impaired Gas Exchange

Defining Characteristics

- Hypoxia
- Decreased oxygen saturation

Nursing Interventions

- Administer medication as ordered
- Monitor changes in cardiorespiratory status
- Monitor and document change in arterial blood gases
- Have available appropriate emergency equipment

Expected Outcomes

- Oxygen saturation improves
- Cyanosis decreases

Nursing Diagnosis
Parental Anxiety

Defining Characteristics

- Verbalization of apprehension, uncertainty, distress, worry
- Expression of concern about change in life events
- Fear of unspecified consequences
- Increased tension

Nursing Interventions

- Encourage verbalization of concerns
- Keep parent informed of rationale for assessments and tests
- Identify and address knowledge needs
- Help parent identify coping resources

Expected Outcomes

- Parent verbalizes that information helped to lessen anxiety
- Parent's questions address specific rather than vague concerns
- Parent identifies coping strategies and uses them

Management

Once it is determined that the cause of this emergently ill infant's cyanosis is a ductal-dependent cardiac lesion, an infusion of prostaglandin E_1 is administered to maintain ductal patency. The infant is admitted to the intensive care unit (ICU) and referred to a pediatric cardiologist for diagnosis and further medical and surgical management.

Nursing responsibilities during administration of prostaglandin E_1 (initial dose of 0.1 μg/kg/minute, which is decreased to half after cyanosis lessens and oxygen saturation is 80–90%) include close monitoring of the infant's response (improved oxygen saturation) and evidence of any untoward side effects such as apnea, systemic hypotension, fever, and other central nervous system effects such as jitteriness. The nurse must be prepared to initiate or assist in emergency measures because it is not uncommon for an infant with cyanosis to require intubation for ventilation or additional venous access for fluid resuscitation (Flynn et al, 1992).

An urgently ill child also is admitted to the hospital and referred to a pediatric cardiologist for further evaluation and determination of a treatment plan.

Psychosocial Support and Patient and Family Education

Parents often are overwhelmed by the flurry of activity that surrounds their infant while the medical staff works to stabilize the infant's condition and at the same time attempt to decipher the physiologic cause for the infant's cyanosis and rapid deterioration. This is an extremely frightening experience for the parents, who feel helpless, useless, guilty, and often fearful that their infant may die. Parents need the presence of a supportive, sensitive nurse who can explain in general why certain procedures are being done and respond to the parents' questions. Parents also need to be reassured that everything possible is being done and that they did the right thing in bringing the infant to the ED. They also need to know that the sudden change in the infant's condition is not related to something the parents did or did not do or to something that could have been prevented. It is important that parents not be left alone or made to feel that they are "in the way." They need the presence of a supportive, reassuring person during this time.

Once the infant's condition is stabilized, it is important that the parents be allowed to see and touch their child. At this time more definitive information can be shared with them as to the treatment plan, which includes hospitalization and usually surgical intervention.

HYPERCYANOSIS

Infants and children whose cardiac disease consists of systemic desaturation caused by right-to-left shunting have some degree of cyanosis. Their body adapts to the lowered oxygenation with accelerated hematopoiesis as evidenced by a hematocrit of 55–70%. They also modify their activity level to accommodate their low oxygen saturations, which are 60–80%. Although they adapt to their limited arterial saturation, these children have no reserve and respond poorly to events that lower their baseline level. About 25% of infants with cyanotic heart disease may be brought to the ED after a hypercyanotic episode (Hazinski, 1992). These episodes usually occur during the first year of life; the peak incidence is between the second and the fourth months of life (Park, 1988). Most episodes occur in the morning during times of feeding, crying, or defecation. Hypercyanosis is also referred to as *hypoxic spell* or *tet spell* because most, although not all, of these infants have tetralogy of Fallot.

Etiology and Pathophysiology

There are a variety of causes of increased cyanosis, including mechanical factors, such as shunt (natural or surgical) obstruction; illnesses, such as fever or dehydration, that siphon blood from the pulmonary to the systemic circulation; or pressure gradient changes between existing pulmonary resistance and systemic resistance so that any increase in pulmonary resistance or decrease in systemic resistance reduces pulmonary flow (Flynn et al, 1992).

Why some infants have hypercyanotic episodes or spells and others do not is unknown. There is no correlation with the degree of cyanosis or hypoxemia at rest or with the infant's hematocrit. These episodes occur during times of increased demand for oxygen which the body is unable to supply because of the relatively fixed pulmonary blood flow that exists because of the arterial, infundibular, or valvular stenosis. The multifactorial cause of hypercyanotic or hypoxic spells involves a decrease in systemic vascular resistance, an increase in pulmonary resistance, and an exaggeration of the right-to-left shunt through the large ventricular septal defect in tetralogy of Fallot or the truncus in persistent truncus arteriosus. This action increases the proportion of desaturated blood in systemic circulation, causing a decrease in PaO_2, an increase in $PaCO_2$, and a decrease in pH. The falling pH produces acidemia, which stimulates the respiratory center to produce hyperpnea. Hyperpnea normally improves cardiac output by increasing systemic venous return. In the presence of fixed pulmonary blood flow, however, it promotes right-to-left shunting and a further decrease in systemic arterial oxygen saturation and increased cyanosis. Acidosis also contributes to further pulmonary vasoconstriction and resistance (Driscoll, 1990) Thus a vicious cycle is established (Figure 14–2), hyperpnea aggravating the situation instead of rectifying it.

Situations that reduce right ventricular filling, such as excessive tachycardia and hypovolemia, also contribute to the effect of right ventricular outflow tract obstruction. Anything that reduces pulmonary blood flow decreases arterial oxygen saturation and stimulates hyperpnea, thus triggering the vicious cycle of hypoxic spells.

The development of hypercyanotic spells is a criterion for immediate surgical intervention to palliate or correct the restricted pulmonary blood flow. Blood gas analysis of infants during hypoxic spells documented arterial oxygen saturations of 15–33% (Hazinski, 1992). Hypoxemia this severe places the infant at risk for cerebral hypoxia and a cerebrovascular accident or even death. Because of the high risk for intracranial complications and the limitations in growth and development associated with cyanotic heart disease, surgical correction is routinely being done within the first 6 months of life.

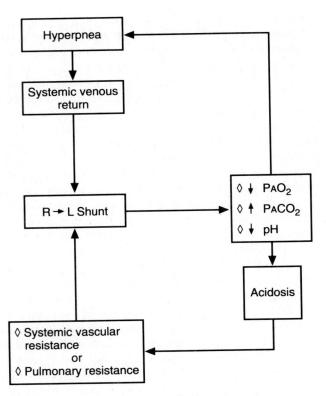

Figure 14–2. Vicious cycle of hypercyanosis.

During a spell, the typical systolic ejection murmur heard along the middle and upper left sternal border becomes decreased in intensity and may even be absent.

The infant needs to be evaluated for concurrent illness. The possibility of a pulmonary process is determined by documenting temperature, breath sounds, adequacy of air exchange, and presence of cough. The presence of gastrointestinal disease is ascertained by assessing the infant's hydration status, appetite, urine output and specific gravity, and report of any nausea, vomiting, or diarrhea.

Laboratory and Diagnostic Tests. The physical appearance of the infant and the known cyanotic cardiac anomaly are all that is needed to confirm the diagnosis of a "tet" spell. Although it is known that arterial oxygen saturation and pH are low, testing is deferred in preference to immediate intervention. A needle stick during an hypoxic spell is an unnecessary stressor that could prolong or worsen the spell.

If the infant also is ill, additional testing includes chest radiography, determination of serum electrolyte levels and arterial blood gases, and other diagnostic tests relevant to presenting signs and symptoms.

Assessment

History. Usually a cardiac anomaly has been diagnosed previously, and the parents have been informed of the high risk for hypercyanotic spells. Upon admission to the ED, it is important to identify the infant's diagnosis as understood by the parents and whether the infant's degree of cyanosis is greater than baseline. If the infant has tetralogy of Fallot, helpful data include the events before the spell, including time of day and activity of the infant; the infant's initial signs and symptoms; and actions that the parents initiated and the infant's response. It is important to document any medications that the infant has been taking or the existence of a concurrent respiratory or gastrointestinal illness.

Physical Assessment. By the time the infant arrives in the ED, the spell frequently has resolved. The infant is no more cyanotic than baseline but is fatigued and wants to sleep. The classic signs and symptoms of an hypoxic spell include progressive irritability and inconsolability, diaphoresis, increasing cyanosis, and hyperpnea (rapid and deep respiration). With continued hypoxemia, the infant becomes hypoxic and limp, loses consciousness, and may have a seizure. In severe cases, a cerebral vascular accident or death may occur.

Nursing Diagnoses
The nursing diagnoses for hypercyanosis are the same as those for infant cyanosis.

Management
The goal of intervention is to break the vicious cycle. The first step is to comfort the infant and place him or her in a knee-chest position. The parents can usually do this best and benefit from being involved with their infant's care. The knee-chest position improves pul-

monary blood flow. It is thought that flexion of the hips and knees increases systemic vascular resistance by slowing, or even blocking, blood flow to the legs while at the same time reducing the systemic venous return by temporarily trapping blood in the legs. Both mechanisms serve to decrease the right-to-left shunting and help propel blood through the narrowed right ventricular outflow tract into the pulmonary circulation.

Intravenous morphine sulfate (0.1 mg/kg/dose) is given slowly (by the physician) to suppress the respiratory center and break the hyperpnic cycle. Sometimes the murmur can be heard to return or increase in intensity during morphine administration.

Oxygen is administered at 5–8 L by face mask or blow-by. Because the problem is the amount of pulmonary blood flow and not the ability to oxygenate, the effect of oxygen administration is minimal. Oxygen does, however, promote pulmonary vasodilatation thereby improving blood flow and increasing arterial oxygen saturation slightly. Parents view oxygen as beneficial and administering oxygen may lessen their anxiety.

If the infant is not fully responsive to the foregoing measures, a bolus of intravenous fluids is given. Because there is a right-to-left intracardiac shunt and blood returning from the body bypasses the filtering system of the lungs, it is critical that no air enter the intravenous system. The intravenous tubing must be equipped with an air filter, and special precautions must be taken to ensure that the tubing remains clear of even tiny air bubbles. It is important to remember that infusion pumps catch large air bubbles but allow some small ones to pass through. In addition, a vasoconstrictor such as phenylephrine (2–5 μg/kg/minute) is administered by continuous infusion to increase systemic vascular resistance and improve pulmonary flow (Shaddy et al, 1989). In addition, the beta blocker, propranolol (0.1–0.2 mg/kg/dose) may be given to reduce cardiac output by prolonging A-V noded conducting and decreasing rate and contractility, thereby slowing somewhat the right-to-left shunting. If surgical treatment must be delayed for a few days, the infant is given maintenance therapy with propranolol to prevent hypoxic spells. Severe spells may require intubation and ventilation. These infants are candidates for emergency surgical treatment.

The usual sequence after a hypercyanotic spell is hospital admission and an operation. Once an infant has a spell, more spells are likely to follow, increasing in both frequency and severity. It is important for preventing potential morbidity or even mortality that a corrective surgical procedure be performed as soon as possible.

Infants who have a concurrent illness should be treated vigorously to reduce the fever and to correct any dehydration. Antipyretic medication should be given around the clock for at least the first 24 hours; then the infant should be reevaluated. The pulmonary process should be treated both symptomatically and with antibiotics as indicated. Even mild dehydration from poor oral intake or gastrointestinal upset is treated with a bolus of fluid. If the infant has clinically significant dehydration or active vomiting or diarrhea, admission and intravenous rehydration are advised.

Patient and Family Teaching and Psychosocial Support

Parents need much reassurance because it is a very frightening experience to see their infant turn so deeply cyanotic and then become limp. They need a thorough explanation of interventions being done and the infant's anticipated response. Once the spell has resolved and the infant's condition is stable, the parents need time to hold and caress their son or daughter. They need the opportunity to ask questions and to be comforted as they express their fears and concerns. They also need to know that the infant's condition has returned to baseline, although the child is exhausted from the experience.

Usually an infant whose spell is sufficiently severe to warrant an ED visit is admitted. A pediatric cardiologist discusses the infant's condition and management plan with the family. Unless surgical intervention is contraindicated, which is exceedingly rare, the infant is scheduled for an operation within a day or two. Parents need time and support to adjust to the sudden change in plans and to make the necessary arrangements at home and work so they can be with their infant.

Even though the parents may know that their infant will require an operation in the future, the emergency nature of the situation leaves them feeling numb and confused. The nurse needs to be sensitive to these feelings and to encourage verbalization of questions, concerns, and fears.

If an infant's worsening cyanosis is related to an illness, the nurse carefully explains signs and symptoms of the illness and the effect of the illness on the infant's cardiac disease. The parents are instructed to notify the infant's health care provider for even a mild illness and to expect more vigorous intervention, such as round-the-clock medication for fever control.

SHOCK

An infant or child who presents or who progresses to a state of shock in the ED is one whose survival depends on the nurse's quick recognition of signs and symptoms, skill and speed in initiating and monitoring treatment, and knowledgeable, precise implementation of subsequent nursing measures. A multiplicity of etiologic events are responsible for shock. Shock is manifested by hypotension from altered hemodynamics, resulting in inadequate tissue perfusion to meet the oxygen and nutrient demands of metabolism and which may result in the death of cells and of the organism (Rimar, 1988a). Some of the etiologic events include hemorrhage, plasma loss, or water loss, which produce hypovolemic shock, overwhelming sepsis, anaphylaxis or drug overdose, leading to distributive shock and insufficient cardiac output in spite of adequate ventricular preload, left ventricular outflow obstruction, systemic to pulmonary shunting, myocardial insufficiency from dysrhythmias, or conditions related to cardiomyopathy leading to cardiogenic shock.

Etiology and Pathophysiology

Whatever the specific cause of shock, there are some common physiologic responses to the phenomenon. Characteristic of all early shock syndromes is inadequate oxygen consumption to meet increased tissue demands secondary to the accelerated metabolic activity. Shock is a progressive condition of circulatory dysfunction that entails compromised cardiac output in the form of hypotension and its potential consequences. This imbalance between supply and demand of oxygen leads to impaired function of cells, tissues, organs, and, if not reversed, entire body systems (Rice, 1991a).

Immediately after the shock-producing event, several compensatory mechanisms are activated in an effort to maintain the functional capacity of vital organs. The initial drop in blood pressure and decrease in cardiac output stimulate the cardiac centers in the brainstem to instigate the compensatory responses. As long as these intrinsic measures support systemic blood flow, they enable cardiorespiratory values to remain within normal limits. The response mechanisms involve sympathetic reflex actions and the activation of various humoral and hormonal secretions aimed at increasing the cardiac output and blood pressure and increasing oxygen extraction through enhanced alveolar ventilation. The efficacy of these responses is greatly determined by the child's prior cardiac and pulmonary status. It is important to remember that a child can lose 25% of total blood volume before symptoms appear. Compensatory mechanisms fail with the loss of 25–30% of blood volume (Kitt and Kaiser, 1990).

The continued lack of availability of sufficient oxygen for tissue use means that cellular processes occur without the benefit of oxygen. When anaerobic metabolism occurs, lactic acid accumulates, leading to metabolic acidosis. As compensatory mechanisms fail and

established shock progresses, minute ventilation rises. The increase in rate and depth of breathing creates a respiratory alkalosis that attempts to compensate for the metabolic acidosis.

It is important to note that respiratory alkalosis may occur as part of the initial response to the shock event. As a nonspecific stress response, it is the first respiratory reaction to the body's increased need for available oxygen for tissue metabolism. This increase in alveolar ventilation occurs even before any change in arterial blood gases is evident. The presence of respiratory alkalosis during early shock may mask the severity of the child's condition (Rimar, 1988a).

As the shock state progresses in the uncompensated phase, microvascular perfusion is impaired, leading to low perfusion pressures, increased arteriolar constriction, and decreased venous capacity, which allows blood to stagnate. Continued anaerobic metabolism and release of vasoactive substances exacerbates myocardial depression. Platelet aggregation and the release of tissue thromboplastin fosters coagulopathies such as disseminated intravascular coagulation (DIC). Thus, with prolonged shock and underperfusion comes cellular damage, individual organ dysfunction, and eventually multisystem organ failure (Rice, 1991b). When damage to vital organs such as the heart and brain occurs and therapeutic measures are ineffective in staying or reversing the damage, shock becomes irreversible and death eventually results.

Assessment

History. Because shock is the result of another etiologic event and the management plan must address that event as well as the physiologic manifestations of shock, a thorough history is imperative. The most common causes for shock are hypovolemia, sepsis, anaphylaxis, and cardiac dysfunction. The nurse therefore ascertains the presence or absence of conditions that may generate fluid loss or shift. Some of these conditions are vomiting, gastroenteritis, nephrosis, diabetes mellitus, diabetes insipidus, inflammatory bowel disease or other gastrointestinal bleeding disorders, recent trauma with blood loss or internal injury, and burns, including severe sunburn.

Any prior signs and symptoms of infection must be identified and carefully described because gram-negative organisms are frequently responsible for shock in infants and young children. The child's medication history is important, especially if the child has access to barbiturates, tranquilizers, or antihypertensive agents; excessive intake of these drugs results in abnormal distribution of blood. Exposure to potential offending antigens must be assessed. The most common offenders are insect stings (bees, hornets, yellow jackets, or wasps); foods, such as nuts, shellfish, eggs, or berries; and medications, especially penicillin but also cephalosporins, sulfonamides, streptomycin, and others. Finally, any history of cardiac disease, cardiac surgery, syncopal episodes, palpitations, or decreased exercise tolerance and shortness of breath either after a viral illness or in general must be defined.

Age is another factor to be considered. A neonate with severe left ventricular outflow obstruction does not appear distressed until late in the first week of life as the ductus closes. When this occurs, the blood flow to the lower body is obstructed and symptoms develop rapidly. Older children are more likely to have anaphylactic reactions because repeated exposure to the offending antigen is needed to form the reaginic antibodies. It is this interaction of antigen and antibody that precipitates the profound pulmonary and vascular response of shock.

Physical Assessment. The onset of physical signs and symptoms is unique to the child and occurs some time after cellular changes and the activation of compensatory mechanisms. Indices of impaired peripheral perfusion include cool, clammy, pale, gray, or mottled skin; prolonged capillary refill; and diminished intensity and quality of peripheral pulses. The reverse is true in early septic shock. Instead of decreased cardiac output, there is an initial increase in normal cardiac output. The children present well perfused with warm and dry skin even though their condition is life-threatening.

A discrepancy between the right arm and lower extremities in regard to pulses, oxygen saturation, and blood pressure in a neonate (usually 5–10 days of age) signifies a ductal-dependent lesion. The degree of discrepancy is related to the severity of the obstruction and the dependence of the lower extremities on the ductus arteriosus for its systemic blood supply. The neonate is pale, lethargic, clammy, and may have a dusky color to the lower body and pink color to the upper body. In more extreme cases, the neonate is cyanotic, has extremely poor perfusion, and has a hyperdynamic precordium.

Changes in vital signs such as tachycardia, tachypnea, narrowing pulse pressure, and hypotension also reflect circulatory dysfunction. Often an early sign of impending shock is a slight increase in diastolic blood pressure while the systolic pressure remains normal. Jugular veins are flat in hypovolemic shock but bulging in cardiogenic shock. Dysrhythmias, which further interfere with cardiac function, may occur in response to electrolyte imbalance, metabolic acidosis, and hypoxemia.

Decreased cerebral perfusion is manifested early by delayed response to stimuli, decreased alertness,

and presence of anxiety, irritability, or lethargy. Subtle indicators during infancy are poor feeding, weak cry, and listlessness. Pupils are dilated and react appropriately to light, but as shock progresses to the uncompensated phase, reaction becomes sluggish and in the final stage absent. As shock progresses, the child's level of consciousness diminishes to somnolence and finally obtundation.

Children in a state of hypovolemic shock also present with signs of dehydration such as poor skin turgor and dry mucous membranes. Infants younger than 1 year have a sunken fontanelle.

Urine output is reduced in response to decreased renal perfusion. This reduction occurs even though the child is adequately hydrated; it is part of the compensatory response to insufficient cardiac output. Guideline parameters are an output of less than 0.5–1.0 ml/kg/hour for infants and children and less than 1.0–2.0 ml/kg/hour for neonates. Again, it is important to note that in sepsis, urine output initially may be normal or even increased in spite of relative hypovolemia.

Children in a state of anaphylactic shock manifest immediate symptoms including urticaria, laryngeal edema with stridor, bronchospasm, abdominal cramping, weak peripheral pulses, and hypotension.

Laboratory and Diagnostic Tests. Extensive blood studies are done to aid in discerning the compensatory status and to monitor metabolic acidosis, respiratory alkalosis, electrolyte imbalance, hypoglycemia, coagulation abnormalities, infection, renal dysfunction, and hepatic dysfunction. Additional tests related to the underlying cause are also done.

During the compensated phase, laboratory abnormalities include increased blood glucose and serum sodium levels. Arterial blood gases show a decrease in oxygen and carbon dioxide tension and an increase in arterial pH. Complete blood count values vary according to the underlying cause; if sepsis is present, the white blood count is elevated, if hypovolemia is present, the hematocrit reflects the hemoconcentration. If the cause is uncertain, a toxic screen (blood and urine) is ordered to rule out a drug overdose.

As shock progresses, additional abnormalities become evident in blood and urine tests. Because pulmonary capillary blood flow is decreased, gas exchange is impaired, leading to decreased arterial oxygen levels and increased carbon dioxide levels and a decreased pH. The liver is no longer able to metabolize waste products, and continued ischemia contributes to liver cell death, which is reflected in elevated levels for all liver function studies. As renal dysfunction progresses, the serum blood urea nitrogen (BUN) and creatinine levels are elevated; urine sodium level is variable and urine osmolality is fixed or dilute. Increased levels of serum amylase and lipase come from ischemic pancreatic cells.

Depending on the child's presentation, use of chest x rays, electrocardiography, echocardiography, and additional laboratory studies may be warranted.

T R I A G E
Shock

Emergent
Neonates with rapidly deteriorating cardiac output. Infants and children with failing compensatory mechanisms and a progressive decrease in cardiac output (hypotension), poor systemic perfusion (weak or absent peripheral pulses), increased lethargy (coma), and minimal urinary output. Anaphylaxis is life-threatening and perhaps is the most emergent of the shock syndromes. Older infants and children whose state of compensation is unstable as evidenced by rapidly changing signs and symptoms as their body attempts to compensate for decreased cardiac output with tachycardia, tachypnea, decreased urine output, restlessness, and hypoactive bowel sounds.

Urgent
An older infant or child with adequate compensatory mechanisms in place, regardless of the cause of shock.

Nursing Diagnosis
Decreased Cardiac Output

Defining Characteristics

- Variations in blood pressure
- Jugular vein distention
- Decreased peripheral pulses
- Dysrhythmias
- Color changes in skin and mucous membranes
- Cold, clammy skin
- Oliguria
- Dyspnea
- Restlessness
- Change in mental status

Nursing Interventions

- Monitor cardiorespiratory status
- Monitor and interpret laboratory results
- Administer medication as ordered
- Monitor hydration status
- Measure and document hourly output

- Place child in semi-Fowler position
- Monitor indwelling pressure lines
- Interpret and document changes in mental status
- Prevent complications

Expected Outcomes

- Tissue perfusion improves
- Cardiorespiratory status stabilizes
- Blood pressure improves
- Child responds appropriately to environment

Nursing Diagnosis
Impaired Gas Exchange

Defining Characteristics

- Somnolence
- Restlessness
- Irritability
- Hypercapnea
- Hypoxia
- Decreased oxygen saturation

Nursing Interventions

- Administer medication as ordered
- Monitor changes in cardiorespiratory status
- Monitor and document change in arterial blood gases
- Maintain fluid and electrolyte balance
- Have appropriate emergency equipment available
- Assist in establishment and maintenance of patent airway

Expected Outcomes

- Arterial blood gases improve
- Cardiorespiratory status stabilizes
- Child is alert and responsive

Nursing Diagnosis
Altered Tissue Perfusion

Defining Characteristics

- Cold extremities
- Diminished arterial pulsations
- Pale or dusky extremities
- Blood pressure changes in extremities

Nursing Interventions

- Monitor vital signs including blood pressure and distal pulses
- Measure intake and output

- Monitor for changes in skin temperature or color
- Monitor for neurologic changes
- Administer medications as ordered
- Maintain intravenous line or fluid administration

Expected Outcomes

- Vital signs return to normal
- Skin color and temperature return to normal
- Peripheral pulses are strong and capillary refill brisk

Nursing Diagnosis
Fluid Volume Deficit

Defining Characteristics

- Decreased urine output
- Decreased venous filling
- Hemoconcentration
- Hypotension
- Increased pulse rate
- Decreased pulse volume and pressure
- Dry skin
- Dry mucous membranes

Nursing Interventions

- Monitor circulatory status
- Monitor hydration status
- Measure intake and output
- Monitor and interpret laboratory values
- Maintain intravenous fluid administration

Expected Outcomes

- Urine output increases in response to fluid administration
- Child has improved skin turgor and moist mucous membranes
- Child's circulatory status improves with fluid administration

Nursing Diagnosis
Knowledge Deficit

Defining Characteristics

- Verbalizations indicating inadequate understanding, misinterpretation, misconception
- Inappropriate or exaggerated behaviors (hysteria, agitation, hostility)

Nursing Interventions

- Review parent's level of knowledge about child's condition

- Determine if there are any ambiguities in the parents' minds
- Identify and address knowledge needs relative to procedures, policies, diagnosis, and prognosis
- Encourage parents to express concerns or fears about child
- Provide collaboration with health team members as needed

Expected Outcomes

- Parent verbalizes understanding of information provided
- Parent verbalizes satisfaction in resources provided
- Parent's behavior is under control; they are able to ask questions without hostility and to converse in a calm manner

Management
When a child arrives in the ED in a state of shock, the first concern is to ensure a patent airway. For many patients this means insertion of an endotracheal tube (ET) and mechanical ventilation with 100% oxygen. Special considerations must be made for neonates because of the documented relation between retrolental fibroplasia and exposure to environments with concentrated oxygen.

Of equal importance is the establishment of intravenous lines for the administration of fluids and medications. Because some of the medications are toxic to the tissues if they infiltrate, a central venous line is ideal; however, in the ED placement of a central venous line usually is not possible, so peripheral venous lines are used. Fluid replacement is critical because it increases preload and thereby enhances cardiac output. Replacement must be carefully monitored to prevent pulmonary edema or cardiac decompensation from fluid overload. An immediately available balanced salt solution such as Ringer lactate is the fluid of choice. Unless a predisposing condition indicates otherwise, 10 mL/kg of body weight is infused over several minutes (Rimar, 1988b). If there is no improvement in vital signs or perfusion, a second bolus can be given. If improvement is still lacking, pharmacologic interventions are added. Table 14–1 presents the medications most commonly used in the treatment of pediatric shock. It is essential that the nurse be knowledgeable about these medications and how to titrate the infusions to achieve the desired results while also monitoring for side effects.

In neonates with ductus-dependent lesions, prostaglandin infusion and monitoring as described earlier is a life-saving intervention. Inotropic medications also are needed to stabilize the condition of the neonate,

TABLE 14–1. PEDIATRIC SYMPATHOMIMETIC AND OTHER INOTROPIC DRUGS[a]

Drug	Dose	Effects	Cautions
Dobutamine	2–20 μg/kg/minute	Selective beta-adrenergic effects; increases cardiac contractility and also increases heart rate (the latter effect is variable). Beta-2 effects produce peripheral vasodilatation. No dopaminergic or alpha-adrenergic effects.	Extreme tachyarrhythmias have been reported (particularly in infants); hypotension may develop; many produce pulmonary venoconstriction
Dopamine	1–5 μg/kg/minute	Dopaminergic effects predominate (including increase in glomerular filtration rate and urine volume).	Can produce extreme tachyarrhythmias; can result in increase in pulmonary artery pressure; inhibits thyroid stimulating hormone and aldosterone secretion
	2–10 μg/kg/minute	Dopaminergic effects persist and beta-1 effects are seen (especially an increase in heart rate).	
	8–20 μg/kg/minute	Alpha-adrenergic effects dominate.	
Epinephrine	0.05–0.15 μg/kg/minute	Alpha, beta-1 and beta-2 adrenergic effects; at low doses, beta-1 effects dominate.	Increases myocardial work and oxygen consumption at any dose; splanchnic constriction occurs at even low doses
	0.2–0.3 μg/kg/minute	Alpha-adrenergic effects dominate.	
Isoproterenol	0.05–0.1 μg/kg/minute	Beta-adrenergic effects; beta-1 effects may result in rapid increase in heart rate; beta-2 effects may produce peripheral vasodilatation and also may effectively treat bronchoconstriction.	Monitor for tachyarrhythmias, hypotension. Increases myocardial oxygen consumption
Norepinephrine	0.05–1.0 μg/kg/minute	Alpha- and beta-adrenergic effects; produces potent peripheral and renal vasoconstriction; can increase blood pressure.	May produce tachyarrhythmias, increased myocardial work, and increased oxygen consumption; may result in hepatic and mesenteric ischemia
Amrinone	0.75–5 mg/kg (Loading, slowly) 5–10 μg/kg/minute	Phosphodiesterase inhibition and increase in intracellular cyclic-AMP; intracellular calcium uptake delayed. These effects result in improved cardiac contractility and vasodilatation.	Arrhythmias may occur (especially accelerated junctional rhythm, junctional tachycardia, and ventricular ectopy); may produce hypotension (especially if patient is hypovolemic), liver and gastrointestinal dysfunction, thrombocytopenia, and abdominal pain; experience in children is limited

[a] Infusion rate (mL/hr) = $\dfrac{\text{wt (kg)} \times \text{Dose (μg/kg/min)} \times 60 \text{ min/hr}}{\text{Concentration (μg/mL)}}$

(Reproduced with permission from Hazinski MF. [1990]. Shock in the pediatric patient. Critical Care Nursing Clinics of North America *2:309)*

who is then transferred to the ICU. Upon transfer, a pediatric cardiologist and cardiac surgeon with the aid of additional testing provide a definitive diagnosis and treatment plan.

While the patient is in the ED, the nurse places electrodes on the child for continuous monitoring of cardiac rhythm and documents the child's blood pressure at least every half hour. If an arterial line is present, it is used to provide a continuous display of systemic blood pressure, including the diastolic pressure, which in turn conveys systemic vascular resistance. The pulse pressure, which relates to stroke volume, is also monitored.

Renal perfusion is monitored by hourly output.

The nurse therefore inserts a urinary catheter so accurate measurements can be obtained. Respiratory function is monitored either by a continuous pulse oximeter or transcutaneous oxygen and carbon dioxide monitors. The nurse also monitors the infant's or child's response to stimuli, level of alertness, and quality of cry as indicators of cerebral perfusion.

Once his or her condition is stabilized, the child is admitted to a pediatric ICU for further testing and treatment of the underlying disorder.

When the cause of shock is anaphylaxis, epinephrine (1:1000) 0.01 ml/kg (maximum dose of 0.4 mL) is administered subcutaneously. Immediate improvement often follows, but the child may experience the uncomfortable side effects of rapid heart beat and palpitations. The nurse informs the child and parents that these sensations and possible hyperactivity are related to the epinephrine and will subside.

Psychosocial Support and Parent Education

Shock, whatever its cause, is a terrifying experience for both parents and child. The nurse helps to reduce anxiety by listening attentively and calmly to parents and explains procedures and the child's response to the treatments. The nurse encourages parents to verbalize their questions, thoughts, and feelings. The parents should be allowed to remain with the child as much as possible. The nurse provides support by combining technical skills with tender compassion for the child and family.

If the child has experienced anaphylactic shock, the parents are encouraged to obtain a medical alert bracelet and information card for the child. When the antigen is related to insect stings, the parents and child may be provided with an anaphylaxis kit and instructions in its use. When food or medications are the offending agent, the child and parents are given careful instructions about avoiding these substances by reading labels and asking questions about ingredients.

CONGESTIVE HEART FAILURE

Congestive heart failure, like shock, is not a condition in and of itself but is the manifestation of an underlying disease. The etiologic factors responsible may be classified as those that cause (1) increased volume, (2) obstruction to outflow, (3) ineffective myocardial function, (4) dysrhythmias, or (5) excessive demand for cardiac output. In children, the most common cause of CHF is increased volume secondary to one of several congenital cardiac defects that result in altered hemodynamics and increased pulmonary blood flow. This redirection of blood to the pulmonary from the systemic circulation increases the workload of the heart as it attempts to supply a sufficient volume of oxygenated blood to meet the metabolic needs of the tissues.

Infants with undiagnosed cardiac disease may present in the ED with a history of decreased feeding, increased fatigue, poor weight gain, and tachypnea. This visit sets in motion the process that results in a diagnosis and treatment plan. At other times an infant or child with a known left-to-right shunt anomaly comes to the ED because of symptoms suggestive of exacerbation of CHF. In reality the symptoms may be caused by a respiratory tract or gastrointestinal illness or a combination of illness and failure. It is also possible that the child has outgrown the medication dosages, allowing failure to recur.

Etiology and Pathophysiology

As with shock, impending failure causes the body to initiate compensatory mechanisms that temporarily maintain adequate cardiac output and blood pressure. However, with every effort to improve myocardial contraction and blood flow to vital organs, there is a cost. At some point, these mechanisms are no longer effective, and the child presents with signs and symptoms of CHF.

Congestive heart failure originates from inadequate pumping action and therefore incomplete or insufficient emptying of either the left or the right ventricle. Because both sides ultimately work together, when one side fails, there is reciprocal failure of the other side. Ineffective pumping and decreased blood pressure stimulate the baroreceptors and vascular stretch receptors in the aorta and carotid arteries, which in turn trigger the compensatory mechanisms of the sympathetic nervous system. Sympathetic stimulation releases catecholamine and activates beta receptor sites to increase the rate and force of myocardial contractions. Venous tone also is increased by catecholamines, thereby enhancing blood return to the heart. At the same time circulation is redirected from the skin, viscera, extremities, and kidneys to maximize the blood flow to the heart, lungs, and brain. In addition, decreased renal perfusion instigates the release of renin, which activates angiotensinogen to produce angiotensin I, which is converted in the lungs to angiotensin II and III, which when they circulate, cause the adrenal cortex to release aldosterone, resulting in retention of sodium and water. The result of these compensatory actions are tachycardia, pallor, sweating, cool extremities, weak peripheral pulses, low urine output, and hypervolemia.

Mechanical changes also occur in response to the hypervolemia and consequent increased cardiac workload. The myocardium thickens and the fibers lengthen to accommodate increased volume and temporarily improve force of contraction. However, as muscle mass increases, compliance decreases and eventually the muscle either weakens and fails or outgrows its blood supply and suffers ischemia.

When elevated systemic resistance or inadequate contractility of the left ventricle prevents complete emptying during systole, end-diastolic pressure and volume increase. This impedes forward flow of blood and eventually causes fluid to leak from the capillaries into the interstitial spaces, resulting in pulmonary edema. Likewise, the hindrance of venous return secondary to elevated pulmonary pressures contributes to incomplete right ventricular emptying and end-diastolic pressure. This phenomenon in turn elevates right atrial pressure and systemic venous pressure, causing systemic congestion and edema.

Lesions that cause increased pulmonary pressure and blood flow primarily through large left-to-right shunts are associated with CHF during infancy. Although present at birth, these lesions do not become symptomatic for 6–8 weeks or until the pulmonary vascular resistance falls low enough to allow the shunting to occur and symptoms to develop. Associated murmurs do not appear until the infant is 2 weeks to 2 months of age (Flynn et al, 1992).

Other causes of CHF include acquired heart disease, such as rheumatic fever, myocarditis (Kawasaki disease), cardiomyopathy, pericarditis, endocarditis, and cor pulmonale from obstructive respiratory conditions. In addition, CHF may be present as part of the clinical manifestations of certain metabolic or endocrine states, such as electrolyte imbalance, hypoglycemia, severe or chronic anemia, and sepsis.

Assessment

History. The onset of CHF is insidious, and early signs and symptoms may be overlooked. The mother usually reports a normal pregnancy and that the infant was discharged from the hospital after delivery, normal and healthy. Critical data gathered by the nurse include the infant's growth, especially weight gain, feeding pattern, and sleeping pattern. An infant with CHF demonstrates poor weight gain, gradually increasing fatigue with feedings and decreased total intake, long naps, often having to be awakened for feedings, and the presence of diaphoresis on the forehead and nape of neck during sleep and feeding. The parents may or may not have observed rapid breathing on the part of the infant.

A child may have a history of increased fatigue, dyspnea on exertion, and orthopnea. The parent may have observed a gradual decrease in the child's energy and exercise tolerance and appetite over 2–3 weeks.

Not infrequently, the infant presents in the ED with signs and symptoms of a respiratory illness. The concurrent illness has increased the infant's fussiness and aggravated the other symptoms sufficiently to alarm the parents. This scenario also occurs with children with known cardiac disease. It is often difficult to decipher whether the presenting symptoms are evidence of illness or of cardiac decompensation. Of critical importance is the onset of symptoms. The child with a worsening cardiac status has demonstrated a gradual decline from baseline over 2 weeks, whereas a child with an illness has been in a stable condition until 2 days before the symptoms started.

Physical Assessment. The child generally is pale with cool, clammy skin. A striking feature of many infants with CHF is that although the respiratory rate is very rapid (60–100 breaths per minute), the infant does not appear distressed. This is evidence of the infant's precarious state of balance and ability to adapt to physiologic stress. It is important to observe for the presence and degree of other indicators of respiratory effort such as nasal flaring, intercostal and subcostal retractions, head bobbing, and expiratory grunting. An infant also compensates for this increased work of breathing by limiting involvement with the environment and engaging in few motor or energy-requiring activities. On auscultation, it is important to note that rales are almost never present in infants with CHF. Crepitant rales may be present in children older than 3 years during the early stages of failure; there may be an increased expiratory phase and wheezing in advanced pulmonary edema (Reece, 1984).

On inspection, there may be a hyperactive precordium and prominent precordial bulge of the left chest. A thrill may also be palpated. Tachycardia (150–180 beats per minute at rest) is always present. Sometimes it may be accompanied by a low-pitched third heart sound heard during early diastole. The presence of this sound during tachycardia causes a gallop rhythm. A murmur may be auscultated; its timing within the cardiac cycle is related to the specific lesion. In most cases the peripheral pulses are present but weak.

Temperature and blood pressure complete the assessment of vital signs. Temperature is a necessary piece of data in evaluating cardiac rate. Tachycardia in the absence of fever is more important and helps to focus the assessment. Blood pressure may be elevated or low depending on the defect. It is important in relation to the child's baseline state.

Additional findings vary. Some are age-related, and others depend on the cardiac disease. Older children, but never infants, may have distended jugular veins with right-sided failure. Edema from systemic venous congestion is manifested by infants and young children as periorbital and eyelid puffiness and occasionally as sacral edema and dorsal swelling of the feet and hands. Older children have ankle edema. Hepatomegaly may or may not be present depending on the stage of the illness; it is rare in early left-sided failure. The child also demonstrates failure to thrive, showing poor growth below the fifth percentile or evidence of regression from the initial percentile curve.

Laboratory and Diagnostic Tests. The most valuable diagnostic aid is a chest x ray. The presence of cardiomegaly is a critical piece of data that provides evidence of cardiac compensation. The appearance of hazy lung fields and increased vascular markings confirms the presence of pulmonary arterial or venous congestion, which often eludes conclusive findings in physical examinations of infants.

An echocardiogram provides additional data about the size of the ventricles and adequacy of function. The echocardiogram along with an electrocardiogram (ECG) helps determine the cause of the CHF. The ECG is not helpful in determining the presence of failure, but it does help in the treatment plan.

Laboratory tests may include a complete blood count (CBC), serum electrolyte measurement, and blood gas determination. A white blood count and differential rule out an infectious process; a low hematocrit level generally is attributable to hemodilution. Serum electrolyte concentrations are measured to determine baseline levels, which are low because of dilutional effects. In prolonged tissue hypoperfusion, metabolic acidosis may be evident.

TRIAGE
Congestive Heart Failure

Emergent

An infant or child with severe respiratory distress (rales, wheezing, severe intercostal retractions and markedly prolonged expiration, extreme pallor or cyanosis, and air hunger) from pulmonary congestion.

Urgent

An infant or child with moderate tachycardia, tachypnea, history of fatigue and diaphoresis with feedings, poor growth, hepatomegaly, and cardiomegaly.

Non-urgent

An infant with new murmurs but no tachycardia, tachypnea, or hepatomegaly.

Nursing Diagnosis
Decreased Cardiac Output

Defining Characteristics

- Fatigue
- Decreased peripheral pulses
- Tachycardia
- Gallop rhythm
- Color changes in skin and mucous membranes
- Cold, clammy skin
- Oliguria
- Tachypnea
- Diaphoresis
- Edema (periorbital in infant, extremity in older child)

- Jugular vein distention (older child)
- Orthopnea (older child)

Nursing Interventions

- Monitor cardiorespiratory status
- Place child in semi-Fowler position
- Monitor and interpret laboratory results
- Administer medication as ordered
- Measure and document output
- Monitor peripheral pulses and capillary refill
- Weigh child
- Prevent chilling
- Minimize stress and energy output from crying

Expected Outcomes

- Tissue perfusion improves
- Cardiorespiratory status stabilizes
- Urine output improves
- Child responds appropriately to medications.

Nursing Diagnosis
Ineffective Airway Clearance

Defining Characteristics

- Tachypnea
- Use of accessory muscles of respiration
- Changes in rate or depth of respiration
- Dyspnea
- Rales (older child)
- Hazy lung fields on x ray

Nursing Interventions

- Monitor respiratory status
- Place the child in a semi-Fowler position and change the position every 2 hours
- Administer humidified oxygen
- Perform chest physiotherapy
- Administer medications and monitor effect
- Monitor peripheral perfusion by pulse oximetry

Expected Outcomes

- Respiratory rate decreases.
- Respiratory effort decreases.
- Ventilation improves.
- Child has a positive response to medications.

Nursing Diagnosis
Fluid Volume Excess

Defining Characteristics

- Edema (periorbital in infant, extremity in child)
- Pulmonary congestion

- Shortness of breath
- Change in respiratory pattern
- Decreased hemoglobin and hematocrit levels
- Altered serum electrolyte levels
- Oliguria
- Weight gain

Nursing Interventions

- Monitor and document edema
- Measure intake and output
- Administer medications
- Note changes in laboratory values of electrolytes and hematocrit
- Monitor respiratory pattern

Expected Outcomes

- Output increases
- Edema decreases
- Respiratory pattern improves

Nursing Diagnosis

Fatigue

Defining Characteristics

- Inability to maintain usual routines
- Lack of interest in surroundings
- Decreased performance, especially during feeding
- Lethargy
- Verbalization of lack of energy

Nursing Interventions

- Modify procedures to decrease stress
- Monitor tolerance for activity (feeding)
- Provide undisturbed periods of rest
- Meet needs promptly to limit anxiety and crying

Expected Outcomes

- Infant's intake of formula increases
- Child's interest in environment improves
- General tolerance for activity increases
- Complaints of fatigue decrease

Management

The primary method of treatment of CHF is medication, namely a combination of digoxin to decrease the rate of contractions and to improve myocardial contractility and diuretics to reduce preload volume by preventing sodium and fluid retention and promoting diuresis, thus reducing the cardiac workload.

Often furosemide is the first medication administered. It is given intravenously at a dose of 1 mg/kg. There should be marked clinical improvement and di-uresis within 15–30 minutes. The nurse documents the child's response by measuring output and monitoring respiratory rate and effort and pulse. The infant or child will be more comfortable in a semi-Fowler position. If dyspnea is present, the patient may benefit from cool, humidified oxygen either by mask or blow-by while awaiting hospital admission.

Sometimes digitalization is initiated in the ED under the direction of a pediatric cardiologist. If the infant is in severe heart failure, loading doses are generally given intravenously and the infant's response is carefully monitored. An initial ECG is obtained for baseline comparison. The child is monitored continuously because changes in rhythm and PR interval are the most sensitive indicators of therapeutic effect versus toxicity. Sinus slowing and a prolonged PR interval are positive outcomes, whereas excessive sinus slowing, second-degree block, or a prolonged QRS complex are evidence of toxicity. The digitalizing dose for neonates is 0.02–0.03 mg/kg; for infants younger than 2 years, it is 0.02–0.04 mg/kg; and for children older than 2 years, it is 0.015–0.035 mg/kg. The first dose is 50% of the total calculated dose; the second one follows 6–8 hours later and is 25% of the total; the final 25% of the dose is give 6–8 hours after the second dose. Thereafter the child is maintained on a dose 25–35% of the total digitalizing dose; the maintenance dose is given orally in two divided doses. When an infant is in mild congestive heart failure, the loading dose may be omitted and the oral maintenance dose started.

The nurse needs to monitor serum electrolyte concentrations as the infant's body responds to the medications. With diuresis, the original hemodilution effects change and a more accurate electrolyte profile emerges. Potassium is the electrolyte most likely to be low. This is clinically significant because hypokalemia enhances the action of digoxin and may precipitate toxicity. Potassium replacement may be needed if urinary output is adequate.

In infants with severe distress and compromised cardiac output, rapidly acting catecholamines may be given in place of digoxin. These drugs include dopamine, isoproterenol, and dobutamine. The short duration of action of these drugs makes them preferable for CHF complicated by renal dysfunction.

Patient and Family Teaching and Psychosocial Support

The parents need much support during the process of diagnosis and decision making relative to a treatment plan. Sometimes, because the infant's condition has worsened gradually over time, the parents are not aware how distressed the infant has become and feel guilty that they did not seek treatment sooner. Some infants tolerate a certain degree of failure but become rapidly distressed when their function decreases even slightly. Children with known cardiac disease, who are well maintained with medication, may experience CHF when they have a fever secondary to an infection. The child and parents may question if they erred in the medication regimen, thereby contributing to the CHF.

It is frightening to parents to see their child in respiratory distress. Parents often state that they feel helpless, and they become angry when procedures are done that upset the child or precipitate crying. It is important to reduce parental anxiety because the parents' anxiety is often transferred to the child, who already feels vulnerable. Parents need information about procedures and tests as they apply to their child, and they need to have the freedom to ask questions and the reassurance that concerns will be addressed.

The ED is not the place to pass judgment, but rather to inform and support the family. It is important to explain the purpose and action of the medications the infant is given and to identify signs of improvement, no matter how minor. The nurse also seeks to allay the parents' anxiety by explaining procedures and suggesting ways in which the parents can assist in calming the infant, thus helping the parents feel useful and involved. If a child is older, the nurse uses appropriate play and diversional activity to explain the procedures to the child and to distract the child during stressful events. Children need to be reassured that everyone is trying to help them, not punish them. To assist school-aged children to gain some sense of control over the situation, the children can be involved in decisions, such as which arm to use for the blood test. They can also be given tasks, such as holding the gauze in place after blood is drawn.

Unless he or she has mild CHF, a child is admitted for further evaluation and adjustment of medications or for surgical intervention. The nurse prepares the family for hospital admission, answering questions and explaining the process. Children with mild failure are referred to a pediatric cardiologist for additional monitoring. If digoxin is prescribed, the nurse teaches the parents about the action, purpose, and side effects of the drug and how to measure the dose and administer it every 12 hours. It is important to emphasize the potential toxicity of digoxin, safe storage, and immediate reporting of any side effects.

ENDOCARDITIS

Children who have cardiac disease are at risk for infective endocarditis, an infection of the valves and endocardial lining of the heart. Those most at risk are children whose defect involves turbulent blood flow, such as mitral valve deformities, ventricular septal defects, aortic stenosis, patent ductus arteriosus, tetralogy of Fallot, and postoperative repairs involving prosthetic valves, conduits, or aortopulmonary shunts (Malinowski and Yablonski, 1986). In addition, valvular lesions from acquired cardiac disease such as rheumatic fever may be the site of infection in older children.

Knowledge about endocarditis is important for the ED staff for two reasons. First, a child may present with vague signs and symptoms that may be overlooked if the child's cardiac disease is unknown. Prompt diagnosis and treatment of endocarditis is vital to prevent damaging sequelae. Second, some of the diagnostic and injury-related procedures performed in the ED are of high risk for introducing bacteria and subsequent infection in children with cardiac disease (Table 14–2). Most of these children must receive adequate antibiotic prophylaxis to prevent infective endocarditis. There are some exceptions both pre and post surgical repair (Table 14–3).

Etiology and Pathophysiology

Although endocarditis affects children of all ages, it is found more frequently in children older than 10 years and rarely in infants younger than 2 years. The offending bacterium most commonly responsible is *Streptococcus viridans*. Eighty percent of the bacteria identified in cases of endocarditis are either *S. viridans* or *Staphylococcus aureus*, *S. aureus* presenting the greater risk for complications. The more virulent but much less common fungal organisms tend to invade neonates and immunologically compromised children (Kaplan and Schulman, 1989). The sources of these organisms vary and sometimes are never identified. In most cases, however, bacteria enter the bloodstream

TABLE 14–2. EMERGENCY DEPARTMENT PROCEDURES REQUIRING PROPHYLAXIS

Dental procedures with potential for bleeding
Minor surgical procedures such as biopsies, incision and drainage of infected site, wound debridement
Rigid bronchoscopy
Urethral catheterization when infection is suspected

TABLE 14–3. RECOMMENDATIONS FOR REQUIRED PROPHYLAXIS OF INFECTIVE ENDOCARDITIS

Most congenital cardiac anomalies, especially tetralogy of Fallot and aortic or mitral valve anomalies
Postoperative systemic-to-pulmonary shunts
Prosthetic cardiac valves
Hypertrophic cardiomyopathy
Previous diagnosis of infective endocarditis

secondary to another event, for example, dental work, invasive procedures such as urethral catheterization or prolonged intravenous infusions, incision and drainage of infected tissue, or surgical procedures.

The continuous turbulent blood flow from the cardiac defect erodes the endocardial or intimal lining while depositing platelets and fibrin and allowing thrombi to form. Bacteria that are already in the blood stream become entrapped in the fibrin network, multiply, and may form vegetative growth on the valves or invade the conduction system. The colonies of bacteria become encased in this fibrin network, preventing destruction by phagocytosis or circulating antibodies. Vegetation growing on the valves interferes with complete closure, causing regurgitation and producing a high risk for CHF. The vegetation also is friable; fragments can break off and be carried by either pulmonary or systemic circulation and lodge in other organs as emboli. These emboli block local circulation, causing pulmonary infarctions if the infected area is on the right side; on the left side they cause neurologic, renal, splenic, or extremity dysfunction or arthralgia.

Assessment

History. A careful review of the child's past provides the key to diagnosis. First, the child's cardiac history must be defined. Second, any recent illnesses, injuries, or procedures must be identified, and it must be determined whether or not the child received adequate prophylaxis. Next, the presence and progression of the child's signs and symptoms are documented.

Endocarditis is a condition without specific clinical features. Most children do have fever, often low-grade but prolonged, and a new or changed heart murmur. Other vague complaints may include malaise, anorexia, weight loss, fatigue, or headache. Some children have additional symptoms that stem from the effects of microemboli. Therefore, some have pulmonary symptoms, such as dyspnea and cough, whereas others have musculoskeletal symptoms, such as arthralgia, or neurologic symptoms, such as headache, delirium, and coma.

Physical Assessment. The physical assessment includes documentation of vital signs, careful auscultation of heart sounds with a notation of any irregular beats, tachycardia, and the presence, type, and location of any murmurs. Breath sounds are auscultated to identify areas of decreased or absent air exchange caused by pulmonary infiltrates. The child's abdomen should be palpated for evidence of hepatomegaly or splenomegaly. A child's arms, legs, and mucous membranes should be examined for petechiae; an adolescent's hands should be checked for splinter hemorrhages under the nails.

In addition, any manifestation of embolic phenomena, such as acute chest, abdominal, or flank pain, paralysis, visual disturbance or sudden blindness, hematuria, or acute vascular insufficiency, must be thoroughly explored. The child also must be assessed for any evidence of right- or left-sided heart failure or both.

Children frequently have a less acute form of endocarditis, known as subacute bacterial endocarditis (SBE). The clinical signs and symptoms differ because the children are not acutely ill. They have a persistent low-grade fever, pallor, anorexia, fatigue, and generalized weakness. The vagueness of these symptoms makes diagnosis difficult. Whenever cardiac disease exists, however, SBE must be suspected until proved otherwise.

Laboratory and Diagnostic Tests. The most important laboratory tests for endocarditis are blood cultures. At least two, and preferably three, sets of blood cultures are drawn before treatment is started. In 80–85% of the patients, the responsible organism is identified. Additional blood studies are a complete blood count (CBC) and erythrocyte sedimentation rate (ESR). The white blood count is elevated with a shift to the left, and the red blood count may be low, especially if symptoms have been present for a time. The ESR is elevated.

Urine is checked for hematuria, which if present may indicate renal microemboli provided there is no genitourinary tract infection. Urine and sputum cultures are done to rule out additional sites of infection.

The only other diagnostic test that offers any assistance is echocardiography. It can identify vegetative growth on the valves and the competency of valvular function.

T R I A G E
Endocarditis

Emergent ─────────────────────
A child with severe CHF (pulmonary congestion or marked hepatomegaly, edema, and visible jugular venous pressure). A child with high fever or severe pain from the effects of emboli.

Urgent ─────────────────────
A child who appears acutely ill with fever, chills, pallor, weight loss, petechiae, and a new or changing heart murmur.

Non-urgent ─────────────────────
A child with low-grade fever, anorexia, fatigue, and general lack of interest in activities.

Nursing Diagnosis
Decreased Cardiac Output

Defining Characteristics

- Dysrhythmias
- Fatigue
- Decreased peripheral pulses
- Tachycardia
- Color changes in skin and mucous membranes
- Tachypnea
- Diaphoresis
- Jugular vein distention (older child)
- Cough
- Weakness

Nursing Interventions

- Monitor cardiac rate and rhythm (prolonged PR interval and evidence of heart block)
- Monitor vital signs, including blood pressure and peripheral pulses
- Document type and location of murmurs and any changes
- Group procedures to allow periods of rest
- Explain and assist with diagnostic tests

Expected Outcomes

- Vital signs stabilize
- Child tolerates diagnostic testing

Nursing Diagnosis
Hyperthermia

Defining Characteristics

- Increase in body temperature above normal range
- Warm to touch
- Tachycardia

Nursing Interventions

- Monitor temperature
- Gather data relevant to contributory factors
- Explain and support child during venipunctures
- Assist with obtaining serial blood cultures (2–3 sets)
- Administer antipyretic agents as ordered
- Medicate with antibiotics *after* all blood work is drawn

Expected Outcomes

- Child's temperature returns to normal
- Child copes with venipunctures without undue stress
- Child is more comfortable

Nursing Diagnosis
Fatigue

Defining Characteristics

- Disinterest in activities, eating
- Lethargic or listless
- Verbalization of lack of energy
- Inability to maintain usual routines

Nursing Interventions

- Modify procedures to decrease stress
- Monitor tolerance for activity
- Provide undisturbed periods of rest

Expected Outcomes

- Child's interest in environment improves
- Child's general tolerance for activity increases
- Child's complaints of fatigue decrease

Nursing Diagnosis
Knowledge Deficit

Defining Characteristics

- Inaccurate follow-through of previous instruction
- Misinterpretation, misconception of information

Nursing Interventions

- Explain chronic aspects of cardiac lesion
- Discuss increased risk for infection
- Discuss purpose of prophylaxis
- Identify when and for what events prophylaxis is necessary
- Encourage verbalization of questions, concerns, misperceptions
- Discuss responsibility to inform other health care providers about need for prophylaxis
- Provide written material about prophylaxis of endocarditis

Expected Outcomes

- Parents and child verbalize knowledge about the purpose and necessity for prophylaxis
- Parents and child identify times when prophylaxis is needed
- Parents and child state that their questions and concerns have been addressed

Management
Initial treatment is oriented to the child's symptoms, such as CHF or pain from an embolic event. The child is positioned for comfort and ease in breathing. Medications such as diuretics and analgesics are administered. A peripheral intravenous line is inserted for

medication. Caution must be taken to ensure sterile technique during insertion of the intravenous line and giving of medications because the child already is at high risk for infection.

When a child has a fever of unknown origin, blood cultures are drawn to determine whether or not bacteremia is present. This is especially true if the child has a known cardiac defect. The first set of blood cultures is drawn in the ED and the remainder after the child is admitted to the hospital. The nurse prepares the child and family for the procedure, explains the rationale for serial cultures, and supports the child during the procedure. After the cultures have been drawn, parenteral antibiotic therapy consisting of some form of penicillin and an aminoglycoside is instituted and continued for 4–6 or even 8 weeks, depending on the organism. Once the organism is identified, antibiotic therapy may need to be adjusted.

When a prosthetic valve or conduit is the site of infected vegetation, surgical removal often is necessary. Surgical intervention may be necessary for worsening CHF unresponsive to medications, for recurrent septic emboli, or for progressive cardiac damage.

Of equal importance for the ED staff is providing prophylaxis to a child with known cardiac disease before diagnostic or treatment procedures are performed for an unrelated illness or injury. Prophylactic treatment is especially important before dental procedures that involve bleeding and before minor operations. According to the American Heart Association (AHA), antibiotic prophylaxis for children at risk entails medication a half hour to an hour before the procedure and 6 hours after the first dose (Table 14–4).

Patient and Family Teaching and Psychosocial Support

Parents and children often experience a variety of emotions in response to infective endocarditis. Initially, there is the uncertainty and anxiety associated with vague, inconclusive symptoms. Early symptoms resemble those of minor viral or bacterial illnesses and

TABLE 14–4. ANTIBIOTIC RECOMMENDATIONS FOR PROPHYLAXIS OF ENDOCARDITIS[a]

■ FOR DENTAL, ORAL, OR UPPER RESPIRATORY TRACT PROCEDURES	
Amoxicillin	50 mg/kg (3 g) po 1 hour before procedure
	25 mg/kg (1.5 g) po 6 hours after first dose
(if unable to take oral medications)	
Ampicillin	50 mg/kg (2 g) IV 30 minutes before procedures
	25 mg/kg (1 g) IV 6 hours after first dose
■ FOR PATIENTS ALLERGIC TO PENICILLIN	
Erythromycin	20 mg/kg (800 mg) po 2 hours before procedure
	10 mg/kg (400 mg) po 6 hours after first dose
or	
Clindamycin	10 mg/kg (300 mg) po 1 hour before procedure
	5 mg/kg (150 mg) po 6 hours after first dose
(if unable to take oral medications)	
Clindamycin	10 mg/kg (300 mg) IV 30 minutes before procedure
	5 mg/kg (150 mg) IV 6 hours after first dose
or	
Vancomycin	20 mg/kg (1 g) IV over 1 hour, starting 1 hour before procedure
	No repeat dose needed
■ FOR GENITOURINARY AND GASTROINTESTINAL PROCEDURES	
Ampicillin	50 mg/kg (2 g) IV 30 minutes before procedure
and	
Gentamycin	2 mg/kg (80 mg) IV 30 minutes before procedure
then	
Amoxicillin	50 mg/kg (1.5 g) po 6 hours after first dose
■ FOR PATIENTS ALLERGIC TO PENICILLIN	
Vancomycin	20 mg/kg IV over 1 hour, starting 1 hour before procedure
and	Repeat 8 hours after first dose
Gentamycin	2 mg/kg (80 mg) IV 1 hour before procedure
	Repeat 8 hours after first dose
■ ALTERNATIVE REGIMEN FOR PATIENTS CONSIDERED AT LOW RISK	
Amoxicillin	50 mg/kg (3 g) po 1 hour before procedure
	25 mg/kg (1.5 g) po 6 hours after first dose

[a]For pediatric patients. Maximum adult doses in parentheses.
(*From Flynn PA, Angle MA, Ehlers KH. [1992]. Cardiac issues in the pediatric emergency room. Pediatric Clinics of North America* 39:969)

are often treated by antibiotics. The symptoms are relieved temporarily but return once administration of the antibiotic is discontinued. Some children who become ill after cardiac surgery assume they are supposed to feel lethargic, fatigued, and anorexic. Being unaware that these feelings are not part of normal recovery, the parents do not seek medical attention but are discouraged by their child's slow response.

Once the diagnosis is made, the child and family must adjust to the length of treatment and, for some, the need for an operation. Families require a great deal of understanding as they cope with this complication. They need clear explanations as to why the child is at risk, what the condition entails, and how it is managed. They need time and encouragement to ask questions and express concern and even anger. The implications of the length of treatment must be addressed, especially for children in school because arrangements need to be made for a tutor.

For children whose condition is stable, who have not required surgical care, and who have no clinical manifestations of embolisms, the last 2–4 weeks of treatment may be carried out at home. Numerous home care agencies provide staff and equipment for home intravenous antibiotic therapy. This option has many advantages, but it requires thorough teaching and preparation of the family by the nurse.

The nurse must review with the family all aspects of prophylaxis of endocarditis. Children need to be taught good oral hygiene and infection prevention. They and their parents must be able to list the various signs and symptoms of infective endocarditis and the importance of seeking health care for even minor symptoms.

MYOCARDITIS

Most of the time when a child comes to the ED with chest pain, the cause is related to musculoskeletal trauma, pulmonary infections with or without cough, or even psychological stress. Cardiac causes are rare, accounting for only 5% of the total. These children are acutely ill, however, and for some the condition is life-threatening. Myocarditis is an inflammation of the myocardium that ranges from mild and often undiagnosed to severe, resulting in cardiac decompensation and sudden death in children. The causative agent can be any pathogen (bacteria, virus, fungus, parasite, protozoa), systemic infection (varicella, herpes zoster, hepatitis), infective endocarditis, or systemic disease (lupus erythematosis or polyarteritis nodosa). The most frequent causative agent is viral. It is rare for myocarditis to occur without a preceding illness.

Etiology and Pathophysiology

Inflammation of the myocardium interferes with the normal function of the myocardium at both the cellular and the structural level. The myocardium becomes edematous, soft, flabby, and pale with patches of necrosis (Park, 1988). In addition, the body responds to inflammation by infiltrating the area with leukocytes and available antigen-antibody complexes. Over time, the necrotic muscle area is absorbed and replaced by scar tissue. Children with a mild, acute episode recover completely with no sequelae. Some children have chronic myocarditis with persistent cardiomegaly with or without progressive atrioventricular (AV) valve insufficiency, ventricular dysfunction, and CHF. A few previously healthy children experience dramatic decompensation that occurs so rapidly it results in sudden death.

Assessment

History. Children with myocarditis do not have any prior cardiac condition. They do have a history of an upper respiratory infection or flu-like symptoms. Some have a recent or concurrent communicable illness or systemic condition such as rheumatic fever. Children with mild, chronic myocarditis may have no symptoms or have a gradual accumulation of vague, minor symptoms. Others, especially infants, may have an acute onset of vomiting, fever, myocardial dysfunction, poor systemic perfusion, or shock.

Physical Assessment. Physical signs and symptoms may range from a cough, malaise, fatigue, and myalgias through tachypnea, dyspnea, and chest pain without any evidence of pneumonia to palpitations, tachycardia, a gallop rhythm, and a new, systolic murmur. Congestive heart failure may be present, as may hepatomegaly and cardiomegaly.

Myocarditis should be considered whenever a previously healthy child presents with tachycardia out of proportion to the fever. This is especially true if there also is an irregular rhythm or pericardial friction rub.

Laboratory and Diagnostic Tests. The diagnosis is made on the basis of the findings of the ECG, chest x ray, and echocardiogram. The chest x ray may range from normal to showing varying degrees of cardiomegaly and, in severe cases, pulmonary edema. The ECG typically shows a low-voltage QRS complex, ST depressions, and flat or inverted T waves as well as irregular rhythms, such as premature atrial or ventricular contractions. The echocardiogram provides information about the size of the cardiac chambers and myocardial contractility; thus information aids in the evaluation of ventricular function. The results of these diagnostic tests also serve as baseline data.

TRIAGE
Myocarditis

Emergent
An infant or child with cardiac decompensation, signs of severe CHF, or shock.

Urgent
An infant or child with tachycardia, systolic murmur, irregular rhythm, cardiomegaly, or mild or no evidence of CHF.

Non-urgent
A child with mild, chronic myocarditis whose only symptoms may be fatigue, lethargy, anorexia, and myalgia.

Nursing Diagnosis
Decreased Cardiac Output

Defining Characteristics

- Dysrhythmia
- Dyspnea
- Fatigue
- Tachycardia, gallop rhythm
- Weakness
- Variations in blood pressure

Nursing Interventions

- Attach cardiac monitor, note rate, premature contractions, changes in ST segment or T waves
- Place child in semi-Fowler position
- Monitor vital signs
- Monitor for worsening of CHF
- Medicate with diuretics as prescribed and note effects
- Medicate with inotropic agents and monitor child's response
- Provide oxygen as symptoms indicate
- Encourage rest to conserve oxygen consumption
- Space procedures to provide uninterrupted rest in between

Expected Outcomes

- Child's cardiac and respiratory status stabilizes
- Child's cardiac output improves

Nursing Diagnosis
Anxiety

Defining Characteristics

- Apprehension
- Uncertainty
- Feeling scared
- Facial tension
- Restlessness
- Glancing about

Nursing Interventions

- Provide ongoing information during process of diagnosis
- Identify and address knowledge needs
- Identify ways to assist parents and child in coping with anxiety
- Encourage verbalization of concerns
- Involve parents in caregiving and comforting activities
- Reassure child and parents that everything is being done to help the child recover

Expected Outcomes

- Child and parents state that anxiety is under control
- Parents participate in care of their child
- Facial expressions relax

Management

The initial management of myocarditis depends on the degree of cardiac decompensation present. In infants and with severe forms, it is life-threatening. A pediatric cardiologist is consulted, and the child is hospitalized in a unit that provides telemetry and close observation. Treatment is directed at maximizing ventricular function and supporting the cardiovascular system. Aggressive measures are prescribed to reverse CHF and to increase cardiac output. These measures include intravenous administration of furosemide 1 mg/kg/dose every 4–6 hours and inotropic agents such as dopamine or isoproterenol. Digoxin is used with care because many children with myocarditis have an increased sensitivity to the drug, and signs of toxicity develop easily. Antidysrhythmic drugs are used cautiously because many of them decrease contractility, thus working against the other therapies. If rhythm-controlling drugs are needed, the child must be monitored closely, and any decrease in systemic perfusion must be reported immediately.

Of equal importance are bedrest and limitation of activity in an effort to reduce demands on cardiac output. Research with laboratory animals that had myocarditis showed that those that rested were more likely to recover, whereas those that engaged in strenuous activity usually died. The same phenomenon has been validated with military recruits (Denfield and Garson, 1990). Care must be supportive; the child's physical needs must be anticipated or met promptly.

Fever should be treated with antipyretics because fever increases oxygen demands and thus cardiac work. The underlying infection or systemic disease, if identified, is treated appropriately. Controversy surrounds the use of corticosteroids because these drugs suppress the child's immune system and ability to fight the original infection. If the myocardial inflammation however, is causing life-threatening dysrhythmias that are not responsive to medication, steroids may be tried.

Although most children recover completely, there are a few whose initial signs of cardiac dysfunction progress rapidly to complete cardiac decompensation and death. Myocarditis is a diagnosis that places the child at risk. The nurse must be alert and respond quickly to early signs of deterioration in the child's cardiac function. Subtle changes in the child's cardiac output indicating a fall in systemic pressure and loss of peripheral pulses demand immediate intervention, sometimes including overdrive pacing for malignant dysrhythmia or even cardiopulmonary resuscitation.

Patient and Family Teaching and Psychosocial Support

The initial diagnosis of acute myocarditis is frightening for all concerned. The child and parents require sensitive support and continual update of information. The parents need to know that the course for myocarditis is erratic and unpredictable, including the potential for sudden death.

To alleviate the feelings of frustration and helplessness, parents should be involved in the child's care whenever possible. Their presence and continuation of routine caregiving actions reduce the child's anxiety and promotes rest, which is an important component for recovery.

PERICARDITIS

Precordial pain ranging from dull, aching to sharp, stabbing and occasionally radiating to the left shoulder is characteristic of pericardial disease. This pain tends to worsen on inspiration or on lying flat but is decreased by sitting upright and leaning forward. A variety of conditions may be responsible for this inflammatory or infectious process, including viral, bacterial, autoimmune, postpericardiotomy syndrome, tu-

berculosis, a collagen vascular or renal disease, or a complication of oncologic disease or its therapy. Rarely does pericarditis present without prior infection, most commonly an upper respiratory infection.

Although the intensity of pain varies, a child with pericarditis demands careful assessment. Fluid accumulation has the potential to cause sudden cardiac decompensation, known as cardiac tamponade.

Etiology and Pathophysiology

Viral and autoimmune causes of pericarditis are probably the most common; with neither one does the child appear toxic. Bacterial causes are generally responsible for more fulminant disease and are more frequent in children younger than 2 years (Fleisher, 1985). Although less common since the advent of antibiotics, *S. aureus* and *Haemophilus influenzae* are two of the bacteria that invade the pericardium either by direct extension or by bronchial circulation because of pneumonia or a more distal focus of infection.

The invasion of a pathogen produces inflammation of the parietal and visceral layers of the pericardium resulting in fibrin deposition and accumulation of fluid or purulent exudate in the pericardial space. This fluid may be absorbed, but the rubbing of the inflamed layers produces a characteristic friction rub. The fluid also may accumulate so rapidly that there is clinically significant hemodynamic compromise from restricted ventricular filling. Two factors determine whether or not decompensation will occur: rapidity of fluid accumulation and competence of the myocardium. If the myocardium is not inflamed, it tolerates a slow increase of a large volume of fluid. If the myocardium is not intact, it is unable to expand to adapt to any increase in fluid and the condition quickly becomes symptomatic. Also, a slow increase in pericardial fluid allows compensatory responses to occur, whereas a rapid increase causes decreased cardiac output and a high risk for cardiac tamponade.

Assessment

History. The child most often either has or has had an upper respiratory infection; however, a remote bacterial infection or viral syndrome is also a possibility. For some children the significant event was an open heart operation 7–21 days before the development of signs and symptoms. A few children have a history of an autoimmune or collagen systemic condition as the probable responsible agent.

Fever of varying degrees is present; it is low grade except in bacterial pericarditis, in which it is high (39°C). The child indicates pain and, if old enough, is able to describe the classic precordial pain and position changes that worsen or alleviate it.

Physical Assessment. Some of the child's signs and symptoms are general while others are related to the causative factor. The general ones include a pericardial friction rub heard best at the left sternal border during held inspiration. (Pleural friction rubs are either muted or not heard during held inspiration.) On auscultation, the heart is hypodynamic and the sounds are somewhat decreased in the presence of pericardial effusion. Heart murmurs are absent unless the causative factor is rheumatic fever.

Additional signs and symptoms during assessment relate to the size of the effusion. As the effusion compromises cardiac function, tachycardia, tachypnea, and dyspnea appear and blood pressure decreases. Of importance is the appearance of a pulsus paradoxus 10 mm or greater, neck vein distention, muffled heart sounds, and the inability to lie flat. These signs may herald the onset of cardiac tamponade.

Laboratory and Diagnostic Tests. If the causative factor is viral, the white blood count is normal with increased lymphocytes; if the cause is bacterial, the white blood count is elevated with leukocytosis and a left shift in the differential. The ESR may be elevated. A chest x ray may be normal or show varying degrees of cardiomegaly depending on the size of the effusion.

The ECG findings include elevation of ST segments, and as effusion increases, the QRS voltage becomes diffusely decreased. An echocardiogram is the most useful diagnostic tool because both anterior and posterior effusions can be visualized.

TRIAGE
Pericarditis

Emergent ————————————————
A child with evidence of hemodynamic compromise as evidenced by tachycardia, dyspnea, neck vein distention, pulsus paradoxus, and decreased heart sounds. A child with suspected bacterial pericarditis who appears toxic, has grunting respirations, and a fever 39°C or greater.

Urgent ————————————————
A child who has precordial chest pain, pericardial friction rub, and a low-grade fever.

Nursing Diagnosis
Pain

Defining Characteristics
- Guarding behavior, refusal to lie down
- Communication of pain
- Distraction behavior—crying, restlessness

Nursing Interventions
- Place child in position of comfort
- Provide distraction and reassurance
- Administer medications—nonsteroidal anti-inflammatory medications and antibiotics if infection is bacterial
- Explain cause of pain and treatment plan to alleviate it

Expected Outcomes
- Child states that pain is less
- Child responds to therapy with evidence of decreased inflammation and effusion

Nursing Diagnosis
Decreased Cardiac Output

Defining Characteristics
- Variations in blood pressure
- Jugular vein distention
- Tachycardia
- Dyspnea
- Restlessness
- Decreased peripheral pulses

Nursing Interventions
- Monitor cardiovascular status
- Monitor respiratory status
- Have child maintain Fowler or semi-Fowler position
- Provide blow-by oxygen as indicated
- Maintain bedrest
- Group procedures to facilitate uninterrupted rest
- Provide calm reassurance to promote relaxation and rest

Expected Outcomes
- Child's cardiopulmonary status stabilizes
- Child cooperates with bedrest
- Child sleeps or rests quietly during designated quiet times
- Child appears relaxed and comfortable

Management
The treatment plan depends on the type and severity of symptoms. Most children have viral or idiopathic peri-

carditis, which is relatively benign and self-limiting. Nursing care is directed at comfort measures for pain and reassurance concerning outcome. Nonsteroidal anti-inflammatory medications such as aspirin and indomethacin are given to relieve the inflammation. Bedrest is critical and may be required for several weeks. Healing is verified by laboratory tests that indicate no further evidence of inflammation. In rare cases, steroids, although controversial because of their rebound effect, may be tried.

A child with postpericardotomy also requires symptomatic treatment and supportive nursing care with bedrest, analgesia, prophylactic antibiotics because of the recent operation, antipyretic agents for elevated temperature, and distraction. If there is a pleural effusion, drainage through a chest tube may be needed. Unless the pericardial effusion is large and cardiac function is threatened, conservative treatment is given. If cardiac tamponade is imminent, emergency pericardiocentesis is done. For most children, however, the pericarditis is self-limiting, lasting about 2–3 weeks with no further sequelae.

When bacteria are the causative agent, the child's condition is toxic and at risk for hemodynamic compromise from advancing pericardial effusion secondary to the pericarditis. In addition to the preceding treatment plan, these children require 4–6 weeks of intravenous antibiotic therapy; if the effusion is large, they may need subsequent pericardiocentesis. Initial pericardiocentesis is done to identify the responsible bacteria and appropriate antimicrobial agents. It is best for pericardiocentesis to be done by a cardiothoracic surgeon, either in an ICU with sophisticated monitoring capabilities or under fluoroscopy in the cardiac catheterization laboratory. There are many risk factors associated with the procedure, including myocardial puncture, pneumothorax, and ventricular fibrillation.

Patient and Family Teaching and Psychosocial Support

The child and family must be prepared for hospital admission and diagnostic procedures. The more thoroughly the family's questions are answered and their concerns addressed, the better they can cope with these procedures. It is important to explain events simply and slowly because the family feels stress because of the diagnosis and its implications. For many, this is the first time that they have encountered a problem involving the child's heart, so there is added fear and dread about the meaning of the diagnosis and potential future effects.

It is important to inform the family that close monitoring of the child is routine and does not imply that the child's condition is deteriorating. Many parents and older children appreciate knowing the purpose and information obtained from the monitoring equipment. It is also helpful to prepare them initially for a long hospitalization. Even in viral pericarditis, it often takes a week or longer for the inflammation to subside. When long-term intravenous antibiotic therapy is necessary, it may be completed at home for selected children and families.

PERICARDIAL TAMPONADE

Pericardial tamponade is the complication of fulminant pericarditis. It also may be caused by thoracic operations or traumatic chest injuries in which blood invades the pericardial space. Whatever the cause, the effect is the same, namely, rapid and profound cardiac decompensation requiring emergency intervention.

Etiology and Pathophysiology

Rapid accumulation of blood or fluid within the pericardial space increases the pericardial pressure. This increased pressure interferes with the diastolic expansion and filling of the heart, resulting in decreased cardiac output. There is a subsequent fall in blood pressure with a narrow pulse pressure. With restricted ventricular inflow, there is limited outflow, and the child quickly manifests early signs of hypoxia, such as restlessness. Atrial pressure becomes elevated and is evidenced in distended neck veins. Heart sounds are muffled because the pericardial fluid interferes with conduction of sound. During inspiration, fluid in the pericardium compresses the heart further. This phenomenon causes a sharp reduction in cardiac output and is demonstrated by pulsus paradoxus of 10 mm or more. In an effort to compensate for these effects, the heart rate increases (tachycardia) and peripheral vasoconstriction occurs.

Assessment

History. The child's history is obtained quickly with a focus on any prior flu-like or respiratory illness, thoracic operation, or trauma. Any family history of tuberculosis also is noted. Of most importance is a description of the onset, timing, and intensity of signs and symptoms before arrival in the ED.

Physical Assessment. The child appears acutely ill, tachypneic, and in a shock-like state. Initial vital signs serve as a baseline and often reflect the compensatory effort of tachycardia plus hypotension and a narrow pulse pressure. In addition to a rapid rate, there may be increased respiratory effort and diminished breath sounds. Other evidence of decreased cardiac output may include engorged jugular veins; an enlarged liver; cool, pale, clammy and even mottled skin; weak peripheral pulses; and restlessness, irritability, or lethargy.

It is important to remember that in a young child, it is very difficult to evaluate the jugular veins because of the shorter neck. Likewise, pulsus paradoxus is almost impossible to evaluate for a young child, especially if hypotension already exists.

The child's heart sounds and rate are monitored for change. A previously heard friction rub that disappears as the condition becomes more symptomatic is a sign that the effusion is increasing in size. Heart sounds that become more muffled or distant-sounding also may indicate increasing effusion. A decrease in the child's heart rate may mean impending arrest; intervention to relieve the intrapericardial pressure is needed immediately.

Laboratory and Diagnostic Tests. Often there is little time for diagnostic tests. The diagnosis is based on clinical judgment, history, and presenting signs and symptoms. Echocardiography detects the presence and location of the effusion. The cardiac monitor confirms tachycardia and may reveal some abnormality in the ST segments.

T R I A G E
Pericardial Tamponade

Emergent

A child with signs and symptoms of decreased cardiac output, tachycardia, and faint heart sounds. Hypotension and bradycardia are especially ominous signs.

Nursing Diagnosis
Decreased Cardiac Output

Defining Characteristics

- Variations in blood pressure, hypotension
- Jugular vein distention
- Decreased peripheral pulses
- Rhythm changes—tachycardia changing to bradycardia
- Cold, clammy skin
- Dyspnea
- Change in mental status

Nursing Interventions

- Monitor vital signs closely
- Attach cardiac monitor leads to child
- Monitor cardiac output
- Place child in semi-Fowler position
- Prepare child for diagnostic and therapeutic procedures
- Assist with insertion of intravenous line
- Assist with pericardiocentesis

Expected Outcomes

- Child tolerates procedures
- Child's cardiac output improves

Management
Pericardial tamponade is a true cardiac emergency that requires skilled, immediate intervention to restore cardiac output (Figure 14–3). The ED personnel must be sensitive to signs that indicate even minor changes in cardiac function, which may become life-threatening.

An intravenous line is started immediately to administer fluids if hypovolemia is present because of blood loss from trauma or a surgical procedure. Fluids are also given to oppose intrapericardial pressure and promote more effective ventricular filling. The intravenous line also provides an access site for emergency administration of medications. Although it is an inotropic agent, digoxin is not given because it slows the heart and would work against the body's compensatory mechanism against pericardial tamponade.

A child with obvious cardiac decompensation must undergo emergency pericardiocentesis and not wait for transfer to the ideal situation. The nurse prepares the child and parents for the procedure by explaining in age-appropriate terms what is to be done and why it is necessary. Emphasis is placed on the goal of helping the child feel better and breathe more easily, and to ease the pain. The child is then positioned supine with the head of the bed at a 45° angle.

Throughout the procedure, the nurse monitors the child's vital signs and overall condition while providing emotional support. Emergency equipment, including a defibrillator, is at hand. After the procedure, a chest x ray is done to assess for any evidence of pneumothorax or changes in the cardiac silhouette. The nurse continues to monitor the child closely for any evidence of dysrhythmia, recurrence of tamponade, or other complications.

Patient and Family Teaching and Psychosocial Support
Because pericardial tamponade is an emergency, assessment and intervention are often occurring at the

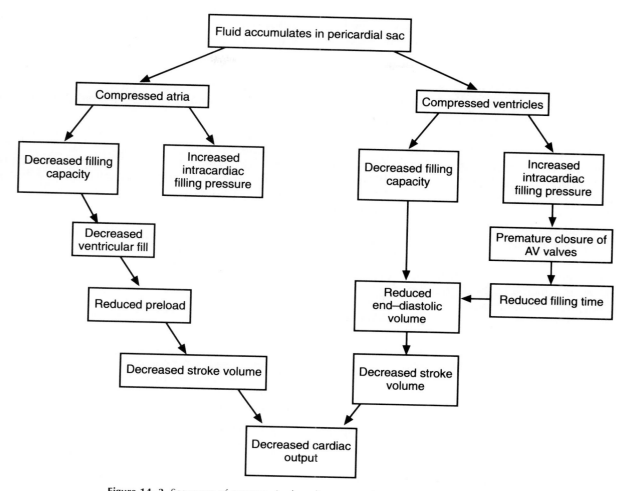

Figure 14–3. Sequence of compromised cardiac output during pericardial tamponade.

same time, which can be anxiety-producing for the child and parents. It is important that the nurse remember to offer explanations and to answer questions. It is essential for the nurse to remain calm and to provide supportive reassurance to the child and family.

After pericardiocentesis, the child is admitted for observation and further treatment as indicated. It is important to spend time with the child and family and to help them verbalize through words or play their fears and feelings during the emergency situation. This enables the nurse to clarify any misperceptions and for the family members to work through their fears. The sudden invasive procedures have the potential to stimulate fears about needles, pain, doctors, and death. It is most helpful to identify and deal with those fears immediately so they can be resolved and not interfere with health care needs in the future.

HYPERTROPHIC CARDIOMYOPATHY

Hypertrophic cardiomyopathy is a primary cardiac disease that involves the heart muscle itself. It is one of the conditions that accounts for the sudden death of children older than 1 year. Premature sudden death shows a predilection for adolescence and young adults. It is believed to have both familial and nonfamilial forms and a myriad of patterns of distribution of left ventricular hypertrophy and mitral valve morphology. Diagnosis requires a high degree of suspicion because physical findings are variable. Often the child or adolescent enters the ED because of exercise-induced chest pain, dizziness, or dyspnea.

Etiology and Pathophysiology
The muscular hypertrophy that occurs within the left ventricle causes abnormal stiffness and impaired fill-

ing. In addition, this massive hypertrophy of the left ventricle, particularly the interventricular septum, causes a potential outflow tract obstruction. This condition was formerly identified as idiopathic hypertrophic subaortic stenosis (IHSS) or muscular subaortic stenosis because the hypertrophied interventricular septum dramatically narrows the outflow tract. In some children the actual obstruction occurs late in systole as an anterior motion of the mitral valve causes the valve and the septum to meet. This obstruction is variable and occurs after 80% of the stroke volume has been ejected (Park, 1988).

The degree of obstruction is variable and is constantly influenced by the left ventricular systolic volume. Any factor, such as positive inotropic agents (digoxin), vasodilators, reduced blood volume, or decreased systemic vascular resistance, that reduces the systolic volume increases the obstruction. On the other hand, negative inotropic agents such as propanolol, calcium channel blockers, raising the legs, blood transfusion, or increased systemic vascular resistance increase the left ventricular systolic volume and decrease the obstruction (Panza et al, 1990).

Assessment

History. The familial history is extremely important because hypertrophic cardiomyopathy is an autosomal dominant condition; about a third of the time, there is a positive family history. Although they may appear at any age, symptoms are rare during infancy and early childhood. Clinically significant data are any prior complaint of palpitation, anginal pain, syncope, or fatigue with exercise.

Physical Assessment. The physical examination often reveals a normal S_2 and a late systolic ejection murmur along the left sternal border or at the apex. There may be a sharp upstroke of the arterial pulse that marks the stroke volume ejected before obstruction. Of interest is that the presence and intensity of the murmur varies from examination to examination. Peripheral pulses usually are prominent and the precordium is hyperdynamic.

Laboratory and Diagnostic Tests. The ECG is abnormal; it demonstrates left ventricular hypertrophy, ST-T changes, left atrial enlargement, and deep Q waves with diminished or absent R waves in the lateral precordial leads. A chest x ray depicts a globular-shaped heart with left ventricular enlargement. The echocardiogram is diagnostic and reveals asymmetric septal hypertrophy of the interventricular septum.

T R I A G E
Hypertrophic Cardiomyopathy

Emergent —————————————————
A child with any evidence of dysrhythmias, especially ventricular.

Urgent —————————————————
A child who has had an episode of exercise-induced chest pain or dyspnea and has a systolic ejection murmur.

Nursing Diagnosis
Anxiety

Defining Characteristics

- Verbalization of apprehension, uncertainty, fear
- Concern about change in life events
- Increased wariness, concern for own life

Nursing Interventions

- Explain symptoms and their meaning
- Offer support and encourage questions
- Discuss necessary changes in activities
- Refer to support group

Expected Outcomes

- Child and parent verbalize acceptance of change in life events
- Child and parents verbalize ability to cope with anxiety

Nursing Diagnosis
High Risk for Activity Intolerance

Defining Characteristics

- Presence of circulatory problems
- History of previous intolerance to activity

Nursing Interventions

- Discuss implications of diagnosis
- Discuss necessity of restricting physical activity
- Suggest alternative activities and hobbies
- Administer medications and monitor effect

Expected Outcomes

- Child modifies activity
- Child and parents verbalize action, purpose, and importance of medications

Management

Management consists primarily of medication and a change in lifestyle. Because most sudden deaths occur during strenuous activity, it is important to restrict such activity. A beta-adrenergic blocker (propranolol) is usually prescribed to reduce the extent of outflow tract obstruction and to control dysrhythmias. In addition, calcium channel blockers such as verapamil may help to improve diastolic filling.

Once a child receives the diagnosis of hypertrophic cardiomyopathy, all family members should have a thorough diagnostic evaluation for the condition. Early identification and referral of any child with exercise-induced symptoms may reduce the incidence of sudden death.

Patient and Family Teaching and Psychosocial Support

The role of the nurse is teaching lifestyle changes and supporting the child and family during initial acceptance and transition. The nurse also teaches the child and family about the medications and their importance, even when the child is feeling well. Although infective endocarditis is rare, prophylaxis is indicated. The nurse provides the child and family with information and written material relative to events and standard medication regimens for the prophylaxis of endocarditis.

The diagnosis carries much potential for guilt and fear for the child's life. There could be the tendency on the part of parents to be overly protective and restrictive of the child's activities. It is important to address these issues with the parents and openly discuss what are and what are not appropriate activities. Growth and developmental issues also play a role because many of these children do not demonstrate symptoms until late childhood or adolescence. Both child and parents need support and counseling as they struggle to adapt to the many lifestyle changes that the diagnosis demands.

REFERENCES

Denfield SW, Garson A (1990). Sudden death in children and young adults. *Pediatric Clinics of North America* 37:215–231

Driscoll DJ (1990). Evaluation of the cyanotic newborn. *Pediatric Clinics of North America* 37:1–23

Fleisher G (1985). Life-threatening infections. In Ludwig S (ed), *Pediatric Emergencies*. New York: Churchill Livingstone, pp 45–78

Flynn PA, Engle MA, Ehlers KH (1992). Cardiac issues in the pediatric emergency room. *Pediatric Clinics of North America* 39:955–986

Hazinski MF (1992). Cardiovascular disorders. In Hazinski MF (ed), *Nursing Care of the Critically Ill Child* (2nd ed). St. Louis: Mosby Year Book, pp 117–394

Kaplan EL, Schulman SR (1989). Bacterial endocarditis. In Adams FH, Emmanouilides GC, Riemenschneider TA (eds), *Moss' Heart Disease in Infants, Children, and Adolescents* (4th ed). Baltimore: Williams & Wilkins, pp 565–574

Kitt S, Kaiser J (1990). *Emergency Nursing: A Physiologic and Clinical Perspective*. Philadelphia, Saunders, pp 523–544

Malinowski P, Yablonski C (1986). Congenital heart disease in infants: Nursing assessment. *Critical Care Quarterly* 9:6–23

Panza JA, Maris TJ, Maron BJ (1990). Morphologic determinants of the development of subaortic obstruction in hypertrophic cardiomyopathy during childhood. *Circulation* 82 (Suppl 3):25–59

Park MK (1988). *Pediatric Cardiology for Practitioners* (2nd ed). Chicago: Year Book, pp 108–109; 217–224; 226–232; 309–317

Reece RM (1984). *Manual of Emergency Pediatrics* (3rd ed). Philadelphia: Saunders, pp 12–13; 66–72; 305–307; 409–411; 501–505

Rice V (1991a). Shock, a clinical syndrome: An update. Part 2. The stages of shock. *Critical Care Nurse* 11:74–85

Rice V (1991b). Shock, a clinical syndrome: An update. Part 4. Nursing care of the shock patient. *Critical Care Nurse* 11:28–43

Rimar JM (1988a). Recognizing shock syndromes in infants and children. *American Journal of Maternal/Child Nursing* 13:32–37

Rimar JM (1988b). Shock in infants and children: Assessment and treatment. *American Journal of Maternal/Child Nursing* 13:98–105

Shaddy RF, Viney J, Judd VE (1989). Continuous intravenous phenylephrine infusion for treatment of hypoxemic spells in tetralogy of Fallot. *Journal of Pediatrics* 114:468–469

CHAPTER 15

Cardiac Dysrhythmias

MARTHA A.Q. CURLEY

INTRODUCTION

Improved survival rates among critically ill children and widespread monitoring have heightened nurses' awareness of cardiac dysrhythmias in the pediatric population. The role of the emergency department (ED) nurse in caring for pediatric patients with a cardiac dysrhythmia is multifaceted. The nurse is responsible for identifying pediatric patients at risk for cardiac dysrhythmias, correctly identifying the dysrhythmia using maturational dependent norms, assessing the hemodynamic effect of the dysrhythmia, assisting in the initiation and evaluation of treatment, and for providing child and family education.

Unlike for adults, normal parameters of pediatric rhythm strips vary according to the patient's level of maturation. Also, cardiac dysrhythmias are seldom primary events in the pediatric population. Most often, cardiac dysrhythmias occur secondary to an abnormal quality, not quantity, of coronary artery blood flow. This necessitates a change in the focus of the ED nurse because both of these factors—maturation and patent coronary arteries—must be considered whenever assessing a pediatric rhythm strip for normalcy, dysrhythmias, electrolyte imbalance, and drug effects.

CLINICAL SIGNIFICANCE OF DYSRHYTHMIAS

As for adults, the risks posed by cardiac dysrhythmias in the pediatric population include further deterioration in cardiac rhythm and decreased cardiac output. Figure 15–1 shows the rapid deterioration in cardiac rhythm that occurred in a 9-month-old infant. This

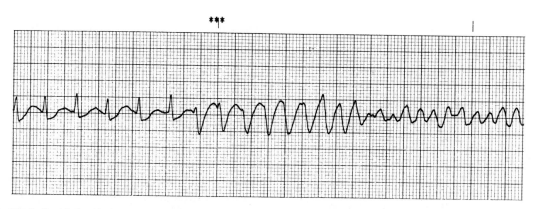

Figure 15–1. Rapid electrical compromise in a 9-month-old infant. Supraventricular tachycardia to ventricular tachycardia to ventricular fibrillation.

rhythm strip illustrates the equable lethality and high risk for rapid electrical compromise in a pediatric patient.

The risk of dysrhythmia-related, decreased cardiac output is high in the pediatric population. Cardiac output is the product of stroke volume multiplied by the heart rate. Stroke volume is determined by three factors: preload, afterload, and contractility. Preload is determined by ventricular end-diastolic pressure; the quantity of blood in the ventricle just before systole. Starling's law demonstrates the positive relation between contraction force and end-diastolic pressure or volume. Afterload refers to the resistance or impedance faced by the ventricle just before systole; contractility is the speed and efficiency of myocardial shortening independent of preload and afterload.

Like adults, young children and adolescents are capable of increasing stroke volume to maintain cardiac output when the heart rate decreases. (Cardiac output is maintained by an increase in stroke volume, ie, bradycardia increases diastolic filling time, thus increasing preload and the resultant contraction.) Infants younger than 6 months have relatively fixed stroke volumes, so their cardiac outputs depend almost entirely on their heart rate and rhythm. The limited capacity to increase stroke volume in this age group is related to decreased ventricular compliance. This phe-

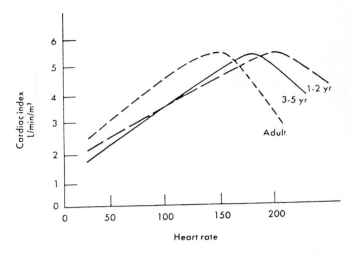

Figure 15–3. The impact of changes in heart rate on cardiac index in various age groups. (Reproduced with permission from Daily EK, Schroeder JS [1985]. *Techniques in Bedside Hemodynamic Monitoring.* St. Louis: Mosby, p 142)

nomenon can be attributed to the greater proportion of noncontractile myocardial tissue to contractile myocardial mass in infants (Zaritsky and Chernow, 1984). Ventricular compliance and stroke volume increase with growth and development (Figure 15–2). The child becomes less dependent on heart rate for cardiac index (Figure 15–3).

Although they are very much dependent on heart rate and rhythm, ironically infants are, at the same time, sympathetically immature. Infants have decreased sympathetic receptor density and responsiveness and thus are more sensitive to parasympathetic or vagal stimulation (Zaritsky and Chernow, 1984). Sympathetic stimulation provides a positive chronotropic, inotropic, and dromotropic (speed of impulse conduction) effect, whereas parasympathetic stimulation provides a negative chronotropic and dromotropic effect. For this reason procedures such as suctioning, obtaining rectal temperatures, and invasive procedures, that may induce vagal stimulation or valsalva induction are always to be performed with care in infants. Maturation of sympathetic innervation occurs with time, as noted by an improved response to catecholamine administration.

Etiology and Pathophysiology

Immaturity of the conduction system and its autonomic innervation are contributing factors in the pathogenesis of cardiac dysrhythmias in newborns and infants. Cardiac dysrhythmias are not infrequent in the first week of life. This phenomenon can be attributed to the numerous metabolic and functional alterations

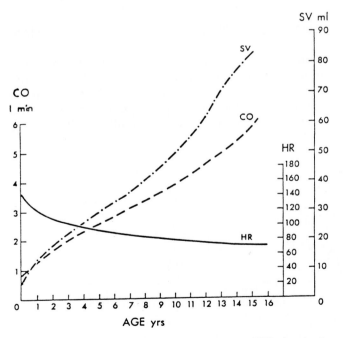

Figure 15–2. Postnatal changes in cardiac output (CO), heart rate (HR), and stroke volume (SV) from birth to 16 years. (Reproduced with permission from Rudolf AM [1974]. *Congenital Diseases of the Heart.* Chicago: Year Book, p 27)

taking place during the transition from intrauterine to extrauterine life. The parasympathetic dominance in this population also places newborns and infants at greater risk for vagally-induced dysrhythmias, such as sinus bradycardia, sinus arrest with junctional escape rhythms, first-degree heart block, and second-degree type 1 atrioventricular (AV) block.

Cardiac dysrhythmias occur more frequently in pediatric patients with structurally normal hearts. Cardiac dysrhythmias are *seldom* primary events but occur secondary to an abnormal quality of blood delivered to the myocardium and conduction system. Abnormalities may include an electrolyte imbalance, especially of potassium and calcium, hypoxia, hypercapnia, acidosis, which is the usual case during pediatric arrests, and alterations in temperature (both hyperthermia and hypothermia). Drug-related problems also may induce cardiac dysrhythmias in the pediatric population; these include digoxin toxicity, excessive use of beta-adrenergic blocking agents or catecholamines, and ingestion of toxins (both accidental or intentional).

Pediatric patients for whom cardiac dysrhythmias are a special risk are children who arrive at the ED after surgical repair of congenital heart defects. Surgical injury can alter impulse initiation and conduction around the site of the surgical repair. Bradycardias may occur after cardiac operations involving the atria, such as repair of an atrial septal defect or repair of an endocardial cushion defect. Ventricular dysrhythmias may be present in pediatric patients with ischemic or hypertrophied ventricles, such as those with aortic ste-

nosis or tetrology of Fallot; those who have had a right ventriculotomy; those who were older at the time of the cardiac operation; and especially in pediatric patients with residual intracardiac defects (Krongrad, 1984).

Cardiac dysrhythmias also may be the first indication that a problem exists. This is the case in acquired heart disease, such as myocarditis and myocardiopathy.

ASSESSMENT: NORMAL SINUS RHYTHM

Normal cardiac rhythm depends on repetitive impulse initiation at a single site in the heart, the sinoatrial (SA) node, and an orderly sequence of propagation and repolarization. Tremendous electrocardiographic changes occur during cardiac system maturation. It is imperative that normal maturational changes be considered when assessing a pediatric rhythm strip (Table 15–1). In addition, the patient's activity level, medication history, and possible positive cardiac history are also important.

In the assessment of a rhythm strip, a systematic approach is essential so that nothing is overlooked. Assessment includes the heart rate and rhythm, P wave, P:QRS relationship, PR interval, QRS duration, ST segment, T wave, QT_c interval, and U wave. To apply the following parameters, a standardized lead II rhythm strip is used. That is, the paper speed is 25 mm/second, and a 1-mv stimulus equals a 10-mm stylus deflection.

TABLE 15–1. PEDIATRIC NORMS

Age	Heart Rate Mean (Range) (per minute)	P Wave Height/Duration (mm/second)	Maximum PR Interval Heart Rate/Interval (per minute/second)	QRS Duration (seconds)	QT_c Interval (seconds)
0–24 hours	119 (94–145)	<3.0/0.6	<0.11	0.04–0.05	<0.45
1–7 days	133 (100–175)				
8–30 days	163 (115–190)				
1–3 months	154 (124–190)	<2.5/0.08	91–110 <0.14		
			111–130 <0.13		
			131–150 <0.12		
			>150 <0.11		
3–6 months	140 (111–179)				
6–9 months	140 (112–177)				
9–12 months			91–110 <0.15	0.05–0.06	
			111–150 <0.14		
			>150 <0.10		
1–3 years	126 (98–163)				<0.44
3–5 years	98 (65–132)			0.06–0.08	
5–8 years	96 (70–115)		<90 <0.18		
			>90 <0.16		
8–12 years	79 (55–107)			0.08–0.10	
12–16 years	75 (55–102)				<0.43

Heart Rate

The heart rate gradually increases during the first week to month of life, then gradually decreases throughout childhood (Table 15–1). Sinus tachycardia and sinus bradycardia are defined as heart rates above and below the norm for the child's age. Individual heart rates reflect the patient's cardiac output requirement. For example, a sinus tachycardia of 200 beats per minute is an expected finding in a febrile, hypovolemic, or crying 1-month-old, whereas a sinus bradycardia of 90 beats per minute is expected in an afebrile, normovolemic, sleeping infant. *Heart rates incongruent with clinical need require further assessment.*

The inherent rates of other pacemaker sites within the heart are, as with adults, slower than that of the sinus node but they also have maturation-dependent faster rates. These accessory pacemaker sites (atrial, junctional, and ventricular) are capable of producing faster escape and accelerated rhythms than seen in the adult population. Pediatric ectopic rhythms cannot be defined on the basis of heart rate alone.

Cardiac Rhythm

The cardiac rhythm is fairly regular. Sinus arrhythmia is common and considered normal because of the parasympathetic dominance experienced by this population. Clinically significant sinus arrhythmia, ie, a doubling of the R to R interval with expiration, is observed frequently in pediatric patients with increased intrathoracic or intracerebral pressures.

P Wave

The P wave is evaluated for configuration, amplitude, duration, and consistency. In pediatric patients the P wave duration is less than 0.08 second and 2.5 mm in height (0.06 second and 3 mm in neonates). The P wave is gently rounded and always consistent in configuration. Right and left atrial hypertrophy can be easily assessed from a standardized lead II rhythm strip. Right atrial hypertrophy may be present when the P wave is consistently taller than the norm, whereas left atrial hypertrophy may be present when the P wave duration is consistently wider than the norm.

P:QRS Relationship

The P:QRS relationship is always 1:1. Sinus node discharge produces atrial depolarization, the P wave, then ventricular depolarization, the QRS complex. All P waves occurring after a T wave should be followed by a QRS complex. If this is not the case, second- or third-degree heart block is suspected.

PR Interval

The PR interval varies according to the patient's age and heart rate (Table 15–1). Reflecting normal maturational vagal tone, a prolonged PR interval is not uncommon in the pediatric population. Prolonged PR intervals also result from ectopic supraventricular rhythms, digoxin effect, fever, myocarditis, and some congenital heart lesions, such as an endocardial cushion defect, Ebstein anomaly of the tricuspid valve, and L-transposition of the great arteries. Short PR intervals (less than 0.08 second to 3 years of age, 0.10 second from 3 to 16 years of age, and 0.12 in children older than 16 years) may be present with junctional rhythms, Wolff-Parkinson-White (WPW) syndrome, and tricuspid atresia.

QRS Duration

Correlating with ventricular mass, the QRS duration can be as short as 0.04 second in a premature infant, less than 0.06 second in infants, and 0.08 second in children (Figure 15–4). Anything wider *than the child's normal* QRS duration is associated with aberrant conduction, which may occur secondary to bundle branch block or premature ectopic contractions.

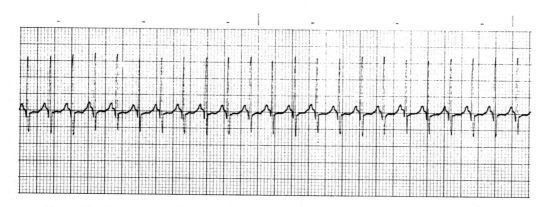

Figure 15–4. Sinus tachycardia in a 2-week-old infant. Note normal QRS duration of 0.04 second.

ST Segment
The ST segment is assessed from the j point, which is identified as the junction of the QRS complex and the ST segment. The ST segment may deviate 1 mm from the baseline and still be considered normal. The ST segment is abnormal if it is horizontal to or slopes downward from the j point. A digoxin effect commonly produces deviation of the ST segment opposite to that of the QRS complex, for example, elevation with negative QRS complexes and depression with positive QRS complexes. Deviation of the ST segment also may be associated with myocardial ischemia, inflammation, and severe hypertrophy. An extra deflection, the J wave, located at the QRS-ST junction is associated with severe accidental hypothermia.

T Wave
The T wave should be directed along the same plane as the QRS complex, that is, positive when the QRS complex is positive and negative when the QRS complex is negative. Deviations may be caused by primary repolarization abnormalities, such as myocarditis, or depolarization abnormalities, such as premature ventricular contractions (PVCs).

QT Interval
The QT interval varies according to heart rate, so a QT_c (a QT interval corrected for heart rate) is calculated in pediatric patients. The QT_c is calculated by dividing the square root of the R to R interval into the measured QT interval (Figure 15–5). The normal interval should not exceed 0.45 second in infants, 0.44 second in children, and 0.43 second thereafter. Calcium and magnesium levels alter the QT_c interval. High calcium or magnesium levels shorten the QT_c interval, whereas low calcium or magnesium levels prolong the

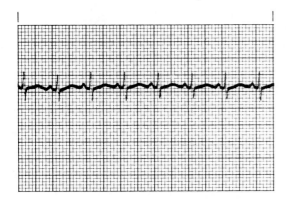

Figure 15–5. Calculation of the QT_c. The R-R interval measures 0.40 second; its square root is 0.632. The QT interval measures 0.28 second. The calculated QT_c is 0.443. (Reproduced with permission from Curley MAQ [1985]. *Pediatric Cardiac Dysrhythmias.* Bowie, Md: Brady Communications, p 158)

QT_c interval. Short QT_c intervals also occur in patients receiving digoxin. Prolonged QT_c intervals occur in patients on receiving quinidine and in those with genetically inherited prolonged QT interval syndrome (Weintraub et al, 1990).

U Waves
Occasionally U waves may be present. The genesis of these waves is thought to reflect delayed repolarization of the terminal Purkinje network. Prominent U waves may occur secondary to hypokalemia.

ASSESSMENT: RHYTHM STRIP

The lead II rhythm strip can be used as a rapid assessment tool to assist in the detection of electrolyte imbalance, toxic tricyclic overdose, and digoxin toxicity. Intracranial hypertension also produces many electrocardiographic changes, such as tall or notched T waves, U waves, or short then prolonged QT_c intervals. These alterations are ominous in that they may occur before neurologic deterioration and the occurrence of lethal ventricular dysrhythmias (Zegeer, 1984). Dysrhythmias pose risk for patients with cerebral hypertension because any dysrhythmia that alters the mean arterial pressure compromises cerebral perfusion pressure. (Cerebral perfusion pressure is a product of the mean arterial pressure minus the intracranial pressure.)

Electrolyte Imbalance
Whereas serum potassium and calcium levels may be misleading, a rhythm strip graphically represents the ionic movement of these two cations across the excitable cardiac cell membrane. Thus, the rhythm strip is a useful tool in the assessment of total body potassium and calcium concentration. Hyperkalemia initially produces tent-shaped T waves then progresses to wide QRS durations, increased PR intervals, broad P waves, atrial arrest, and eventually a sine-wave pattern representing QRS complex and T wave fusion (Figure 15–6). Hypokalemia produces depressed ST segments and flattened T waves and U waves. Hypercalcemia produces a short QT_c interval; the opposite is true with hypocalcemia.

Overdose of Tricyclic Drugs
A rhythm strip also provides more information about the pharmacologic effects of medications at the receptor level than do serum concentrations. Prolonged QRS durations (Figures 15–7 and 15–8) can serve as a guide to predict immediately the incidence of complications of an overdose of tricyclic drugs. These complications include seizures, ventricular dysrhythmias,

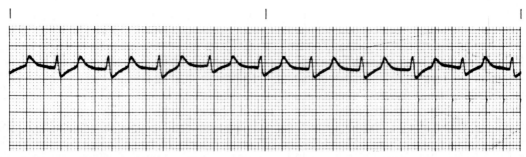

Figure 15–6. Hyperkalemic sine-wave pattern in a 3-year-old child. The serum potassium concentration was 10.0 mmol/L. (Reproduced with permission from Curley MAQ [1985]. *Pediatric Cardiac Dysrhythmias.* Bowie, Md: Brady Communications, p 153)

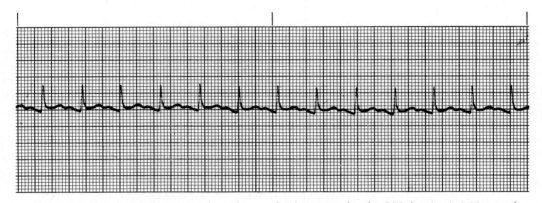

Figure 15–7. Ten hours after an overdose of a tricyclic drug. Note that the QRS duration is 0.08 second.

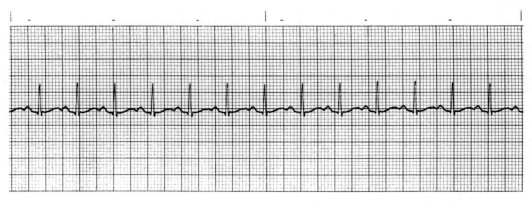

Figure 15–8. Eight hours after the rhythm strip in Figure 15–7 was obtained. Note that the QRS duration is 0.04 second.

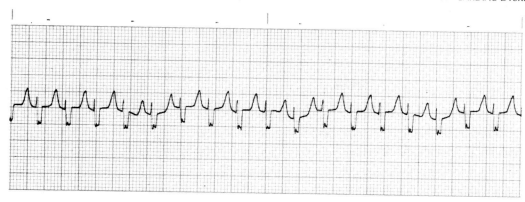

Figure 15–9. Digoxin toxicity in a 7-month-old infant. Junctional tachycardia. (Reproduced with permission from Curley MAQ [1985]. *Pediatric Cardiac Dysrhythmias.* Bowie, Md: Brady Communications, p 161)

and death (Boehnert and Lovejoy, 1985). A patient who comes to the ED with a prolonged QRS interval after ingesting tricyclic drugs is admitted to an intensive care unit (ICU).

Digoxin

Therapeutic digoxin levels are difficult to interpret in infants because of the wide therapeutic range observed in this population. Infants require higher doses of digoxin per kilogram of body weight, and individual levels may be considered toxic if assessed by adult standards. Peak serum digoxin levels of 0.8–2.2 ng/mL are considered normal, but 3.5 ng or higher may be required in selected infants before therapeutic effects are evident.

Inconclusive level assessment necessitates an accurate lead II rhythm assessment. The digoxin effect reflects the normal electrocardiographic changes produced by this drug and are not related to dose, therapeutic range, or toxicity. These changes are minor bradycardia, minor first-degree heart block, short QT_c interval, and ST segment deviation opposite to that of the QRS complex. Digoxin toxicity can be identified as clinically significant sinus bradycardia, ectopic supra-

ventricular activity, junctional tachycardia, AV blocks, and PVCs. Any dysrhythmia present after administration of digoxin is started may be related to digoxin toxicity (Figures 15–9, 15–10, 15–11, 15–12).

Before the administration of digoxin to a pediatric patient, a lead II rhythm strip is obtained and assessed for the presence of digoxin effect and toxicity. The rhythm strip, along with assessment of the patient's heart rate and, more important, cardiac rhythm is documented in the medical record for future reference.

The digoxin effect and toxicity are related to potassium ion concentration. Potassium and digoxin compete for myocardial cell-binding sites. Thus, an increased serum potassium level decreases the effect of digoxin, whereas a decreased serum potassium level increases the potential for digoxin toxicity. Premature infants and children with renal dysfunction have a decreased rate of digoxin excretion, so they are at increased risk for digoxin toxicity.

Symptomatic management of digoxin toxicity includes correcting electrolyte imbalances that enhance the digoxin effect (hypokalemia and hypercalcemia), temporary pacing for second- or third-degree heart block, and dilantin for ventricular ectopy (Walsh and

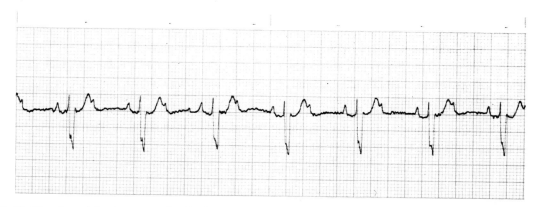

Figure 15–10. Digoxin toxicity in a 7-month-old infant—2:1 type II AV block. (Reproduced with permission from Curley MAQ [1985]. *Pediatric Cardiac Dysrhythmias.* Bowie, Md: Brady Communications, p 137)

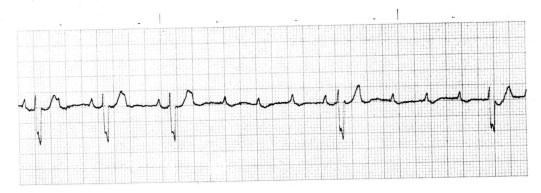

Figure 15–11. Digoxin toxicity in a 7-month-old infant—2:1 type II AV block to third-degree heart block. (Reproduced with permission from Curley MAQ (1985). *Pediatric Cardiac Dysrhythmias.* Bowie, Md: Brady Communications, p 138)

Saul, 1992). Digoxin cannot be removed from the system by dialysis but can be inactivated by digoxin-specific fragment antigen binding (Fab).

Assessment: Hemodynamic Effect

Whenever a dysrhythmia is noted, it is imperative to first assess the hemodynamic effect. These effects or symptoms are understood by noting that to maintain blood pressure when cardiac output ceases, the systemic vascular resistance must increase appropriately. (Blood pressure is equal to the cardiac output multiplied by the systemic vascular resistance.) The increased systemic vascular resistance produces cool, dusky extremities; pallor or mottled skin; poor capillary refill; increased core and decreased surface temperatures; decreased urine output (less than 1 mL/kg/hour or 2 mL/kg/hour in neonates); decreased level of consciousness; and lethargy. Blood pressure is maintained temporarily even when the cardiac output is decreased. Astute nursing assessment and rapid appropriate intervention to improve cardiac output must occur before compensatory mechanisms to maintain cardiac output fail.

Transient sinus bradycardia, sinus arrest with junctional escape rhythms, first-degree heart block, second-degree-type 1 AV block, and premature supraventricular and ventricular contractions have been identified to occur without hemodynamic compromise in healthy pediatric patients (Southall et al, 1981). Dysrhythmias occurring without hemodynamic compromise in patients with morphologically normal hearts are generally considered benign in pediatric patients and do not require treatment.

Nursing Diagnosis

Decreased Cardiac Output

Defining Characteristics

- Heart rate not equal to metabolic need
- Inadequate perfusion to major organs
- Cool, dusky extremities
- Prolonged capillary refill (> 2 sec)
- Low urine output for age
- Decreased level of consciousness or responsiveness
- Hypotension

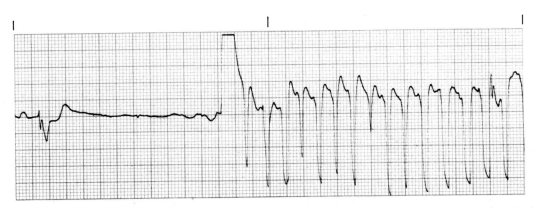

Figure 15–12. Digoxin toxicity in a 7-month-old infant. Ventricular tachycardia. (Reproduced with permission from Curley MAQ [1985]. *Pediatric Cardiac Dysrhythmias.* Bowie, Md: Brady Communications, p 122)

Nursing Interventions

- Eliminate or modify etiologic factors
- Monitor for dysrhythmias
- Titrate antidysrhythmic medications collaboratively with the physician
- Monitor and treat electrolyte abnormalities collaboratively with the physician
- Monitor arterial blood gases, venous blood gases, and oxygen saturations for hypoxemia
- Titrate supplemental oxygen therapy collaboratively with the physician
- Monitor for hypovolemia, which is characterized by decreased right atrial pressure and a normal or decreased systolic arterial pressure
- Titrate volume expanders collaboratively with the physician
- Monitor for inappropriate afterload, eg, increased systemic vascular resistance
- Maintain normothermic environment
- Titrate positive inotropic agent administration collaboratively with the physician after addressing factors that contribute to a negative inotropic state, eg, hypoxemia, acidosis, electrolyte abnormalities, and hypoglycemia
- Decrease the workload of the heart, eg, plan care to allow for rest periods. Promote stress reduction.
- Position patient for comfort
- Titrate analgesics and sedatives within the guidelines established collaboratively with the physician
- Teach patient adaptive techniques necessary to deal with the effects of decreased cardiac output, stress reduction techniques, and how to cope with and learn about related health problems

Expected Outcomes

- Normal sinus rhythm
- Perfusion to major organs is adequate
- Extremities are warm and pink
- Capillary refill is brisk (< 2 seconds)
- Urine output is normal for the patient's age
- The level of consciousness and responsiveness is at baseline
- Arterial blood pressure is within normal limits for the patient's age

Parent and Family Teaching and Psychosocial Support

Much fear is associated with any cardiac dysfunction. Parents and children need information and support. The parents' baseline knowledge is frequently oriented toward adult coronary artery disease, so many fear sudden death of a heart attack. The nurse can be instrumental in providing appropriate reassurance and easily comprehended information to both child and family. A parent-teaching booklet that specifically addresses pediatric cardiac dysrhythmias is available from the American Heart Association (1983). This teaching aid contains illustrations that can be used, in part, to facilitate individualized family instruction.

SPECIFIC DYSRHYTHMIAS

Supraventricular Tachycardia

Supraventricular tachycardia (SVT) is the most common tachydysrhythmia in pediatrics. This disorder occurs most often in boys younger than 4 months of age with structurally normal hearts. Occasionally, associated congenital heart defects, such as Ebstein anomaly, L-transposition of the great arteries, or tricuspid atresia are identified.

Etiology and Pathophysiology

Supraventricular tachycardia is thought to be the result of either increased automaticity of a single focus above the bundle of His or the re-entry mechanism. The first is uncommon, is associated with a gradual onset and end, and is frequently noted to be interspersed with sinus tachycardia. The re-entry mechanism is thought to be the most common cause of SVT. In this situation rapid ventricular rates are perpetuated over a re-entry circuit consisting of two functionally distinct pathways or limbs (Figure 15–13). Both limbs have different repolarization times and allow bidirectional (normal antegrade or retrograde) impulse travel.

Supraventricular tachycardia is initiated by a premature supraventricular contraction (PSVC) that can-

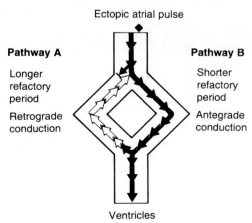

Figure 15–13. Schematic representation of the reentry mechanism. (Reproduced with permission from Curley MAQ [1985]. *Pediatric Cardiac Dysrhythmias.* Bowie, Md: Brady Communications, p 84)

not conduct through one of the limbs (A) because it is still in a refractory period from a previous contraction, but the impulse is able to conduct slowly in a normal antegrade manner through the other limb (B). By the time the slow antegrade conduction is complete through pathway B, pathway A has had time to complete repolarization, so it is ready to accept an impulse. The *same* impulse is then conducted in a retrograde manner along pathway A *and* down to the ventricles, causing ventricular depolarization. When the impulse completes retrograde travel through pathway A, pathway B is again ready to accept another impulse, so the process repeats itself and the re-entry circuit is established. The re-entry process requires unidirectional block and perfect reciprocal timing of the refractory periods of both limbs.

Intranodal or extranodal re-entry circuits can be established. Intranodal re-entry frequently occurs within the AV node, because this node contains a dense network of fibers that can facilitate alternate-pathway conduction. Extranodal re-entry occurs when an active accessory pathway outside the AV node exists, such as in WPW syndrome.

Tachycardia effectively increases cardiac output only to a certain point. Excessive tachycardia (SVT) shortens the rapid ventricular filling time that occurs during diastole and thus compromises stroke volume and cardiac output (Figure 15–14). Excessive tachycardia also limits diastolic coronary artery filling; thus myocardial perfusion is compromised at a time of increased need.

Assessment

History. The clinical presentation of SVT depends on the ventricular rate, duration, and the underlying condition of the patient's myocardium. Supraventricular tachycardia is considered a medical emergency in infants younger than 1 year because if the rapid ventricular rates, 260–320 beats per minute, are allowed to continue for more than 24 hours, congestive heart failure (CHF) and then cardiogenic shock will develop. The patient's history usually contains the parents' descriptions of poor feeding, pale skin color, and irritability followed by lethargy. Supraventricular tachycardia is better tolerated by older children, whose ventricular rates are much slower, approximately 160 beats per minute, than by infants. Older children may come to the ED complaining of chest pain, feeling "sick," palpitations, or abdominal pain with or without vomiting. Those with congenital heart disease exhibit a decreased hemodynamic tolerance to SVT. These children usually decompensate rapidly and present in severe CHF or cardiogenic shock.

Physical Assessment. The findings are consistent with those of CHF or cardiogenic shock. The heart rate is often too fast to count. The respiratory rate also is fast, and symptoms of inadequate tissue perfusion are present, ie, cool, dusky, mottled extremities; prolonged capillary refill (> 2 seconds); decreased urine output for age; and decreased level of consciousness or responsiveness. If compensation is effective, blood pres-

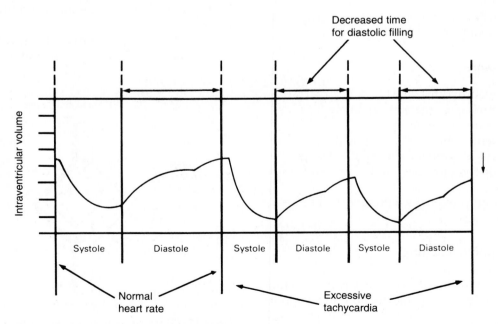

Figure 15–14. Excessive tachycardia shortens the rapid ventricular filling phase that occurs during diastole. This mechanism limits stroke volume.

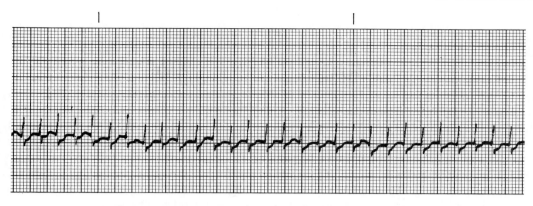

Figure 15–15. Supraventricular tachycardia in a 2-week-old infant.

sure is normal for the patient's age. If compensation fails, hypotension (defined as a systolic blood pressure less than 70 mmHg + 2 × the age in years) occurs.

Rhythm Strip. In addition to the patient's history, definitive electrophysiologic criteria for SVT due to the re-entry mechanism include an abrupt onset and a monotonously regular rhythm because each QRS complex is an exact replication of the previous one (Figures 15–15, 15–16). The P waves usually cannot be identified because they are either located on top of the preceding T wave or buried in the previous QRS complex. If visualized, the P waves are different from the patient's normal ones. If measured, the PR interval is longer than the child's normal interval. Most often there is a 1:1 P:QRS ratio. The QRS complexes are usually normal, but rarely a rate-related aberrancy, most often right bundle-branch block (RBBB), may be present. Aberrant QRS complexes also may be present when bypass tracts, congenital heart disease, or surgical RBBB is present. In these patients the wide QRS complex SVT may resemble ventricular tachycardia. Depression of the ST segment, indicating myocardial ischemia, is a frequent finding during SVT or after conversion to normal sinus rhythm.

TRIAGE
Supraventricular Tachycardia

Emergent
Child with signs or symptoms of low cardiac output.

Management

The treatment goal centers on what is known about the mechanism of this dysrhythmia. For example, it is known that SVT most frequently is initiated by a PSVC and maintains itself through a re-entry mechanism involving the AV node. The goal of treatment is break the re-entry circuit by interrupting the reciprocating refractory periods of the re-entry limbs. Before medical management begins, nursing priorities include obtaining a high-quality cardiac tracing, starting an adequate intravenous line, giving appropriate doses of resuscitation drugs, and preparing the defibrillator.

Vagal maneuvers, which induce a negative dromotropic effect through the AV node, are usually at-

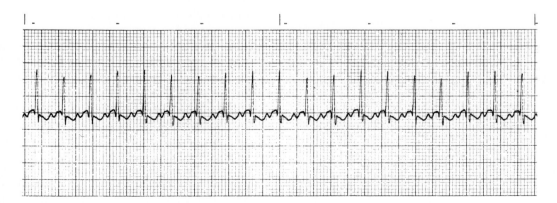

Figure 15–16. Supraventricular tachycardia in a 10-week-old infant. Note the slower rate than in Figure 13–15.

tempted first because they are the least invasive. As anticipated, the vagal maneuvers induce an all-or-none response in SVT while only slowing a sinus tachycardia. Vagal maneuvers include unilateral carotid massage, induction of a gag reflex, rectal stimulation, and ocular pressure. Ocular pressure is avoided in neonates because it may precipitate retinal detachment. The diving or mammalian reflex has gained popularity because of its effectiveness. The diving reflex is present at birth and produces strong vagal stimulation and sympathetic withdrawal. To induce the diving reflex, an ice-cold (4°C–5°C), wet facecloth is placed abruptly on the infant's face for approximately 6–7 seconds. An older child's (over 8 years of age) face is immersed in an ice-cold water bath (Figure 15–17). As anticipated, nursing care includes instruction, coaching, and supporting the older child to help the patient accomplish this maneuver with as little fear as possible.

Pharmacologic management of SVT includes adenosine, verapamil, and digoxin. Adenosine, an endogenous nucleoside, is a new antidysrhythmic agent. Adenosine decreases automaticity and blocks AV node conduction directly, yet briefly, so it is highly effective in rapidly terminating SVT due to the re-entry mechanism. Adenosine is administered by rapid intravenous bolus at 50–100 μg/kg. If this dose is not effective, the dose may be increased by 50 μg/kg and readmin-istered at 2-minute intervals to a maximum total dose of 350 μg/kg or 12 mg. Because adenosine is immediately metabolized and removed from the circulation, side effects—which include shortness of breath, bronchospasm, hypotension, flushing and irritability—are transient.

Verapamil is also very effective in the treatment of SVT. Verapamil slows both antegrade and retrograde conduction through the AV node by prolonging its effective refractory period. Like adenosine, verapamil breaks the re-entry circuit by interrupting the reciprocating refractory periods of the re-entry limbs. Because of its negative inotropic effects, verapamil is not the drug of choice if CHF is present. Side effects include AV block, extreme bradycardia, hypotension due to the smooth-muscle-relaxant effect of the drug, and asystole. These side effects occur more frequently in infants younger than 1 year and in patients receiving beta-blocker therapy (Perry and Garson, 1989). Treatment of the side effects includes administration of calcium chloride, atropine, and isoproterenol. Verapamil is administered very slowly, over 1 minute. The onset of its effect is rapid, 3–5 minutes after administration.

Digoxin is also effective in the medical management of SVT, but it may take up to 10 hours to be effective. The vagotonic action of digoxin directly affects the conductivity and refractoriness of the AV node. One may administer digoxin, wait a few hours, then retry vagal maneuvers.

Cardioversion is the treatment of choice if altered hemodynamic stability or CHF is present. Mild anesthesia with diazepam or thiopental is necessary before this procedure. The largest paddle size that provides the best chest wall contact is used. The dose is 0.2–1.0 joules (J)/kg. The *lowest possible* number of joules must be used if the patient is receiving digoxin because this procedure may induce irreversible cardiac arrest (American Heart Association, 1990).

Parent and Family Teaching and Psychosocial Support

Supraventricular tachycardia can be frightening to a child and his or her family. All require nursing support and information. Patients arriving at the ED in SVT are admitted to a monitored pediatric unit for further study. Patient and family teaching includes use of the cardiac monitor with specific information about the alarm systems. Because parents are not socialized to the hospital environment, they consider all alarms worrisome.

Infants usually continue to receive digoxin for at least 1 year after conversion to a normal sinus rhythm. After that time the drug can usually be discontinued without recurrence of SVT. Families need to know that

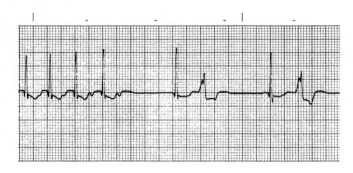

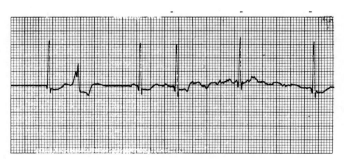

Figure 15–17. Rhythm changes induced by the diving reflex. Supraventricular tachycardia to ventricular bigeminy to atrial fibrillation then normal sinus rhythm in the same 10-year-old child as in Figure 15–15.

until the patient's condition is stabilized by medication, recurrences of SVT are common. Parents of infants are able to rest more comfortably at night if they are informed of the 24 hours or more it takes for SVT to progress to cardiogenic shock. Older children are assessed on an individual basis. Children usually do not require long-term pharmacologic therapy but are taught vagal maneuvers to control their symptoms.

Wolff-Parkinson-White Syndrome

Etiology and Pathophysiology

Normally the atria and the ventricles are separated by a fibrous structure called the trigone, which prevents supraventricular impulses from being conducted to the ventricles except through the AV node and bundle of His. In WPW syndrome, additional muscle links capable of impulse conduction penetrate the trigone that connects the atria to the ventricles. Infants with WPW syndrome usually arrive at the ED in SVT. The activity through bypass fibers is enhanced by the infant's predominant parasympathetic activity. With maturation of sympathetic innervation, these bypass fibers frequently become quiescent, so one can then expect the episodes of SVT to decrease in the first year of life or to disappear spontaneously by the second year. The incidence of WPW syndrome is greater in boys at a 3:2 ratio. There is also a greater incidence of WPW syndrome in children with congenital heart defects, such as Ebstein anomaly, L-transposition, and familial cardiomyopathy.

Electrophysiologic studies have identified various bypass tracts such as Kent, James, and Mahaim fibers. The AV bypass tracts, or Kent bundles, are the most common. They appear along the free wall and septal regions of both left and right ventricles. They present electrophysiologically as a short PR interval, indicating AV node bypass; a delta wave, indicating pre-excitation or premature activation of the ventricular myocardium; and an abnormal QRS complex because of the delta wave. The delta wave (Figure 15–18) can be identified as a slurred upstroke of the QRS complex that prolongs the QRS duration, therefore resembling an interventricular conduction delay. The AV nodal bypass tracts, or James fibers, associated with Lown-Ganong-Levine syndrome connect the atrium to the bundle of His. Their course is perinodal or intranodal, and they produce a short PR interval and normal QRS complex. The nodoventricular bypass tract (connecting the AV node to the ventricles) and fasciculoventricular bypass tract (connecting the bundle of His to the ventricles) are Mahaim fibers. They are uncommon and produce a normal PR interval, a small delta wave, and thus an abnormal QRS complex.

The SVT of WPW syndrome is of two types: an antegrade or a retrograde impulse that travels through the AV node. Normally the accessory pathway has a longer refractory period, so the PSVC first conducts normally through the AV node, then in a retrograde manner through the accessory pathway, producing a normal QRS configuration. This is referred to as orthodromic re-entry. Occasionally the PSVC first conducts through the accessory pathway, then back up in a retrograde manner through the AV node, producing an abnormal QRS configuration. This is referred to as antidromic re-entry. This type is more serious because of the loss of the protective filtering mechanism of the AV node.

Assessment

History and Physical Assessment. Clinical presentation to the ED is the same as for SVT. The findings of physical assessment are consistent with those of CHF and cardiogenic shock.

Rhythm Strip. The defining electrophysiologic criteria for the SVT of WPW syndrome are the same as those

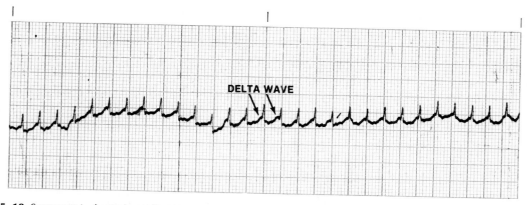

Figure 15–18. Supraventricular tachycardia associated with Wolff-Parkinson-White syndrome. Note the delta waves. (Reproduced with permission from Curley MAQ [1985]. *Pediatric Cardiac Dysrhythmias.* Bowie, Md: Brady Communications, p 87)

for non-WPW SVT—abrupt onset and end, rapid regular rhythm, P waves different from the patient's normal waves, and a 1:1 P:QRS ratio. The PR interval is longer than the patient's normal interval with orthodromic re-entry and shorter than the patient's normal interval with antidromic re-entry. The QRS complexes are normal with orthodromic re-entry and widened by delta waves with antidromic re-entry. Supraventricular tachycardia occurring secondary to antidromic WPW syndrome may resemble ventricular tachycardia. Depression of the ST segment, indicating myocardial ischemia, also may be present.

After conversion to a normal sinus rhythm, sinus impulse conduction to the ventricles may alternate between the AV node and the accessory pathway. This is usually first identified by nurses who observe normal cycles (with normal PR intervals and QRS complexes) interspersed with abnormal cycles of short PR intervals and wide QRS complexes. When observed, the rhythm is documented by a 12-lead electrocardiogram (ECG) and is brought to the attention of the physician.

TRIAGE
Wolf-Parkinson-White Syndrome

Emergent ————————————————
Child with signs and symptoms of low cardiac output.

Management
Treatment includes pharmacologic ablation of either limb, so it is the same for SVT except for a few precautions. Digoxin and verapamil are used cautiously if bypass tracts are suspected because, while increasing the AV node refractory period, they may also decrease the refractoriness of the bypass tracts, thus enhancing conduction to the ventricles. If the patient were to develop atrial flutter or fibrillation with antidromic re-entry, all impulses would rapidly conduct to the ventricles, causing ventricular flutter or fibrillation. This effect is uncommon in infants but poses a great risk in older children and adolescents.

Propranolol is useful in WPW syndrome because it decreases conduction velocity through the AV node. Propranolol also decreases the automaticity of ectopic atrial pacemaker sites and thus decreases the frequency of PSVCs. Side effects include high-degree AV block, bradycardia, asystole, and hypotension. Treatment of these side effects is with isoproterenol. Propranolol may be used alone or in combination with quinidine, which prolongs the refractory period of the bypass tract. Other drugs that prolong the refractory period of bypass tracts include procainamide and amiodarone. Patients are admitted to a monitored pediatric unit for further study. Recurrences of WPW SVT are common. Patients with WPW syndrome usually remain on antidysrhythmic therapy longer than 1 year.

Psychosocial Support and Parent Education
Psychosocial support and education are fundamentally the same as for SVT.

Ventricular Dysrhythmias

Etiology and Pathophysiology
Most PVCs in pediatric patients are benign, yet fear accompanies them because of their ominous nature in the adult population. Idiopathic PVCs with uniform fixed coupling, a constant interval from the last normal QRS to the premature QRS, are common in adolescents. Premature ventricular contractions without fixed coupling, multiform PVCs, bigeminy, or couplets in pediatric patient with a normal heart and no symptoms also may be idiopathic, but consultation with a pediatric cardiologist is warranted.

Table 15–2 provides a summary of the pathogenesis of PVCs in the pediatric population. A severe metabolic or electrolyte imbalance is the most frequent cause of PVCs in the pediatric population.

Management
Treatment depends on the severity of the ventricular dysrhythmia, as evidenced by an altered hemodynamic effect. Concern that PVCs will initiate an

---

TABLE 15–2. ETIOLOGY OF PREMATURE VENTRICULAR CONTRACTIONS IN THE PEDIATRIC POPULATION

Severe metabolic or electrolyte imbalance
    Hypoxia, acidosis
    Hypoglycemia
    Hyperkalemia or hypokalemia
    Hypercalcemia or hypocalcemia
Cardiac manipulation
    Insertion of a central line
Congenital heart disease
Cardiomyopathy and myocarditis
Pediatric coronary artery disease
    Kawasaki disease
    Anomalous origin of the left coronary artery
Prolonged QT interval syndromes
Toxic drug levels
    Digoxin
    Class I & III antidysrhythmics
    Tricyclic antidepressant
    Organophosphate poisoning
Cerebral hypertension
Cardiac tumors
No identifiable cause

unstable ventricular tachydysrhythmia may be warranted in the following situations.

Circumstances in Which PVCs Initiate Unstable Ventricular Tachydysrhythmia

- Structural heart disease is present. This is related to areas of potential slow conduction or unidirectional block, which can sustain a ventricular tachydysrhythmia.
- Variable or short coupling intervals are present, especially in a child with structural heart disease. The R-on-T phenomenon is rare among pediatric patients with a normal heart.
- Multiform PVCs are present.
- The child has a prolonged QT interval syndrome. A prolonged QT interval represents prolongation of a vulnerable period in the cardiac cycle; thus the patient is more susceptible to malignant ventricular dysrhythmias and sudden death.
- A family history of lethal dysrhythmias is present.
- The PVCs increase with exercise. The opposite also is true, ie, no treatment is indicated if the dysrhythmias decrease with exercise. Increases may be secondary to endogenous catecholamine release or subendocardial ischemia.
- A possible history of related dysrhythmia side effects is present, ie, syncope, idiopathic seizures.

Acute treatment always takes place concurrently with correction of acid-base and electrolyte imbalances. Correction of these disturbances alone may convert the ventricular dysrhythmia. Use of antidysrhythmic medications in pediatric patients still involves a great deal of empiricism. Lidocaine is effective 85% of the time, so it is the drug of choice. The dose of 1.0 mg/kg is administered by intravenous push. Lidocaine is rapid-acting but of short duration, so a repeat bolus is necessary every 3–5 minutes until a continuous intravenous infusion is prepared. To prepare the infusion, 120 mg of lidocaine is added to 5% dextrose in water (D_5W) to make a total volume of 100 mL. This solution is infused at a rate of 1–2.5 mL/kg/hour to deliver 20–50 µg/kg/minute. Therapeutic levels are not clear in a developing heart, so it is difficult to extrapolate adult values to children. Lidocaine is totally metabolized in the liver, so liver function studies are followed carefully.

Procainamide is the second drug of choice, but it is used with caution because severe peripheral vasodilatation, and thus profound hypotension, can occur. The negative inotropic effects of procainamide are more significant in patients with an already depressed myocardium. This drug also may enhance or induce AV block. The PR, QRS, and QT intervals are assessed and should not increase more than 25% over pretreatment values.

Bretylium can be used when lidocaine and procainamide are ineffective. The side effect is severe hypotension. Bretylium is not used if digoxin-related dysrhythmias are suspected because it may enhance the dysrhythmias.

Other drugs include propranolol, which is effective in children with prolonged QT interval syndrome, mitral valve prolapse, or obstructive cardiomyopathy; phenytoin, which is effective for patients for whom digoxin is toxic or patients who are recovering from cardiac surgery and have residual hemodynamic lesions; and amiodarone, which is effective in patients with ventricular tumors and cardiomyopathies.

All cases of wide QRS complex tachycardia in pediatric patients should be managed as ventricular tachycardia until proved otherwise (Garson, 1987). Unlike in adults, wide QRS complex SVT is rare in infants and children.

Both SVT and ventricular tachycardia are rapid rhythms of abrupt onset. Ventricular tachycardia that exceeds 250 beats per minute may occur, especially in infants. While SVT is monotonously regular, ventricular tachycardia may be irregular with varied beat-to-beat QRS configurations that are different from the patient's normal supraventricular-originated beat.

Factors that favor SVT aberrancy include a past history of RBBB, presence of bypass tracts (WPW syndrome), preceding premature ectopic supraventricular activity, and no compensatory pause. Previous rhythm strips, if available, can be scanned for premature supraventricular or ventricular beats; the QRS configuration in the current rhythm may be similar. Fusion complexes, those that resemble both a supraventricular and a ventricular beat, frequently appear at the onset or end of the run of ventricular tachycardia.

The P:QRS relationship is 1:1 in SVT, whereas atrial-to-ventricular dissociation is common in VT. The P:QRS relation can be difficult to determine during rapid tachycardia, but it can be facilitated by changing the lead system or by using an esophageal lead. The midportion of the esophagus lies posterior to the left atrium (Figure 15–19). A properly positioned esophageal lead provides excellent atrial recordings, which allow rapid identification of atrial activity and its relation to ventricular activity. The same catheter can be used to provide rapid overdrive pacing of the atria to convert SVT to a normal sinus rhythm (Benson, 1987). Nursing care is similar to that for cardioversion. For example, emergency medications and equipment are readied and the patient's level of comfort and sedation are monitored.

Dysrhythmias Related to Pediatric Cardiac Arrest

Unlike in the adult population, asystole and bradydysrhythmias account for 90% of all pediatric car-

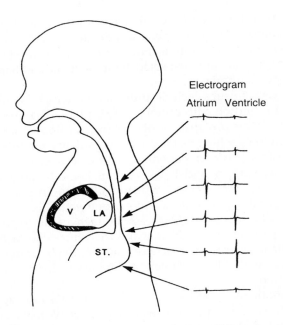

Electrogram

Atrium Ventricle

Figure 15–19. The anatomic relationship between the esophagus and the cardiac chambers in infants. The ideal electrogram at mid-esophagus has an atrial spike which is equal to, or larger than, the ventricular signal. V, ventricle; LA, left atrium; ST, stomach. (Reproduced with permission from Walsh EP [1992]. Electocardiography and introduction to electrophysiological techniques. In Fyler DC (ed), *Nadas' Pediatric Cardiology.* St. Louis: Mosby, p 147)

diac arrest dysrhythmias; ventricular dysrhythmias account for the remaining 10% (American Heart Association, 1990). Ventricular dysrhythmias are observed more frequently in patients with congenital heart disease, in those who experience prolonged resuscitation attempts, in those who are beyond the neonatal period, and in patients who weigh more than 2.23 kg (Walsh and Krongrad, 1983). Pediatric arrest dysrhythmias most often occur secondary to hypoxia, acidosis, and electrolyte disturbance, so primary correction is of utmost importance. Figures 15–20 and 15–21 illustrate the American Heart Association recommendations for collaborative management of arrest-related dysrhythmias.

Defibrillation. The basic procedure for defibrillation in infants and children is the same as that for adults. The defibrillation dose is 2 J/kg; then the dose is doubled and delivered twice in rapid succession. If defibrillation is unsuccessful, additional correction of metabolic dysfunction is warranted. Epinephrine may be used to enhance the likelihood of successful defibrillation. Bretylium has been found to be effective in managing both ventricular tachycardia and ventricular fibrillation that are refractory to conventional therapy, ie, lidocaine and repeated defibrillation. Defibrillators capable of measuring the number of delivered joules

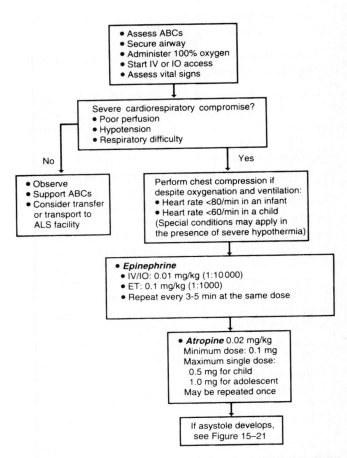

Figure 15–20. Bradycardia decision tree. ABCs, airway, breathing, and circulation; ET endotracheal; IO, intraosseous; IV, intravenous; ALS, advanced life support. (Reproduced with permission from American Heart Association [1992]. Standards and guidelines for cardiopulmonary resuscitation and emergency cardiac care. Part VI. Pediatric advanced life support. *JAMA* 268:2266)

are essential in pediatrics because of the small doses used. More than usual precautions are necessary to prevent arcing of the electrical current over the small pediatric patient's chest wall. That is cross-paddle and conduction-medium contact is to be avoided. Paddle size and digoxin precautions have already been discussed.

Transcutaneous Pacing. Because most slow rhythms in the pediatric population occur secondary to hypoxia and acidosis, transcutaneous pacing during cardiopulmonary resuscitation is rarely successful. Even if atrial capture can be accomplished, oxygenation and ventilation is the better therapy to improve myocardial contractility and systemic blood flow. Transcutaneous pacing may be helpful when managing symptomatic slow rhythms secondary to primary cardiac disease, such as heart block in a patient with congenital heart disease (American Heart Association, 1992).

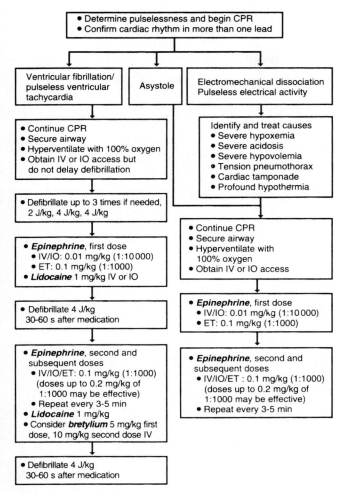

Figure 15–21. Asystole and pulseless arrest decision tree. CPR, cardiopulmonary resuscitation; ET, endotracheal; IO intraosseous; IV, intravenous. (Reproduced with permission from American Heart Association [1992]. Standards and guidelines for cardiopulmonary resuscitation and emergency cardiac care. Part VI. Pediatric advanced life support. *JAMA* 268:2266)

REFERENCES

American Heart Association (1983). Abnormalities of Heart Rhythm: A Guide for Parents. Publication No. 50-058-A/11-83-75M. Dallas: American Heart Association's Office of Communications

American Heart Association (1990). Cardiac rhythm disturbances. In Chameides L (ed), *Textbook of Pediatric Advanced Life Support*. Dallas: American Heart Association, pp 61–67

American Heart Association (1992). Standards and guidelines for cardiopulmonary resuscitation and emergency cardiac care. Part V. Pediatric basic life support; Part VI. Pediatric advanced life support. *JAMA* 268:2251–2275

Benson DW (1987). Transesophageal electrocardiography and cardiac pacing: State of the art. *Circulation* 75(Suppl III):III86–III89

Boehnert MT, Lovejoy FH (1985). Value of the QRS duration versus the serum drug level after an acute overdose of tricyclic antidepressants. *New England Journal of Medicine* 313:474–478

Garson A (1987). Medicolegal problems in the management of cardiac arrhythmias in children. *Pediatrics* 79:84–88

Krongrad E (1984). Postoperative arrhythmias in patients with congenital heart disease. *Chest* 85:107–113

Perry JC, Garson A (1989). Diagnosis and treatment of arrhythmias. *Advances in Pediatrics* 36:177–199

Southall DP, Johnson PGB, Shinebourne EA, Johnston PGB, Vulliamy DG (1981). Frequency and outcome of disorders of cardiac rhythm and conduction in a population of newborn infants. *Pediatrics* 68:58–66

Walsh CK, Krongrad E (1983). Terminal cardiac activity in pediatric patients. *American Journal of Cardiology* 51:557–561

Walsh EP, Saul JP (1992). Cardiac arrhythmias. In Fyler DC (ed), *Nadas' Pediatric Cardiology*. St. Louis: Mosby-Year Book, p. 147

Weintraub RG, Gow RM, Wilkinson JL (1990). The congenital long QT syndromes in childhood. *Journal of the American College of Cardiology* 16:674–680

Zaritsky A, Chernow B (1984). Medical progress: Use of catecholamines in pediatrics. *Journal of Pediatrics* 105:341–350

Zegeer LJ (1984). Systemic cardiovascular effects of intracranial disorders: Implications for nursing care. *Journal of Neurosurgical Nursing* 16:161–167

SUGGESTED READING

Denfield SW, Garson A (1990). Sudden death in children and young adults. *Pediatric Clinics of North America* 37:215–231

Kombol P (1988). Dysrhythmias in infancy. *Neonatal Network* 6:41–52

Zeigler VL, Gillette PC, Crawford FA, Wiles HB, Fyfe DA (1990). New approaches to treatment of incessant ventricular tachycardia in the very young. *Journal of the American College of Cardiology* 16:681–685

CHAPTER 16

Respiratory Emergencies

ANNE PHELAN

INTRODUCTION

Difficulty breathing is a frequent presenting complaint of children in the emergency department (ED). Conditions that alter the normal breathing patterns of a child of any age are stressful to both child and parents. This factor must be considered when providing emergency nursing care to a child with respiratory distress. Nursing interventions must be directed toward normalizing air exchange and oxygenation, minimizing respiratory effort, providing adequate hydration, and easing anxiety. Careful attention must be paid to giving parents and children adequate, understandable explanations of all procedures, treatments, and signs of improvement throughout the ED visit.

It should be noted that the most common causes of cardiorespiratory failure and arrest in children are respiratory in origin. In children with severe respiratory distress, especially if they are becoming tired, it is advantageous to anticipate and prepare for elective intubation to secure the airway (Table 16–1).

ASSESSMENT OF THE RESPIRATORY SYSTEM

When a child first arrives in the ED with any respiratory problem, a rapid but thorough assessment to determine the nature and severity of the problem must be performed. It is best to develop an organized, systematic approach to assessment, including the four steps of observation, palpation, percussion, and auscultation. It must be kept in mind that with young children the best results are obtained by performing the least intrusive procedures first. Figure 16–1 reviews the anatomy of the respiratory system.

Observation

Although observation is the simplest assessment tool, it gives the nurse a high yield of information about the possible origins and severity of respiratory difficulty. The child's bare chest is inspected for structural abnormalities, symmetry of movement during both inspiration and expiration, and use of accessory muscles. Careful documentation is made of the location and severity of retraction; the intercostal areas, the areas above the manubrium and clavicles and below the xiphoid process are most common (Figure 16–2). Any movement of the head in association with respiratory effort indi-

TABLE 16–1. RAPID SEQUENCE INTUBATION

1. Preoxygenate, place intravenous lines, monitor, perform oximetry, prepare equipment
2. Premedicate if indicated, with lidocaine, 1 mg/kg and/or atropine, 0.01 mg/kg IV
3. Administer muscle relaxant
   Atracurium, 0.5 mg/kg/dose IV
   Pancuronium, 0.1 mg/kg/dose IV
   Vecuronium, 0.1 mg/kg/dose IV
   Succinylcholine, 1.5 mg/kg/dose IV
4. Begin Sellick maneuver
5. Administer sedative
   Fentanyl, 1–5 μg/kg/dose IV
   Midazolam, 0.05–0.1 mg/kg/dose IV
   Pentobarbital, 2–3 mg/kg/dose IV
6. Intubate
7. Assess tube placement

Steps 1–7 should be completed in 3 minutes.

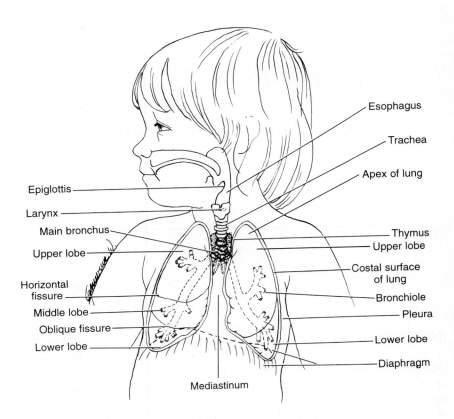

Figure 16-1. Respiratory system.

cates severe distress. Paradoxic or diaphragmatic (abdominal) breathing is normal in infants.

Palpation

In addition to its use in the detection of abnormal growth, palpation is used in instances of known or suspected trauma to detect the presence of bony abnor-

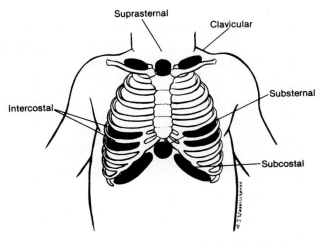

Figure 16-2. Location of retractions. (Reproduced with permission from Whaley LF, Wong DL [1991]. *Nursing care of infants and children* [4th ed]. St Louis: Mosby)

malities and areas of tenderness and swelling. Crepitant swelling most often indicates the free air of subcutaneous emphysema or pneumomediastinum. The trachea should be palpated for the deviation from midline associated with unilateral pneumothorax. Tactile fremitus may be elicited by placing the whole hand over various thoracic sites to detect abnormalities in sound transmission during the cries of an infant and during conversation with an older child. Abnormalities in sound transmission may indicate atelectasis or consolidation in that area.

Percussion

Percussion may be performed on infants by tapping with a single finger. The normal percussion note is hyperresonant over all lung fields. Any variations, excluding the sternal area, connote possible lobar consolidation, intrathoracic mass, or presence of pleural fluid.

Auscultation

The bell or small diaphragm of the stethoscope is used to listen for normal bronchovesicular breathing. Any adventitious breath sounds must be localized and documented. Infants and small children normally have irregular rate and depth of respiration. This necessitates a full minute of auscultation during a quiet time to obtain an accurate respiratory rate.

Respiratory Distress

The signs and symptoms of respiratory distress are summarized in Table 16–2.

The situation of a child presenting with a respiratory problem should be considered urgent if any of the following factors are present, either alone or in combination.

Urgent Respiratory Problems

- Asymmetric movement of the chest wall during the respiratory cycle
- Crepitant swelling
- Dullness of the percussion note
- Retractions or nasal flaring
- Adventitious breath sounds, ie, rales (high-pitched crackles), rhonchi (coarse rattles), wheezes (inspiratory or expiratory, not cleared by coughing), stridor, or decreased air movement

BRONCHIOLITIS

Bronchiolitis is best defined as an inflammatory process affecting the bronchioles and alveoli. It is seen in infants and is most common in the winter and spring months because of its viral etiology.

Etiology and Pathophysiology

The most common causative organism of bronchiolitis is the respiratory syncytial virus (RSV). Other viruses have been implicated in bronchiolitis, including influenza, parainfluenza, rhinovirus, and adenovirus. Al-though healthy infants typically shed RSV for about 10 days, Toltzis and Brooks (1992) found that immunocompromised infants may continue to shed the virus for several months.

The viral agent settles in the mucosal lining of the bronchioles, causing the cells of the lining to slough. During this process the bronchial mucosa become edematous and secretes copious amounts of mucus, which adds to the debris of dead cells, causing irregular patterns of obstruction and plugging. The irregularity of obstruction leads to air trapping and may cause patchy or segmental atelectasis and hyperinflation as seen on an x ray. The wheezing, heard clinically, is caused by air attempting to flow through these partially obstructed passages. A bronchoconstrictive component may be present in these infants. Air trapping distal to the point of obstruction causes abnormal ventilation or perfusion at the alveolar level, leading to hypoxemia. Hypercapnia is a late sign in infants and should be taken as a sign of impending respiratory failure.

History

The history of an infant with bronchiolitis typically includes symptoms of a cold, cough, and coryza for a few days before the onset of dyspnea. The infant may have a low-grade fever, and there may have been prior episodes of bronchiolitis.

Careful history taking elicits the point at which dyspnea began. Because the critical period of bronchiolitis usually occurs during the first 24–72 hours after the onset of dyspnea, this information becomes important in predicting the course. An infant who exhibits cyanosis, areas of decreased air flow, and tiredness on the first day of the illness should be consid-

TABLE 16–2. SIGNS AND SYMPTOMS OF RESPIRATORY DISTRESS

Clinical Feature	Infants	Children
Respiratory rate (breaths per minute)	Newborn: 60 1–12 months: 40	1–4 years: 32 5–18 years: 28 10–14 years: 24
Respiratory observations	Nasal flaring Substernal retracting Seesaw abdominal breathing Subcostal retraction	Nasal flaring Substernal retraction Supraclavicular retraction Intercostal or subcostal retraction
Breath sounds	Expiratory grunt Inspiratory stridor Inspiratory or expiratory wheezes Diminished breath sounds	Expiratory grunt Inspiratory stridor Inspiratory or expiratory wheezes Diminished breath sounds
Color	Palor, circumoral or general cyanosis, mottled, dusky	Palor, cyanosis, dusky
Behavior	Irritability Lethargy Refusal to drink fluids Weak cry	Irritability Lethargy Refusal to eat or drink

ered to be in a far more critical condition than an infant with moderate wheezing who is tolerating oral fluids well on the third day of the illness. Obtaining a history of the infant's normal feeding pattern and a history of any decrease in urination or onset of vomiting or diarrhea is important in assessing the hydration status of the infant. Poor tolerance of oral feeding, including refusal to eat or drink, and choking spells are indicative of respiratory distress.

Physical Assessment

Physical assessment of an infant with bronchiolitis must always include a full set of vital signs. Tachycardia may indicate impending failure, so an infant with an apical pulse rate approaching 200 beats per minute should be carefully observed. The respiratory rate, usually 50–80 breaths per minute, in these infants is more valuable when assessed for a full minute when the infant is at rest. Also, the location and severity of any nasal flaring or retractions should be documented cautiously because they may change over short periods of time. Infants with bronchiolitis typically have retractions in the intercostal and substernal areas. Profound tachypnea or a reduction in respiratory rate associated with increased retractions, including head bobbing at rest, are signs of exhaustion and are worrisome.

Restlessness should be viewed as a sign of hypoxemia; cyanosis, pallor, and lethargy may herald respiratory failure. Palpation for tactile fremitus should be performed in a gentle manner. Any areas of decreased sound transmission usually indicate areas of consolidation or atelectasis and provide the nurse with a valuable clue as to where areas of decreased air movement will be heard on auscultation. Gentle palpation of the neck and supraclavicular areas and chest wall elicit any deviation of the trachea from midline or the presence of any crepitant swelling associated with a pneumomediastinum or subcutaneous emphysema. Dullness of the percussion note in any area other than the sternal region indicates fluid accumulation or consolidation.

Auscultation of the chest of an infant with bronchiolitis should be performed with careful attention to the quality and character of the wheezing and to the presence of any asymmetry in air movement. An infant with loud, moist wheezing and good air movement throughout is in a far less worrisome condition than an infant with dry crackles and decreased air flow in sections of lung fields.

Assessment procedures should be performed frequently and should be carefully documented to provide a basis for evaluating improvement or worsening of condition and response to any interventions. Upon arrival in the ED and at completion of the initial as-

sessment, the child should be brought to the acute care area, where nursing observations can be made frequently.

Laboratory and Diagnostic Tests

Laboratory and diagnostic tests for an infant with bronchiolitis usually include a posteroanterior and a lateral chest x ray. The chest x ray typically shows hyperinflation with peribronchial cuffing and flattened diaphragms indicative of the air trapping of lower airway obstruction and the presence of a concurrent pneumonia. Nasopharyngeal cultures or wash specimens may be obtained in an effort to isolate the causative viral agent. Frequent monitoring of oxygen saturation by pulse oximetry is a noninvasive method of evaluating the need for supplemental oxygen. Persistently low oxygen saturation (< 95%) in babies receiving supplemental moist oxygen indicates the need for an arterial blood gas determination to evaluate for possible hypercapnea.

TRIAGE
Bronchiolitis

Emergent

An infant with cyanosis or pallor; decreased breath sounds; marked retractions; tachypnea (more than 80 breaths per minute); tachycardia (resting heart rate more than 180 beats per minute); severe respiratory distress; tacky or dry oral mucosa.

Urgent

An infant with areas of decreased air movement; pink color; moist mucous membranes; moderate level of nasal flaring and retractions as indicators of degree of distress; mild to moderate tachypnea and tachycardia; tolerance of oral fluids.

Nursing Diagnosis
Ineffective Airway Clearance

Defining Characteristics

- Abnormal breath sounds
- Cough
- Change in rate or depth of respiration
- Tachypnea
- Dyspnea
- Cyanosis

Nursing Interventions

- Administer supplemental moist oxygen
- Administer medications as ordered
- Monitor vital signs and oxygen saturation

Expected Outcomes

- Respiratory rate normalizes
- Retractions and nasal flaring are absent or decreased
- Air movement increases
- Oxygen saturation rises
- Frequency of cough decreases

Nursing Diagnosis
Ineffective Breathing Pattern

Defining Characteristics

- Retractions or nasal flaring
- Dyspnea
- Tachypnea
- Cough
- Prolonged expiratory phase

Nursing Interventions

- Administer oxygen
- Administer medications as ordered
- Monitor vital signs and oxygen saturation

Expected Outcomes

- Tachypnea resolves
- Retractions or nasal flaring are decreased or absent
- Air movement increases
- Oxygen saturation improves
- Frequency of cough decreases

Nursing Diagnosis
High Risk for Fluid Volume Deficit

Defining Characteristics

- Excessive fluid loss through tachypnea
- Inability to take in fluids because of respiratory distress

Nursing Interventions

- Monitor hydration status
- Administer intravenous fluids as ordered

Expected Outcomes

- Oral mucosa is pink and moist

- Secretions are moist and easily removed
- Urine output normalizes

Nursing Diagnosis
Knowledge Deficit (Caring for Bronchiolitis)

Defining Characteristics

- Deficiency in knowledge related to home management of bronchiolitis
- Inadequate demonstration of nasal bulb suctioning

Nursing Interventions

- Review signs of improved condition contrasted with signs of increased distress as infant's respiratory distress improves
- Explain and demonstrate procedure for nasal bulb suctioning and have parent return demonstration

Expected Outcomes

- Parent verbalizes signs of increased respiratory distress and when to return for further treatment
- Parent returns demonstration of nasal bulb suctioning

Management
Several authors have noted a bronchoconstrictive component to bronchiolitis and an ability for infants to respond to bronchodilators (Alario et al, 1992; Barkin and Rosen, 1990). Therefore the use of aerosolized bronchodilators has become quite common in providing symptomatic relief of wheezing in these infants. Albuterol has emerged as the drug of choice (0.01–0.03 mL/kg in 2 mL of normal saline solution, nebulized), although isoetharine (0.25–0.5 mL of 1% solution in 2 mL of normal saline solution, nebulized) is still in occasional use. Infants receiving bronchodilators in the ED should be monitored carefully for signs of poor tolerance of the drug, such as tachycardia, tremors, and vomiting. If complications develop a lower dose or less frequent dosing may be helpful. It is important to document any signs of clinical improvement or deterioration reflected in accessory muscle use, quality of breath sounds, ability to feed, and ability to retain a good oxygen saturation (> 95%) on room air.

An infant with bronchiolitis may be treated by outpatient follow-up care if the following conditions are met.

Conditions for Outpatient Follow-Up Care of Bronchiolitis

- The respiratory rate is below 60 breaths per minute.

- The hydration status is inadequate and the infant demonstrates a good tolerance of oral fluids and oral medications.
- Oxygen saturation rates on room air remain consistently above 95% even while the patient is feeding.
- The infant maintains good color and is not fatigued.
- The parent or caretaker feels comfortable caring for the infant at home.

An infant who is admitted to the hospital usually receives regular bronchodilator nebulizations and may receive antiviral therapy. Aerosolized ribavirin is sometimes used to treat hospitalized infants with viral pneumonia or bronchiolitis. Toltzis and Brooks (1992) noted the best results using the drug 18–20 hours per day over 3–5 days. Ribavirin is reportedly well tolerated and has no serious side effects aside from mild mucosal irritation. Ribavirin therapy is used for those hospitalized infants with underlying chronic health problems such as bronchopulmonary dysplasia (BPD), congenital cardiac lesions, or immunodeficiency problems.

Parent and Family Teaching and Psychosocial Support

When an infant with bronchiolitis is to be cared for at home, the parents must have an understanding of the signs of increased respiratory distress, ie, increased respiratory rate and effort (retractions), color changes, inability to feed, and inability to rest well. The baby will have to return for admission if these problems occur. The parents also must understand how to administer oral albuterol if prescribed. Nasal bulb suctioning helps to remove the copious secretions associated with this viral infection. A review of fever control is helpful for these parents.

ASTHMA

Asthma may be best described as recurrent reactive airway disease. It is characterized by bronchospasm, mucosal edema, and increased production of mucus as well as the reversal of bronchospasm in response to beta-adrenergic agonists. It is estimated that 5–10% of children in the United States experience asthmatic episodes at some time in their youth. Table 16–3 differentiates asthma from bronchiolitis.

Etiology and Pathophysiology

When a child with asthma is exposed to allergens, respiratory infections, emotional trauma, exercise, or the inhalation of an irritating substance, the smooth muscles of the bronchioles react by constricting. The narrowing of the air passages results in a decreased ability to move air out of the lungs and causes the first feeling of tightness. This feeling is followed by excessive production of mucus and eventually edema of the lining of the bronchioles, which causes further obstruction to air flow and gas exchange. In general, the longer an asthmatic attack is allowed to progress without intervention, the more medication is required to reverse the process.

A typical child with asthma arrives in the ED with some degree of respiratory distress, such as audible wheezing, decreased air movement, shoulder lifting on inspiration, retractions of accessory muscle groups, nasal flaring, and frequent spasmodic cough. The child may have difficulty speaking or color changes.

History

The history of a child with asthma usually reveals other evidence of atopic problems such as eczema or hay fever. The family history usually shows that other members have asthma. When taking the history of a patient with previously diagnosed asthma, the ED nurse should include time of onset of the present epi-

TABLE 16–3. DIFFERENTIATION BETWEEN BRONCHIOLITIS AND ASTHMA

Clinical Feature	Bronchiolitis	Asthma
Etiology	Viral	Allergic and infectious
Occurrence	12 months or younger	After 1 year of age
Respiration	Expiratory or inspiratory wheezes	Expiratory or inspiratory wheezes
	Shallow	Shallow
	Tachypnea	Tachypnea
	Retractions	Retractions
	Hyperinflation	Hyperinflation
Chest x ray findings	Hyperinflation with or without scattered infiltrate	Hyperinflation
Response to beta-adrenergic drugs or theophylline	Varies	Reversal of bronchospasm

sode of wheezing, cough, and dyspnea; medications taken before arrival at the ED and the frequency of any treatments; the presence of a recognized trigger for the attack, such as exposure to a known allergen, an upper respiratory infection, or prolonged exercise. Noting the time of the last attack or admission also is helpful.

Physical Assessment

The assessment of a child with asthma initially shows some degree of tachypnea and tachycardia, which should gradually resolve with therapy. Vital signs should be obtained and recorded frequently, usually between treatments. This assessment, along with intermittent auscultation of the chest and observations of respiratory effort, provides a valuable indication of the effectiveness of therapy.

The blood pressure in an older child with asthma may exhibit a phenomenon called pulsus paradoxus. Pulsus paradoxus may be described as the fluctuation of arterial pressure with the respiratory cycle. During severe respiratory distress, the arterial pressure may rise with expiration and fall with inspiration. The ED nurse can measure this pressure by stopping the fall of mercury at the point of the first systolic sound and observing for variations of the mercury level during the respiratory cycle. If the difference in aterial pressure is equivalent to 30 mmHg, the patient is said to have a pulsus of 30 mmHg. Pulsus paradoxus disappears as intrathoracic pressures resolve.

Observe the child's bare chest for the presence, location, and depth of retractions. The presence of nasal flaring, shoulder lifting, tripod stance, pallor, or cyanosis should be carefully documented.

Auscultation of the chest over all lung fields yields a wealth of information. The characteristic wheezing may vary in intensity from a loud musical wheeze with other coarse sounds present to a tight squeaking wheeze or the localized areas of absent breath sounds usually indicative of markedly decreased air flow through the narrowed bronchioles. Auscultation should always be performed comparing the same site on both sides alternately with an ear toward detecting any inequality of breath sounds indicative of decreased air flow. Because a child with asthma has difficulty expelling air, auscultation should include a timed value for the inspiration to expiration ratio. Initially the expiratory phase may be quite prolonged.

The supraclavicular and intercostal areas and neck should be palpated for the crepitant swelling indicative of a pneumomediastinum or interstitial emphysema. The trachea should be palpated for any deviation from midline associated with a unilateral pneumothorax.

It is important to remember that wheezing does not always mean asthma, and an asthmatic attack may occur when wheezing is not noted. An asthmatic attack also may manifest itself by a persistent cough, usually occurring in spells, or the feeling of tightness associated with decreased air flow. A child with no personal or family history of asthma should therefore be assessed for the possibility of an aspirated foreign body, pulmonary edema, pulmonary contusion, or, for infants, a tracheoesophageal fistula or vascular ring.

Laboratory and Diagnostic Tests

Laboratory tests include a complete blood count (CBC) and blood culture if the child has a fever. If the blood samples are drawn after the administration of beta-adrenergic drugs, it must be understood that these drugs can produce artificially elevated white blood cell counts. A child who is taking prophylactic or maintenance medications and who may need a dosage adjustment should have a serum sample drawn to determine the level of the drug. The time elapsed since ingestion of the medication should be noted.

Oxygen saturation measured by pulse oximetry is a valid, noninvasive method of assuring adequate tissue perfusion when a good correlation exists between the pulse rate displayed and the child's apical pulse rate. Arterial blood gas sampling is usually reserved for severe attacks that do not respond well to therapy. A chest x ray during an asthmatic attack usually shows flattened hemidiaphragms, hyperinflation and gas trapping; areas of consolidation or atelectasis also may be present. Ideally, the child's pulmonary function should be measured directly on initial presentation in the ED and periodically throughout treatment through the use of a peak flow meter. The forced expiratory volume at 1 second (FEV_1) together with O_2 saturation or arterial blood gas levels provide the best objective indication of bronchiolar smooth muscle relaxation and improved gas exhange.

TRIAGE
Asthma

Emergent —————————————————
A child with pallor or cyanosis; decreased breath sounds; marked retractions; inability to speak; severe respiratory distress.

Urgent —————————————————
A child whose color is pink; who has diffuse wheezing; some decreased air movement; mild retractions; and moderate to minimal distress.

Non-urgent —————————————————
A child with occasional expiratory wheeze; good air movement; no retractions; who is able to speak well; and is in no distress.

Nursing Diagnosis
Ineffective Airway Clearance

Defining Characteristics

- Inability to effectively clear secretions from respiratory tract, ineffective cough
- Tachypnea
- Adventitious or decreased breath sounds

Nursing Interventions

- Administer supplemental oxygen as needed
- Administer medication as ordered
- Monitor vital signs
- Monitor oxygen saturation

Expected Outcomes

- Cough decreases in frequency
- Respiratory rate and rhythm return to normal
- Air movement increases
- Adventitious breath sounds decrease

Nursing Diagnosis
Ineffective Breathing Pattern

Defining Characteristics

- Use of accessory muscles, retractions
- Tachypnea and dyspnea
- Assumption of three-point position
- Pallor or cyanosis

Nursing Interventions

- Administer supplemental oxygen as needed
- Administer medications as ordered
- Monitor vital signs and oxygen saturation

Expected Outcomes

- Patient's color returns to normal
- Retractions decrease or are absent
- Patient is able to assume comfortable position
- Respiratory rate returns to normal

Nursing Diagnosis
Impaired Gas Exchange

Defining Characteristics

- Hypoxia
- Confusion or restlessness
- Pallor or cyanosis
- Decreased air movement

Nursing Interventions

- Administer supplemental oxygen as needed
- Administer medications as ordered
- Monitor vital signs

Expected Outcomes

- Patient's color returns to normal
- Patient is alert and oriented
- Breath sounds become symmetric with good air movement
- Oxygen saturation remains above 95%

Nursing Diagnosis
Knowledge Deficit (Asthma)

Defining Characteristics

- Deficiency in knowledge related to home management of asthma
- Medication regimen not followed

Nursing Interventions

- Assist family in identifying triggers of the asthma attacks and signs of respiratory distress that is not responding to home management
- Review proper administration and schedule for medications
- Have child return demonstration of inhaler

Expected Outcomes

- Parents and child verbalize knowledge related to allergens in the home and activities that may precipitate wheezing
- Parents and child demonstrate proper administration of oral medications and use of inhalers and verbalize knowledge of schedule for medications

Management

Upon presentation in the ED, a child with asthma is assessed for degree of respiratory distress. The initial vital signs may show some tachypnea and tachycardia. If the child requires it, supplemental oxygen (O_2 saturation < 95% on room air) should be delivered in a manner comfortable for the child.

The medication regimens for children with asthma in the setting of the ED have changed considerably in a short time. Subcutaneous epinephrine is usually reserved for only the most acute attacks of asthma, and the use of intravenous aminophylline has declined. The use of inhaled steroids is becoming more widespread.

Typically, a child with moderate to severe distress is given inhaled beta-adrenergic agents with oxygen. Nebulized albuterol treatments are usually given every 20 minutes for three doses and the child is re-evaluated for the need for further therapy or admission. Terbutaline nebulized with normal saline solution is frequently used when the child does not respond to the albuterol treatments. Oral and inhaled steroids are usually well tolerated in children who do not require an intravenous line for other therapies. Table 16–4 summarizes the medications most often used in the ED for the treatment of asthma.

Hydration status in a child with asthma is important because these children are prone to insensible fluid loss due to hyperventilation. If the severity of the attack interferes with the child's ability to tolerate sufficient oral fluids, intravenous fluids should be administered, usually calculated at 1½ times the maintenance requirement over the first several hours. Hypotonic solutions such as dextrose in 0.45 normal saline (D_5 0.45 NS) or in 0.25 normal saline (D_5 0.25 NS) are preferable for young children (Thompson, 1990).

Admission to the hospital should be considered when (1) the wheezing and respiratory distress persist after a series of nebulized treatments; (2) tachypnea, retractions, or pallor or cyanosis continue in the absence of wheezing; (3) the child has required frequent recent visits to the ED; (4) parental exhaustion or apprehension exist to such a degree that the provision of adequate home care is questionable.

Criteria for admission to an intensive care unit (ICU) may vary widely from hospital to hospital. In general, intensive care should be considered for patients with asthma who (1) require treatment with more advanced agents, such as terbutaline or isoproterenol in nebulizer or drip form; (2) require placement of an arterial line for frequent blood gas monitoring; (3) exhibit clinically significant persistent hypoxemia and hypercapnia ($pO_2 < 70$ mm Hg, $pCO_2 > 35$ mm Hg); (4) require individual attention because of the patient's level of fear or exhaustion secondary to the increased work of breathing.

Patient and Family Teaching and Psychosocial Support

A child with asthma and his or her family require teaching about what happens in the lungs during an attack that causes the difficulty in breathing. They also need to be aware of the things that most often trigger attacks in children, ie, exposure to an allergen, an upper respiratory infection, pneumonia, or an emotional upset. A referral for allergy testing may be helpful if the child is 4 years of age or older. Careful instructions on administration of medication and scheduling are needed. If the child is using inhalers at home, a spacing device may be helpful. The child should be able to demonstrate an ability to use the inhaler before discharge. The parents or child should be able to verbalize the signs of increased repiratory distress and to return to the ED if the distress recurs.

CROUP

Croup (laryngotracheobronchitis) is a viral inflammation of the subglottic area, including the trachea and bronchi. Croup occurs most frequently in infants and children 6 months–3 years of age. It is slightly more prevalent in boys, and it may recur in older children. Croup is most frequently seen in the cooler months.

Etiology and Pathophysiology

The most common viral agent isolated in croup is parainfluenza types 1 to 3. Rhinoviruses, RSV, and influenza A are also viral etiologic considerations. Bacterial suprainfection, although rare, may be caused by *Streptococcus pneumoniae* or *Haemophilus influenzae*. Spasmodic or allergic recurrent croup also occurs suddenly at night and is managed similarly to viral croup.

The inflammatory process of viral croup produces edema of the trachea and surrounding structures (Figure 16–3). The edematous airways secrete tenacious mucus, which, along with a sloughing or ciliated epithelial lining, leads to problematic removal of secretions. The child's efforts to inspire air through these edematous structures produce the characteristic stridor.

History

The history typically reveals an upper respiratory infection for a few days followed by the late night onset of the characteristic barking cough. The cry or voice may also have a hoarse quality. It is important to elicit whether the child has a history of croup and whether admission or intubation was required. This helps in uncovering parental impressions or apprehensions about the disease. A history of fever and of medications taken also should be determined.

Physical Assessment

The nursing assessment should be performed carefully. The goal is to keep the child calm because the stress of crying increases the work of breathing, and both stridor and retractions markedly increase. The assessment should focus on the child's cardiorespiratory status, hydration, anxiety or fatigue level, and parental anxiety.

The child's face is observed for the classic open-mouth gulp breathing, the amount of drooling, expres-

TABLE 16–4. DRUGS USED IN THE MANAGEMENT OF ACUTE ASTHMA

Drug	Dosage and Route	Frequency	Nursing Implications
Albuterol	Nebulized: 5 mg/mL 0.01–0.03 mL/kg Max dose 1 mL in 2 mL NS Tabs: 2 mg and 4 mg Elixir: 2 mg/15 ml Aerosol inhaler: 90 μg.dose	q 20 minutes to q 4 hours prn 0.1 mg/kg/dose tid q 8 hours Max dose 8 mg/dose 1–2 puffs q 4–6 hours	Usually well tolerated May cause tachycardia, tremor, nervousness, GI upset, and headache
Aminophylline	Tabs and capsules: 50 mg– 300 mg Elixir: 105 mg/5 mL Injectable: 25 mg/mL	Oral: 3–6 mg/kg/dose q 6 hours IV loading: 6 mg/kg bolus over 20–30 minutes IV maintenance drip: 0.8– 1 mg/kg/hour	Usually used in children currently receiving oral maintenance; usually poorly tolerated, causes GI upset. Monitor for tachyarrhythmias, restlessness, tremors, tachycardia. Monitor serum levels Therapeutic range, 10–20 mg/L
Atropine sulfate	Nebulized: 2% or 5% (0.5 mL)	0.05 mg/kg/dose in 2.5 mL NS Max dose 1 mg	May cause dry mouth, blurred vision, tachycardia, and CNS signs (dizziness, restlessness)
Aqueous epinephrine 1:1000	0.01 mL/kg/dose Max 0.3 mL/dose	1 dose usually if in severe distress	Monitor for signs of cardiac irritability, nausea and vomiting, headache, hypertension
Isoetharine	1% solution (10 mg/mL)	Nebulized: 0.25–0.5 mL in 2 mL NS q 20 minutes–q 40 hours prn	May cause tachyarrythmias, headache, anxiety, hypertension
Isoproterenol	Nebulized: 0.01 mL/kg/dose with 2 mL NS or 0.25–0.5 mL of 1:1000 with 2 mL NS IV: 0.1–1.5 μg/kg/minute; increase by 0.1 μg/kg/ minute until desired effect	Nebulized: 0.01 mL/kg/ dose 1:200 with 2 mL NS q 20–60 minutes in severe respiratory distress Dose increased only q 5– 10 minutes of constant infusion	May cause tachycardia, especially when used with epinephrine Monitor continuously May cause hypertension and profound tachycardia
Metaproterenol	5% solution for inhalation	Nebulized: 0.1–0.3 mL in 2.5 mL NS q 1 hour for severe distress	May cause tachycardia, arrhythmias, hypertension, increased O_2 consumption, nausea, tremors, palpitations
Methylprednisolone	IV or IM loading dose: 1–2 mg/kg/dose. Max 250 mg/dose Tabs: 2, 4, 8, 16, 24, 32 mg Elixir: 15 mg/5 mL po 1 mg/kg loading dose	1 loading dose then 0.5 mg/kg q 6 hours	For IM use acetate (Depomedrol) for less local irritation at injection site. Complications occur with prolonged use Long onset of action
Prednisone	Tabs: 1, 5, 10, 20 mg Elixir: 0.5 mg/mL	0.5–2 mg/kg/day Max 40 mg/dose	Methylprednisolone usually preferable now that oral preparations are readily available Complications occur with long-term use

(continued)

TABLE 16–4. (*Continued*)

Drug	Dosage and Route	Frequency	Nursing Implications
Terbutaline	1 mg/mL Tabs: 2.5–0.5 mg IV drip: 0.08 μg/kg/minute after bolus of 2 μg/kg	Nebulized: 0.5–1.5 mL in 2.5 mL NS q 20–120 minutes prn May increase by 0.02-μg increments	Used more commonly than isoproterenol for severe bronchospasm not responding well to albuterol nebulization. May cause restlessness, tremor, tachycardia, headache, arrhythmias. Monitor constantly; injectable solution used for nebulization.

NS, normal saline solution; GI, gastrointestinal; CNS, central nervous system.

sions of anxiety, and cyanosis or pallor in the areas around the mouth, nose, or ears. The presence and depth of chest wall retractions should be carefully noted. The quality of the cough must be recorded, and vital signs should be taken frequently. Exhaustion, tachycardia, and changes in respiratory effort may signal impending respiratory failure.

Auscultation of all lung fields should be performed frequently to ascertain the amount of air movement and prolongation of the inspiratory phase. The importance of frequent assessments and meticulous documentation cannot be overemphasized, because just as rapid improvement may be noted in a humidified environment, rapid deterioration is a possibility.

The presenting symptoms of croup vary in severity according to the degree of inflammation and the amount of exhaustion experienced by the child. In mild croup, the child may appear comfortable and have a hoarse cough on occasion; stridor may only be heard on auscultation or may be audible when the child is upset. In more severe cases, air hunger is evident; inspiratory stridor is audible at rest; the cough is more intense and frequent; retractions are visible, notably in the suprasternal area; and substernal depression may be present. In moderate to severe croup, the child may appear frightened and restless and may exhibit tachycardia and tachypnea, which are characteristic of hypoxia. Cyanosis, hypercapnea, and acidosis are late signs and along with increased respiratory effort, air

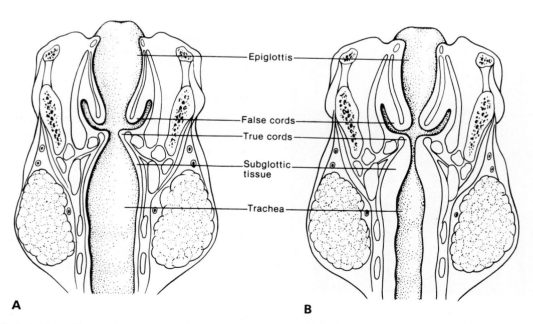

Figure 16–3. A. Normal larynx. B. Obstruction and narrowing caused by the edema of croup. (From Mott SR, James SR, Sperhac AM [1990]. *Nursing care of children and families* [2nd ed]. Menlo Park, Calif: Addison-Wesley)

hunger and inability to take in calories may be an indication for artificial airway support.

The clinical grading of croup divides the illness into three classifications based on observable data.

Clinical Grading of Croup

- Grade I—Child is quiet at rest; barking cough and stridor occur when child is disturbed or agitated.
- Grade II—Child has stridor and mild sternal retraction when quiet.
- Grade III—Child has profound inspiratory stridor at rest; deep sternal retraction; restlessness; cyanosis.

Grade III is indicative of severe disease. These children require aggressive airway management.

Laboratory and Diagnostic Tests

It is advisable to keep intrusive procedures to a minimum, because crying and fear increase the work of breathing. In croup many physicians forgo the visualization of the epiglottis in favor of anteroposterior and lateral neck chest x rays as the primary diagnostic studies. An x ray of a child with croup usually demonstrates the characteristic steeple sign, narrowing of the tracheal diameter (Figure 16–4). Any attempt to visualize the epiglottis by direct examination may cause severe laryngospasm, necessitating immediate intubation or tracheostomy. Measuring oxygen saturation by

pulse oximetry is a less invasive means of assuring adequate oxygenation and tissue perfusion. Arterial blood gas sampling may be avoided if the child maintains an oxygen saturation greater than 95% on room air and has mild to moderate croup.

T R I A G E
Croup

Emergent
A child with profound inspiratory stridor at rest; deep sternal retractions; restlessness; pallor or cyanosis; inability to take oral fluids or handle secretions; markedly prolonged inspiratory phase.

Urgent
A child with stridor and mild sternal retractions at rest; is able to tolerate oral fluids; is pink in color.

Non-urgent
A child who is quiet at rest; has stridor, a barking cough only when agitated; is pink in color; has no retractions; is able to take fluids well; is able to play.

Nursing Diagnosis
Ineffective Breathing Pattern

Defining Characteristics

- Stridor on inspiration
- Retractions
- Hypoxia, restlessness
- Cough, barking

Nursing Interventions

- Obtain baseline oxygen saturation and administer humidfied supplemental oxygen as needed
- Administer medications as ordered
- Administer cold oral fluids
- Provide a calm environment

Expected Outcomes

- Stridor decreases or resolves
- Retractions decrease or resolve
- Patient is able to relax and appears well perfused
- Cough decreases in frequency and intensity

Nursing Diagnosis
Sensory-Perceptual Alteration: Input Excess or Sensory Overload

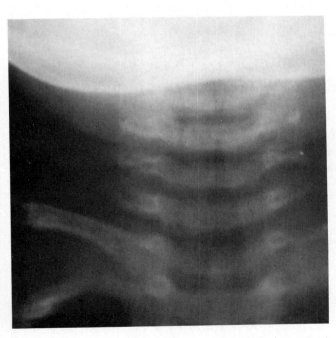

Figure 16–4. A 3-year-old boy with laryngotracheobronchitis (croup). Note the airway steeple sign and the narrowing of the tracheal diameter. (Photo courtesy of Richard DeNise, MD, and the Pediatric Radiology Department of Boston City Hospital)

Defining Characteristics

- Anxiety
- Restlessness
- Sleeplessness
- Amount or complexity of stimuli exceeds cognitive capabilities to handle sensory input

Nursing Interventions

- Speak in quiet comforting tones
- Provide simple explanations of all procedures before the procedure
- Allow child constant contact with parent
- Provide soft lighting if preferable to child

Expected Outcomes

- Child is able to relax in a comfortable position
- Child is able to cooperate with assessment and interventions

Nursing Diagnosis

Knowledge Deficit Related to Symptoms of Distress and Comfort Measures

Defining Characteristics

- Verbalization of fear and confusion regarding the sudden onset of cough and distress
- Verbalization of inadequate understanding of comfort measures parents can provide at home

Nursing Interventions

- Provide clear oral and written explanations of the symptoms of croup and signs of increased respiratory distress
- Provide oral and written explanations for home care

Expected Outcomes

- Parents are able to verbalize instructions for home care.
- Parents are able to verbalize signs of increased distress and to return if these develop.

Management

The nursing interventions in croup are focused on relieving anxiety and reducing the work of breathing. On completion of the initial assessment, cool humidified oxygen should be provided in a manner comfortable for the child. Racemic epinephrine is usually reserved for severe, or grade III, croup. It may be administered by nebulizer in a dose of 0.25–0.5 mL in 3 mL of normal saline solution. The use of subcutaneous epinephrine 1:1000, nebulized in normal saline solution is a cost effective alternative. Racemic epinephrine has been noted to reduce mucosal edema and laryngospasm. Children receiving this therapy experience profound relief of stridor and retractions, but they should be observed carefully for a rebound worsening of their condition. The rebound effect is thought to be caused by actual clinical deterioration rather than the waning effects of the drug. The need for management with racemic epinephrine may be an indication for hospital admission.

The use of steroids in croup remains controversial. Currently dexamethasone (Decadron) in a dose of 0.6–1.2 mg per kg is given IM for children with grade II to grade III croup who are to be cared for at home. The same dose is given IV or IM to children who require hospital admission. Skolnik (1990) reported that steroids act by reducing the local subglottic inflammation, usually about 6 hours after administration. No studies have shown any adverse effects of the use of this single dose of dexamethasone.

Antibiotics are of little use in uncomplicated cases of croup. Sedation should be avoided because restlessness, in addition to the oxygen saturation rate, is used as an indicator of the degree of hypoxia. As anxiety and dyspnea resolve, the child may want to lie down, but keeping the head of the bed elevated is advisable.

The decision for hospital admission rests on the degree of respiratory distress, the ability to maintain adequate hydration, the child's ability to rest, and the degree of parental apprehension.

Parent and Family Teaching and Psychosocial Support

If the child's croup is judged to be mild to moderate and the parents feel comfortable caring for the child at home, the parents should be given careful instructions for home care. These instructions should include comfort measures aimed at easing the child's respiratory effort, such as, the use of a cool mist vaporizer; keeping the windows open at night; offering frequent, cold oral fluids; and fever control. The parents also need to become familiar with the signs of increased respiratory distress (retractions, dyspnea, inability to take liquids, inability to rest) and seek immediate attention if these occur. Croup may reccur in the same child in subsequent seasons.

EPIGLOTTITIS

Epiglottitis, or supraglottic laryngitis, is the most emergent type of acute airway obstruction of childhood. This disease produces rapid onset inflammatory edema of the epiglottis and supraglottic structures. Epiglottitis occurs throughout the year, is seen in boys and girls with equal frequency, and usually affects older children and teenagers.

When a child with epiglottitis presents in the ED, an aura of heightened anxiety usually surrounds him or her. The anxiety on the part of the child and parents usually stems from the fact that the child appeared well until about 2–4 hours before arrival. The child typically has a fever, drools excessively, exhibits signs of air hunger (open-mouthed, gulping respirations, tachypnea, stridor, retractions, and a prolonged inspiratory phase), refuses or chokes on oral fluids, and refuses to lie down. Coughing is not as frequent as in croup. Nemes et al (1988) described the pathognomonic signs of epiglottitis as the four Ds—drooling, dysphonia, dysphagia, and distressed inspiration.

Etiology and Pathophysiology

Epiglottitis is bacterial in origin. *H. influenzae* type B is by far the most common organism involved; there is an occasional streptococcal, pneumococcal, or staphylococcal infection. The frequency of occurrence of epiglottitis is declining due to use of the *hemophilus influenzae* vaccine in infancy and early childhood.

After the colonization with *H. influenzae*, the onset of symptoms is rapid. Copious supraglottic edema is usually evident within 2 hours of onset (Figure 16–5). The edema is followed by increased mucosal secretion that may lead to secondary bronchopneumonia, atelectasis, pulmonary edema, or pleural effusion. The difficulty inspiring air past inflamed supraglottic structures causes inspiratory stridor, air hunger, retractions, tachypnea, and anxiety. Because of the fulminant nature of this bacterial infection, the temperature is usually high, more than 39°C. As clinical hypoxia progresses, cyanosis may become apparent.

History

The history of a child with epiglottitis typically reveals that the child appeared well until approximately 2–4 hours before arrival in the ED. The parent usually describes a rapid onset of fever, inability to eat or drink, drooling or choking, and difficulty breathing. Older children may have complained of a sore throat and have a muffled voice. Some children have an infrequent barking cough and an episode of vomiting.

Physical Assessment

The nursing assessment must be detailed and rapid, and invasive or disturbing techniques should be avoided. If the child is comfortable while sitting in the parent's lap he or she should remain there. The child's crying or attempts to make the child lie down may lead to severe laryngospasm and airway obstruction. The goal for this child is to protect the airway.

The most valuable assessment tools with this child are observation and auscultation. Only those vital signs that cause no discomfort to the child are obtained, and any signs of air hunger are carefully documented. Such observations include the presence and extent of stridor relative to the respiratory cycle; any timed prolongation of the inspiratory phase; the presence and depth of chest wall muscle retractions; the presence and location of cyanosis; and the degree of tachypnea and tachycardia. Such observations must be made continually to provide early detection of any changes.

Croup is the condition most closely resembling epiglottitis (Table 16–5). Differentiation should occur rapidly in light of the fulminant course of the symptomalogy of epiglottitis. Aspiration of a foreign body lodged in the upper airway and asthma also may be diagnostic considerations.

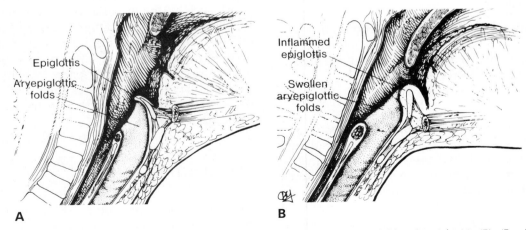

A   **B**

Figure 16–5. Appearance of the lateral neck region in a healthy child (**A**) and in a child with epiglottitis (**B**). (Reprinted with permission from Fleisher GR, Ludwig S [eds] [1993]. *Textbook of pediatric emergency medicine.* Baltimore: Williams & Wilkins)

TABLE 16–5. DIFFERENTIATION BETWEEN CROUP AND EPIGLOTTITIS

Clinical Feature	Croup	Epiglottitis
Etiology	Viral agent, usually one of the para-influenza type	Bacterial agent—usually *Haemophilus influenzae* type B
Occurrence	Seasonal, late fall and late spring; age 6 months to 3 years; recurrent	Not seasonal; seen in older children frequently
Respirations	Inspiratory stridor; varying degrees of substernal retractions may involve suprasternal notch; inspiratory phase usually prolonged	Inspiratory stridor; deep substernal retractions; unable to manage oral secretions (drooling is constant)
Assessment findings	History reveals a few days of upper respiratory infection with slow progression to hoarse, barking cough; may have low-grade fever; will accept fluids	Sudden onset of high fever (102°F–105°F); rapid development of hoarse barking cough; drooling; refusal to lie down. Symptoms usually heighten over 2–4 hours after onset. Intervention must be immediate.
Chest x rays	Laryngotracheal narrowing is the hallmark steeple sign	Inflamed epiglottis causing partial airway obstruction
Response to antibiotic therapy	None	Once a patent airway is established, intravenous antibiotics should be started as second priority

Laboratory and Diagnostic Tests

Laboratory data are minimal in suspected epiglottitis because of the need to avoid intrusive procedures. Oxygen saturation determinations using pulse oximetry may be obtained. If x ray studies of the neck are to be taken, the child must be accompanied by personnel and equipment necessary to perform emergency intubation and a tracheostomy. Typically an otorhinolaryngologist, an anesthesiologist, and an emergency nurse accompany the patient to the x ray suite. When the x rays confirm the diagnosis, the child and parents are escorted directly to the operating room. The drawing blood for a baseline CBC and cultures and the establishment of an intravenous line and visualization of the cherry-red epiglottis are deferred until the patient is in the operating room and a patent airway is assured.

The initial arterial blood gases usually show some degree of hypoxemia. The results of the CBC usually show an elevation of the leukocyte count indicative of a bacteriologic infection. Blood cultures often are positive for *H. influenzae* type B. X rays usually reveal a marked increase in the size of the epiglottis and edema of the supraglottic structures (Figure 16–6).

TRIAGE
Epiglottitis

Emergent

A child with suspected epiglottitis; a child with fever, sore throat, excessive drooling, muffled voice, dysphagia, and inspiratory stridor; cough may or may not be present.

Nursing Diagnosis
Impaired Swallowing

Defining Characteristics

- Inability to swallow food or fluids
- Inability to handle oral secretions manifested by drooling

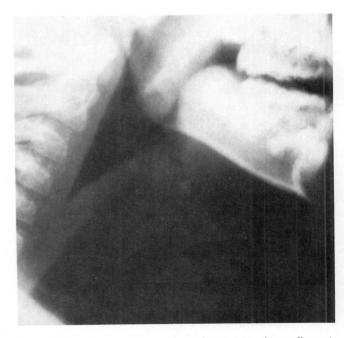

Figure 16–6. A 5-year-old boy with epiglottitis. Note the swollen epiglottis almost completely obstructing the airway. (Photo courtesy of Richard DeNise, MD, and the Pediatric Radiology Department of Boston City Hospital)

Nursing Interventions

- Provide nonintrusive means of emptying oral cavity
- Assure patent airway

Expected Outcomes

- Patient is able to remove oral secretions
- Patient is able to maintain a patent airway

Nursing Diagnosis
Anxiety

Defining Characteristics

- Apprehension about child's sudden onset of distress.
- Questions about child's outcome
- Restlessness

Nursing Interventions

- Provide calm simple explanations of every procedure before it is performed
- Provide careful explanations of what can be expected during ED visit
- Allow child to maintain comfortable position close to parents

Expected Outcomes

- Parents are able to verbalize understanding of ED procedures
- Child does not cry and is able to keep airway open

Nursing Diagnosis
Ineffective Airway Clearence

Defining Characteristics

- Inability to clear secretions
- Dyspnea on inspiration
- Tachypnea

Nursing Interventions

- Provide noninvasive method of clearing oral cavity
- Provide supplemental oxygen in a manner comfortable for the child

Expected Outcomes

- Child is able to clear secretions from mouth
- Child maintains pink color

Management
Nursing intervention must take place swiftly. At the same time a concerted effort is made to explain the procedures and treatments to the child and parents. The primary focus is to maintain a patent airway. Efforts must be directed toward keeping the child calm and comfortable. If the child is quiet while sitting in a parent's lap, he or she should be allowed to remain there during the brief history and physical assessment.

As soon as epiglottitis is suspected, the nurse must gather all of the equipment necessary to perform emergency intubation and a tracheostomy. It is imperative that the anesthesiologist, otorinolaryngologist, or emergency pediatrician who is prepared to perform these procedures have the appropriate equipment at hand at all times and that the child is never left unattended.

Ideally the establishment of an artificial airway should occur rapidly and in a controlled environment, such as an operating room. The child should be carried to the operating room in an upright position, preferably by the parent.

Hospital admission is always necessary for known or suspected epiglottitis. Intravenous fluid maintainence is necessary until oral fluids are easily tolerated after extubation. This is also the preferred route for the administration of antibiotics. Ampicillin (50–100 mg/kg/dose) is the drug of choice to combat *H. influenzae,* but there are strains of this organism known to be ampicillin-resistant. Dual coverage with chloramphenicol (20 mg/kg/dose) or one of the second- or third-generation cephalosporins, such as ceftriaxone (50 mg/kg/dose), is usually desirable until the culture and sensitivity results are available. The initial doses are administered as soon as possible in the operating room. Epiglottitis seldom recurs in the same child. Because most young children are now being vaccinated against *H. influenzae,* there may be a decreased incidence of epiglottitis in the future, especially in the younger age groups.

PNEUMONIA

Pneumonia may be best defined as an acute inflammation of the lungs. It may be caused by a variety of agents, including bacteria and viruses as well as fungi and other agents. Pneumonia is one of the most common infections of the lower respiratory tract in children and may occur at any age.

Etiology and Pathophysiology
A variety of organisms cause pneumonia in children. Respiratory viruses are the most common. The bacte-

rial organisms most frequently associated with pneumonia in children are *S. pneumoniae* in children of all ages and *H. influenzae*. In preschool-aged children, *Streptococcus pyogenes*, *Staphylococcus aureus*, *Pseudomonas aeruginosa*, *Klebsiella pneumoniae*, *Escherichia coli*, and *Mycobacterium tuberculosis* also are known causative agents.

The viral agents that have been identified as causative in childhood pneumonia include RSV, enteroviruses, adenoviruses, influenza, varicella, rubeola, and reoviruses. Also implicated are *Mycoplasma pneumoniae*, *Chlamydia*, Q fever, and protozoa, as well as several types of fungi. Pneumonia also may manifest itself after an aspiration episode or as a sequela of some chemical ingestions.

Causative agents of pneumonia in children may vary with the age of the child or area of infiltration on an x ray. Segmental or lobar pneumonias are usually caused by *S. pneumoniae* and may be associated with empyema. Staphylococcal pneumonia occurs in young infants, is less common than streptococcal pneumonia, and is often associated with empyema. Pneumonia is a frequent occurrence in children younger than 2 years and may be associated with a pleural effusion. Klebsiella pneumonia has a fulminant course and is seen in young infants or children with chronic pulmonary problems such as cystic fibrosis. Bronchopneumonias may be of mixed viral and bacterial etiology. Mycoplasma pneumonia is usually seen in older children and adolescents. Chlamydial pneumonia is usually found in infants from birth to 3–4 months of age. It occurs as a sequela of vaginal delivery by an infected mother and is usually seen in conjunction with conjunctivitis in the infant.

In children infected with the human immunodeficiency virus (HIV), the most common opportunistic infection is *Pneumocystis carinii* pneumonia (PCP). Another common problem in children with HIV is lymphoid interstitial pneumonitis (LIP), which may resemble tuberculosis, PCP, or viral pneumonia on a chest x ray.

History

The history of a child with pneumonia varies according to age, the causative organism, and the duration of evident symptoms. A young infant often has a history of fever and dyspnea that may have been preceded by symptoms of a cold, such as a cough, coryza, and irritability. There are also generalized symptoms associated with pneumonia in an infant. They include poor feeding, vomiting, and diarrhea. Extensive or fulminant pneumonia should be suspected when an infant has tachypnea, high fever, circumoral cyanosis, nasal flaring, retractions, and the hallmark expiratory grunt.

Adventitious breath sounds are not always present in infants with pneumonia.

An older child with pneumonia often has fever, chills, a cough (may be productive), headache, abdominal pain, and chest pain that is not necessarily localized to the area of infection. Tachypnea, tachycardia, dyspnea, retractions, and circumoral pallor or cyanosis also may be present.

A careful tracing of the onset of symptoms, beginning when the child last appeared well and continuing to the present should be obtained and recorded. The progression of symptoms over time may be an important factor in determining the possible causative agent. For young infants a history of conjunctivitis or maternal vaginitis around the time of delivery should be carefully documented. A history of any prior hypersensitivity to antibiotics in this child should be carefully elicited. The history or presence of any related symptoms, such as vomiting, headache, chest or abdominal pain, and lethargy, should be carefully documented.

Physical Assessment

An infant should be assessed in terms of the quality of respirations (tachypnea with minimal distress as opposed to slower but more labored respirations); the presence, location, and depth of retractions; the presence of a cough; the presence and location of cyanosis, including assessment of capillary filling in the distal portions of limbs; nasal flaring; and the presence of expiratory grunting. The location of any adventitious sounds, or areas of decreased breath sounds and the quality of the infant's cry are documented. Some assessment of the infant's ability to tolerate oral fluids should be made to determine the infant's ability to maintain adequate hydration.

An older child may exhibit increased vocal tactile fremitus, a dull percussion note over the affected area, and rales on auscultation. Careful documentation must also be made of the child's respiratory effort as a baseline to assess improvement as opposed to deterioration of the condition. Such assessment should include the presence, location, and depth of retractions; the presence and location of pallor or cyanosis; and the degree of lethargy.

A child who arrives in the ED with a primary episode of wheezing and dyspnea should be considered to have pneumonia as a precipitating factor. The aspiration of a foreign body also must be considered.

Laboratory and Diagnostic Tests

Blood studies for a child with suspected pneumonia usually include a CBC and blood cultures. A bedside cold agglutinin also may be performed on an older child or adolescent with pneumonia to detect *Mycoplasma pneumoniae*. Oxygen saturation is measured by pulse oximetry. More invasive arterial blood gas sampling is reserved for the most severe cases of pneumonia. Sputum for culture and sensitivity also may be obtained as may a smear for microscopic examination in the ED. Anteroposterior and lateral chest x rays are most helpful in confirming the diagnosis of pneumonia and in identifying areas of involvement (Figure 16–7). The clinical symptoms of pneumonia may be present for up to 72 hours before x ray evidence is visible.

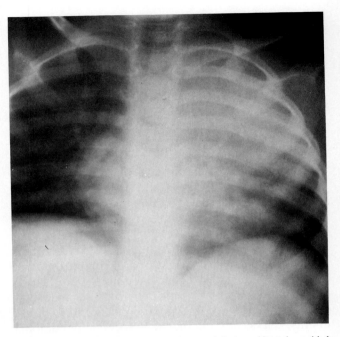

Figure 16–7. A 2-month-old girl with consolidation of lingula and left upper lobe. Diagnosis: left upper lobe pneumonia. (Photo courtesy of Richard DeNise, MD, and the Pediatric Radiology Department of Boston City Hospital)

TRIAGE
Pneumonia

Emergent —————————————————
An infant or child with cyanosis or pallor; decreased breath sounds; profound dyspnea (retractions flaring); tachypnea; in severe respiratory distress.

Urgent —————————————————
An infant or child with pink color; mild to moderate retractions; tachypnea; areas of rales or decreased breath sounds; in mild to moderate distress.

Non-urgent —————————————————
An infant or child with rales on auscultation; no flaring or retractions; pink color; good air movement; tolerating oral fluids well; alert and able to play.

Nursing Diagnosis
Ineffective Airway Clearance

Defining Characteristics

- Abnormal breath sounds
- Cough
- Tachypnea
- Dyspnea
- Cyanosis

Nursing Interventions

- Administer supplemental oxygen if needed
- Administer medications as ordered
- Offer oral fluids as tolerated
- Monitor vital signs and oxygen saturation

Expected Outcomes

- Respiratory effort decreases
- Child's color is normal
- Tachypnea resolves
- Frequency of cough decreases

Nursing Diagnosis
Ineffective Breathing Pattern

Defining Characteristics

- Retractions and nasal flaring
- Dyspnea and tachypnea
- Cough
- Cyanosis

Nursing Interventions

- Monitor vital signs and oxygen saturation
- Administer supplemental oxygen as needed
- Administer medications as ordered

Expected Outcomes

- Respiratory effort normalizes
- Respiratory rate returns to normal
- Color improves
- Cough decreases in frequency

Nursing Diagnosis
Impaired Gas Exchange

Defining Characteristics
- Restlessness
- Cyanosis
- Lethargy
- Irritability

Nursing Interventions
- Monitor vital signs and oxygen saturation
- Administer supplemental oxygen
- Administer medications ordered

Expected Outcomes
- Color and perfusion return to normal
- Level of awareness improves
- Child or infant is consolable

Management
Treatment varies according to the age of the child, the suspected causative agent, the severity of symptoms, and the immune status of the host. Infants younger than 2 months usually require hospital admission for IV antibiotic therapy. Table 16–6 contains the antibiotics used in the treatment of pneumonia.

Children from infancy to 6 years of age usually contract viral pneumonia. If the white blood cell count is above 20,000, however, *S. pneumoniae* or *H. influenzae* should be suspected as the causative agent in this age group. Intravenous ampicillin may be administered to children who are in great distress or are refusing or not tolerating oral fluids. Dual coverage with one of the second- or third-generation cephalosporins (cefuroxime or ceftriaxone) to combat ampicillin-resistant strains of *H. influenzae* may be ordered. Therapy if the child is allergic to penicillin may include trimethoprim-sulfamethoxazole. Children with minimum distress who are tolerating oral fluids well can usually be treated at home with oral antibiotic therapy. Aerosolized bronchodilators may be a helpful adjunct at any age.

In addition to a viral or bacterial etiology, in school-aged children and adolescents, *Mycoplasma pneumoniae* should be considered. Erythromycin is the drug of choice to combat *Mycoplasma,* as well as *Chlamydia* and bronchopneumonias. Parents should be instructed always to give erythromycin with food because gastric irritation may be severe. If intravenous erythromycin is to be given the ED nurse should prepare the parents and child by informing them that the medicine is irritating to veins and the IV site may need to be changed often.

Pneumocystis carinii pneumonia is the most common opportunistic infection seen in children infected with HIV. These children usually present with fever and tachypnea and may have infiltrates seen on an x ray. The drug of choice is trimethoprim-sulfamethoxazole; occasionally aerosolized pentamidine and steroids are given. Hospital admission is necessary for any child with great distress or a supplemental oxygen requirement or who is unable to tolerate oral hydration. Children with PCP who require artificial airway support and ventilation have a poor prognosis. Lymphoid interstitial pneumonitis is also seen in children with HIV. These children usually have an oxygen requirement and may be treated with home oxygen and oral steroids if distress is not severe.

Hospital admission is recommended when (1) respiratory distress is severe; (2) supplemental oxygen is needed (room air saturation < 95% by pulse oximetry); (3) the child is unable to tolerate oral fluids or medications because of respiratory distress or vomiting; (4) the infant is younger than 2 months of age; (5) underlying disease is present (eg, cardiac disease, sickle cell disease, cystic fibrosis); (6) the parents or caretakers are unable to care for the child.

Parent and Family Teaching and Psychosocial Support
In addition to specific instructions for administering the medications prescribed, parents should be advised to complete the course of antibiotics even if the child's condition improves greatly in a few days. The parents or caretakers need reinforcement about the importance of oral hydration and oral hygiene. Humidification using a cool mist vaporizer may be recommended. Families need to be aware of the signs of increased respiratory distress (retractions, tachypnea, intolerance of oral fluids, inability to rest). They should be advised to contact their primary provider or return to the ED if these signs occur. Families also require instructions on the management of fever.

PERTUSSIS

Pertussis, or whooping cough, is a bacterial infection of the respiratory tract. It may occur at any age but is most common in infants younger than 1 year who have not been immunized properly. Pertussis has an incubation period of 7–21 days and occurs most frequently in late summer and early fall.

TABLE 16–6. COMMON ANTIBIOTICS USED IN THE TREATMENT OF PNEUMONIA

Drug	Dosage, Route, and Frequency	Nursing Implications
Amoxicillin	Suspension: 125 mg/5 mL and 250 mg/5 mL Capsules: 250-mg 50 mg/kg/day up to 250–500 mg (every 8 hours)	May cause mild diarrhea; allergic reactions may include a rash
Amoxicillin and clavulanic acid	Tabs and chew tabs: 125 mg and 250 mg Suspension: 125 mg and 250 mg/5 ml 20–40 mg/kg/day dosed as amoxicillin every 8 hours Max 250–500 mg/dose	Causes more diarrhea than amoxicillin
Ampicillin	Suspension: 125 mg and 250 mg/5 mL Capsules: 250–500 mg IV solution: 250 mg, 500 mg, 1 g 50–100 mg/dose	May cause diarrhea Allergic reactions include rash
Ampicillin sulbactam	Vial: 1 g dosed as ampicillin	Diarrhea, allergic rash
Cefaclor	Suspension: 125–250 mg/5 mL Capsules: 250–500 mg 40 mg/kg/day q 8 hours	Not recommended for newborns. Allergic reactions often severe, including erythema multiformae and serum sickness
Cefotaxime	Vials: 1–2 g IV 20–50 mg/kg/dose every 4–6 hours Max 12 g/24 hours	Toxic reactions include neutropenia, thrombocytopenia, eosinophilia, elevated BUN, creatinine, and liver function tests
Ceftriaxone	Vials: 250 mg, 500 mg, 1 g, 2 g 50 mg/kg/dose every 12–24 hours	May cause elevated liver function tests and diarrhea
Cefuroxime	Vials: 750–1500 mg Tabs: 125 mg, 250 mg, 500 mg 50 mg/kg/dose every 6–8 hours	May cause thrombophlebitis at IV site. Toxicities similar to cefotaxime
Erythromycin	Suspension: 200 mg, 400 mg/5 mL Tabs: 200 (chew), 250 mg, 500 mg IV vial: 500 mg, 1 gm 20/50 mg/kg/day q 6 hours PO or IV	Give after meals; GI upset common; may enhance levels of other medications such as digoxin, methylprednisolone, or theophylline
Tetracycline	Tabs: 250 mg, 500 mg Capsules: 100 mg, 250 mg, 500 mg Suspension: 125 mg/5 mL Injection: 250 mg, 500 mg po: 25–50 mg/kg/day q 6 hours IV: 10 mg/kg/dose q 8–12 hours	Not given to children younger than 8 years. May cause GI upset, hepatotoxicity rash, photosensitivity Do not give with dairy products Give 1 hour before or 2 hours after meal
Trimethoprim/sulfamethoxazole	6–12 mg TMP/kg/day q 12 hours orally In pneumocystis: 15–20 mg/kg/day q 6–8 hours po or IV	Not used in children younger than 2 months May cause bone marrow suppression, GI upset

BUN, blood urea nitrogen; GI, gastrointestinal.

Etiology and Pathophysiology

Pertussis is caused by *Bordetella pertussis*, which primarily affects the bronchi and bronchioles. It is spread by droplet nuclei and can be cultured from the nasopharynx early in the disease process.

There are well-defined stages of pertussis. The initial catarrhal stage resembles a simple upper respiratory tract infection with sneezing and a cough that usually occurs at night. Over the initial stage, the child's condition slowly worsens; a low-grade fever and a cough develop.

The paroxysmal phase is marked by the onset of prolonged coughing spasms that end with the hallmark inspiratory whoop. The effort expended by the child in these spasmodic coughing episodes is such that vomiting, sweating, neck vein distention, confusion, and convulsions may occur in the aftermath. During this phase mucus becomes thick and tenacious and may cause obstructive emphysema or atelectasis through plugging. In very young infants choking spells may be observed instead of a whoop. It should be remembered that coughing spasms are exacerbated by the inhalation of irritants and by excitement or sudden changes in activity or temperature.

The convalescent phase lasts approximately 2 weeks. During this time the severity of the paroxysms decreases, while the interval between spasms gradually increases until resolved.

If a child presents in the ED during the first phase of pertussis, the diagnosis will probably be missed. Pertussis is usually indistinguishable from a common cold until the paroxysmal stage. The child at this stage may have fever, hypoxia, and the paroxysmal cough. The child also may have petechiae above the nipple line, otitis media, atelectasis, vomiting, pneumothorax, and the sudden appearance of hernias as a result of exertion during coughing.

History

The history typically reveals the progression of the symptoms of an upper respiratory tract infection with gradual worsening of the cough until the onset of the spasms with an inspiratory whoop. The child may not have been fully immunized.

Assessment

Because excitement and crying tend to worsen the coughing paroxysms, care should be taken to keep the child as calm as possible. The child is observed for cyanosis before, during, and after a paroxysm. The depth of substernal retraction during the inspiratory whoop is noted. The frequency and length of the coughing spasms should be timed. Auscultation should be performed during a quiet time with careful attention to the detection of adventitious breath sounds or diminished breath sounds over an area of atelectasis, since pertussis may be complicated by pneumonia.

Other types of respiratory infections may mimic pertussis. These include RSV, influenza, adenoviruses, and chlamydial infections. The possibility of an inhaled bronchial foreign body also must be considered.

Laboratory and Diagnostic Tests

Laboratory data may reveal an elevated white blood cell count with leukocytosis. A nasopharyngeal swab may be obtained for culture or a fluorescent antibody stain. A chest x ray usually shows peribronchial cuffing with patchy infiltrates and a "shaggy" heart border. Oxygen saturation measured by pulse oximetry should be monitored to determine trends both at rest and during coughing paroxysms.

TRIAGE
Pertussis

Emergent ————————————————————
An infant or child with pallor or cyanosis during coughing paroxysms; deep retraction during an inspiratory whoop; or seizure activity.

Urgent ————————————————————
An infant or child with prolonged coughing paroxysms not associated with color change; vomiting; petechiae; and areas of decreased breath sounds.

Non-urgent ————————————————————
An infant or child with brief and infrequent coughing paroxysms; pink color; ability to tolerate oral fluids well; clear breath sounds with good air movement over all fields.

Nursing Diagnosis
Ineffective Airway Clearance

Defining Characteristics

- Abnormal breath sounds
- Cough
- Cyanosis
- Excessive thick secretions

Nursing Interventions

- Administer humidified oxygen
- Administer medication as ordered
- Suction nose and oral cavity as needed
- Monitor vital signs and oxygen saturation rate

Expected Outcomes

- Color improves
- Secretions are removed
- Air movement improves
- Coughing spasms are less frequent

Nursing Diagnosis
Impaired Gas Exchange

Defining Characteristics

- Restlessness
- Irritability
- Inability to remove secretions
- Hypoxia

Nursing Interventions

- Administer humidified oxygen
- Administer medication as ordered
- Use bulb to suction nasal and oral cavity as needed
- Monitor vital signs and oxygen saturation

Expected Outcomes

- Child is consolable and able to rest
- Airway is clear
- Color improves

Nursing Diagnosis

Sleep Pattern Disturbance

Defining Characteristics

- Interrupted sleep
- Restlessness
- Frequent yawning

Nursing Interventions

- Provide a quiet, softly lit environment
- Keep intrusive procedures to a minimum

Expected Outcomes

- Child is able to nap for longer periods
- Child is aware of surroundings and is interactive when awake

Management

Airway clearance is the first step in managing pertussis. Gentle suctioning may be necessary to clear thick secretions from the nasopharynx. Humified oxygen should be readily available for administration during and after coughing episodes.

Although strict isolation is difficult to achieve in an ED, a private room with a closed door is helpful in protecting other patients. In addition to universal precautions, masks should be worn by all persons in the room and care must be taken when handling and disposing of secretions. Isolation is typically maintained for at least the first 5 days of antibiotic therapy.

The antibiotic of choice for pertussis is erythromycin, 50 mg/kg/day, every 6 hours, orally whenever possible, for 10–14 days. Antibiotic therapy is effective in the decontamination of secretions but cannot be relied upon to shorten the course of the disease or lessen the severity of the coughing spasms.

Ongoing assessment and documentation of the child's condition should be made. These include the frequency, duration, and sequelae of paroxysms as well as observations of color changes and oxygen saturation during these events. Supplemental oxygen and suctioning may be required, and these children require close monitoring.

Hospital admission is usually recommended for infants with pertussis, especially those who exhibit respiratory distress in association with paroxysms. Arrangements must be made to treat exposed persons. Exposed children younger than 7 years who have had a primary series of pertussis vaccine should receive a booster vaccine, preferably as diphtheria-pertussis-tetanus (DPT), as well as prophylaxis with erythromycin. Older children and other adults also may be provided prophylaxis with erythromycin. Pertussis immune globulin has not proved helpful.

Parent and Family Teaching and Psychosocial Support

Because most children with pertussis require admission to the hospital, the ED nurse may provide the parents with information about the expected course of the illness. Helping the parents position the child and administer oxygen during a coughing paroxysm may provide them with a way to give extra comfort to the child. Parents also may have questions about the visiting or rooming-in policy at the hospital and how to arrange treatment for other exposed family members.

PNEUMOTHORAX

Aside from the neonatal period, spontaneous pneumothorax occurs most often in adolescents and young adults. It is defined as a collection of air in the pleural space caused by rupture of an alveolar bleb on the surface of the pleura and results in partial collapse of one or both lungs.

Mild unilateral or bilateral pneumothorax may be asymptomatic and remains undetected unless specifically sought. Extensive (> 40%) pneumothoraces are painful and cause tachypnea and dyspnea. Older children may complain of being unable to take a deep breath.

Etiology and Pathophysiology

Pneumothoraces may occur spontaneously or secondary to bronchial obstruction, trauma, ruptured abscesses or cysts, a fungal process, cancer, or tuberculosis. The leakage of small amounts of air unilaterally or bilaterally may be asymptomatic. By contrast, a large amount of displaced air prevents full expansion of the lung on the side involved. This causes tachypnea, dyspnea, grunting, hypoxia, and cyanosis. Contrary to most respiratory problems that cause retraction of the chest wall musculature, pneumothorax may cause bulging of these muscles, especially the intercostal muscles over the affected area. Unilateral tension pneumothorax causes tracheal deviation and a shift of the mediastinum toward the affected side.

Pneumomediastinum differs from pneumothorax in the location of trapped extrapleural air. The free air of a pneumomediastinum is located between the lungs, around the heart anteriorly or posteriorly. This condition may manifest itself with dyspnea, crepitant swelling in the precordial and supraclavicular area, neck vein distention, and distant heart sounds. Breath sounds may appear normal.

History

A history of events leading to the current problem should be obtained as should a subjective and objective description of the symptoms. A history of a pneumothorax increases the likelihood that this is a recurrence of the problem. It is important to note whether there was a sudden onset of symptoms or whether progressive respiratory illness has preceded the problem. A history of trauma to the chest should be elicited.

Physical Assessment

The chest is observed for symmetry of movement during inspiration and expiration, presence of retractions or bulging of intercostal muscles, neck vein engorgement, and change in coloring. The neck and chest are palpated for crepitant swellings. The trachea is palpated for deviation from midline. Auscultation of the chest is performed to check distant heart or breath sounds. With pneumothorax the breath sounds seem distant or diminished over affected areas, and the location of heart sounds may have shifted. Conversely, with pneumomediastinum the breath sounds are usually normal, whereas heart sounds are muffled or distant. The percussion note over affected areas is hyperresonant.

Laboratory and Diagnostic Tests

Determination of oxygen saturation is a noninvasive method of monitoring interference with gas exchange. A child who has symptomatic pneumothorax never should be sent to the radiology department unaccompanied. Anteroposterior and lateral upright x rays may be obtained in the ED before intervention, or the child may be accompanied to the radiology department by the ED nurse or physician.

TRIAGE
Pneumothorax

Emergent
A child with dyspnea at rest; cyanosis; tracheal deviation; absent breath sounds unilaterally; and distended neck veins.

Urgent
A child with normal color; mild to moderate shortness of breath; an area of diminished breath sounds; trachea at midline.

Nursing Diagnosis
Fear

Defining Characteristics

- Fear of procedure
- Increased information-seeking
- Perceived inability to control event

Nursing Interventions

- Explain procedure in a calm manner
- Offer only realistic choices

Expected Outcomes

- Child tolerates procedure without panic
- Child participates in decision when applicable

Nursing Diagnosis
Ineffective Breathing Pattern

Defining Characteristics

- Dyspnea
- Use of accessory muscles
- Altered chest excursion
- Cyanosis

Nursing Interventions

- Administer supplemental oxygen
- Monitor vital signs and oxygen saturation
- Assist with and coach patient through chest tube insertion
- Monitor functioning of chest tube drainage system

Expected Outcomes

- Respiratory effort normalizes
- Chest excursion become symmetric
- Color improves

Management

Hospital admission is recommended for any child who has the symptoms of a pneumothorax. Bedrest and the administration of oxygen are the only treatments necessary for partial, mildly symptomatic pneumothorax. Serial chest x rays and assessments are usually performed to detect any evidence of further collapse or re-expansion.

Tension pneumothorax is a life-threatening emergency requiring immediate intervention. The child may be placed in a sitting position while a large-bore needle or catheter is introduced between the second and third ribs on the anterolateral portion of the chest for immediate relief. Chest tube insertion always follows the needle thoracotomy. Children with more than a 40% pneumothorax usually require chest tube insertion with closed drainage to evacuate the pleural space and to re-expand the lung. The chest tube typically is inserted using local anesthesia and a blunt dissection technique at the space between the fourth and fifth ribs on the midaxillary line of the affected side. The surgeon inserts the tube along the top edge of the fifth rib because of the location of nerve bundles along the bottom edge of each rib. The chest tube must be attached at all times to a closed-seal drainage system with the air fluid level clearly marked and each connection taped separately. Symptoms are relieved as the lung re-expands.

Parent and Family Teaching and Psychosocial Support

It is important that the ED nurse anticipate the need for a closed thoracotomy and assemble all necessary equipment for insertion and prepare the closed drainage system in a sterile manner. The child and parents should be given a clear, understandable explanation of the procedure. If a parent elects to stay with the child, it will usually be the parent and the ED nurse who provide coaching and verbal encouragement during the procedure. Once inserted and sutured in place, the chest tube is connected to the drainage system by the ED nurse, who is then responsible for taping each connection separately and monitoring the system to assure proper functioning. The parents and child should be provided with an explanation of signs of improvement and of signs of increased respiratory distress so this information can be communicated to the care providers.

FOREIGN BODY ASPIRATION

Aspiration of a foreign body occurs when material is inhaled and becomes lodged in the upper or lower respiratory tract. This phenomenon is usually seen in children younger than 4 years with a peak incidence among children 1–2 years of age.

Etiology and Pathophysiology

The most common foreign body aspirated is food—nuts most frequently, followed by sunflower seeds, beans, popcorn, fruit and vegetable peels, and pieces of hot dog. Coins and inorganic objects also have been aspirated.

In the period immediately following the aspiration there is usually an episode of choking, coughing, gagging, wheezing, or stridor. Then symptoms may subside for days, weeks, or months without recurrence unless the object becomes dislodged and moves. This cessation of symptoms occurs as the lining of the respiratory tract adapts to the presence of the foreign material. Disturbance of ventilation distal to the foreign body, however, continues over time. Although aspiration of organic foreign bodies is by far more common than that of inorganic materials, the identification of organic materials on an x ray is often more difficult because these objects are radiolucent.

Bronchial foreign body aspiration is most common. The usual site of lodging is the right mainstem bronchus; the left mainstem bronchus is the second most frequent site. When a child arrives in the ED in the period immediately following bronchial aspiration of a foreign body, he or she may exhibit paroxysmal coughing, dyspnea, wheezing, rales, and cyanosis. Over time, the wheezing may persist with rales and intermittent fever, making differentiation between aspiration, asthma, and pneumonia difficult. The most common radiographic finding is obstructive emphysema, although as time goes on, a secondary pneumonia, atelectasis, or air trapping distal to the location of the foreign body may be seen. If the foreign body goes undetected for a period of weeks to months, the child may experience recurrent bouts of pneumonia.

Laryngotracheal foreign body aspirations are more rare than bronchial aspirations and are usually more difficult to detect. A chest x ray on inspiration and expiration may appear normal, necessitating a fluoroscopic examination for detection. The fluoroscopic examination may also yield normal findings, placing the emphasis on the history and clinical features. The signs of a laryngotracheal foreign body include dyspnea, cough, stridor, and cyanosis.

History

The history of an observed aspiration or choking spell is the single most important diagnostic tool. When the child has exhibited periods of intermittent wheezing, stridor, dyspnea, or cyanosis over time, the nurse must exact a meticulous history of events leading up to the primary episode. The parent may recall witnessing the aspiration or the immediate sequelae, then negating its importance in light of the rapid resolution of symptoms.

Physical Assessment

Because the emphasis of detection of an inhaled foreign body is usually placed on the history and clinical signs and symptoms rather than on radiologic or laboratory tests, careful attention must be paid to documentation of physical findings. The child is observed for respiratory effort and presence of cyanosis, pallor, or retractions. The trachea is palpated for any deviation from midline associated with mediastinal shifting when lobar collapse secondary to obstruction exists.

Auscultation must be performed with careful attention to minute details. The presence of adventitious or decreased breath sounds must be noted with description of their exact location and intensity. The most frequent complications of aspiration of foreign bodies are pneumonia, atelectasis, bronchiectasis, and pneumothorax.

Any infant or toddler who arrives in the ED with clinical signs and symptoms resembling those of asthma, bronchitis, pneumonia, or croup must be assessed for an aspirated foreign body. The history of the respiratory problem should be elicited carefully for any correlation with an aspiration. As previously discussed, this may involve retracing events as far back as a few months.

Laboratory and Diagnostic Tests

Oxygen saturation should be measured using pulse oximetry. When a child presents with symptoms of pneumonia, a CBC and a blood culture may be helpful. Although the chest x rays may be inconclusive, every attempt should be made to obtain high-quality anteroposterior and lateral views of the chest during inspiration and expiration (Figure 16–8).

Fluoroscopy may be necessary to determine the location of a bronchial foreign body, but children with laryngotracheal foreign bodies also may have normal fluoroscopic examinations. A lung scan may be needed to localize the object in such patients.

TRIAGE
Foreign Body Aspiration

Emergent
An infant or child with cyanosis; dyspnea; profound tachypnea or distress; decreased breath sounds.

Urgent
An infant or child with pink color; mild to moderate retractions and dyspnea; fairly good air movement.

Nursing Diagnosis
Impaired Swallowing

Defining Characteristics

- Difficulty swallowing, excessive drooling
- Coughing or choking when swallowing
- Evidence of aspiration

Nursing Interventions

- Provide calm explanations of x rays and expected procedures
- Provide a means of gently removing oral secretions

Expected Outcomes

- The child will tolerate x rays and procedures without increased distress
- The child or parent will remove secretions in a comfortable manner

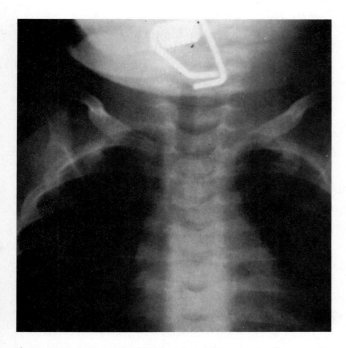

Figure 16–8. A 7-month-old infant found lying on the floor gasping and coughing. Diagnosis: clothespin in the hypopharynx. (Photo courtesy of Richard DeNise, MD, and the Pediatric Radiology Department of Boston City Hospital)

Nursing Diagnosis
Ineffective Airway Clearance

Defining Characteristics

- Abnormal breath sounds
- Cough
- Dyspnea
- Cyanosis

Nursing Interventions

- Administer oxygen
- Provide a calm atmosphere
- Monitor vital signs and oxygen saturation

Expected Outcomes

- Color improves
- Respiratory effort eases
- Oxygen saturation remains above 95%

Nursing Diagnosis
Knowledge Deficit Relative to Child Safety

Defining Characteristics

- Verbalization of child's consumption of inappropriate foods for age or toys
- Low readiness for reception of information secondary to anxiety

Nursing Interventions

- Provide explanations of all procedures to identify and correct the current problem
- Provide simple, nonthreatening information about the common choking hazards to children and child-proofing the home once babies become mobile

Expected Outcomes

- The parent verbalizes an understanding of age-appropriate foods and toys
- The parent verbalizes an understanding of the steps needed to child-proof the home

Management
A child who has aspirated a foreign body that completely occludes the airway is in an acute emergency. This child probably is in respiratory arrest by the time he or she reaches the ED. A history of such an aspiration necessitates immediate delivery of age-appropriate maneuvers to dislodge the object, ie, chest or abdominal thrusts. If these measures fail to restore a patent airway, an immediate tracheostomy must be per-

formed to open the airway before cardiopulmonary resuscitation (CPR) can be effective.

Hospital admission is always recommended for suspected foreign body aspiration because of its high mortality. Attempts to dislodge and remove laryngotracheal or bronchial foreign bodies that cause partial airway obstruction should be reserved for a controlled environment such as an operating room. The foreign bodies are usually removed using general anesthesia with laryngoscopy, tracheoscopy, or bronchoscopy. Emergency attempts at removal may simply relocate the object and cause additional respiratory compromise.

Management in the ED is focused on supportive measures to promote more effective respiration. Humidified oxygen is desirable when any cyanosis is present, when wheezing or stridor are severe, and to maintain oxygen saturation above 95%. An intravenous line should be established for administration of fluids and medications. Antibiotics are necessary with pneumonia and at times are used prophylactically before removal of the foreign body. Steroids may be helpful in reducing edema before removal of the foreign body and after removal. As is true with esophageal foreign bodies, after the removal of a single foreign body, the child must be assessed for the presence of another.

Parent and Family Teaching and Psychosocial Support
The ED nurse can ease parental anxiety by providing calm, objective information on expected ED and operative procedures. In a nonjudgmental manner, the ED nurse may supply the parents with information on child-proofing the home.

CARBON MONOXIDE POISONING

Carbon monoxide poisoning is a toxic condition produced when carbon monoxide gas is inhaled, usually in a fire, from car exhaust fumes, space heaters, barbeque grills, or furnaces.

The clinical features differ according to the extent of toxicity. Symptoms may be generalized in children, making diagnosis in the absence of known exposure difficult. At the lower spectrum of toxicity, nausea, vomiting, headache, dizziness, or blurred vision may be present. One may anticipate a carboxyhemoglobin level of 20–40% when the child is irritable and tired and has muscle weakness, nausea or vomiting, and palpitations. Children with carboxyhemoglobin levels above 40%, if conscious, are ataxic and manifest central nervous system damage, which may progress to coma and death.

Etiology and Pathophysiology

Carbon monoxide is a colorless, odorless gas that, when inhaled, combines with hemoglobin at a rate 240 times faster than oxygen. This greatly reduces the amount of oxygen available for transport, producing tissue hypoxia. The body responds to this tissue hypoxia by increasing the respiratory rate, which leads to increased inspiration of the gas and a further decrease in available oxyhemoglobin.

Because the brain and heart have the highest need for oxygen, these organs often demonstrate the ill effects of carbon monoxide poisoning. Early symptoms include irritability, headache, fatigue, weakness, confusion, ataxia, and nausea. Tachycardia and tachypnea are common; children with cardiac lesions are often unable to compensate well for the increased cardiac demands. Cherry-red skin is a late sign of severe carbon monoxide poisoning and is often a poor prognostic indicator.

History

The history of a known or possible exposure to carbon monoxide gas provides the emergency nurse with the best possible indication for the immediate intervention necessary. When the clinical index of suspicion is high, the parents should be questioned closely for relevant history. Llano and Raffin (1990) discussed the importance of obtaining any history of similar problems in other family members and also in pets because they often experience symptoms sooner than people. The time of onset of symptoms and their progression must be carefully noted.

Physical Assessment

A brief but thorough assessment should be performed, including baseline determinations of vital signs, observations of respiratory pattern and effort, nausea and vomiting, and manifestations of central nervous system alterations.

Laboratory and Diagnostic Tests

An arterial blood gas determination with carboxyhemoglobin level is mandatory and should be repeated as treatment progresses to ensure resolution. Chest x rays may be helpful in providing baseline data that later aid in detecting complications, but radiographs should be deferred until adequate treatment has been provided.

TRIAGE
Carbon Monoxide Poisoning

Emergent ————————————————
A child with altered mental status, tachypnea, ataxia, and palpitations.

Urgent ————————————————
A child with nausea and vomiting, headache, dizziness, visual disturbance.

Nursing Diagnosis
Impaired Gas Exchange

Defining Characteristics

- Increased respiratory rate
- Increased pulse rate
- Confusion, irritability, somnolence

Nursing Interventions

- Administer high concentration of oxygen
- Monitor vital signs
- Monitor alterations in level of consciousness

Expected Outcomes

- Respiratory rate returns to normal
- Patient becomes more alert and is consolable
- Vital signs are normal

Nursing Diagnosis
Altered Tissue Perfusion

Defining Characteristics

- Gas exchange problems
- Delayed capillary refill
- Weak distal arterial pulse

Nursing Interventions

- Administer high-concentration oxygen
- Provide a warm environment

Expected Outcomes

- Perfusion improves and capillary refill is brisk
- Distal pulses are strong

Management

The primary treatment is the administration of 100% oxygen, which should be initiated immediately in any case of suspected carbon monoxide poisoning. In children with evidence of central nervous system impairment, elective intubation ensures adequate ventilation with 100% oxygen. For patients with carboxyhemoglobin levels above 60%, a hyperbaric oxygen chamber may be used to reduce the carboxyhemoglobin level quickly. Intravenous maintainence fluids should be administered with caution to avoid cerebral edema. Efforts should be made to reduce the body's oxygen requirements by keeping the child quiet and calm. In some cases acidosis may need to be corrected by administration of intravenous sodium bicarbonate.

Children with known or suspected inhalation of carbon monoxide are usually admitted for close observation and oxygen therapy. Because carbon monoxide has a half life of approximately 2 hours, oxygen therapy is needed for a prolonged period of time. Initial carboxyhemoglobin levels may be misleading in that tissues continue to release the carbon monoxide molecules stored for up to 7 days. Pulmonary complications occur in 15–20% of children with severe burns and are frequently seen in fire victims who suffer no thermal burns.

Parent and Family Education and Psychosocial Support

Common causes of carbon monoxide poisoning are a faulty home heating system and faulty exhaust systems in automobiles. Families should be encouraged to obtain at least annual inspections to ensure proper functioning. The ED nurse may be of assistance to families who must persuade their landlords to inspect and repair faulty equipment in the home.

SMOKE INHALATION

Smoke inhalation can be described as the breathing in of particles and gases, often the products of combustion, that produce some degree of damage to the structures of the airway.

Children exposed to fires or explosions should be treated as if smoke inhalation has occurred until it is proved otherwise. A high index of suspicion for smoke inhalation is present when there are burns of the head, neck or chest; singed facial or nasal hairs; soot in the nasal secretions, oral mucosa, or sputum; edema of the oropharynx or trachea; a history that the exposure took place in a closed environment; a history of a lapse of consciousness during the fire; extensive dermal burns; or any history of prior pulmonary or cardiac problems.

The structures of the upper airway may suffer actual burns. These result in edema of the oropharynx

and trachea, which have the potential to obstruct the airway. Early intubation to ensure a patent airway is critical to these children. Similarly, severe burns of the chest may limit the expansion needed for adequate ventilation. These children may require escharotomies in the ED as a life-saving measure.

Etiology and Pathophysiology

The extent of damage to the bronchial lining and smaller tributaries is difficult to assess immediately upon the child's arrival in the ED. Chest x rays may show no apparent abnormalities in the first 48 hours. The damage caused by smoke inhalation begins with the destruction of the ciliated epithelium and mucosal edema. The gaseous products of combustion may extend their damage to structures of the lower respiratory tract, affecting the lining of the bronchioles and alveoli. The linings of the trachea and bronchi may actually become necrotic. When the child comes to the ED with auscultatory abnormalities such as stridor, wheezing, or rhonchi, it is assumed that major inhalation injury has occurred.

The appearance of a child who has suffered smoke inhalation varies widely with the degree of injury. That a child arrives in an alert state with an effective cough and adequate air movement does not necessarily preclude serious respiratory damage. These children should be treated as if an insult has occurred until an adequate history, physical examination, and laboratory investigation have proved otherwise. To err on the side of safety very well may minimize delayed complications.

History

Obtaining a meaningful and reliable history when a child arrives after a fire is often a difficult task because of the possible injuries to and anxiety of persons who witnessed the event. One person from the ED should be designated to gather whatever facts are available while immediate intervention is begun with the child. Pre-hospital providers are often the best source of information from the scene.

Physical Assessment

The most reliable criteria for intervention in known or suspected smoke inhalation is determined during the physical assessment. The face and neck are evaluated for color, edema, or blistering indicative of a dermal burn. The nares are inspected for singed hair or mucosal edema and the presence of soot. The bare chest is examined for evidence of burns and assessed for adequate excursion of the chest during a few deep breaths. The oral cavity is palpated for degree of dryness, and the trachea is palpated gently for any evidence of edema. Auscultation of the lung sounds may yield normal bronchovesicular breath sounds on initial presentation, and indeed breath sounds may remain normal for up to 2 days after the injury. The presence of adventitious breath sounds on presentation to the ED signifies that a moderate to extensive insult has occurred. Ongoing assessment of the child's vital signs with frequent temperature readings is essential.

Laboratory and Diagnostic Tests

Because carbon monoxide is a by-product of the combustion of several common materials, such as polyvinylchloride (in synthetic rubber) and polystyrene (in foam cushions), the level of toxicity should be assessed. A baseline determination of arterial blood gases, pH, and carboxyhemoglobin level should be obtained immediately upon arrival. Because results may reflect near-normal values initially, it is important to repeat them periodically throughout treatment. Baseline chest x rays should be obtained but should be deferred until the patient's condition is stable. Xenon lung scanning or fiberoptic bronchoscopy may be desirable tools to evaluate the extent of lung tissue damage.

T R I A G E
Smoke Inhalation

Emergent
Child with facial burns; chest burns; dyspnea; altered level of consciousness.

Urgent
Child who is alert; has good air movement; effective cough; and normal respiratory rate and effort.

Nursing Diagnosis
Impaired Gas Exchange

Defining Characteristics

- Increased respiratory rate
- Increased pulse rate
- Confusion, irritability, somnolence

Nursing Interventions

- Administer high concentration of oxygen
- Monitor vital signs
- Monitor alterations in level of consciousness

Expected Outcomes

- Respiratory rate returns to normal
- Patient becomes more alert and is consolable
- Vital signs are normal

Nursing Diagnosis
Altered Tissue Perfusion

Defining Characteristics

- Gas exchange problems
- Delayed capillary refill
- Weak distal arterial pulsations

Nursing Interventions

- Administer high concentration oxygen
- Provide a warm environment

Expected Outcomes

- Perfusion improves and capillary refill is brisk
- Distal pulses are strong

Management

Provision of, or protection of, a patent airway is the first priority. Oxygen therapy with 100% oxygen using a snug-fitting non-rebreather mask should be begun in the field and continued on arrival in the ED. In the presence of laryngeal edema, hypoxemia, copious secretions or clearly audible stridor, nasotracheal intubation should be performed to ensure airway maintenance and the delivery of appropriate oxygen concentrations. When facial burns are evident, the nasotracheal route is preferred for intubation because anchoring the tube becomes difficult with the oral route. When wheezing or stridor are present, bronchodilator nebulizers or intravenous administration of steroids may be desirable. Steroids, however, should not be given when the child has dermal burns. Intravenous fluids should be administered in amounts determined by the extent of the dermal burns. In the absence of dermal burns, rates of intravenous administration should be adjusted to provide maintenance of fluids for body weight.

All children with smoke inhalation injuries should be admitted for careful observation because of the likelihood of delayed onset of complications. The child and family members are often frightened by the fire and need much support and reassurance while in the ED.

DROWNING AND NEAR DROWNING

Drowning is defined as death resulting from submersion asphyxia anytime within 24 hours of the submersion. *Secondary drowning* is death resulting from the complications of the submersion more than 24 hours after the episode. *Immersion syndrome* is sudden death in which extremely cold water enters the nasopharynx, vagally inducing arhythmias and cardiac arrest. In *near drowning* the person survives after a submersion incident and has varying degrees of sequelae.

It is estimated that more than 7000 deaths per year in the US are the result of drowning. Adolescent males account for the peak incidence, although 40% of victims are younger than 4 years. Drowning incidents typically involve children who are inadequately attended in or near swimming pools, bathtubs, lakes, hot tubs, and other bodies of water, even those as small as a bucket or toilet. The increased risk among adolescents is usually attributed to overestimation of ability. The use of alcohol or drugs, trauma, and seizure disorders also may be risk factors. Most incidents of drowning and near drowning occur close to the victim's home.

Etiology and Pathophysiology

A variety of factors, either alone or in combination, contribute to injury and death after a submersion injury. *Dry drowning* accounts for about 10% of all deaths and is so named because no fluid is aspirated—laryngospasm causes the asphyxiation. The remaining 90% of victims suffer *wet drowning* when the victims either inhale or swallow large amounts of water and then vomit and aspirate during the initial period of panic, struggle, and breath holding.

In theory there should be a difference between salt-water and fresh-water near drownings with respect to clinical findings. Salt-water aspiration should cause intravascular fluid to be drawn into the alveoli, leading to hypovolemia and hemoconcentration with resultant higher levels of serum electrolytes. Similarly, fresh-water aspiration should produce osmosis of fluid from the alveoli into the intravascular spaces, causing hemodilution and lower serum electrolyte levels. These changes, however, are seldom noted in patients who survive long enough to reach the ED because these victims have aspirated less than the estimated 11 mL/kg of water necessary to cause serum electrolyte imbalances.

Asphyxia and hypoxia are the common causes of tissue injury and death in submersion incidents. Hypoxia is the result of intrapulmonary shunting caused by the loss of surfactant. Surfactant is rendered inert by fresh water and is diluted by salt water, causing alveolar collapse and atelectasis. The loss of surfactant and intrapulmonary shunting leads to pulmonary edema, which is further aggravated by the inhalation of debris (gastric material, mud, algae, and sewage) that combines to produce a high degree of hypoxia. This may be observed immediately or may have a delayed onset of up to 72 hours after the episode.

As a result of hypoxemia, severe metabolic acidosis and hypercarbia develop, which may lead to central nervous system ischemia, encephalopathy, and seizures. The mechanism of injury must be considered to protect the victim who may have suffered head or neck trauma in addition to the submersion injury. Further insult to the central nervous system may be caused by vigorous fluid resuscitation, which may cause increased intracranial pressure.

Immediately upon rescue, most people who have nearly drowned have a "death-like" appearance. Children, with the possible exception of those submerged in hot tubs or heated baths, also suffer some degree of hypothermia. There is some evidence that cold water submersion may be protective by activating the diving reflex. When the face is submerged in cold water, a neurogenic response shunts blood from the periphery to the brain and heart, leading to bradycardia.

The body's ability to survive a cold water submersion depends greatly on length of exposure, insulation, and the body's ability to balance heat production with heat loss. One of the ways the body produces heat is through exercise. In very cold water, however, exercise may cause more rapid heat loss by constantly stirring the cold water around the body. Exercise also produces exhaustion, increases lactic acidosis, and leads to more rapid loss of consciousness. The body loses heat 25% more rapidly in cold water than in cold air because of conduction differences. A factor that reduces heat loss is insulation from either heavy clothing or body fat.

Submersion for more than 4 minutes begins to produce cerebral hypoxia and decreased cerebral perfusion, leading to cerebral edema and increased pressure. The rate of increasing intracranial pressure and ischemia cause varying degrees of neurologic damage. Neurologic sequelae may develop up to 24 hours after the submersion incident.

History

The history obtained from the pre-hospital providers or family members should include an estimate of the length of submersion, type of water, condition on removal from water, and length of time of resuscitation efforts until first spontaneous breathing effort. If the mechanism of injury suggests a possibility of head or neck trauma, cervical spinal immobilization must be maintained until the integrity of the cervical spine has been confirmed by x rays.

Physical Assessment

Assessment of a child on arrival in the ED must include the status of the airway and breathing, heart rate, rhythm and effective circulation, body temperature (using a hypothermia probe), and mental status. After a submersion accident a child may arrive in the ED with a wide range of symptoms that progress from alertness and apparent recovery to cardiorespiratory arrest. As one might suspect, children who arrive unconscious with fixed, dilated pupils and in sustained cardiorespiratory arrest despite rapid and competent pre-hospital care have the poorest outcomes. Quan et al (1990) found that submersion for at least 10 minutes and resuscitation lasting longer than 25 minutes in their pediatric population predicted either severe neurologic sequelae or death.

TRIAGE
Drowning and Near Drowning

Emergent ———————————————
A child with altered level of consciousness; sustained cardiorespiratory distress or arrest.

Urgent ———————————————
A child who presents alert; with near normal vital signs and temperature; good bilateral air movement.

Nursing Diagnosis
Impaired Gas Exchange

Defining Characteristics

- Hypoxia
- Pulmonary edema
- Respiratory distress or arrest
- Depressed level of consciousness

Nursing Interventions

- Administer 100% oxygen with assisted ventilation if necessary
- Monitor vital signs and arterial blood gases
- Administer medications as directed

Expected Outcomes

- Respiratory status improves
- Heart rate and blood pressure normalize
- Acidosis and cerebral perfusion improve

Nursing Diagnosis
Anxiety

Defining Characteristics

- Verbalization of feelings of guilt and fear about outcome of event
- Concern about equipment and procedures

Nursing Interventions

- Provide calm reassurance and realistic progress reports on the resuscitation efforts
- Explain procedures and equipment

Expected Outcomes

- Family members are able to verbalize support for each other and the victim
- Family members are able to participate in care when appropriate

Nursing Diagnosis
Hypothermia

Defining Characteristics

- Body temperature below 30°C
- Bradycardia or asystole
- Cold skin

Nursing Interventions

- Monitor vital signs and core temperature
- Initiate and continue passive and active rewarming techniques, ie, warming lights, rectal lavage, warmed intravenous fluids
- Check skin perfusion

Expected Outcomes

- Rectal temperature is 30°C or higher
- Heart rate normalizes
- Skin is warmer
- Capillary refill improves

Management

The death-like appearance of most children on initial rescue is caused by apnea, cyanosis or profound pallor; extreme peripheral vasoconstriction; and myocardial depression. Because a higher number of children than adults survive, a child should receive skilled vigorous resuscitative efforts. As in other situations of pediatric cardiorespiratory arrests, the first concern is the airway and the first drug given is oxygen, which is delivered at the highest possible concentration to minimize progressive hypoxemia, correct acidosis, and improve perfusion to the heart and brain.

The initial focus of management is aimed at correction of hypoxemia and metabolic acidosis. The initial arterial blood gas determinations guide the effectiveness of oxygen therapy and carbon dioxide reduction and the need for administration of sodium bicarbonate to correct acidosis.

All child victims should be closely monitored for heart rate and rhythm, blood pressure, respiratory effort, and auscultation of lung sounds. Children with persistent respiratory distress, hypoxemia, hypercapnea, and pulmonary edema may require intubation and ventilation with positive and expiratory pressure (PEEP) or continuous positive airway pressure (CPAP) to maintain lung compliance.

When a child's blood pressure has reached an adequate and stable level, intravenous fluids should be limited to one-half maintenance, and diuretic therapy may be initiated. This may improve oxygenation in lungs with decreased surfactant and compliance while maintaining renal function. Children who remain comatose after submersion often have signs of increased intracranial pressure. Intraventricular catheters are frequently inserted to measure and monitor pressures and the effectiveness of therapy.

Rewarming a child to a minimum core temperature of at least 30°C is essential before pronouncement of death and cessation of resuscitation efforts. Techniques for rewarming children include active rewarming with rectal lavage, gastric lavage, and warmed intravenous fluids and passive rewarming with heat lamps directed at the trunk and warmed blankets. Active rewarming is more effective.

All children who have nearly drowned should be admitted for observation. Children who appear to have no symptoms require monitoring and observation for a minimum of 24–48 hours to assess any delayed onset of symptoms. Admission to the ICU should be considered for children who required advanced life support resuscitation.

Patient and Family Teaching and Psychosocial Support

One of the most important and sometimes difficult roles for nurses in the ED is supporting a family of a child who has nearly drowned. It is important to keep the family updated on the child's progress during resuscitation. The parents should be informed that everything possible is being done for the child. Parents should be prepared for poor outcomes when indicated. A nonjudgmental approach is important—family members may already be experiencing guilt, depending on the circumstances of the accident.

Prevention may be the single most effective method of reducing the morbidity and mortality from submersion accidents. All pools should be properly enclosed to limit access to unsupervised children. Adults must be diligent in their supervision of children, especially infants and toddlers, around water, including the bathtub. Swimming and water safety should be taught to children at early ages. Rules forbidding alcohol and illicit drug use near swimming areas and hot tubs should be strictly enforced.

REFERENCES

Alario AJ, Lewander WJ, Denehey P, Seifer R, Mansell AL (1992). The efficacy of nebulized metaproterenol in wheezing infants and young children. *American Journal of Diseases of Children* 146:412–418

Barkin RM, Rosen P (1990). *Emergency pediatrics: A guide to ambulatory care* (3rd ed). Philadelphia: C. V. Mosby Company, p 634

Gordon M (1991–1992). *Manual of nursing diagnosis*. St. Louis: Mosby Year Book

Llano AL, Raffin TA (1990). Management of carbon monoxide poisoning. *Chest* 97:165

Nemes J, Schmidt E, Kelly L (1988). Epiglottitis: ED nursing management. *Journal of Emergency Nursing* 14:70–75

Quan L, Wentz KR, Gore EJ, Copass MK (1990). Outcomes and predictors of outcome in pediatric submersion victims receiving prehospital care in King County, Washington. *Pediatrics* 86:586–593

Skolnik NS (1990). Strategies for viral croup. *Emergency Medicine* 10:111–114

Thompson SW (1990). *Emergency care of children*. Boston: James and Bartlett, p 141

Toltzis P, Brooks LJ (1992). Bronchiolitis. In Reece R (ed), *Manual of emergency pediatrics*. Philadelphia: Saunders, pp 416–417

SUGGESTED READING

Adams WG, Deaver KA, Cochi SL et al (1993). Decline of childhood *Haemophilus influenzae* type b (Hib) disease in the Hib vaccine era. *JAMA* 269:221–226

Bella LAD (1992). Steroidphobia and the pulmonary patient. *American Journal of Nursing* 2:26–29

Bjerklie SJ (1990). Status asthmaticus. *American Journal of Nursing* 9:521–555

Carlson KL (1989). Assessing a child's chest. *RN* 11:26–31

Erickson RS (1989a). Mastering the ins and outs of chest drainage. Part 1. *Nursing 89* 5:37–43

Erickson RS (1989b). Mastering the ins and outs of chest drainage. Part 2. *Nursing 89* 6:436–449

Halpern JS (1992). Respiratory syncytial virus (RSV): A common health problem. *Journal of Emergency Nursing* 18:61–62

Losek JD (1990). Diagnostic difficulties of foreign body aspiration in children. *American Journal of Emergency Medicine* 8:348–350

Melish ME (1991). The impact of pediatric HIV infection on emergency services. *Emergency Medicine Clinics of North America* 9:655–666

Nelson MS, Hofstadter A, Parket J, Hargis C (1990). Frequency of inhaled metaproterenol in the treatment of acute asthma exacerbation. *Annals of Emergency Medicine* 19:21–25

Pender ES, Pollack CV (1990). Cough-variant asthma in children and adults: Case reports and review. *The Journal of Emergency Medicine* 8:727–731

Shovein JT, Land LP, Richter G, Leedom CL (1989). Near drowning. *American Journal of Nursing* 5:680–684

Spyr J, Preach MA (1990). Pulse oximetry, understanding the concept, knowing the limits. *RN* 5:38–45

Steele RW (1998). Antiviral agents for respiratory infections. *Pediatric Infectious Desease Journal* 7:457–461

Wintemute GJ (1990). Childhood drowning and near-drowning in the United States. *American Journal of Diseases of Children* 144:663–669

Young L (1992). A 22-month-old victim of near drowning. *Journal of Emergency Nursing* 18:197–198

PART 4

Trauma and Environmental Emergencies

CHAPTER 17

Care of the Multiply Injured Child

LISA MARIE BERNARDO
SUSAN J. KELLEY

INTRODUCTION

Injuries, the leading cause of childhood morbidity and disability in the United States, are responsible for 25,000 deaths each year. Among children 1–19 years of age, injuries cause more deaths than all diseases combined. Childhood injuries claim almost five times as many lives as cancer, the second leading cause of death among children. Almost one-half of all deaths of children 1–14 years of age are the result of major trauma, as compared to one death in ten in the general population.

Each year, almost 16 million children are treated for injuries in emergency departments (EDs). An estimated 600,000 children are hospitalized for injuries (Centers for Disease Control, 1990). Injuries are responsible for 20% of all hospitalizations among children; they are second only to respiratory illnesses, which are responsible for 23% of all childhood hospitalizations. Injuries to children lead to more hospital days of care than any disease, cause the highest proportion of admissions to rehabilitation facilities, and result in the highest proportion of children who require home health care after hospital discharge (Centers for Disease Control, 1990). It is estimated that more than 30,000 children suffer permanent disabilities from injuries each year. The costs of injuries to children are estimated to exceed 7.5 billion dollars each year (Centers for Disease Control, 1990). The emotional costs to injured children and their families are enormous, and of course, they cannot be measured.

According to the Centers for Disease Control (1990) 47% of all injury deaths among children involve motor vehicles. Homicide is the second leading cause of injury death among children, accounting for 12.8%; suicide ranks third, accounting for 9.6% of childhood injury deaths. Drowning, the fourth leading cause of injury death among children, accounts for 9.2% of injury deaths. Pedestrian injuries are the fifth ranking cause of injury deaths among children, followed by fires and burns as the sixth leading cause of injury deaths among children. Almost 30% of all childhood injury deaths result from a head injury (Centers for Disease Control, 1990).

The term *injury* has replaced the term *accident* because the term *accident* implies an event that is unexpected and uncontrollable. In reality, injuries occur in highly predictable patterns and are controllable (Centers for Disease Control, 1990; Jones, 1992). Injuries are usually divided into two major categories—unintentional (accidental) and intentional (deliberate) (Jones, 1992). Unintentional injuries include motor vehicle crashes, falls, drowning, burns, and poisonings. Intentional injuries include homicide, child maltreatment, and suicide.

Age and Sex Differences

Injury-related death rates and patterns of injuries vary by age and sex. The peak age range for injuries is 4–12 years; the highest frequency is at age 8. The mortalities for burns, drowning, and pedestrian injuries are highest among children 0–4 years of age. This age group is twice as likely as school-aged children to die from burns and three times as likely as adolescents to die of burns (Guyer and Ellers, 1990).

Trauma to child passengers in motor vehicles is

the leading cause of death among children after the first few months of life. In the age group 0–5 years, fall-related injuries occur at a rate 1½–2 times greater than with older children. One of every 12 children younger than 6 years requires hospital treatment for a fall. Falls occur most frequently in the home and usually are from furniture or down stairs. Outside the home, most falls are from playground equipment or strollers (Guyer and Gallagher, 1985).

The risk among elementary-school-aged children (6–12 years) of a pedestrian injury is twice that of younger children. More than 1 of every 80 elementary-school-aged children requires hospital treatment because of a non-motor-vehicle accident. This injury rate is twice the rate for teenagers and four times that for preschoolers (Guyer and Gallagher, 1985).

Adolescence is associated with an increased injury mortality; 78% of all injury deaths occur in this age group. Fifty-six percent of pediatric injury deaths occur during adolescence, which accounts for only 26% of the pediatric population (Guyer and Ellers, 1990).

Adolescents have a motor vehicle mortality rate ten times that of the younger age groups (Agran et al, 1990). One of every 50 teenagers is injured as a motor vehicle occupant each year. Adolescent drivers have the highest motor vehicle mortalities of all age groups, and 23% of all passengers who die in motor vehicle crashes do so when an adolescent is driving (Agran et al, 1990). Characteristics unique to motor vehicle crashes involving adolescent drivers are an increased likelihood of single vehicle crashes, an excess of crashes at night and on weekends, and a high number of occupants (Agran et al, 1990). Alcohol and drug use among adolescent drivers is thought to make a major contribution to the increased fatality rate among occupants 15–19 years of age, especially among males (Agran et al, 1990).

One of every 14 adolescents requires hospitalization for a sports-related injury. The largest proportion of sports injuries are from football, basketball, roller-skating, and baseball.

Boys sustain fatal and nonfatal injuries more often than girls. Boys have the highest rate of completed suicides; the highest incidence is among adolescents 15–19 years of age (Hollinger, 1990).

Interpersonal Violence

Interpersonal violence, including homicide, child maltreatment, and assault by peers, causes more than 2000 deaths each year of children 0–19 years of age.

Homicide is the leading cause of death among African American males and females 15–19 years of age; for African American males 10–14 years of age, homicide has ranked either third or fourth as a cause of death for several years. Males generally have the highest homicide rate (Ropp et al, 1992). Homicide explains a rapidly growing proportion of the total pediatric mortality; guns, in particular, are involved in a disproportionately large number of homicide deaths (Ropp et al, 1992). Firearm homicides among urban African American males 10–14 years of age and males and females 15–19 years of age have risen dramatically in the past decade (Ropp et al, 1992).

In a study of gun-related violence among inner-city high school students from five urban centers in the United States, researchers found that 23% of students had been victims of gun-related violence (Sheley et al, 1992). Twenty percent of students had been threatened with a gun and 12% had been shot at. Twenty-two percent of the students reported carrying a gun outside of school, and 6% carried a gun at school at least some of the time. Males were more likely than females to carry a gun. Forty-six percent of the high school students reported knowing a schoolmate who had carried a gun to school during the last year.

Mechanisms of Injury

There are seven mechanisms of injury: kinetic; thermal; electrical; chemical; radiant; lack of oxygenation; and lack of thermoregulation. The first mechanism of injury is kinetic forces. Kinetic means motion. Examples of kinetic forces include blunt force, crush, acceleration-deceleration, and penetration. Blunt forces are most often associated with pediatric injuries. A blunt-force injury occurs during a fall from a height or during a motor vehicle crash. A crush injury involves direct energy to a particular body area, as would occur while using shop equipment in school. Acceleration-deceleration forces occur when the body is abruptly stopped but the internal organs continue to move. These organs, such as the spinal cord, liver, and descending thoracic aorta, stretch or rupture, causing tears and lacerations. Penetrating forces are either high or medium energy (M-16s, handguns) or low energy (knives or ice picks). This chapter covers the injuries associated with kinetic forces.

The second mechanism of injury is thermal. A thermal injury occurs when heat absorption is greater than the rate of heat dissipation. Electricity is the third mechanism of injury. When electricity, either through current or lightning, comes into contact with the body, the energy is converted to heat, causing injury. The fourth mechanism of injury is chemical, in which a chemical comes into contact with the body and produces either heat or protein denaturization. Radiant energy, the fifth mechanism of injury, occurs through exposure to the sun or to radiation (nuclear or therapeutic). Lack of oxygenation is the sixth mechanism of injury; it is associated with drowning or hanging. The last mechanism, lack of thermoregulation, occurs during exposure to the elements and results in heat- or cold-related emergencies.

BLUNT FORCE TRAUMA

Injuries to Motor Vehicle Occupants

From 0–19 years of age, injuries to motor vehicle occupants are the major cause of death in the US (Centers for Disease Control, 1990). Three separate events occur in motor vehicle crashes: machine collision; body collision; and organ collision (Creel, 1988). First, the motor vehicle crashes into a moving or stationary object. The occupants, however, are still moving inside the car; they come to rest against the car's interior surfaces, such as the steering wheel or dashboard. Finally, the internal organs, which are still moving, come to rest. This triad of events must be considered later when evaluating the pediatric occupant of a motor vehicle crash.

There are four common types of automobile collisions: head-on collisions; lateral impact collisions; rear-end collisions; and rollover collisions (Creel, 1988). The nature and extent of injury in a motor vehicle crash are a function of the mass of the occupant; the speed of travel; the ability of the affected tissues to tolerate mechanical energy; and the degree of energy absorbed by the impacting surfaces, their configuration, and the area and length of contact (Robertson, 1985).

Most trauma in motor vehicle crashes is associated with the movement of occupants against interior surfaces within the vehicle or from ejection. Children can become pinned under the dashboard or impaled on the gearshift. Collisions among occupants also contribute to injury, particularly among young children. An unrestrained child in a moving vehicle that is stopped by a sudden impact continues to move at the original speed until impact with the interior of the vehicle. Again, the child's organs continue to move inside the child's body. Children seated in improperly secured car seats also can become projectiles. As a result of mandatory use of child car-restraint devices, the number of serious injuries and deaths among children 0–4 years of age has decreased considerably in states with laws that require use of child car-safety devices. The impact of driver-side and passenger-side airbags on reducing pediatric passenger injury is not known.

Injuries from motor vehicle crashes can involve a restrained or an unrestrained passenger. An infant or young child restrained in a car seat is susceptible to high cervical spinal injuries during sudden deceleration (Bernardo and Waggoner, 1992). A child held on an adult's lap can be crushed between the adult and the dashboard, steering column, or front seat.

Although motor vehicle crashes most likely involve cars, other motorized vehicles are associated with pediatric injuries. Farm equipment, trucks, snowmobiles, all-terrain vehicles, and motorcycles all have associated risks for injury to their drivers and occupants.

Pedestrian Injuries

Each year in the US, 50,000 children are injured as pedestrians; 1800 children are fatally injured; 18,000 are admitted to hospitals; and 5000 have serious long-term sequelae (Rivara, 1990). Most fatal and nonfatal pedestrian injuries occur among children between the ages of 4 and 9 years. Collisions between pedestrians and motor vehicles differ from other types of motor vehicle trauma in that few victims escape injury. Whereas 1% of pedestrians struck by cars are uninjured, 94% of all motor vehicle collisions involve no personal injuries (Rivara, 1990).

Eighty percent of pedestrian injuries to children occur during the daylight hours, most between noon and 6 PM Most pedestrian injuries occur on local, through streets in urban area. the mortality for pedestrian injuries increases in proportion to the speed limit at the site of injury. Injuries at intersections account for less than 15% of fatal and less than 30% of nonfatal injuries to children younger than 15 years. Pedestrian injuries most often involve children who dart or run into the street in the middle of a block; the second most common cause is dashing across an intersection. Incidents in which children are run over by a vehicle backing up are limited primarily to young children (Rivara, 1990).

Children usually sustain fractures of the pelvis and femur when struck by a car because they are short and the bumper hits them in these areas. After the first impact with the car, the child can be thrown over the car's hood and into the oncoming lane of traffic. Alternatively, the child can be dragged by the car for a distance. Consequently, a child experiences a triad of injuries: extremity trauma; thoracic and abdominal trauma; and head trauma. This triad of injuries is referred to as Waddell's triad (Halpern, 1989).

Falls

Falls are the second leading cause of death from trauma, excluding drownings and burns, among children in the US. They are the most frequent cause of injury that brings children to the ED. The highest incidence of falls occurs in young childhood and in the elderly. Falls have been found to be more frequent among boys than among girls; the injury ratio of boys to girls living in urban areas increases with age. Falls in the home, for children younger than 1 year, are found more frequently in lower socioeconomic populations. Deficiencies in the environment, such as deteriorating housing, windows that do not close or lock, and windows without secure screens, greatly contribute to the higher rates in low income groups.

The peak time for falls is between noon and early evening. The objects or areas from which children fall vary. Injuries from stairs and steps predominate, but beds, tables, strollers, riding toys, and chairs are also common sites. When children fall from considerable heights, falls from windows predominate. In one study of children who fell from a height greater than 10 feet, most were from falls out of windows. Head trauma was the most common injury, followed by skeletal trauma; all children survived (Musemeche et al, 1991). It appears that infants and small children are unlikely to sustain serious or fatal injuries in falls of less than 10 feet (Williams, 1991). In circumstances in which a young child dies because of a fall of less than 4 feet, the history is incorrect; other plausible causes for the injuries should be investigated (Chadwick et al, 1991). For example, older children and adolescents tend to fall more often from trees, roofs, and ladders.

The surface upon which children land contributes to the prognosis. Concrete and asphalt are associated with more severe injuries than other surfaces. Children who land on hard ground or concrete sustain more severe injury than those who hit grass, even when the heights of the falls are similar. Head trauma is responsible for the most deaths from falls. Multiple trauma also is associated with death from falls.

Bicycle Injuries

More than 600 children and adolescents are killed annually in the US while riding bicycles. An estimated 554,000 injuries are related to bicycle crashes a year that are serious enough to warrant treatment in the ED. One study documented that bicycle-related injuries resulted in serious short- and long-term disabilities (Nakayama et al, 1990a). Boys are at higher risk than girls for bicycle injuries and are 3.6 times more likely to die from a bicycle injury than girls; boys 10–14 years of age have the highest risk of death. Motor vehicles are involved in most deaths of children injured on their bicycles. Most of these fatal injuries involve a head injury; therefore, the use of helmets should be strongly encouraged.

Nonfatal injuries associated with bicycle trauma occur more frequently in boys, most often because of unsafe riding practices; the most common injury that requires hospitalization is a head injury (McKenna et al, 1991). Unfortunately, the results of one study showed that most parents whose children were hospitalized for bicycle-related injuries failed to initiate injury prevention measures with their children. Furthermore,

even though most of these children experienced head injuries, less than one-fourth of them did not use bicycle helmets upon discharge (Nakayama et al, 1990b). Other injuries associated with bicycle crashes include abdominal injuries (from striking the handle bars) and facial and extremity trauma. Skateboards, tricycles, and low-to-ground cycles also are associated with single system and multisystem trauma.

PENETRATING TRAUMA

Although blunt trauma is the leading mechanism of injury associated with pediatric morbidity, the incidence of penetrating trauma is on the rise. Many objects are capable of causing penetrating injuries, including weapons such as knives and firearms as well as children's toys and foreign bodies. Firearms are implicated in drive-by shootings, in which young children are struck by stray bullets while playing in the street or are struck by bullets fired into their homes. Gang violence and botched drug deals are another cause of penetrating trauma. Finally, gun play by young children is implicated in penetrating trauma.

More and more, penetrating injuries among the pediatric population are caused by firearms, such as handguns, rifles, and shotguns. Firearms are classified as either high-velocity or low-velocity. Handguns and some rifles are considered low-velocity because their velocity is below 2000 ft/sec (Creel, 1988). Injuries from low-velocity weapons are generally less destructive than from high-velocity weapons, such as semiautomatic weapons, because high-velocity weapons involve hydrostatic pressure (Creel, 1988).

The injuries inflicted by a firearm include an entry wound, an exit wound, and an internal wound. In general, highly dense organs, such as the liver and muscle, sustain more damage than less dense organs, such as the lungs (Creel, 1988). The damage to body tissues from a bullet or missile is related to shock waves, cavitation, and pulsation of the cavity (Creel, 1988). Bullets may become lodged in the body or exit through a separate wound.

The severity of knife wounds is related to the anatomic area pierced with the knife, the length of the blade, and the angle of penetration (Creel, 1988). An exit wound may or may not be present, and the blade may or may not still be inside the victim.

MULTIPLE TRAUMA

Multiple trauma involves injury to more than one body system. However, any child who presents with obvious traumatic injury to one body system should

TABLE 17–1. RESPONSIBILITIES OF TRAUMA NURSES

■ **TRAUMA NURSE ON RIGHT**
ASSIGNMENT: ED Nurse as Assigned by ED Charge Nurse
ROLE: Assist Physician on Right

Assure room is prepared before patient's arrival
   2 liters lactated Ringer's solution primed with maxi drip tubing (no nonvented Burette sets)
   IV catheter cart at bedside
   Cutdown tray on Mayo stand
   Airway tray at bedside
   Chest tube tray at bedside
   All equipment functional and turned on (except IV pumps)
   Portable oxygen tanks on stretcher; mask appropriate for patient's age and size

Assist with transfer of patient to ED stretcher

Assist with patient immobilization

Assist with clothing removal

Assist with IV access on the right; regulate fluids and provide accurate fluid intake to charting nurse

Provide physician with materials for rectal examination (gloves, lubricant, Hemoccult card, and developer)

Assist with peritoneal lavage if indicated and provide appropriate equipment

Assist with extremity stabilization and splinting on the right

Place patient on an automatic blood pressure machine

Take patient's temperature

Call out vital signs every 5 minutes.

Assist in nasogastric tube and Foley catheter insertion

Assist in surgical intervention on the right as required
   Cutdown
   Thoracotomy
   Insertion of chest tube
   Peritoneal lavage
   Tracheostomy
   Hemorrhage control

Assist with inflation and deflation of MAST as per protocol

Accompany and monitor patient to destination unless otherwise designated by ED charge nurse

Notify receiving unit before departure from ED

Give full report to receiving unit personnel when patient arrives on unit

Ensure all trauma forms accompany patient to unit

■ **Trauma Nurse on Left**
ASSIGNMENT: ED Nurse as assigned by ED Charge Nurse
ROLE: Assist physician on left; provide emotional support; assist with airway management, including intubation

Assure room is prepared before patient arrival
   2 liters lactated Ringer solution primed with maximum drip tubing (no non-vented Burette sets)
   IV catheter cart at bedside
   Cutdown tray on Mayo stand
   Airway tray at bedside
   Chest tube tray at bedside
   All equipment functional and turned on (except IV pumps)

   Portable oxygen tank on stretcher; mask appropriate to patient's age and size

Assist with transfer of patient to ED stretcher

Assist with patient immobilization

Assist with clothing removal

Assist with IV access on left; regulate fluids and provide accurate fluid intake to charting nurse and regulate fluid

Obtain blood for laboratory testing

Attach cardiac monitor and pulse oximeter

Assist with extremity stabilization on the left

Provide patient with supplemental oxygen

Obtain urine specimen and bedside urine testing

Assist with surgical intervention on the left as required
   Cutdown
   Thoracostomy
   Thoracotomy
   Peritoneal lavage
   Hemorrhage control

■ **CHARTING NURSE**
ASSIGNMENT: Chart on Trauma Flow Sheet
ROLE: Trauma Flow Sheet Documentation

Assure videocassette recorder is on and functioning before the arrival of Level I and Level II trauma victims

Assure physician name and time of arrival are on Trauma Flow Sheet

Ensure availability and completeness of requisitions

Call hospital police to obtain elevator

Document calls to computed tomography (CT), time CT is ready, and time patient is sent to CT

Access resources as required

Provide frequent fluid status update

Serve as liaison for secondary team

Facilitate x rays

Remove completed videotape and document appropriate information in video log binder

■ **FLOAT NURSE**
ASSIGNMENT: Prepare Medications and Obtain Additional Equipment
ROLE: Assist Trauma Team as Needed

Prepare medications[a]

Set up chest drainage system for chest tube insertion

Prepare Level I warmer by priming IV tubing with normal saline solution

Administer blood and blood products as needed

Apply appropriate measures to prevent hypothermia, including radiant warmer

Ensure proper personnel and equipment are available before transport of patient, including medications for transport

---

[a]All resuscitation medications are to be drawn up into syringes before the patient arrives (Level I trauma only)
(Reproduced with permission from the Benedum Pediatric Trauma Program, Children's Hospital of Pittsburgh, Pittsburgh, PA)

be treated as having multiple trauma until it is proved otherwise. The first 20 minutes of management is crucial in determining the outcome for a multiply injured child. The prompt assessment and treatment of a multiply injured child require a systematic, coordinated approach. Failure to rapidly assess and treat life-threatening injuries lessens the child's chances for survival. Resuscitation must begin the moment the child arrives in the ED, if it has not already been initiated in the pre-hospital setting.

The trauma team consists of skilled physicians, surgeons, nurses, social workers, and other health professionals. Each person has a specific role during the resuscitation, allowing for an organized approach to the child's and family's care. The specific nursing responsibilities are found in Table 17–1. Table 17–2 summarizes priorities in the nursing management of an injured child.

After notification of the child's pending arrival, preparation of the treatment room begins for the trauma resuscitation. The room temperature is raised or overhead lights are turned on to warm the room. The appropriate-sized equipment and medications are prepared on the basis of the child's age and estimated or actual weight. The equipment includes oropharyngeal airways, endotracheal tubes (ETs) and stylets, laryngoscope blades and handles, suction catheters, oxygen masks, and bag-valve-mask devices, nasogastric tubes, and indwelling bladder catheters—all one size larger and one size smaller than their calculated sizes. These sizes are determined from such published references as the Broselow resuscitation tape (Vital Signs, Inc., Totowa, NJ) or from a quick reference to pediatric emergency equipment (Table 17–3). A blood warmer and O-negative blood should be readily available. Intravenous lactated Ringer solution is primed with trauma tubing, and blood tubes for laboratory studies are arranged nearby. Suction and oxygen sources, a pulse oximeter, a cardiorespiratory monitor, an automatic blood pressure monitor (with the correctly sized cuff), and thermometer should be operating and functional for immediate use. Other equipment, such as thoracotomy and tracheostomy trays and chest decompression equipment, should be readily available. Medications are prepared in advance for any anticipated traumatic arrest, endotracheal intubation, or severe closed-head injury.

ASSESSMENT

History

Upon the child's arrival at the ED, the trauma team accepts the child from the pre-hospital personnel. Table 17–4 summarizes the ED assessment and management of an injured child. The pre-hospital personnel initiate either basic or advanced trauma life support measures in the field. Basic trauma life support measures include the application of oxygen, cervical and spinal immobilization, and monitoring vital signs. Advanced trauma life support measures include all of these plus advanced airway maneuvers (endotracheal intubation), chest decompression, intravenous and intraosseous access, administration of medication, and cardiac monitoring.

The pre-hospital personnel provide information about the injury and about the treatment they initiated. The history is usually obtained from the patient, parent, or witness to the injury. If the child was an occupant of a motor vehicle, the information obtained includes scene fatalities or prolonged extrication. The site of impact (eg, side, rear-end), speed of the motor vehicle at the time of impact, and if the vehicle hit a moving or stationary object should be ascertained. The child's location in the vehicle, use of a safety restraint, or ejection from the vehicle are also important pieces of information.

If the child was hit by a motor vehicle, it should be determined how far the child was thrown, if the child was run over or pinned under the vehicle, on what type of surface the child landed, where the child was struck (such as his or her right side), and how fast the motor vehicle was traveling. If the child was riding a bicycle and was struck by a motor vehicle, the speed of the bicycle, as well as vehicle's position (stationary or moving) should be obtained. Furthermore, it should be noted if the child suffered a loss of consciousness and if a helmet was worn.

If the child fell, the height of the fall and the surface landed on should be determined. In the event of a penetrating injury, information on the type of weapon used should be obtained. The number of bullets fired or the number of stab wounds may be known. If a homicide or suicide is suspected, further information

---

TABLE 17–2. PRIORITIES IN THE NURSING MANAGEMENT OF PEDIATRIC TRAUMA

- PRIMARY SURVEY
  Assess airway and cervical spine, breathing, and circulation; initiate support measures; determine neurologic status; expose patient
  Assess and treat life-threatening injuries

- SECONDARY SURVEY
  Perform head to toe assessment with identification and stabilization of non-life-threatening injuries
  Initiate gastric and bladder decompression; perform diagnostic testing
  Continually monitor vital signs
  Provide ongoing psychosocial support to child and family

TABLE 17–3. QUICK REFERENCE TO PEDIATRIC EMERGENCY EQUIPMENT[a]

Equipment	Premature	Neonate	6 months	1 year	2 years	3 years	4 years	5 years	6 years	7 years	8 years	9 years	10 years	11–18 years
Airway														
Oral airway[b] (size)	Infant	Infant/Small	Small	Small	Small	Small	Med	Med	Med	Med	Med/Lg	Med/Lg	Med/Lg	Large
Endotracheal tube[c] (mm) *cuffed	2.5–3.0	3.0–3.5	3.5–4.0	4.0–4.5	4.0–4.5	4.0–4.5	5.0–5.5	5.0–5.5	5.5–6.0	5.5–6.0	6.0*–6.5*	6.0*–6.5*	6.0*–6.5*	7.0*–8.0*
Laryngoscope blade[b] s = straight c = curved	0 s	1 s	1 s	1 s	1 s	1 s	2 s/c	2 s/c	2 s/c	2 s/c	2–3 s/c	2–3 s/c	2–3 s/c	3 s/c
Suction catheter[c] (French)	5	6	6	8	8	8	10	10	10	10	10	10	10	12
Breathing														
Face mask[b] (size)	Prem NB	NB	NB	Ped	Ped	Ped	Ped	Ped	Ped	Ped	Ad	Ad	Ad	Ad
Bag-valve device[b] (size)	Inf	Inf	Inf	Ped	Ped	Ped	Ped	Ped	Ped	Ped/Ad	Ad	Ad	Ad	Ad
Chest tube[b] (French)	10–14	12–18	14–20	14–24	14–24	14–24	20–32	20–32	20–32	20–32	28–38	28–38	28–38	28–38
Circulation														
Over-the-needle catheter[d] (gauge)	22–24	22–24	22–24	20–22	20–22	20–22	20–22	18–22	18–20	18–20	16–20	16–20	16–20	14–18
Intraosseous device (gauge)	18	15	15	15	15	15	15	15	—	—	—	—	—	—
Gastrointestinal/genitourinary														
Nasogastric tube[e] (French)	5	5	8	8	10	10	10	10	10	12	12	12	12	14–16
Urinary catheter[b] (French)	5 feeding tube	5–8 feeding tube	8	10	10	10	10–12	10–12	10–12	10–12	12	12	12	12–18

[a]Suggested sizes only. Always consider each child's size and health condition when selecting appropriate equipment for procedures.
[b]Committee on Trauma [1989]. *Advanced trauma life support student manual.* Chicago: American College of Surgeons, p 231
[c]Motoyama E [1990]. Endotracheal intubation. In Motoyama E, Davis P (eds) *Smith's anesthesia for infants and children.* St Louis: Mosby, p 275
[d]Chameides L (ed) [1988]. *Textbook of pediatric advanced life support.* Dallas: American Heart Association and American Academy of Pediatrics, 35:105
[e]Skale N [1992]. *Manual of pediatric nursing procedures.* Philadelphia: Lippincott, p. 407
(Reprinted from Bernardo M, Bove M (eds) [1993]. Pediatric emergency nursing procedures. *Boston: Jones & Bartlett*)
Prem, premature infant; NB newborn; Ped, pediatric; Ad, adult; Inf, infant.

TABLE 17–4. Emergency Department Assessment and Management Plan for the Injured Child

Assessment	Diagnosis	Management	Laboratory Study
Airway and breathing		Clear airway Intubate Ventilate	
Cardiac function		External cardiac massage	Cardiorespiratory monitor
Shock	External hemorrhage Internal hemorrhage	Direct pressure Trendelenburg position Establish intravenous access MAST	CBC Cross match for one blood volume
Head/neck injury	Closed head injury Possible cervical spinal fracture	Sand bag splint of neck Hyperventilation	Skull x ray CT of head Lateral neck x ray
Chest injury	Cardiac contusion	ECG Pericardiocentesis	Chest x ray ECG Cardiac ultrasonography Arterial blood gases
	Hemopneumothorax Flail chest Sucking wound	Tube thoracotomy Intubation, ventilation Sterile dressing	
Abdominal injury	Penetrating injury	Nasogastric tube Serial examination	Plain, upright x ray
	Blunt injury	Serial examination Paracentesis with lavage	Tilt table test Amylase Liver function tests Serial CBC
Renal or urinary injury	Renal contusion or laceration	Bladder catheterization	Urinalysis Plain abdominal x ray Intravenous pyelogram
	Bladder or urethral injury	Delayed catheterization	Voiding cystourethrogram
Musculoskeletal injury	Dismembered part	Salvage, irrigate, and cool	Extremity x rays Angiography
	Compound fracture Bone injury	Sterile dressing, splint Splint, traction	
Soft tissue injury		Irrigate, debride Primary as opposed to delayed repair	X ray to exclude foreign body

CBC, complete blood count; MAST, medical antishock trousers; CT, computed tomography; ECG, electrocardiogram.
(*From Fleisher G, Ludwig S (eds) (1993), Textbook of pediatric emergency medicine [3rd ed]. Baltimore: Williams & Wilkins, p. 1100*)

must be obtained. In an attempted homicide, the nature, time, and mechanism of injury should be obtained. Witnesses may be reluctant to provide information, especially if gangs or drugs are involved. In an attempted suicide, the presence of a suicide note and an investigation of the scene provide helpful information.

If the parents have not already been notified, a member of the trauma team should do so. In emergency situations, treatment is not withheld until parental consent is obtained. Information obtained from parents follows the mneumonic AMPLE, which is: *A*llergies to medications; *M*edications the child is currently receiving; *P*ast medical history or illness; *L*ast meal eaten; *E*vents or environment leading to the injury. Finally, the child's special needs, such as vision, hearing, or physical impairments, should be noted.

Primary Survey

The initial assessment of a trauma patient includes primary and secondary surveys. During the primary survey, life-threatening conditions are detected and treated. These life-threatening conditions are unrelieved airway obstruction, open pneumothorax, tension pneumothorax, massive hemothorax, traumatic cardiac arrest, flail chest, cardiac tamponade, and hemorrhagic shock. Life-saving interventions, such as airway management and ventilatory and circulatory support, are initiated simultaneously with the primary survey.

Airway and Cervical Spine. The airway is carefully assessed for patency and is opened using the jaw thrust maneuver. This maneuver is the safest technique for opening the airway of the child with a suspected cervical spinal injury (Chameides, 1990). The jaw thrust technique is performed by placing the child's head in a midline, neutral position; the rescuer stands at the child's head and places two or three fingers under each side of the jaw, displacing it upward and forward (Figure 17–1). The head-tilt, chin-lift method is not used in pediatric trauma patients because of the potential for converting a cervical spine fracture without a neurologic injury into a cervical spine fracture with a neurologic injury.

The jaw thrust technique prevents airway obstruction. In an unconscious child, the tongue is a common cause of airway obstruction; the tongue also may cause airway obstruction in a conscious child with an impaired sensorium (Soud, 1992). The oral cavity in children is relatively small, and the upper airway is easily compromised by the lax oropharyngeal musculature in an obtunded, supine patient. Therefore, the airway is maintained with the jaw thrust technique until airway adjuncts are initiated.

While an open airway is maintained, any foreign material (teeth, vomitus, blood) is carefully cleared from the mouth and oropharynx using a tonsillar tip (Yankauer) suction catheter. Caution should be exercised if the child has an intact gag reflex, because prolonged suctioning may precipitate gagging, vomiting, and aspiration. Blind finger sweeps are not recommended in infants and young children because foreign material could be displaced distally into the oropharynx.

Placement of an oropharyngeal airway may be needed to maintain airway patency. An oral airway should be placed in unconscious children only; placement in a conscious child may precipitate vomiting and aspiration of vomitus. The size of the oral airway is critical: one that is too small may push the tongue backward; one that is too large may damage the delicate, soft intraoral tissues, causing bleeding and swelling and further complicating airway management

(Nakayama et al, 1992). The oropharyngeal airway is measured from the corner of the mouth to the angle of the jaw (Chameides, 1990). This type of airway is inserted directly using a tongue blade to pull the tongue forward (Soud, 1992). Nasopharyngeal airways are not recommended in trauma patients; a basilar or cribiform plate fracture may be present, and during insertion, the nasopharyngeal airway may enter the cranial vault. If prolonged airway maintenance is likely, rapid sequence endotracheal intubation by a skilled practitioner should be performed. Figure 17–2 contains a protocol for intubation of trauma patients. If these actions do not improve airway patency, the obstruction is likely to be in the lower airway, below the larynx. A surgical airway, such as a cricothyroidotomy or tracheostomy, may be required.

A proper-sized cervical collar is used to stabilize the cervical spine. The cervical collar fits properly if the chin rests securely in the chin holder and if the collar is beneath the ears and does not cover the upper part of the sternum (Bernardo and Waggoner, 1992). The front of the collar is opened during the primary survey to inspect the neck for jugular vein distention and tracheal deviation and then is closed; the carotid pulse is palpated at this time. The child should be secured on a pediatric long board with a cervical immobilization device or a manufactured pediatric immobilization device. Care must be taken to avoid unintentional anterior flexion of the cervical spine, which may occur because of a young child's disproportionately large head. Such flexion may jeopardize the airway or aggravate an existing spinal cord injury. A neutral alignment of the cervical spine is maintained continuously. Figure 17–3 illustrates simultaneous cervical spinal stabilization and intubation.

Breathing. Respirations are assessed by looking, listening, and feeling for breathing. The quality of respirations is determined by assessing the presence of bilateral breath sounds high in the axillae and anterior chest. If the child is apneic or if respirations are slow or shallow, artificial ventilation is initiated with a bag-valve-mask and 100% high-flow oxygen until endotracheal intubation is performed. The chest should rise symmetrically when the bag is squeezed; if the chest does not rise, the face mask and head should be repositioned (Nakayama et al, 1992). If the patient is breathing spontaneously, 100% high-flow oxygen by face mask is administered. If the child cannot tolerate a face mask, the oxygen can be administered in a blow-by manner, in which the oxygen mask is held next to the child's face and the oxygen is "blown by" the child for administration.

The chest is exposed and carefully inspected for any surface trauma, penetrating wounds, paradoxic

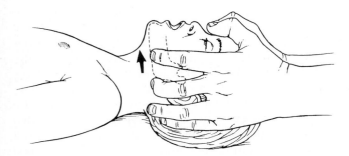

Figure 17–1. Combined jaw thrust–spinal stabilization maneuver for a pediatric trauma victim. (Reproduced with permission from American Heart Association [1992]. Standards and guidelines for cardiopulmonary resuscitation and emergency cardiac care. Part VI. Pediatric advanced life support. *JAMA* 268:2259)

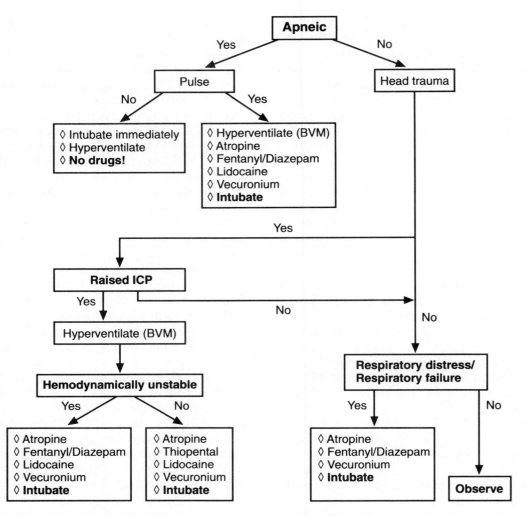

Figure 17–2. Protocol for intubation of trauma patients. Observe cervical spine precautions for all intubations. Use rapid sequence intubation whenever possible. BVM, bag-valve-mask; ICP, intracranial pressure. (Reproduced with permission from the Benedum Pediatric Trauma Program, Children's Hospital of Pittsburgh, Pittsburgh, Pa)

movements, flail segments, and retractions. Unequal bilateral breath sounds indicate a pneumothorax on the diminished or nonmoving side, which may necessitate rapid needle decompression by a physician.

Circulation. Circulation is assessed by auscultating heart sounds for their rate, rhythm and quality and by palpating a carotid pulse and assessing capillary refill. If the pulse is absent, chest compressions are initiated immediately. Muffled heart tones, distended neck veins, and shock may indicate cardiac tamponade, which may necessitate pericardiocentesis or open pericardiotomy (Nakayama, 1991). Major external hemorrhage is controlled by application of direct pressure. Two large-bore intravenous lines of lactated Ringer solution are established. The child is rapidly assessed for signs of hypovolemic shock. The earliest sign of shock is decreased peripheral perfusion (capillary re-

fill greater than 2 seconds, mottled skin, cool extremities, and tachycardia) (Nakayama, 1991).

Disability. A brief neurologic evaluation establishes the patient's level of consciousness and pupillary size and reactivity. Throughout the primary survey, the trauma team talks to the child to determine his or her level of consciousness and to provide emotional support. The AVPU method of evaluation determines the child's response to stimulation: *A*wake; responsive to *V*erbal stimuli; responsive to *P*ainful stimuli; and *U*nresponsive (Committee on Trauma, 1989). Sudden changes in the child's level of consciousness of either agitation or somnolence may indicate decreased oxygenation or perfusion. A more detailed neurologic examination is performed in the secondary survey.

Exposure. To assure that all injuries are located, the child is undressed completely. Overhead warming

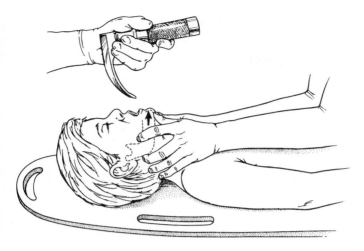

Figure 17–3. Simultaneous cervical spine stabilization and intubation. One rescuer holds the head and neck with both hands, simultaneously lifting the jaw at the angle of the mandible and immobilizing the neck. The second rescuer performs the intubation. (Reproduced with permission from American Heart Association [1992]. Standards and guidelines for cardiopulmonary resuscitation and emergency cardiac care. Part VI. Pediatric advanced life support. *JAMA* 268:221)

lights should help keep the child warm, as should the administration of warmed intravenous fluids and blood. After the primary and secondary surveys are completed, the child should be covered with warm blankets to prevent heat loss. The body areas should be uncovered for examination and then covered again.

Secondary Survey

The secondary survey is a complete head-to-toe examination of the trauma patient in which all non-life-threatening injuries are detected and treated. Again, treatment is initiated in concert with the secondary survey.

Head. The head is examined for hematomas, depressions, lacerations, and impaled objects. The anterior and posterior fontanelles in infants are palpated to detect fullness or bulging. The scalp is palpated for tenderness, pain, crepitance, and deformities.

Face. The face is inspected for lacerations, foreign bodies, impaled objects, facial nerve paralysis, asymmetry, and obvious fractures. Palpation of the orbital and facial bones may reveal pain, crepitance, or deformities. The possibility of LeFort fractures should be entertained in direct blunt force or penetrating trauma to the face. Malocclusion should be noted.

Eyes. The eyes are assessed for pupil responsiveness and symmetry, extraocular movements, hemorrhage, and foreign bodies or penetrating objects. The pres-

ence of contact lenses should be ascertained, and they should be removed. Periorbital bruising, or the raccoon sign, is an indicator of a basilar skull fracture. Scleral hemorrhage may be observed from trauma due to compression forces.

Ears. The ears are examined for the presence of cerebrospinal fluid or bloody drainage. Hemotympanum, or perforation of the eardrum, should be noted. Ecchymoses over the mastoid process, or the Battle's sign, are a late indicator of a basilar skull fracture. The presence of Battle's sign in a child in the ED indicates a head injury that is more than 12 hours old.

Nose. The nose is examined for the presence of cerebrospinal fluid or bloody drainage, nasal flaring, deviated septum, or obvious deformity. Because infants breathe through their noses, the nasal passages of infants should be kept as clear as possible.

Mouth. Any circumoral cyanosis should be noted. The tongue, mucous membranes, and teeth are examined for injury. Loosened teeth can be aspirated, especially during insertion of airways.

Neck. The airway is assessed continually. The front of the cervical collar is opened to allow examination of the neck. The neck is examined for pain, tenderness, lacerations, swelling, deformities, vein distention, subcutaneous emphysema, and impaled objects. The location of the trachea with respect to the midline should be noted. The larynx should be palpated for possible fractures; a fractured larynx is easier palpated than visualized. The cervical collar is removed only after cervical x rays have ruled out any cervical fracture; the child is alert enough to state the presence of any midline cervical pain with palpation; and the child's neurologic examination is normal. The absence of cervical pain, however, does not rule out the presence of a spinal cord injury. If there is any suspicion that a spinal cord injury is present, the cervical collar must remain in place until further neurologic testing is completed.

Chest. The chest is inspected for symmetry of movement, wounds, fractures, and flail segments. The anterior chest is examined for contusions and abrasions that may indicate underlying pulmonary or cardiac injury. The chest is auscultated for equal breath sounds, wheezes, rales, and rhonchi. Auscultation high in the anterior chest detects a pneumothorax, whereas auscultation in the posterior bases detects a hemothorax (Committee on Trauma, 1989). Each rib and both clavicles are palpated.

The heart sounds are auscultated and should be

clear and distinct. The point of maximal impulse (PMI) should be noted.

Abdomen. The abdomen is assessed for pain, rigidity, tenderness, distention, bruising, penetrating wounds, and impaled objects. Bowel sounds should be auscultated. The abdominal girth should be measured as a baseline and then frequently re-measured to note any increase in abdominal distention. A nasogastric tube (or orogastric tube in a patient with a suspected basilar skull fracture, cribiform plate fracture, or multiple facial fractures) should be inserted to prevent gastric distention, vomiting, and aspiration. A guaiac specimen is obtained.

Pelvis. Femoral pulses are assessed for equality and strength. Femoral swelling and hematomas are also assessed. The pelvic girdle is palpated for tenderness and intactness. The bladder is palpated for distention. The genitalia, urinary meatus, perineum, and rectum are inspected for signs of trauma and bleeding. Blood at the urinary meatus is indicative of a urethral tear. If there appears to be no trauma at the meatus, an indwelling urinary catheter may be inserted and connected to a urinary bag, complete with a urometer. The physician performs a rectal examination to assess for the presence of blood or pelvic fractures and for integrity of the rectal wall and quality of sphincter tone (Committee on Trauma, 1989). A guaiac specimen is obtained. A flaccid rectal sphincter is indicative of spinal cord injury.

Extremities. The extremities are carefully inspected for any deformities, lacerations, swelling, contusions, impaled objects, or open fractures. The adequacy of circulation is judged by the strength of the peripheral pulses, skin color, and the time required for capillary refill of the nailbeds. Capillary filling times longer than 2 seconds are considered abnormal. The presence and quality of pulses are assessed, especially those distal to an injury. Capillary filling, sensation, skin color, and temperature must be assessed continually. All suspected fractures should be immobilized. If there are any open fractures, lacerations, or wounds, the child may require tetanus prophylaxis. A check of the child's immunization record indicates if there is a need for tetanus prophylaxis.

Back. The patient is carefully log-rolled to inspect the back for any deformities, lacerations, hematomas, impaled objects, or abrasions on the posterior surface and flank. Each vertebra is palpated for stability and the presence of pain.

Vital Signs. The normal limits for vital signs in pediatric patients can vary appreciably (Table 17–5). It is

TABLE 17–5. NORMAL PEDIATRIC VITAL SIGNS

Age	Pulse (beats per minute)	Respiratory Rate (breaths per minute)	Blood Pressure (mmHg)
Newborn–6 weeks	100–170	30–50	70/40
6 weeks–6 months	100–150	28–40	74/44
6 months–1 year	90–140	24–32	80/50
1 year–3 years	80–130	24–32	90/60
4 years–7 years	80–120	22–28	100/60
8 years–12 years	80–110	20–24	110/60
13 years–16 years	70–100	16–22	120/70

important to be knowledgeable of the normal ranges of vital signs for the different age groups.

Heart rates should always be obtained apically in children and for 1 full minute to detect any irregular beats. Tachycardia may be found in fever, shock, and as an initial response to stress. The heart rate in a crying child can increase as much as 40–80 beats per minute. The heart rate should be obtained again as soon as the child becomes quiet. Bradycardia in children can result from hypoxia, hypoglycemia, increased intracranial pressure, or hypothermia.

Children's respirations are often irregular, especially those of a frightened or crying child. Therefore, the respiratory rate should be obtained for 1 full minute. Tachypnea is a normal response to stress. The respiratory rate should be reassessed once the child has regained composure. When a stressed child presents with a slow respiratory rate, an injury to the brain, spinal cord, phrenic nerve, or diaphragm should be considered.

Obtaining accurate blood pressure readings is critical in monitoring pediatric trauma patients. It is extremely important to use the appropriate size of blood pressure cuff. If a cuff is used that is too large, the reading obtained will be inaccurately low. Likewise, if a cuff is used that is too small, the reading obtained will be inaccurately high. The cuff should cover two-thirds of the extremity. It is often difficult or impossible to auscultate both the systolic and the diastolic blood pressure in infants and toddlers. For these children, it may be possible to obtain only the systolic pressure utilizing a Doppler machine or palpation. The normal diastolic pressure is roughly two-thirds the normal systolic pressure.

Trauma Scoring

After the primary and secondary assessments are completed, a trauma score and pediatric Glasgow Coma Scale (GCS) score are assigned. A trauma score is an adjunct to, not a substitute for, full and ongoing clinical assessments (Reynolds, 1992). Three trauma scores are used in pediatric trauma. The Pediatric

Trauma Score (PTS) assesses six parameters important in the outcome of pediatric trauma: size; airway; blood pressure; central nervous system; fractures; and wounds (see Table 7–4). The Trauma Score (TS) assesses respiratory rate and effort, blood pressure and capillary refill; it also includes the GCS score. The Revised Trauma Score (RTS) comprises the GCS score, blood pressure, and respiratory rate. The TS and RTS are adult scores, but they are used in children. One study demonstrated that the TS was more useful than the PTS in predicting the outcome of pediatric trauma patients in the ED and after hospitalization (Nayduch et al, 1991). Ideally, trauma scores are calculated in the pre-hospital setting, on arrival at the ED, and 1 hour later.

Re-evaluation

A multiply injured child is frequently re-evaluated to assure that treatment is effective and that other signs and symptoms are not missed. A seriously injured child is usually re-evaluated every 5 minutes until the child's condition is stabilized.

TRIAGE
Multiple Trauma

Emergent
Any child with multiple trauma.

Nursing Diagnosis
Ineffective Airway Clearance

Defining Characteristics

- Absent or abnormal breath sounds
- Cyanosis
- Choking, drooling

Nursing Interventions

- Perform jaw thrust maneuver
- Immobilize cervical spine
- Suction oropharynx
- Insert oropharyngeal airway
- Continually assess and support airway

Expected Outcomes

- Airway is patent
- Breath sounds are clear
- Child's color is normal

Nursing Diagnosis
Ineffective Breathing Pattern

Defining Characteristics

- Tachypnea, bradypnea, or apnea
- Cyanosis
- Altered chest excursion
- Adventitious breath sounds

Nursing Interventions

- Provide artificial ventilation if necessary
- Administer high-flow 100% oxygen
- Apply pulse oximeter
- Assist with obtaining arterial blood gases
- Continually assess and support breathing

Expected Outcomes

- Respirations are of adequate rate and quality
- Blood gas values are normal
- Skin color is normal

Nursing Diagnosis
Altered Tissue Perfusion: Cerebral, Cardiopulmonary, Renal, Gastrointestinal, Peripheral

Defining Characteristics

- Normotension or hypotension (late sign)
- Tachycardia, bradycardia (late sign)
- Increased capillary refill time (> 2 seconds)
- Cool, mottled, clammy extremities
- Altered or decreased level of consciousness

Nursing Interventions

- Maintain patent airway
- Administer high-flow 100% oxygen
- Administer warm intravenous fluids and blood products
- Apply PASG as indicated
- Measure fluid intake and urinary output

Expected Outcomes

- Vital signs are normal
- Capillary refill time is normal (< 2 seconds)
- Extremities are warm and color is normal
- Patient is awake, alert
- Urinary output is normal (> 1 mL/kg/hr)

Nursing Diagnosis
Fluid Volume Deficit

Defining Characteristics

- Normotension or hypotension (late sign)

- Tachycardia or bradycardia (late sign)
- Weak peripheral pulses
- Cool, clammy skin

Nursing Interventions

- Maintain airway patency
- Administer high-flow 100% oxygen
- Administer intravenous fluids and blood products
- Carefully monitor vital signs

Expected Outcomes

- Vital signs normal
- Capillary refill normal (> 2 seconds)
- Extremities warm and normal color
- Pulses are strong and palpable

Nursing Diagnosis
Hypothermia

Defining Characteristic

- Decreased body temperature

Nursing Interventions

- Use radiant warmers
- Use warm blankets
- Warm intravenous and blood products before administering them

Expected Outcome

- Body temperature returns to normal

Nursing Diagnosis
Fear

Defining Characteristics

- Verbalization of fear
- Crying, lack of cooperation

Nursing Interventions

- Reassure child
- Talk softly and slowly
- Explain all procedures
- Shield child from viewing any mutilating injuries
- Allow parents to be in trauma room with child as soon as possible

Expected Outcomes

- Child is calm.
- Child verbalizes understanding of procedures
- Parents are at child's bedside as much as possible

MANAGEMENT

Airway, Breathing, and Circulation

As previously dictated, the patient's airway, breathing, and circulation are continually assessed and supported. Supplemental oxygen is administered according to the child's requirements. For children with minimal oxygen requirements, a nasal cannula at a flow rate of 4–6 L/minute is sufficient. For infants and young children, the flow of oxygen should be started after the cannula is inserted into the nares to avoid frightening the child (Bernardo and Waggoner, 1992). A partial rebreathing mask with a flow rate of 10–12 L/minute is used for a child with greater oxygen requirements. The child's oxygen requirements are assessed by skin and mucous membrane color; pulse oximetry is also a useful adjunct in determining the child's level of oxygen saturation. Oxygen saturations should be over 95%.

A patient requiring prolonged airway control is prepared for endotracheal intubation. Rapid sequence intubation is undertaken for a pediatric trauma patient. Medications administered for rapid sequence intubation are pentothal, fentanyl and diazepam or midazolam, lidocaine and vecuronium (see Figure 17–2). These drugs are administered to prevent increased intracranial pressure and to produce adequate states of unconsciousness, pain control, and paralysis (Nakayama et al, 1992). After intubation, a naso- or orogastric tube is inserted because young children are aerophagic, and aggressive ventilation may lead to gastric distention (Semonin-Holleran, 1991).

A cardiorespiratory monitor is placed on the child immediately. An intravenous cannula with the largest diameter possible is inserted into the vein of an upper, preferably uninjured extremity. If intravenous access is unobtainable, intraosseous infusion is considered. If the intraosseous infusion is unsuccessful, central venous cannulation is attempted by an experienced physician. A saphenous vein cutdown by an experienced physician is the last option. Lactated Ringer solution is administered at two-thirds maintenance rate unless the child has signs and symptoms of hypovolemic shock. Overhydration should be avoided until the likelihood of a serious head injury with accompanying cerebral edema has been eliminated.

Resuscitation from Hypovolemic Shock

Shock, or circulatory failure, is characterized by decreased tissue perfusion that is inadequate to meet the metabolic demands of the body. The physiologic consequences of shock include hypotension, hypoxia, and metabolic acidosis. Hypovolemic shock is the most common type of shock in a pediatric trauma patient.

Pediatric patients have an estimated blood volume of 80 mL/kg of ideal body weight. A pediatric patient in hypovolemic shock has lost 25–50% of his or her total blood volume. Early indicators of hypovolemic shock include apprehension, pallor, irritability, slight tachycardia, delayed capillary refill, normal or slightly elevated blood pressure, normal or slightly decreased urine output, and clammy skin. Indicators of advanced hypovolemic shock include a decreased level of consciousness; dusky skin color; cool, clammy extremities; weak, thready pulses; poor capillary filling; tachycardia; tachypnea; and hypotension (a late sign). The blood pressure of the pediatric trauma patient in impending or actual hypovolemic shock often remains stable until the shock state is advanced.

Assessment for shock is ongoing; an initially stable, fully awake multiply injured patient should never be considered immune from sudden deterioration from an evolving hemorrhagic injury (Tepas, 1992). Head trauma alone does not cause shock. Therefore, if shock is suspected in a child with known head trauma, additional injuries such as abdominal hemorrhage are invariably present.

The probability of survival after shock is directly related to its duration; therefore it must be treated promptly. When hypovolemic shock is suspected, a fluid bolus of lactated Ringer solution at 20 mL/kg is rapidly infused with a syringe attached to a stopcock on the intravenous line. The patient's pulse rate, blood pressure and capillary refill are reassessed. If hypotension persists, a second bolus of lactated Ringer solution at 20 mL/kg is again rapidly administered. If the patient does not respond to this second bolus, uncrossmatched O-negative blood (packed cells) is administered at 10 mL/kg. Blood is administered because any further dilution of the patient's remaining blood reduces its oxygen-carrying capacity. Urine output should be 1 mL/kg/hour.

Medical Antishock Trousers

The application of a pediatric pneumatic antishock garment (PASG), often referred to as medical antishock trousers (MAST), may be indicated in hypotension, pelvic or lower extremity fractures, and intraabdominal hemorrhage (David Clark Co., Inc, 1988). The use of the PASG in children is controversial. The current belief is that the PASG is not recommended for fluid replacement because the garment does not displace significant volumes of fluid as was once believed; furthermore, the use of a PASG has been associated with compromised blood flow to the extremities (Yurt, 1992).

Thermoregulation

Major heat losses in an unclothed child during resuscitation may interfere with already compromised metabolic processes. A child left exposed in a cold room can quickly become hypothermic, which may lead to bradycardia and possibly cardiac arrest. Therefore, it is advisable to increase the room temperature or use overhead radiant heaters. Only the portion of the child that is necessary is exposed after the initial assessment. Rapid infusions of cold blood or intravenous fluids can also produce hypothermia. Measures should be taken to warm refrigerated blood and intravenous fluids before infusion is begun.

Pain Management

Pain management is an important part of an injured child's care. Because emotional distress accentuates the child's pain experience (Acute Pain Management Guideline Panel, 1992), efforts to promote the child's comfort should be provided by the emergency nurse.

Assessment of a child's pain is accomplished with age-appropriate methods and by asking a verbal, conscious child if he or she hurts or has pain. For a preverbal or nonverbal child, observing the child's behavior may elucidate his or her experience of pain. Behaviors associated with pain include facial grimacing, guarding, lying still, or resisting movement. Physiologic indicators of pain include increased heart rate, respiratory rate, blood pressure, and perspiration; however, these indicators are not specific for pain and may vary among children (Acute Pain Management Guideline Panel, 1992). Physiologic indicators should be used in conjunction with self-report scales or behavior observations.

The pharmacologic management of pain is not usually initiated for a child with a head injury because of the potential dulling of subsequent neurologic examinations. When invasive procedures, such as chest tube insertion, are undertaken, local anesthesia should be administered. Nonpharmacologic strategies to help children cope with pain include distraction, holding a nurse's hand, holding their stuffed animal or blanket, progressive relaxation, and storytelling. Positive self-talk ("I can make it") also is helpful.

Laboratory and Diagnostic Tests

Venipuncture. A complete blood count (CBC) with differential; coagulation profiles; and levels of serum electrolytes, blood urea nitrogen (BUN), creatinine, and glucose are obtained. Amylase and lipase levels as well as serum glutamic-oxaloacetic transaminase (SGOT) and serum glutamic pyruvate transaminase (SGPT) levels are obtained. A type and crossmatch for two pediatric units of blood is done in cases of impending or actual hypovolemic shock or if operative management will occur. An arterial blood gas sampling is obtained if there are indications of hypovolemic shock or respiratory distress.

Urinalysis. A urinalysis is obtained, usually during urinary catheterization. This first specimen may be urine in the bladder from before the injury; therefore, a second specimen should be tested.

Radiographic Studies. Anteroposterior and lateral cervical spine x rays are obtained for all multiply injured children. An open-mouth view may also be obtained. The x ray must include all seven cervical vertebrae and the first thoracic vertebra to assure the alignment and intactness of the cervical spine. Anterior and posterior chest x rays are obtained to determine the presence of the endotracheal, oro- or nasogastric, and chest tubes; the presence of pneumo- or hemopneumothoraces; rib and clavicle fractures; and intactness of the diaphragm. Abdominal x rays determine the presence of oro- or nasogastric tubes and bladder catheters and intactness of the stomach and intestines. These x rays are obtained in the trauma room with portable x ray machines. If the patient must leave the trauma room to go to the x ray department, at least one emergency nurse and an experienced surgeon should accompany the patient and should bring appropriate equipment in the event of an emergency.

Other x rays are obtained as indicated by history or physical findings. Orthopantomograms are obtained in facial trauma. X rays of the thoracic and lumbar spine may be obtained if a fracture is suspected. Suspected extremity fractures are identified by x rays of both the uninjured and the injured extremity. Computed tomography (CT) is considered if severe head, facial, chest, or abdominal trauma is suspected.

Peritoneal Lavage. In children, peritoneal lavage is rarely performed to diagnose hemorrhage or visceral perforation; CT is the procedure of choice (Donnellan, 1990). Peritoneal lavage is indicated, however, when a multiply injured child requires immediate operative intervention, when CT is unavailable, or when a CT study is normal but an intestinal injury is presumed (Nichols et al, 1991). Abdominal x rays should be obtained before the peritoneal lavage because air may enter the abdomen during the procedure and interfere with the interpretation of later x rays. The bladder is emptied by an indwelling catheter to avoid bladder perforation.

A small incision is made in the midline between the umbilicus and pubis. A pediatric peritoneal lavage catheter is then inserted into the peritoneal cavity.

Next, a syringe is attached and any fluid is aspirated. If gross nonclotted blood returns, the procedure is considered positive, indicative of intra-abdominal bleeding, and the procedure is terminated. If there is no evidence of blood, an intravenous solution of normal saline solution is infused by gravity at a rate of 15 mL/kg. The fluid is then allowed to pool in the abdominal cavity. It may be necessary to roll the patient from side to side to facilitate mixing of the solution with peritoneal fluids. Next, the fluid is drained from the abdominal cavity, the catheter is removed, and the incision site is sutured. If the fluid obtained is clear, the tap is considered negative. However, if the red blood cell count exceeds 100,000 rbc/mm^3, the white blood cell count exceeds 500 wbc/mL, newspaper print cannot be read through the fluid, or stool is present, the procedure is considered to be positive, and operative management may be indicated. Lavage fluid should be sent to the laboratory for a CBC, hematocrit, evaluation for amylase and bile, Gram stain, and culture.

SPECIFIC INJURIES IN PEDIATRIC TRAUMA

Central Nervous System Trauma

Head Trauma. The most frequent cause of death in pediatric trauma is head injury (Billmire, 1992). Seventy-five percent of children with multiple injuries have a concomitant head injury (Donnellan, 1990). Several reasons for this high incidence are that the child's cranium is thin and affords little protection to the less myelinated brain; the head constitutes a greater percentage of body area and weight, making it susceptible to injury; and falls, motor vehicle collisions, and bicycle crashes predispose the child to head injury.

Brain injuries are classified as either primary or secondary. Primary injuries to central nervous system (CNS) tissue occur at the time of initial trauma. These injuries include cerebral contusions, lacerations, skull fractures, and initial neuronal and vascular disruptions: once present, these injuries are seldom influenced by therapeutic intervention (Tecklenburg and Wright, 1991). Secondary brain injuries result from reactive CNS lesions or extracranial disorders after the injurious event. They include cerebral edema, intracranial hemorrhage, altered cerebral vascular tone, and seizures (Tecklenburg and Wright, 1991). Injuries to the cardiovascular or pulmonary systems can lead to hypoxia, hypercarbia, hypotension, and anemia, further compromising the CNS (Tecklenburg and Wright, 1991). Protection from this source of CNS disability is the responsibility of the ED trauma team.

Control of intracerebral pressure, maintenance of adequate CNS perfusion, and prevention of hypoxia are the goals of cerebral resuscitation. The prevention of cerebral edema is achieved by hyperventilation through endotracheal intubation and mechanical ventilation. Destructive increases in intracerebral pressure occur with hypercarbia, and hypoventilation must be corrected. Control of seizures is important because convulsive activity frequently increases carbon dioxide production and impairs respiratory gas exchange.

Once diagnostic testing and the physical examination determine that a spinal cord injury is not present, the head of the bed can be elevated to decrease venous pressure. Intravenous fluids should be restricted to two-thirds of maintenance levels. Corticosteroids are no longer administered to patients with a head injury.

Head injuries are particularly difficult to evaluate in a multiply injured child, who may be anxious, afraid, or combative. Continued neurologic assessment utilizing the modified or infant GCS is critical. See chapter 18 for detailed information on the assessment and treatment of head trauma in children.

Spinal Cord Injuries. A child's spine is hypermobile and has weak vertebral ligaments. Although the vertebral column is capable of considerable elongation, the spinal cord itself is unable to withstand the same degree of trauma. Spinal cord elongation and subsequent injury can occur without x ray evidence of bony malformation. This type of spinal cord injury is called SCIWORA (spinal cord injury without radiographic abnormality). SCIWORA happens not only to unrestrained pediatric motor vehicle passengers but also to those who sustain sports injuries or birth trauma and to pedestrians struck by motor vehicles.

Fracture dislocation is another cause of spinal cord injury. The lower cervical spine is at particular risk for injury because of the marked mobility of the neck. Common sites of spinal cord injuries in children are levels C-1, C-2, C-5, C-6, T-12, and L-1.

Most spinal cord injuries that children sustain in motor vehicle collisions are the result of indirect trauma. These injuries are caused by sudden hyperflexion or hyperextension of the neck, often combined with a rotational force. Seat belt syndrome, or fracture of the lumbar spine with an injury to the small intestine, can occur in younger children wearing a lap belt.

A patient with a possible spinal cord injury is protected from further injury by spinal immobilization. Any injured child who walks into the ED or who arrives by private vehicle whose mechanism of injury may cause a spinal injury must receive immediate cervical and spinal immobilization.

If an infant or child arrives for treatment in a safety seat following a motor vehicle collision, the child should be immobilized in the car seat if the child's airway, breathing, and circulation are stable, if adult spinal equipment is unavailable, and the child safety seat is intact (Widner-Kolberg, 1991). All children with suspected spinal cord injuries remain immobilized with a cervical collar and cervical immobilization device on a long back board until diagnostic evidence assures the presence of an intact spinal cord. If the patient is unconscious, spinal immobilization remains in place until the child is able to respond to neurologic testing. Further diagnostic evaluations, such as flexion-extension studies, CT, myelography and somatosensory evoked potentials (SSEPs), are indicated. The patient's neurologic status is assessed continually.

Chest Trauma

The incidence of thoracic trauma among hospitalized injured children ranges from 1–30% (Newman and Sivit, 1992). Most chest trauma in children is blunt as opposed to penetrating. The severity of thoracic trauma is directly related to its impact on the underlying cardiopulmonary structures. Chest wall mobility is increased in children, making them less susceptible to rib and sternal fractures. Although rib fractures are less common in infants and young children than in adults because of the pliability of the rib cage, cardiac and pulmonary injuries are still possible. When fractures have occurred, a great amount of force was necessary; therefore, a high index of suspicion for underlying pulmonary and cardiac injury must be appreciated.

The heart, great vessels, and mediastinum are less physically shielded from blunt or penetrating forces in children than in adults; consequently, injury is more likely than it is in adults (Messier et al, 1992). However, the flexibility of the mediastinal structures affords some protection from injuries that would cause aortic disruption in adults (Messier et al, 1992). Life-threatening chest injuries in children include open pneumothorax, tension pneumothorax, pneumothorax, hemothorax, and hemopneumothorax, and cardiac tamponade. Flail segments and pulmonary and cardiac contusions also occur.

Pneumothorax. A pneumothorax may occur after blunt chest trauma with or without fractured ribs. Air leaks from the injured lung into the pleural space. The child may have no symptoms if the pneumothorax is small. With a clinically significant pneumothorax, the child demonstrates hypoxemia, asymmetric chest-wall movement, decreased breath sounds on the affected side, and an altered pitch in breath sounds on the affected side (Soud et al, 1992).

Treatment of pneumothorax requires rapid needle thoracentesis. A large-bore needle is inserted in the second intercostal space at the midclavicular line on the side of the pneumothorax; definitive treatment is the insertion of a chest tube at the nipple level (fifth intercostal space) anterior to the midaxillary line (Committee on Trauma, 1989).

Open Pneumothorax. Because penetrating injuries are unusual in the pediatric population, open pneumothorax is relatively rare. An open pneumothorax is characterized by a sucking sound during inspiration and a frothing or bubbling sound with expiration. If the wound is approximately two-thirds the diameter of the trachea, air selectively passes through the chest defect with each respiration (Committee on Trauma, 1989). This air entry eventually compromises lung inflation and leads to hypoxia.

An open pneumothorax is treated by closing the wound with an occlusive dressing. A petrolatum gauze dressing large enough to cover the wound's edges is taped securely on three sides, producing a flutter valve. When the patient inhales, the dressing covers the wound and prevents air entry; when the patient exhales, the open end of the dressing allows the air to escape (Committee on Trauma, 1989). This action should produce immediate improvement in the efficiency of the respiratory gas exchange. A chest tube is then inserted in an area remote from the sucking chest wound (Committee on Trauma, 1989). The wound itself usually requires surgical treatment. A chest x ray confirms the placement of the tube and re-expansion of the lung. A functioning chest tube should fluctuate with respiration.

Tension Pneumothorax. A tension pneumothorax occurs when there is progressive accumulation of air in the pleural space that collapses the lung and shifts the flexible and mobile mediastinum to the opposite hemithorax. The vena cava and pulmonary veins are angulated, decreasing venous return to the heart and compressing the unaffected lung (Nakayama, 1991).

Physical findings typically observed with a tension pneumothorax include dyspnea, anxiety, tachypnea, distended neck veins, decreased breath sounds, hypertympanic percussion on the affected side, and hypotension; tracheal deviation away from the affected side is a late sign (Peitzman and Paris, 1988) and may not be present in young children.

Management of a tension pneumothorax includes rapid needle decompression in the second intercostal space at the midclavicular line on the affected side to relieve the positive intrathoracic pressure. Definitive treatment requires the insertion of a chest tube at the fifth intercostal space anterior to the midaxillary line (Committee on Trauma, 1989).

Hemothorax. A hemothorax occurs as a result of blunt or penetrating trauma when large amounts of blood accumulate in the pleural space and compress the lung. Massive hemothorax produces both circulatory collapse and respiratory failure.

Indicators of hemothorax include signs of shock, then difficulty breathing, decreased or absent breath sounds on the affected side and dullness to percussion on the affected side. The neck veins are usually flat, and tracheal deviation is usually not present (Peitzman and Paris, 1988).

Management includes rapid fluid resuscitation and evacuation of the hemothorax. Thoracotomy is frequently required, especially if the hypotension does not improve with fluid resuscitation (Newman and Sivit, 1992). The chest tubes are placed in the fifth intercostal space in the anterior midaxillary line on the affected side. The chest tubes are connected to underwater seal drainage and 10–20 cm suction.

Flail Chest. Flail chest is rare in younger children (Newman and Sivit. 1992). Flail chest occurs from blunt trauma and is present when three or more adjacent ribs are fractured in at least two places (Peitzman and Paris, 1988). The fractured segment moves paradoxically relative to the intact chest wall. Underlying lung tissue is damaged during the injury, leading to pulmonary contusions. Impaired gas exchange is possible; with a large flail segment, severe respiratory distress may occur. Clinical indicators include tenderness over the ribs with petechiae, crepitus and ecchymoses, tachycardia, tachypnea, hypotension, and paradoxic chest movements. The possibility of associated pulmonary and myocardial contusions should be considered. Management includes stabilization of the flail segment with bulky dressings taped over the chest. Intubation and mechanical ventilation are usually required to achieve sufficient respiratory gas exchange.

Pulmonary Contusion. Pulmonary contusions result from blunt force trauma to the chest. Kinetic energy is transferred through the chest wall to the lung. A high mortality is associated with massive pulmonary contusions (Newman and Sivit, 1992). Signs of pulmonary contusion may not be present in the ED. However, x ray changes may be seen in subsequent hours or days (Newman and Sivit, 1992). Pulmonary contusions should always be suspected in children who sustain blunt force trauma to the chest; these children must receive oxygen and frequent respiratory assessments while in the ED.

Cardiac Tamponade. Cardiac tamponade is usually the result of a penetrating or crushing thoracic injury. It is characterized by an accumulation of blood in the pericardial sac (as little as 25–50 mL) (Soud et al, 1992). This accumulation of blood compresses the heart, preventing cardiac filling and decreasing cardiac output.

The patient typically presents with Beck's triad—an elevation of venous pressure, a decrease in arterial pressure, and muffled or distant heart sounds. Jugular vein distention may be present unless the patient is in hypovolemic shock. The patient is often agitated, hypoxic, and has poor peripheral circulation. Pulsus paradoxis, an 8–10 mm Hg decrease in systolic blood pressure with inspiration, may be observed if the patient is not in a state of shock (Soud et al, 1992).

Cardiac tamponade must be relieved immediately with pericardiocentesis, which involves a needle aspiration of the pericardial sac by the subxyphoid route (Figure 17–4). During this procedure continuous cardiac monitoring is essential. Open thoracotomy and inspection of the heart are required if the pericardiocentesis is positive (Committee on Trauma, 1989).

Traumatic Diaphragmatic Hernia.

Blunt trauma to the upper abdomen or lower chest can cause a tear in the diaphragm, resulting in herniation of intra-abdominal contents into the chest cavity and severe respiratory distress. The patient may complain of abdominal and chest pain, nausea, and vomiting. Tachycardia, hypotension, abdominal distention, or tachypnea may be present. A diaphragmatic hernia on x ray can be mistaken for hemothorax, pneumothorax, or pneumomediastinum.

Morbidity and mortality are usually related to an associated injury, such as head trauma, pulmonary contusion, or intra-abdominal organ injury, rather than to the diaphragmatic lesion itself. Management includes airway support and treatment of hypotension and respiratory distress; decompression of the stomach with a nasogastric tube; and a surgical procedure.

Myocardial Contusion.

Myocardial contusion is caused by blunt trauma to the anterior midchest from motor vehicle collisions, falls, or other blunt trauma. The injury causes a cardiac contusion with sudden disruption of cardiac activity, ventricular fibrillation, or arrhythmia from edema. The diagnosis is often difficult because of the presence of other conditions, such as hypovolemic shock and pneumothorax.

Clinical indicators of myocardial contusion include tachycardia, dysrhythmias, chest pain, murmur, rales, hypotension, contusion, or tenderness over the precordium.

Treatment includes administration of oxygen and intravenous fluids, cardiac monitoring, and treatment of dysrhythmias.

Abdominal Trauma

A large number of pediatric deaths are the result of abdominal trauma. Figure 17–5 illustrates some possible consequences of blunt abdominal trauma. The spleen is the most commonly injured abdominal organ, followed by the liver (Billmire, 1992). Ninety percent of these abdominal injuries are caused by blunt force trauma from direct impact, deceleration, and shearing forces (Billmire, 1992). Blunt force trauma is

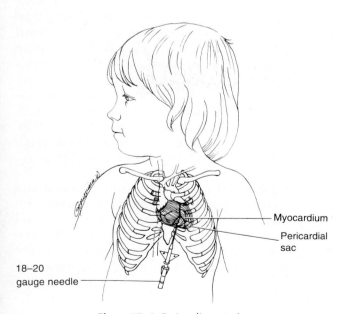

18–20 gauge needle

Myocardium

Pericardial sac

Figure 17–4. Pericardiocentesis.

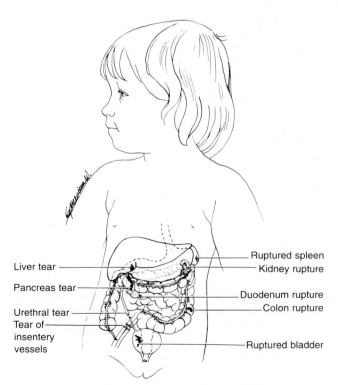

Liver tear
Pancreas tear
Urethral tear
Tear of insentery vessels

Ruptured spleen
Kidney rupture
Duodenum rupture
Colon rupture
Ruptured bladder

Figure 17–5. Possible consequences of blunt abdominal trauma.

not always accompanied by cutaneous lesions such as bruises and abrasions; therefore, a high index of suspicion for abdominal organ injury should be present.

In general, injury to the abdominal organs is associated with pain and guarding, rebound tenderness, decreased or absent bowel sounds, and nausea and vomiting; the child appears quite ill (Donnellan, 1990). Management includes the administration of oxygen, fluid resuscitation, gastric decompression, and close observation.

Liver. Trauma to the liver is a leading cause of morbidity and mortality in pediatric trauma. Although partially protected by the elastic rib cage, the liver remains vulnerable to blunt force trauma injury because of its large size and fragility. A child's thoracic cage is elastic. A firm blow to the right upper quadrant can cause injury to the liver. The absence of localized bruises or abrasions does not rule out the possibility of serious laceration or rupture. Even such seemingly minor trauma as falling against a rigid object or falling from low heights and landing on the right side can cause major hepatic injury and blood loss.

Children with trauma to the liver often complain of right upper quadrant pain or diffuse abdominal pain. Although peritoneal lavage is useful in diagnosing intraperitoneal bleeding, it does not localize the source of bleeding or indicate the need for surgical intervention in hemodynamically stable children (Billmire, 1992). Abdominal CT is the most sensitive, accurate, and expeditious diagnostic tool for detecting the presence of injuries, such as subcapsular hematomas, linear fractures, and stellate or burst fractures (Billmire, 1992).

Management is aimed at prevention or treatment of hypovolemic shock. Vital signs should be assessed frequently. Gastric and urinary output, as well as IV fluid administration, is closely monitored. The child is observed for increasing abdominal distention, pain, or tenderness. An ongoing evaluation for signs of hypovolemic shock is essential. Although about 60–65% of hepatic injuries are managed successfully without surgical intervention (Nakayama, 1991), children with known or suspected liver trauma should be rapidly resuscitated and transferred to a medical facility equipped to perform major hepatic surgical procedures and to provide pediatric intensive care.

Spleen. The spleen is the intra-abdominal organ most commonly injured during blunt abdominal trauma. An injured spleen usually causes intraperitoneal hemorrhage, which produces pain and nausea. The most common physical finding in splenic injury is left upper quadrant tenderness with occasional referred pain to the shoulder, known as Kehr's sign. As in liver injuries, CT is the diagnostic tool of choice.

Bleeding from splenic injuries often ceases spontaneously, obviating the need for surgical intervention 90–95% of the time (Nakayama, 1991). Children whose hemodynamic condition is stable can be safely observed with frequent monitoring of vital signs, hemoglobin and hematocrit values, and intake and output. If an operation is necessary, it is directed toward preservation of the spleen.

Pancreas. Although pancreatic trauma is relatively infrequent in children, as compared with liver and splenic injuries, it remains a cause of morbidity and mortality. The pancreas lies in a retroperitoneal location and is relatively protected from abdominal trauma. However, the pancreas is susceptible to anterior blows to the abdomen, which compress it against the rigid vertebrae. Injury to the pancreas is difficult to diagnose because of the retroperitoneal location and the difficulty of CT diagnosis (Nakayama, 1991).

Contusion is the most frequent pancreatic injury. The clinical presentation may include midepigastric pain, diffuse abdominal pain, nausea, vomiting, and back pain. Laceration of the pancreas produces a much more serious injury; pancreatic juice leaks into the retroperitoneum. Unrecognized pancreatic injuries can progress to pancreatic pseudocyst formation. Trauma is the leading cause of pancreatic pseudocysts in children, which may occur days or even months after trauma.

Pancreatic injury is often associated with injury to the spleen, liver, and duodenum. The most reliable tests for determining pancreatic injury are serial serum amylase and lipase levels, which are elevated. Also, urinary amylase levels are of value in diagnosing pancreatic trauma and may be elevated even with normal serum values. Other injuries that can be detected from elevated serum or urinary amylase levels are injuries to the salivary glands and small-intestinal perforation.

The radiologic evaluation of a child with suspected pancreatic or duodenal trauma should include flat and upright abdominal x rays and CT. Surgical intervention is usually not necessary unless major ductal or glandular injury is present (Nakayama, 1991).

Stomach and Intestines. Injuries to the stomach and intestines usually result from blunt-force trauma, such as lap belt injuries, bicycle handlebar injuries, and child abuse. There may be free air under the diaphragm or air and fluid in the peritoneal cavity. The child usually exhibits signs of peritonitis (abdominal distention, tenderness, leukocytosis and acidosis) (Nakayama, 1991).

Management includes careful monitoring of vital signs and intake and output and observation for worsening of symptoms. Surgical intervention is not usually required.

Abdominal Vascular Injury. The most common intra-abdominal great-vessel injury in children is to the hepatic veins; it is associated with severe liver laceration. Injury to retroperitoneal vessels, particularly rupture of the pelvic vein associated with a pelvic fracture, can cause copious blood loss. Because of the closed space involved, the bleeding usually stops spontaneously by tamponade.

Renal System Trauma

Renal Trauma. After the CNS, the kidneys are the most commonly injured organ (O'Connor and Gibbons, 1992). Children are more susceptible to renal injuries than adults because their kidneys are larger relative to their body size. The kidneys are more mobile and not as well protected by the large quantity of perinephritic fat found in adults. Children also have weaker abdominal muscles and an elastic rib cage, both of which afford little protection to the kidneys. Ectopic kidneys, abnormally positioned kidneys (pelvic or horseshoe), kidneys distended by obstruction, and those affected by tumors or other infiltrative processes are vulnerable to traumatic injury (O'Connor and Gibbons, 1992). Most renal injuries are caused by blunt trauma, including acceleration and deceleration mechanisms. Penetrating trauma to the kidneys, such as gunshot or stab wounds, occur much less frequently in children than in adults.

The volume per minute of blood flow to the kidney is greater than that to any other abdominal organ. The blood flow to the kidney is 25% of the cardiac output. Consequently, injury to a kidney may cause rapid blood loss. Therefore, signs of hypovolemic shock should be carefully monitored.

Children with renal trauma may present with abrasions, ecchymosis, and pain or tenderness over the lower back or abdomen. Hematuria is usually present; however, the absence of hematuria does not exclude renal injury. Associated injuries, especially to the abdomen, are often present.

Renal injuries are classified as either minor or major or into five grades (Karp et al, 1986). Eighty to 85 percent of renal injuries are diagnosed as minor (O'Connor and Gibbons, 1992). Grade 1 injuries include intrarenal contusions or subcapsular hematomas. Grade 2 injuries are minor parenchymal lacerations of the capsule or cortex. The collecting system is not involved, and there is no extravasation of blood.

Grade 3 injuries are major parenchymal lacerations that involve the collecting system; extravasation of urine is present. Grade 4 injuries involve a fractured or shattered kidney with lacerations and disruptions. Vascular structures remain intact. Grade 5 injuries are major vascular or pedicle disruptions in which the kidney is not functioning.

Diagnostic testing for renal injuries includes an intravenous pyelogram, ultrasonography, radionuclide scanning, arteriography, and CT. Management of minor renal injuries includes bedrest and limited activity for 6 weeks; surgical intervention is reserved for major renal injuries in a child in a hemodynamically unstable condition who has evidence of sepsis or an abscess (O'Connor and Gibbons, 1992). Accurate measurement of intake and output, frequent assessment of vital signs, and monitoring for hypovolemic shock constitute nursing care.

Ureter, Bladder, and Urethra. There are few acute manifestations of ureteral, bladder, or urethral injuries. When trauma does occur to these structures, it is rarely life-threatening. It is therefore of secondary concern in the management of a multiply injured child with life-threatening injuries.

Ureteral injuries are usually caused by penetrating trauma. However, in pediatric patients, because of the increased mobility of the renal unit, a forceful blow to the abdomen or flank can separate the ureter from the renal pelvis. Symptoms of ureteral injuries may not be present for several days. Ureteral injuries are often associated with a fracture of a vertebral transverse process.

The bladder of a child is less vulnerable to injury than that of an adult because of its higher position. However, it is frequently ruptured because it is often full and is located high in the abdomen (Donnellan, 1990). Considerable blood loss may result from trauma to the bladder. Blood may accumulate in the bony pelvis and lead to hypotension. Hematuria is not always present with a ruptured bladder. The diagnosis is based on the findings of a cystogram.

Trauma to the urethra can be a serious problem. Complete or partial transection of the urethra can result from direct trauma to the perineum or a crush injury to the pelvis. Urethral injuries are more common in boys. When urethral injuries occur in girls, they are usually the result of penetrating trauma. Blood may or may not be evident at the urethral meatus. Other indicators of urethral trauma include bladder distention, inability to void, irregularity of the pubic bone because of a fracture, ecchymosis over the perineum and buttocks, and a pelvic fracture. If any of these indicators is present, a urethral catheter should not be inserted until a retrograde urethrogram can be performed. Catheterization of a traumatized urethra may convert a lesser injury into a complete disruption.

Musculoskeletal Trauma

The musculoskeletal system is frequently involved in multisystem pediatric trauma. Three common musculoskeletal injuries—pelvic fractures, fractures of the femur, and open fractures—warrant close monitoring and immediate intervention.

Pelvic fractures in children most often result from motor vehicle crashes, including pedestrian–motor vehicle crashes (Bond et al, 1991). As in adults, multiple pelvic fractures in children are associated with abdominal and genitourinary injuries. Unlike in adults, these multiple fractures are not associated with increased mortality from hemorrhage and its complications (Bond et al, 1991). Bleeding may be reduced in children because their periosteum adheres more tightly to the bone than the periosteum of an adult and because the blood vessels of children are more vasoreactive than those of adults (Bond et al, 1991).

Even with these protective mechanisms, children can still lose enough blood into the pelvis to cause exsanguination (Nakayama, 1991). Children with pelvic fractures are closely observed for changes in vital signs, urinary output, level of consciousness, and laboratory values to monitor hemodynamic changes and prevent hemorrhagic shock.

Femoral fractures can result in significant blood loss. For example, a closed fracture of the femur can be responsible for 300–400 mL of lost blood. This amount may be 15–25% of the total circulating blood volume of a child and can contribute to hypovolemic shock. Femoral fractures are associated with pain, redness, and swelling at the fracture site; they can be open, closed, displaced or nondisplaced, comminuted, shattered, or greenstick. Operative treatment may include the placement of an external fixation device, internal fixation or tibial pinning, and 90°–90° traction. Displaced fractures of the femoral neck require emergent closed or open reduction to avoid nonunion, varus deformity, and avascular necrosis of the femoral head (Neustadt, 1992). Ongoing assessments of sensory and motor function are indicated, as is close observation for signs of hemorrhagic shock.

Open fractures require debridement, irrigation and stabilization. To prevent the development of osteomyelitis, all open fractures should be managed surgically as soon as possible, at least 6 hours after the injury (Neustadt, 1992). External fixation devices, plaster casts, and, occasionally, internal fixation devices are applied to facilitate healing. Again, ongoing neurovascular assessment is imperative.

PATIENT AND FAMILY TEACHING AND PSYCHOSOCIAL SUPPORT

During the initial phase of resuscitation, the trauma team may overlook the child's emotional needs in order to save the child's life. Therefore, the important role of emotional support by the emergency nurse cannot be understated.

A multiply injured child experiences fear, apprehension, and pain. During resuscitation, the child is subjected to sensory overload from staff conversing loudly and moving about hurriedly, from invasive and painful procedures, and from unfamiliar surroundings. Therefore, a pediatric trauma patient requires the emotional support of a calm, reassuring emergency nurse. Although it is probably most beneficial if providing emotional support is the nurse's only responsibility, the trauma nurse on the left usually is charged with this important role. The nurse providing emotional support to an immobilized child should stand at the child's chest level so the child is able to see the nurse without turning his or her head (Bernardo and Waggoner, 1992). Standing directly over the child's face may be frightening, especially when different faces keep appearing and reappearing (Bernardo and Waggoner, 1992).

The emergency nurse can hold the child's hand and explain in simple terms what is happening ("The doctor is listening to your heart beat"; "You will feel a pinch in your left hand"). Speaking softly and calmly and using language the child understands should help the child focus on the nurse's explanations and instructions, thereby facilitating the child's coping. Even with an unresponsive or comatose child, the emergency nurse should continue to offer emotional support; it is not known what these children may remember afterward.

Parents are usually not permitted in the trauma room until a seriously injured child's condition is stabilized. If the parents are permitted in the trauma room, a health professional, such as an emergency nurse or social worker, must remain with the family to provide emotional support and to explain the treatment to them. The emergency nurse must reassure the child that his or her parents are nearby in the ED or en route to the hospital. If the parents have also been injured, the emergency nurse may tell the child that he or she will remain with the child until a relative or friend arrives.

Because childhood injuries are unexpected, parents do not have time to prepare for or adjust to their child's serious condition. Parents often experience feelings of shock, denial, disbelief, and guilt. They often fear that their child will die or be permanently disabled. Parents need reassurance that everything possible is being done for their child and that their child is not suffering. They should be kept constantly informed of the child's condition and of all procedures and treatments. Ideally, a member of the trauma team, such as a nurse or social worker, is assigned as the liaison to the parents, providing them with as much information as possible.

Once the child's condition has been stabilized, the parents should be allowed in the trauma room to visit the child. This visit is reassuring to both the child and the parents. Before the parents enter the trauma room, the emergency nurse should prepare them for what they will see, such as monitors and intravenous lines. The emergency nurse should remain with the family and should encourage them to talk with and to touch their child. When possible, parents should be allowed to accompany the child during transportation to places such as the radiology suite or the operating room.

The trauma team caring for a critically injured child also needs emotional support. Critical incident stress debriefing by qualified professionals should be offered to the team after resuscitations, especially if the child dies.

Most childhood injuries are preventable. Therefore, the ED nurse has an ongoing responsibility to teach injury prevention to parents at every possible opportunity. After a child has been seriously injured, however, is not the appropriate time for teaching injury prevention. Not only are parents incapable of absorbing information during this time of crisis but also such information increases their existing feelings of guilt and responsibility. Instead, injury prevention teaching should be done at every opportunity when children are treated in the ED for minor injuries or acute health problems. Finally, the emergency nurse can be involved in pediatric safety education by teaching parents, children, and community members about injuries and how to prevent them (Bernardo and Gardner, 1992).

REFERENCES

Acute Pain Management Guideline Panel (1992). *Acute pain management: Operative or medical procedures and trauma. Clinical practice guideline.* AHCPR Pub. No 92-0032. Rockville, Md: Agency for Health Care Policy and Research, Public Health Service, U.S. Department of Health and Human Services

Agran P, Castillo D, Winn D (1990). Childhood motor vehicle occupant injuries. *American Journal of Diseases in Children* 144:653–662

Bernardo LM, Gardner MJ (1992). Implementing a pediatric safety education program. *Nursing Management* 23:82–83

Bernardo LM, Waggoner T (1992). Pediatric trauma. In Sheehy SB (ed), *Emergency nursing: Principles and practice.* St. Louis: Mosby Year Book, pp 683–690

Billmire DF (1992). Pediatric splenic and hepatic trauma. *Trauma Quarterly* 8:59–67

Bond SJ, Gotschall CS, Eichelberger MR (1991). Predictors of abdominal injury in children with pelvic fracture. *Journal of Trauma* 31:1169–1173

Centers for Disease Control (1990). Childhood injuries in the United States. *American Journal of Diseases in Children* 144:627–646

Chadwick DL, Chin S, Salerno C, Landsverk J, Kitchen L (1991). Deaths from falls in children: How far is fatal? *Journal of Trauma* 31:1353–1355

Chameides L (ed) (1990). *Textbook of pediatric advanced life support.* Dallas: American Heart Association and American Academy of Pediatrics, pp 11; 25

Committee on Trauma, American College of Surgeons (1989). *Advanced trauma life support course for physicians.* Chicago: American College of Surgeons, pp 75–77

Creel JH (1988). Mechanisms of injuries due to motion. In Campbell JE (ed), *Basic trauma life support: Advanced prehospital care* (2nd ed). Englewood Cliffs, NJ: Prentice-Hall, pp 1–20

David Clark Co, Inc. (1990). Medical Anti-Shock Trousers (MAST). Product information booklet. Worcester, Ma: David Clark Company

Donnellan W (1990). Pediatric trauma. In Kitt S, Kaiser J (eds). *Emergency nursing: A physiologic and clinical perspective.* Philadelphia: Saunders, pp 545–574

Guyer B, Ellers B (1990). The causes, impact, and preventability of childhood injuries in the United States: The magnitude of childhood injuries—an overview. *American Journal of Diseases in Children* 144:649–652

Guyer B, and Gallagher SS (1985). An approach to the epidemiology of childhood injuries. *Pediatric Clinics of North America* 32:3–15

Halpern JS (1989). Mechanisms and patterns of trauma. *Journal of Emergency Nursing* 15:380–388

Hollinger PC (1990). The causes, impact, and preventability of childhood injuries in the United States: *Childhood suicide in the United States. American Journal of Disease in Children* 144:670–676

Jones NE (1992). Childhood injuries: An epidemiologic approach. *Pediatric Nursing* 18:235–239

McKenna PJ, Welsh DJ, Martin LW (1991). Pediatric bicycle trauma. *Journal of Trauma* 31:392–394

Messier RH, Marmon LM, Hoy GR (1992). Chest wall and pulmonary injuries in children. *Trauma Quarterly* 8:51–58

Musemeche CA, Barthel M, Cosentino C, Reynolds M (1991). Pediatric falls from heights. *Journal of Trauma* 31:1347–1349

Nakayama DK (1991). *Pediatric surgery: A color atlas.* Philadelphia: Lippincott, pp 112–135

Nakayama DK, Gardner MJ, Rogers KD (1990a). Disability from bicycle-related injuries in children. *Journal of Trauma* 30:1390–1394

Nakayama DK, Pasieka KB, Gardner MJ (1990b). How bicycle-related injuries change bicycling practices in children. *American Journal of Diseases in Children* 144:928–929

Nakayama DK, Venkataraman SG, Orr RA, Thompson AE (1992). Emergency airway management in pediatric trauma. *Trauma Quarterly* 8:22–34

Nakayama DK, Waggoner T, Venkataraman ST, Gardner M, Lynch JM, Orr RA (1992). The use of drugs in emergency airway management in pediatric trauma. *Annals of Surgery* 216:205–211

Nayduch DA, Moylan J, Rutledge R, et al (1991). Comparison of the ability of adult and pediatric trauma scores to predict pediatric outcome following major trauma. *Journal of Trauma* 31:452–458

Neustadt JB (1992). Pediatric skeletal injuries. *Trauma Quarterly* 8:11–21

Newman KD, Sivit CJ (1992). The imaging of pediatric thoracic trauma. *Trauma Quarterly* 8:44–50

Nichols DG, Yaster M, Lappe DG, Buck JR (eds) (1991). *Golden hour: The handbook of advanced pediatric life support.* St. Louis: Mosby Year Book, p 340

O'Connor KP, Gibbons MD (1992). Pediatric renal injuries. *Trauma Quarterly* 8:79–90

Peitzman AB, Paris P (1988). Thoracic trauma. In Campbell JE (ed), *Basic trauma life support: Advanced prehospital care* (2nd ed). Englewood Cliffs, NJ: Prentice-Hall, pp 91–106

Reynolds EA (1992). Trauma scoring and pediatric patients: Issues and controversies. *Journal of Emergency Nursing* 18:205–210

Rivara FP (1990). Child pedestrian injuries in the United States. *American Journal of Diseases in Children* 144:692–696

Robertson LS (1985). Motor vehicles. *Pediatric Clinics of North America* 32:87–94

Ropp L, Vistainer P, Uman J, Treloar D (1992). Death in the city: An American tragedy. *Journal of the American Medical Association* 267:2905–2910

Semonin-Holleran R (1991). Pediatric trauma patients: Differences and implications for emergency nurses. *Journal of Emergency Nursing* 17:24–31

Sheley JF, McGee ZT, Wright JD (1992). Gun-related violence in and around inner-city schools. *American Journal of Diseases of Children* 146:677–682

Soud T (1992). Airway, breathing, circulation, and disability: What is different about kids? *Journal of Emergency Nursing* 18:107–116

Soud T, Pieper P, Hazinski MF (1992). Pediatric trauma. In Hazinski MF (ed), *Nursing care of the critically ill child* (2nd ed). St. Louis: Mosby Year Book, pp 829–873

Tepas JJ (1992). Hemorrhagic shock in the child. *Trauma Quarterly* 8:69–77

Widner-Kolberg M (1991). Immobilizing children in car safety seats: Why, when, and how. *Journal of Emergency Nursing* 17:427–428

Williams RA (1991). Injuries in infants and small children resulting from witnessed and corroborated free falls. *Journal of Trauma* 31:1350–1352

Yurt RW (1992). Triage, initial assessment, and early treatment of the pediatric trauma patient. *Pediatric Clinics of North America* 39:1083–1091

CHAPTER 18

Head, Neck, and Spinal Cord Trauma

RENEÉ SEMONIN-HOLLERAN

INTRODUCTION

Approximately 500,000 Americans, both adults and children, sustain a head injury each year (Stein and Ross, 1992). Head injuries are the most common type of injury seen in pediatric patients who have sustained trauma. The mortality among children who are injured and have head trauma is 26 times greater than in trauma without a head injury (Reynolds, 1992). Mechanisms of injury vary from falls to being thrown about because of improper restraint in a motor vehicle. Injury to the CNS is the most common cause of death in children. The addition of a head injury to other, even minor, injuries may have serious consequences. The automobile continues to be one of the primary causes of head injury to children (Tepas et al, 1990).

Spinal cord trauma accounts for 10,000 injuries annually in the United States (Gerhart, 1991). The most common causes of spinal cord injuries include automobile crashes, falls, diving accidents, hangings, and violent assaults. Spinal cord injuries are not as common among infants and children as they are among adults.

Head injuries account for about 600,000 emergency department (ED) visits each year (Pediatric Alert, 1993). It is estimated that about 250,000 children younger than 14 years are hospitalized because of head injury each year. Twenty-five thousand of these children either die of or are permanently disabled by the injury (Dolan, 1992). Head injuries may cause devastating consequences, including functional disabilities and diminished quality of life (Tepas et al, 1992).

Although head injuries are common among injured children, spinal cord injuries are not. Two to three percent of very young children who are injured sustain cervical spinal injuries (Haley and Baker, 1993; Medina, 1992). Less than 5% of all spinal cord injuries occur in children younger than 16 years (Massagli and Jaffe, 1990). Even though spinal cord injuries are not frequently seen in pediatric patients, the consequences of an injury to the spinal cord—dramatic disturbances of motor, sensory and autonomic functions —alter every aspect of the child's life (Massagli and Jaffe, 1990). Because the child is in the process of growing and developing, even minor head injuries may impact the child's future development (Wesson et al, 1992).

INTENTIONAL HEAD INJURIES

Children depend on their adult caretakers for care and protection. Unfortunately, head and spinal trauma may not always be the result of an accidental injury (Duhaime et al, 1992). In a study conducted by Duhaime et al (1992), 25 of the 100 children younger than 2 years who were admitted for head injury suffered an inflicted injury. Identifying the risk for an inflicted head injury is an important part of pediatric neurologic assessment.

MECHANISMS OF INJURY

The mechanisms of injury that may cause head and spinal cord injuries vary according to the child's age, physical and mental development, and social and physical environment. A child's natural curiosity, sense of immortality (particularly in adolescence), peer pressure and the desire to fit in also contribute to the risk of being injured as children place themselves in an unsafe environment, such as skateboarding in traffic, or do not wear protective devices, such as a helmet. An important component to consider when examining the cause of a head or spinal cord injury is whether the injury was intentional or unintentional. The emergency nurse should consider the educational needs of the child and family related to the prevention of head trauma when evaluating the source of the trauma.

Head Injuries

Tepas et al (1990) reviewed the records of more than 10,000 children who had been entered into the National Pediatric Trauma Registry. They identified falls (37.5%), motor vehicle crashes (18.3%), and bicycle falls or crashes (9.9%) as the most common mechanisms of injury. Most fatal head injuries occurred in automobile crashes.

Peclet et al (1990) found that falls, traffic-related injuries, and burns accounted for 75% of all admissions to urban pediatric trauma centers across all pediatric age groups. Most of these children had head injuries.

Duhaime et al (1992) studied the mechanisms of injury for head injury in children younger than 2 years. Their study found that falls, motor vehicle crashes, and abuse accounted for most of the head trauma in this age group.

Because infants and toddlers are extremely dependent on their caregivers for safety and protection, unsafe environments and lack of protective devices have been implicated as contributing to head injuries in this age group. Examples of unsafe practices include the use of baby walkers (Duhaime et al, 1992); not restraining vehicle occupants (Duhaime et al, 1992; Peclet et al, 1990; Tepas et al, 1990); and not padding coffee tables (Sternbach, 1992).

Partington et al (1991) reviewed 129 charts of children younger than 2 years who had mild head injuries. Fourteen percent of these children suffered baby-walker-related injuries, one-half of them experiencing a skull fracture.

Another source of pediatric head injuries is the use of wheeled vehicles, such as bicycles, all-terrain vehicles (ATVs), and skateboards. Head injuries are seen in all age groups because children could either be operating the wheeled vehicle or be a passenger on the vehicle. Bicycles account for about 600,000 ED visits each year; approximately 1200 of these patients die. Two-thirds of the patients admitted to the hospital as the result of bicycle injuries have head injuries (Spaite

et al, 1991). Spaite et al (1991) evaluated the mortality among bicyclists who either wore helmets or did not at the time of injury. The largest group of injured patients in the study was infants through 19-year-old adolescents. The most common injury was to the head, and head injuries were the primary cause of death. The mortality was higher for bicyclists who did not wear helmets. McKenna et al (1991) found that the most common reason for admission to the hospital because of bicycle trauma was head injury (49%). Injuries included skull fractures and epidural and subdural hematomas.

Additional mechanisms of injury that cause pediatric head trauma are farming accidents and falls from pick-up trucks. Steuland et al (1991) found that more than half of the farm injuries among children younger than 6 years were head injuries. These were frequently caused by falls from farm vehicles and buildings. These falls occasionally resulted in spinal cord trauma in addition to head trauma. Bucklew et al (1992) looked at injuries that resulted from falls from pick-up trucks in New Mexico. The largest age group injured were infants to 19-year-old adolescents. Head injuries accounted for 68% of the injuries sustained in a fall.

Spinal Cord Injuries

Massagli and Jaffe (1990) identified motor vehicle crashes (41.5%); sports (27%), mostly diving, followed by football, skiing, sledding, surfing, bouncing on a trampoline, wrestling, gymnastics, and horseback riding; violence (20.5%), assaults and penetrating trauma; and falls (9.4%) as the major causes of spinal cord injuries. Boys are more frequently injured than girls.

Neonates are also susceptible to spinal cord injuries. These can result from forceful traction and angulation of the spine during delivery (Massagli and Jaffe, 1990).

PATHOPHYSIOLOGY OF HEAD AND SPINAL TRAUMA

Anatomic Variations

Young children have specific anatomic variations that affect their response to head and spinal cord injury. The tissues of the head and neck of children are thinner, softer, and more flexible than those of adults (Wider-Kolberg and Maloney-Harmon, 1988). In infancy and early childhood the brain is less myelinated and can be more easily injured than an adult brain because of the lack of additional protection (Mayer, 1985). During early infancy, the cranial sutures remain open. The anterior fontanelle remains open for the first 10–18 months of the child's life. The elasticity of the infant's skull allows for increased tolerance of changes in intracranial pressure (ICP) (Soud, 1992).

Children's heads are the largest parts of their bodies; in younger children the neck muscles are poorly developed. This makes them more vulnerable to acceleration-deceleration injuries (Johnson, 1988). A relatively large proportion of total blood volume of a young child is contained in the head (Widner-Kolberg and Maloney-Harmon, 1988). In addition, the surface area of the scalp of a child is large and quite vascular; a child may lose a great deal of blood from a serious scalp wound.

The specific anatomic features of the pediatric cervical spine that increase its susceptibility to injury are the interspinous ligaments and joint capsules are lax; the horizontal orientation of the articulating vertebral facet joints makes subluxation easier; the anterior portion of the vertebral body is wedged forward on the vertebra below, making slippage easier; the uncinate process of the vertebral body is flat and ineffective at withstanding rotational forces; and the large heads and poorly developed neck muscles of smaller children leave them more vulnerable to injury (Bohn et al, 1990; Massagli and Jaffe, 1990). Because of these anatomic characteristics, the site of injury in children younger than 12 years is at C-1, C-2, or the atlanto-occipital junction (Bohn et al, 1990).

Pathophysiology of Head Injury

The pathophysiology of brain injury has been classified as primary or secondary (Dolan, 1992). A primary injury is the initial injury, which may result from penetrating (gunshot wounds) or blunt (falling and striking the head) trauma. Blunt impact is more common among pediatric patients. Primary injuries include skull fractures, vascular injuries resulting in hematomas, brain contusions, and subarachnoid hemorrhage (Reynolds, 1992).

A secondary injury follows the initial injury. It is the consequence of a systemic physiologic response to the primary injury. Secondary injuries include hypercapnia, hyperemia, and increases in ICP. If the increasing ICP cannot be controlled, ultimately herniation and death occur (Dolan, 1992; Reynolds, 1992). Secondary injury in a head-injured child has been found to contribute to the loss of autoregulatory mechanisms. Cerebral hyperemia is an increase in blood flow that results in an increase in ICP (Dolan, 1992). The reasons for this development in a pediatric patient with a head injury are still not clear (Dolan, 1992). Controversy remains as to whether children completely lose their autoregulation mechanisms because of secondary brain injuries (Reynolds, 1992).

Changes in ICP are reflected in the neurologic assessment of a pediatric patient. These include changes in the child's level of consciousness, pupillary function, motor movement, sensory responses, and vital signs. Changes in vital signs involve changes in respiration, pulse rate, systolic blood pressure, and temperature. A late and rather ominous change in vital signs that signals impending herniation is known as the Cushing triad—changes in respiration and heart rate accompanied by systemic hypertension.

Pathophysiology of Spinal Cord Injuries

The pathophysiology of spinal cord injury is not completely understood (Dolan, 1992). After injury, the spinal cord may be functionally disrupted. The neurotransmitters no longer perform as they previously did. Ischemia and tissue hypoxia play a role in dysfunction of the cord. In addition, certain neurotransmitters such as endorphins, free catecholamines, and free radicals may play a role in the injury process (Dolan, 1992).

Injuries to the spinal cord may be partial or complete. If the spinal cord injury is complete, there is immediate loss of motor reflexes and sensory function below the level of the injury.

ASSESSMENT

The neurologic assessment of a pediatric patient is a part of the initial assessment of an injured child. The emergency nurse needs to recognize that certain factors play an important role in the assessment. Age, growth, and development influence a child's ability to provide a history of what happened and the child's ability to respond to and follow commands.

A thorough neurologic assessment has six parts: history; level of consciousness; pupillary response; motor response; sensory response; and vital signs. The neurologic assessment of an infant or child is an ongoing process. Once baseline data have been collected, the emergency nurse needs to constantly reassess the child's neurologic status.

History

As previously noted, several factors make it difficult to obtain an accurate history from a pediatric patient: The age and cognitive development of the child may not be advanced enough for the child to respond. There may be no witnesses. The parents themselves may be injured. The emergency personnel performing the assessment are usually strangers to the child (Semonin-Holleran, 1991; Shapiro, 1990; Wagner, 1992a).

The history taken for head and spinal cord trauma should include the following elements.

TABLE 18–1. INDICATIONS OF POSSIBLE INTENTIONAL HEAD AND SPINAL CORD INJURIES

Circumstances of the injury are unclear.
Reported historical information is inconsistent with the extent of the injury.
Injury is to child younger than 1 year.
Child is younger than 1 year, is comatose, and has a bulging fontanelle.
Retinal hemorrhages are present.

(From Shapiro K [1990]. Emergency care of the head injured child. Topics of Emergency Medicine *11:36–40)*

Questions to Ask in Taking History of Head and Spinal Cord Trauma

- How did the injury happen? Was it in a motor vehicle crash? Was the child hit by a vehicle? Did the child fall? From how far? Is there a penetrating injury?
- How long has it been since the injury occurred?
- Were safety devices used? Was the child appropriately restrained? Did he or she use a helmet?
- Was there any loss of consciousness? For how long?
- Is there any nausea, vomiting, headache, or blurred vision?
- What was the child's behavior after the injury?
- Has the child's behavior changed? Is the child lethargic or irritable?
- If the child is newly born, when and where was the child born?
- What is the child's medical history? Was there a premature birth? Have there been seizures, developmental disabilities, or physical handicaps?
- Does the child have any allergies?
- Is the child taking any medications?
- Has the child ingested drugs or alcohol?
- When was the last time the child ate or drank?
- What is the child's immunization history?

Children with shunts in place for hydrocephalus and children with chronic diseases such as hemophilia and leukemia are at greater risk for complications of head injuries than are other patients (Shapiro, 1990).

An important component of the history of a child who has sustained either head or spinal cord trauma is whether the injury was accidental or intentional. Table 18–1 contains a summary of the indications of possible intentional head or spinal cord injuries.

PHYSICAL ASSESSMENT

The physical assessment of a child who has suffered a head or spinal cord injury always begin with a primary survey. During the primary survey it is imperative that spinal immobilization be maintained. The primary survey is discussed in Chapter 17.

The component of the primary survey that is carefully evaluated in a child with head or spinal trauma is disability or neurologic function. The neurologic assessment begins with the history and continues with level of consciousness, pupillary response, motor and sensory response, and vital signs.

Level of Consciousness. When assessing a child's level of consciousness, some baseline growth and development information should be obtained by the emergency nurse. Table 18–2 contains examples of growth and development parameters that may be of use in an evaluation of level of consciousness (Semonin-Holleran, 1991).

Two methods have been used successfully to assess the level of consciousness of pediatric patients (Dolan, 1992; Semonin-Holleran, 1991). Table 18–3 contains the AVPU method for pediatric assessment and Table 18–4 contains the modified Glasgow Coma Scale (GCS).

Additional methods to assess a child's level of consciousness include evaluating how the child interacts with the environment and his or her recognition of and interaction with parents or caretaker. Wagner (1992a) pointed out that infants 2–3 months of age should follow an object with their eyes; children 3–4 months of age should try to reach for the object; 1-year-olds imitate expressions of emotions, such as a smile; and 18-month-olds can follow simple commands, but may choose not to. If a child makes a concerted effort to ignore the emergency nurse or displays discomfort around a stranger, it can be safely assumed that this may be indicative of a normal mental status (Wagner, 1992a).

Changes in a child's level of consciousness are the first sign of changes in ICP (Lower, 1992). Lower (1992) noted that one problem nurses have when performing a level-of-consciousness assessment on an unconscious patient is that the nurse does not adequately stimulate the patient. The suggested sequence is voice first; if no response, shout; then shake (always being careful of the cervical spine); and finally use a painful stimulus (trapezius squeeze, sternal rub).

Another problem is the length of time a stimulus is applied. Lower (1992) suggested that a 5-second stimulus may elicit one type of response, but application of the stimulus for 20–30 seconds may actually elicit the brain's true response. It is important not only to document the child's response to the painful stimulus but also to indicate what type of stimulus was used to elicit the response.

TABLE 18–2. GROWTH AND DEVELOPMENT

Age	Physical Development	Psychosocial Development	Major Fears
Infant	Initially has primitive reflexes (such as Babinski); may grasp objects; responds to pain. During first year sits up, crawls, and begins to walk.	Should interact with environment, recognize parents	Separation from primary caregiver
Toddler	Climbs; can ride a tricycle; has bowel and bladder control	Curious; has a simple vocabulary; still depends on parents	Separation from parent; needs security objects (such as stuffed animal or blanket)
Pre-school-aged	Jumps a rope; ties shoelaces; opens windows and doors	Vocabulary increases; can give some history about what has happened; should know name and address; honesty important	Loss of control; the dark; mutilation
School-aged	Rides a bicycle; involved in sports; mobile from home environment	Begins logical thinking; identifies with peer group; can care for things such as pets; understands illness and its effects	Mutilation; death
Adolescent	Menses or nocturnal emission begins; sexual activity may begin; drives a car	May experiment with drugs and alcohol; peer group important; abstract thinking present	Loss of control; altered body image

(*Modified with permission, from Semonin-Holleran R [1991]. Pediatric trauma patients: Differences and implications for emergency nurses. Journal of Emergency Nursing 17:25*)

Pupillary Response. The child's pupils should be evaluated for size, shape, reaction, and equality. A brightly colored object can be used to attract the child's attention so that the eyes can be assessed. Wagner (1992a) suggests using a pacifier to get a child to open his or her eyes. When babies suck, they usually do so with their eyes open.

An early pupillary change indicative of injury is unilateral hippus (Lower, 1992). The pupil initially constricts to the light stimulus but then dilates without regard to light. Another subtle indication of change occurs when the pupils constrict with light stimulation, but one reacts more sluggishly than the other (Lower, 1992). Pupillary changes usually occur on the same side as the lesion.

The size, shape, and equality of the pupils should be documented in concrete terms. Subjective terms such as small, medium, and large should be avoided. Ingestion of any drugs that may influence pupillary changes, such as atropine or narcotics, should be documented.

TABLE 18–3. AVPU METHOD FOR PEDIATRIC LEVEL OF CONSCIOUSNESS ASSESSMENT

Letter	Status
A	Alert
V	Responds to verbal stimuli
P	Responds to painful stimuli
U	Unresponsive

Motor and Sensory Response. The motor and sensory responses are assessed at the same time, especially if the child is unconscious. Because a child may not be able to follow commands because of age or may not want to because of fear, observation plays an important role in evaluating a child's motor and sensory responses.

One of the first things the emergency nurse should observe is the posture of the child. Full-term healthy infants hold their extremities in flexion. Using a brightly colored object, the nurse evaluates the child's use of the upper extremities. The child should be evaluated for any asymmetric movement of the extremities. To test the lower extremities, the nurse may rub the bottom of the child's foot and watch the child's response. It is important to remember that a Babinski is present in children younger than 18 months (Cardona, 1994; Dolan, 1992; Wagner, 1992a).

Older children may be asked to move their arms and legs. If the child refuses, the nurse may have to elicit a response by gently rubbing the extremity. Young children may not know which is the left or the right side. Using a gentle stimulus on an awake child also provides information about the child's sensory response.

Abnormalities that may be noted in a child with a head or spinal cord injury include decorticate posturing (flexion of the arms, wrists, and fingers with abducted upper extremities and extension, internal rotation, and plantar flexion of the lower extremities); decerebrate posturing (pronounced rigidity of the

TABLE 18–4. MODIFIED PEDIATRIC GLASGOW COMA SCALE

Eye opening			Best Motor Response			Best Verbal Response			
Score	>1 year	<1 year	Score	>1 year	<1 year	Score	>5 years	2–5 years	0–24 months
4	Spontaneously	Spontaneously	6	Obeys	Spontaneous movement	5	Oriented and converses	Appropriate words and phrases	Smiles, coos appropriately
3	To verbal command	To shout	5	Localizes to pain	Localizes to pain	4	Disoriented and converses	Inappropriate words	Cries, but consolable
2	To pain	To pain	4	Flexion—withdrawal	Flexion—withdrawal	3	Inappropriate words	Persistent cries or screams	Persistent inappropriate crying or screaming
1	No response	No response	3	Flexion—abnormal (decorticate rigidity)	Flexion—abnormal (decorticate rigidity)	2	Incomprehensible sounds	Grunts	Grunts, agitated, restless
			2	Extension (decerebrate rigidity)	Extension (decerebrate rigidity)	1	No response	No response	No response
			1	No response	No response				

Data from Janes HE [1985]. Brain insults in infants and children. Orlando: Grune and Stratton Publications)
(Reproduced with permission from Semonin-Holleran R [1991]. Pediatric trauma patients: Differences and implications for emergency nurses. Journal of Emergency Nursing *17:28)*

extremities, arms and legs extended); and flaccidity (Dolan, 1992). Wrist posturing can be a subtle sign of neurologic deterioration (Lower, 1992).

The motor and sensory assessment of a child with a possible spinal cord injury helps identify the amount of injury sustained by the cord. If the injury is complete, loss of motor and sensory function occurs below the level of the lesion. If the injury is incomplete, the bulbocavernosus and anal wink reflexes are evaluated. The bulbocavernosus reflex is elicited by squeezing the base of the penis or vulva, which should produce contraction of the internal anal sphincter. The anal wink reflex is seen in response to painful stimulation around the anus. The presence of these reflexes indicates an incomplete injury to the cord (Haley and Baker, 1993).

As a part of the motor and sensory survey, the cranial nerves may be assessed. Wagner (1992a) suggests that when appraising the second cranial nerve (optic) in a child, the nurse should shine a light in the child's eyes and test for a direct and consensual pupillary reflex. The third (oculomotor), fourth (trochlear), and sixth (abducens) cranial nerves can be tested by making a game out of visual field assessment. A brightly colored object or toy or a parent can be used to elicit a response. Finally the seventh cranial nerve can be tested by observing the child while he or she is crying or conversing (Wagner, 1992a).

Vital Signs. The child's blood pressure, pulse, respiration, and temperature need to be closely monitored.

An accurate temperature is particularly important because hypothermia can produce signs and symptoms of neurologic injury. As already mentioned, the classic changes in vital signs seen in impending cerebral herniation is known as the Cushing triad or response. The Cushing response includes changes in respiratory patterns (ataxic respiration, bradypnea), bradycardia, and systemic hypertension (Dolan, 1992).

A child with a spinal cord injury may have changes in blood pressure (hypotension) and pulse (bradycardia) due to sympathectomy from the spinal cord injury (Medina, 1992). Depending on the level of the injury (especially injuries to C-3, C-4, and C-5), the potential for respiratory difficulty and arrest exists. Bohn et al (1990) identified a group of children with sudden cardiac arrest after a traumatic injury. On autopsy, the authors found that most of these children had suffered a high cervical cord injury.

Inspection and Palpation. While performing the six-part neurologic assessment, the emergency nurse inspects and palpates the head, neck, and spinal column of the child. The nurse should inspect for the presence of facial injuries, mandibular fractures, calcaneal injuries, or seat belt signs that may indicate a head or spinal cord injury. The fontanelle of an infant should be inspected for bulging. Signs of a skull fracture include periorbital ecchymosis (raccoon eyes), bleeding behind the ear (Battle sign), hemotympanum, and leakage of cerebrospinal fluid (CSF). Cerebral spinal fluid may be detected by checking any drainage from the nose and ears for the presence of glucose. In addition, the nurse may observe whether the fluid separates, forming a halo sign.

A child's scalp and skull should be palpated for the presence of lacerations and any depressions. Hair can easily hide severe wounds and depressed skull fractures. Infants who suffer a skull fracture may have a "ping-pong" effect because the skull is malleable (Shapiro, 1990). The neck and spinal column should be palpated for tenderness, crepitus, or deformity. Extreme care should be used so that the cervical spine is not moved. Most cervical collars allow the nurse or physician to evaluate the child without removing the collar. However, whenever there is the possibility that the neck may be moved, manual immobilization should be applied by one member of the trauma team.

Laboratory and Diagnostic Tests

In addition to the routine studies that would be performed for an injured child, the specific diagnostic procedures performed for head and spinal trauma include a portable cross-table lateral-view x ray of the cervical spine, computed tomography (CT), and, when indicated, skull x rays (Dolan, 1992; Medina, 1992). Because hypoxia, hypotension, and drugs alter a child's level of consciousness, laboratory tests including arterial blood gases, hemoglobin and hematocrit, and a drug screen help in the initial evaluation. Drugs such as alcohol, cocaine, and PCP can contribute to an altered mental status and make it difficult to evaluate the child's level of consciousness.

There continues to be some controversy as to what type of head injury calls for CT. About 70% of head injuries that occur each year are classified as mild (GCS 13–15) (1991; Stein and Ross, 1992). Stein and Ross (1992) identified that the risk of an intracranial lesion rose from 13% with a GCS score of 15 to 40% with a GCS score of 13. They recommended routine and immediate CT for any patient who suffered a loss of consciousness or who could not recall the event. If CT is not immediately available, a skull x ray may be useful if there is a CSF leak, pneumocephalus, or the possibility of a depressed skull fracture.

TRIAGE
Head and Spinal Cord Injuries

Emergent ——————————————
An infant or child with severe head injury; Pediatric GCS (PGCS) score less than 8; spinal cord injuries with motor or sensory deficits.

Urgent ——————————————
An infant or child with a PGCS score of 9 to 12; spinal cord injuries without motor or sensory deficits.

Non-urgent ——————————————
An infant or child with a PGCS score of 13 to 15; alert with stable vital signs.

Nursing Diagnosis
Ineffective Breathing Pattern

Defining Characteristics

- Apnea
- Cheyne-Stokes respirations
- Central neurogenic hyperventilation
- Apneustic breathing
- Cluster breathing
- Ataxic breathing

Nursing Interventions

- Administer oxygen
- Prepare for intubation
- Assist with rapid sequence intubation
- Hyperventilate patient as indicated
- Monitor vital signs
- Monitor pulse oximetry
- Monitor CO_2 level
- Monitor blood gas levels

Expected Outcomes

- Patient's breathing is controlled with bag-mask-valve ventilation or with a ventilator
- Respiratory patterns improve with oxygenation
- Neurologic status improves with hyperventilation
- PCO_2 remains below 25 mmHg
- Vital signs are normal for the child's age
- Oxygen saturation is greater than 94%

Nursing Diagnosis
Altered Thought Processes

Defining Characteristics

- Irritable, inconsolable crying
- Lack of recognition of parents or caretakers
- Lack of response to verbal or painful stimuli

Nursing Interventions

- Decrease stimulation
- Provide child with familiar objects
- Administer sedation as indicated and ordered
- Talk to and touch the child; encourage the parents and caretakers to do so as well

Expected Outcomes

- Child's crying decreases or stops
- Blood pressure and pulse change with comfort measures and decreased stimulation in an unresponsive child
- Child's agitation or anxiety decreases

Nursing Diagnosis
Knowledge Deficit (Head Injury)

Defining Characteristics

- Verbalization of deficiency in knowledge
- Complications of head trauma not recognized by parents or caretakers

Nursing Interventions

- Provide family with information about neurologic assessment of minor head injury
- Explain what each of the components of the evaluation means and what the parent or caretaker should look for

Expected Outcomes

- Parents, caretakers, or child verbalize knowledge of neurologic assessment for minor head injury
- Parent or caretaker demonstrates how to perform a neurologic assessment for minor head injury

Nursing Diagnosis
High Risk for Injury

Defining Characteristics

- Child not appropriately immobilized after injury
- Seizure activity after head injury
- Inappropriate administration of medication

Nursing Interventions

- Immobilize child with appropriate equipment to protect the cervical spine
- Monitor child for seizure activity
- Provide safety mechanisms, such as side rails, for protection
- Check drug dosage and indications before administration

Expected Outcomes

- Child is appropriately immobilized with a cervical collar, backboard, and head immobilizer
- Respirations are not impaired with immobilization devices
- Seizure activity is immediately recognized and treated
- Drugs are appropriately administered and their effects documented

MANAGEMENT

The initial treatment of a child who has sustained a head or spinal cord injury is based on the assessment and management of the child's airway, breathing, circulation, neurologic disability, and cervical spinal immobilization. It is important to identify and treat any life-threatening injuries, particularly those that cause hypotension. Normotension provides much-needed blood flow to the brain. Systemic hypotension should not be ascribed to head injury in general except in the case of a severe scalp laceration in a young child (Shapiro, 1990).

Indications for admission for a child who has suffered a head injury include mechanism of injury, continuous abnormal neurologic findings, post-traumatic seizures, persistent vomiting, suspicion of child abuse, and a skull fracture in an infant (Wagner, 1992b). A child who displays any type of spinal cord deficit after the injury needs to be admitted.

Immobilization
Spinal immobilization of a pediatric patient may pose a challenge to the emergency nurse. Cervical spinal immobilization includes application of a cervical collar; a headblock or cervical immobilization device (CID); and a backboard. The manufacturer's directions should be closely followed in the application of any of these devices. It is not recommended that chin straps be used to secure the headblock or CID because they may interfere with the child's airway. Pre-hospital care providers are an excellent source of advice on the appropriate immobilization of a child (Bernardo and Bove, 1993).

Head Injury

Classification. Head trauma has been classified into three major categories using the Pediatric Glasgow Coma Score (PGCS) (Dolan, 1992; Johnson, 1988). Table 18–5 contains a summary of these categories.

Minor Head Injury. A PGCS score of 13 to 15 has been classified as a minor head injury. Children who have

TABLE 18–5. CLASSIFICATION OF HEAD INJURY BASED ON GLASGOW COMA SCALE (GCS)

- MINOR HEAD INJURY
  GCS score 13 to 15
  Associated injuries
    Superficial scalp or facial injuries
  Transient loss of consciousness
  Normal neurological exam
  Need for observation
  Potential complications
    Pediatric concussion syndrome
    Posterior fossa syndrome
    Vertebrobasilar occlusion

- MODERATE HEAD INJURY
  GCS score 9 to 12
  Associated injuries
    Subdural hematoma
    Epidural hematoma
    Intracranial hemorrhage
  Loss of consciousness
  Post-traumatic anesthesia
  Confusion and disorientation
  Seizures
  CT needed
  Complications
    Secondary brain injury

- SEVERE HEAD INJURY
  GCS score 8 or less
  Associated injuries
    Depressed skull fractures
    Penetrating skull injuries
    Compound skull fractures
  Airway and circulatory management required
  Management of intracranial pressure required
  Complications
    Secondary brain injury

suffered a minor head injury may have experienced a momentary or transient loss of consciousness. The child may complain of a mild headache or dizziness and may feel nauseated. On neurologic examination and after a period of observation (usually about 6 hours), no focal neurologic deficits are identified.

A child who has suffered a minor head injury is at risk for a problem unique to childhood known as pediatric concussion syndrome (Wagner, 1992b). Symptoms of this syndrome range from generalized seizures after injury (with normal CT findings) to complaints of irritability, lethargy, and persistent vomiting. The child is treated on the basis of the severity of the syndrome.

Two injuries of which the emergency nurse must be aware that may not be clearly identified in a child with a minor head injury are posterior fossa hematoma and vertebrobasilar occlusion (Wagner, 1992b). These injuries should be suspected in a child with a history of minor head trauma who has suffered trauma to

the occipital area or has any abnormal cerebellar function (Wagner, 1992b).

Moderate Head Injury. A moderate head injury is associated with a PGCS score of 9 to 12. Symptoms of moderate head injuries include a loss of consciousness for more than 5 minutes, post-traumatic amnesia, agitation, combativeness, and seizures. Injuries commonly associated with moderate head injuries include subdural and epidural hematomas, intracranial hemorrhages, and basilar skull fractures (Dolan, 1992).

The child with a moderate head injury requires CT and repeated neurologic examinations to detect any focal neurologic deficits. Depending on the symptoms of the injury, management of ICP may be necessary. Specific interventions are discussed later in this chapter.

Severe Head Injury. A PGCS of 8 or less is considered a severe head injury. A child with a severe head injury has focal neurologic deficits, such as pupillary changes and posturing. Injuries associated with severe head trauma include a depressed palpable skull fracture, a penetrating skull injury, and a compound skull fracture (Dolan, 1992).

These children require the most aggressive management to keep their ICP under control. Airway management and oxygenation are crucial first steps in the care of a child who has suffered a severe head injury.

Interventions. Emergency nursing care of a child who has suffered a moderate or severe head injury is directed at decreasing the effects of secondary brain injury. Mitchell and Ackerman (1992) noted three nursing interventions that are directed at this. They are promotion of cerebral perfusion pressure; ongoing monitoring of the child's physiologic status; and decreasing or controlling stimuli in the child's environment.

Management of Intracranial Pressure. Once the type of head injury has been identified, the focus of care should be on management of ICP. A child who has suffered a moderate or severe head injury should be aggressively treated to decrease the potential damage that can occur from increasing ICP.

The first step in management of ICP is intubation and controlled hyperventilation. Intubation helps prevent aspiration, provides adequate oxygenation, reduces cerebral blood flow, and offers a secured airway if the child has to be transferred. If the child is still conscious, rapid sequence intubation is indicated. Table 18–6 contains a protocol for this procedure. Because CO_2 is a powerful vasodilator, the child's pCO_2 is usually maintained at 27–30 mmHg (Mitchell and Ackerman, 1992). A nasogastric or orogastric tube

TABLE 18–6. RAPID SEQUENCE INTUBATION PROTOCOL FOR A PEDIATRIC PATIENT WITH A HEAD INJURY

1. Identify the need for intubation, eg, controlled ventilation for ICP management.
2. Assist the child's ventilation with appropriate-sized bag-mask-valve.
3. Be sure that the child's neck is immobilized throughout the procedure.
4. Perform a neurologic assessment before administration of medication.
5. Premedicate the child with atropine sulfate 0.01 mg/kg IVP if using succinylcholine. Perform and document pupil assessment before administration of atropine.
6. Premedicate the child with lidocaine 1 mg/kg to help decrease the transient increase in ICP that can occur with intubation.
7. If the child is alert, use a sedative agent for amnesia and to decrease anxiety and agitation.
8. Administer paralyzing agent and assist with ventilation until intubation completed.
9. Assist with intubation by immobilization of cervical spine and applying cricoid thyroid pressure (Sellick maneuver).
10. Confirm tube placement by assessing presence and equality of the child's breath sounds, listening over the child's stomach, checking for fogging in the tube and improvement in the child's physiologic status, and using a CO_2 detector.
11. Talk to and touch the child.
12. Remember that the child may be sedated or paralyzed, but the child can still experience pain and may require pain medication.

should be inserted for gastric decompression and to decrease the chances of vomiting and aspiration.

Keeping the child normotensive or possibly increasing the mean arterial pressure (MAP) slightly may help keep the ICP as normal as possible (Bruce, 1993). A child with only a head injury should receive two-thirds maintenance with such fluids as 0.5 normal saline solution, saline solution, or lactated Ringer solution. Fluids with sugar are not recommended because hyperglycemia has been found to contribute to additional injury to the brain. Glucose levels should be closely monitored and glucose administered as the child's condition indicates (Bruce, 1993).

Medications. Some pharmacologic interventions for head injury and seizure management are listed in Table 18–7. The type and amount of drugs used vary according to the neurologic protocols used at individual institutions. Additional medications that may be administered to a child with a head injury include tetanus immunization and antibiotics, particularly for a child who has a CSF leak.

Seizure Precautions. Post-traumatic seizures are more common in pediatric patients than in adults and generally may not be an indication of a serious head injury (Reynolds, 1992). However, a child may be at risk for injury from aspiration and striking his or her extremities against side rails or from falling during a seizure. The emergency nurse should perform frequent

neurologic assessments and provide a safe environment such as a padded crib or bed, raised side rails, and someone to monitor the patient. Medications used for seizure management are listed in Table 18–7.

Surgical Intervention. Emergency decompression of a child's head may be indicated in the most severe cases of increasing ICP. About 20–30% of children with head injuries require surgical intervention, including a craniotomy, burr holes, and a fontanelle tap (Bruce, 1993). Evans and Billittier (1990) noted that the indications for burr holes in the ED included severe head injuries that continued to deteriorate neurologically and displayed evidence of brainstem dysfunction or herniation.

For an infant with a severe head injury whose condition continues to deteriorate, the emergency physician may elect to perform a fontanelle tap. A needle is inserted into the lateral area of the fontanelle. Fluid should come out by itself; one should never aspirate it (Wagner, 1992b).

Ongoing Monitoring. The ongoing monitoring of a child's physiologic status involves the continuous

TABLE 18–7. MEDICATIONS USED FOR THE TREATMENT OF A CHILD WHO HAS SUFFERED A HEAD INJURY

Medication	Dosage and Route	Indications
Acetaminophen	1g/yr of age 10 mg/kg/dose 300 mg/kg day rectally or orally	Analgesia after minor head injury Fever reduction
Fentanyl	0.002–0.003 mg/kg IV	Short-acting anesthetic used for sedation
Furosemide	0.5–1.0 mg/kg IV	Diuretic used to decrease ICP
Lidocaine	1 mg/kg IV	Helps decrease the transiently high ICP that occurs with intubation
Lorazepam	0.05 mg/kg IV	Sedation, amnesia, and seizure control
Mannitol	0.25–0.5 g/kg IV	Osmotic diuretic to decrease ICP
Midazolam	0.1 mg/kg up to 5 mg maximum dose IV	Sedation and amnesia for intubation and painful procedures. Useful for sedation when child placed in CT scanner.
Phenytoin	10–20 mg/kg infused at 1 mg/kg/minute	Control of postinjury seizures
Vecuronium	0.2 mg/kg IV	For intubation and to keep patient paralyzed for mechanical ventilation or hyperventilation. Useful for procedures such as CT

ICP, intracranial pressure; IV, intravenous.

TABLE 18–8. ADVANTAGES AND DISADVANTAGES OF INTRACRANIAL PRESSURE MONITORING DEVICES

Type	Advantages	Disadvantages
Intracranial bolt	Provides direct measurement; useful for small ventricles; easy to insert	Requires a closed skull; cannot drain CSF
Ventricular catheter	Provides direct measurement; can drain CSF	Very invasive, difficult to place in tight ventricles; increased potential for infection
Epidural probe	Minimally invasive; fiberoptic system does not depend on patient position for accuracy	CSF cannot be drained; fiberoptic system requires a special monitor

CSF, cerebrospinal fluid.
(*From Reynolds E [1992]. Controversies in caring for the child with a head injury.* American Journal of Maternal/Child Nursing *17:249*)

monitoring of the child's vital signs and neurologic status. In addition, the emergency nurse should monitor and document the effects of specific treatments used to manage moderate and severe head injuries.

Some hospitals now insert ICP monitoring devices in the ED. Devices that may be used to monitor and manage ICP include an intracranial bolt, ventricular catheter, and an epidural probe. It is recommended that if the GCS score is less than 6 an ICP monitor be inserted in the ED (Bruce, 1993). If ICP monitors are to be used in the ED, the emergency nurse should become familiar with their use, the normal readings, and the complications that may occur with the use of these devices. Table 18–8 contains a list of some of the ICP monitoring devices and their advantages and disadvantages (Reynolds, 1992).

Finally, the emergency nurse needs to control and decrease the stimuli in the child's environment. This is not always easy in the frenzied environment of an ED. Sequencing of care has been shown to help decrease excessive patient stimulation (Mitchell and Ackerman, 1992). When possible, the child's family should be involved in care.

Spinal Cord Injury
A child with a head and spinal cord injury needs to be immobilized appropriately. Appropriate immobilization entails the use of a proper-fitting cervical collar, a head immobilizer, and a spinal board. Several pediatric collars are available. It is important that no matter what collar is chosen, each comes with specific instructions that indicate how to determine the right size for a particular child. There are also pediatric spinal boards that meet the needs of young children (Figure 18–1). Sandbags and taping have been recommended to prevent neck rotation by an awake, active child. However,

improper taping and placement of the sandbags can leave the child at risk of being injured.

Schafermeyer et al (1991) demonstrated that the functional vital capacity (FVC) of healthy children decreased markedly when the children were restrained on a spinal board. Straps placed around a child's chest and abdomen for spinal immobilization can restrict chest wall movement and diaphragmatic excursion. A child who is immobilized must be closely observed.

The child needs to be thoroughly evaluated for injuries to other sites, including the chest and abdomen. If a child has lost function below the level of the lesion, a Foley catheter should be inserted. A nasogastric tube may be needed for prevention of aspiration.

If the child has suffered a severe head injury, it may be difficult to identify an associated cervical spinal injury. Physical clues that may indicate a spinal cord injury include a dermatomal pattern of sensory loss, a symmetric absence of reflexes, flaccidity, an absence of sacral reflexes, incontinence of bowel and bladder, and, in a boy, priapism (Massagli and Jaffe, 1990).

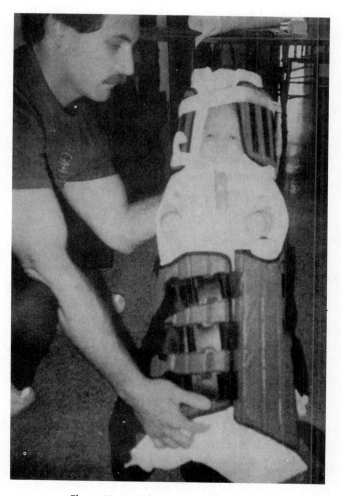

Figure 18–1. Pediatric immobilization.

TABLE 18–9. MEDICATIONS USED FOR TREATMENT OF A CHILD WHO HAS SUFFERED A SPINAL CORD INJURY

Medication	Dosage and Route	Indications
Methylprednisolone	30 mg/kg initial dose mixed in 50 mL of normal saline Administered IV piggyback over 15 minutes 5.4 mg/kg/hour over 23 hours	Treatment of isolated spinal cord injuries
Dopamine	1–5 μg/kg/min	Treatment of hypotension due to spinal shock

Interventions. As with the head injured child, the airway, breathing, and circulation are assessed and maintained. If intubation is required and a cervical spinal injury is suspected, Bohn et al (1990) recommend that nasotracheal intubation not be attempted. Enlarged adenoids and soft tissue in the child's upper airway could make intubation a traumatic and dangerous procedure for a pediatric patient.

If a child has an isolated spinal cord injury, it is recommended that the child be treated with high-dose methylprednisolone just as an adult patient would be (Medina, 1992). A child who has spinal shock also requires pharmacologic intervention. The medications used in the treatment of a child with a spinal cord injury are listed in Table 18–9.

If required to treat a spinal cord injury, traction may be applied in the ED. Just as with pharmacologic intervention, the protocol varies among institutions.

SPECIFIC INJURIES

Pediatric Concussion Syndrome

A concussion is generally classified as a minor head injury. The child may have a transient loss of consciousness, complain of a headache and dizziness, and experience nausea and vomiting after the injury.

A child who has suffered a minor head injury is at risk for a problem unique to childhood known as pediatric concussion syndrome (Wagner, 1992b). Symptoms of this syndrome range from generalized seizures after the injury (with normal CT findings) to complaints of irritability, lethargy, and persistent vomiting. The child is treated according to the severity of the syndrome.

Research has demonstrated that sequelae of pediatric concussion syndrome include learning difficulties, behavioral changes, and emotional disturbances (Allison, 1992; Reynolds, 1992). Symptoms may not occur until 8 weeks after the injury (Allison, 1992). When teaching parents about home care, it is impor-

tant to emphasize that the child may have some problems later related to the injury and to always be sure that the information about past head trauma be provided to health care providers. One educator suggested that for a school-aged child who has sustained a head injury, the parents may want to keep a record of any problems with attention, memory, fatigue, irritability, or concentration up to a few weeks after the injury (Allison, 1992).

Skull Fractures

Skull fractures in children are generally the result of blunt trauma. Skull fractures can be either open or closed. The malleable skull of a child is also susceptible to penetration from objects such as scissors, needles, and kitchen implements (Shapiro, 1990). If a child has a hematoma or laceration on the scalp or forehead, the wound should be palpated for a fracture. Fractures also can be identified on skull x rays and CT scans and by specific signs such as periorbital hematomas, Battle's sign (bruising behind the ear), hemotympanum, and leakage of CSF.

Linear and Depressed Skull Fractures. A skull fracture may be linear or depressed. Linear skull fractures are the most common ones seen in children (Dolan, 1992). Linear skull fractures that may indicate more serious injury include those that cross the middle meningeal artery and extend into the paranasal sinuses (Dolan, 1992; Shapiro, 1990).

A depressed skull fracture occurs because of a direct impact on the skull, as when a child falls and hits the edge of a coffee table. Many times depressed skull fractures are hidden under a scalp hematoma (Paul and Fahner, 1991). A unique type of depressed skull fracture called a "ping-pong" defect—a round depression in the frontal area—may be seen in infants because of their malleable skull bones.

The treatment of a depressed skull fracture is elevation of the depressed area. This is usually done surgically. However, a recent patient report by Paul and Fahner (1991) suggested the use of a vacuum extractor to elevate the depressed part of the skull. Depressed skull fractures may be associated with underlying contusions and lacerations.

Basal Skull Fracture. Basal skull fractures are suspected when a child has periorbital ecchymosis, hemotympanum, a Battle sign, or CSF leakage. Antibiotics may be used to prevent the development of meningitis (Dolan, 1992).

Epidural and Subdural Hematomas. Intracranial hemorrhages may result from tears related to skull fractures, blunt impact, and shearing forces that cause vessels to rupture in the head (Duhaime et al, 1992). It was previously thought that the presence of a skull fracture was not as likely to indicate an intracranial hemorrhage in a child as it was in an adult. It has been found, however, that the presence of a skull fracture may indicate a serious intracranial injury, such as an epidural or a subdural hematoma (Luerssen, 1993).

About 3% of children who are admitted to the hospital for head trauma have an epidural hematoma. These hematomas may have devastating, even fatal consequences. An epidural hematoma is usually the result of a tear in the middle meningeal artery or in a vein. Skull fractures that cross the path of a major vascular structure should lead one to suspect the development of an epidural hematoma.

In a study conducted by the Children's Hospital of Boston, it was found that epidural hematoma was diagnosed by CT in 53 children during the 10-year period from 1980 to 1990. Twenty-four of these children incurred the epidural hematoma after a fall of less than 5 feet; 13 of the 53 children had a history of post-traumatic loss of consciousness. Symptoms displayed by 51 of the 53 children with an epidural hematoma were vomiting, headache, and lethargy. Many of the children did present initially alert and with normal vital signs. Skull fractures were present in 35 of the 53 children (Pediatric Alert, 1993).

Subdural hematomas usually are venous bleeds. The source of this bleed is usually the bridging veins across the dura. Subdural hematomas are frequently associated with the shaken baby syndrome of child abuse (Dolan, 1992; Duhaime et al, 1992; Shapiro, 1990). Subdural hematomas that occur in children after infancy carry the same mortality as those that occur in adult patients, about 40% (Luerssen, 1993).

Signs and symptoms of subdural hematoma include a full fontanelle, vomiting, irritability, and lethargy. Infants with the shaken baby syndrome may have retinal hemorrhages (Dolan, 1992).

Intracranial hemorrhages are diagnosed by CT. Treatment is usually by neurosurgical intervention followed by control of ICP (Dolan, 1992). It is important to emphasize that the signs and symptoms of intracranial bleeds may not appear immediately after the injury. The emergency nurse must be sure that family members receive detailed, but simple instructions about head injury and that they express an understanding of the need to return to the ED if there are any changes in the child that could indicate complications of the head injury.

Pediatric Spinal Cord Injury

As previously pointed out, spinal cord injuries are relatively uncommon in younger children. There is, however, a "juvenile" type of injury that occurs in children before adolescence. The injury involves the high cervical spine and may show no radiologic abnormality

(Bohn et al, 1990; Medina, 1992; Shapiro, 1990). The name for this phenomenon is SCIWORA (spinal cord injury without radiologic abnormality). It may be the result of the anatomic differences between children and adults previously discussed. SCIWORA occurs almost exclusively in young children, usually those younger than 8 years of age (Dickman and Rekate, 1993). Injury is frequently to the cervical and thoracic levels of the spine, the cervical spine being affected more commonly. Deficits range from brief motor or sensory changes to a complete neurologic injury.

TRANSPORT OF A NEUROLOGICALLY INJURED PEDIATRIC PATIENT

A child who has sustained a moderate or severe head injury or a spinal cord injury with deficits should be in a facility that can appropriately assess, intervene, and provide rehabilitation. Wesson et al (1992) identified the long-term devastating impact of severe head injury on both the child and the family. Inappropriate management of head and spinal cord trauma affects not only the acute phase of a child's injury but also the rest of the child's life. Pediatric centers skilled in the care of children with head or spinal cord injuries should be identified by the emergency nurse and the child transferred as needed.

PATIENT AND FAMILY TEACHING AND PSYCHOSOCIAL SUPPORT

Because head injuries are the most common type of injury suffered by pediatric patients, prevention of further injury should be an important focus for the emergency nurse. Many studies have documented a decrease in the rate of injury or the severity of injury when helmets are used (McKenna et al, 1991; Spaite et al, 1991; Thompson et al, 1993). Appropriate use of seat belts and car seats helps keep children from being thrown in automobile crashes (Tepas, 1990). Thompson et al (1993) used a hypothetical model to demonstrate that the use of bicycle helmets for children 5–9 years of age would save $84,000 in hospital care per year. Helping communities with unique needs, such as farm communities, develop ways to prevent falls would decrease the incidence of falls and the consequent head injuries (Steuland et al, 1991).

When a child is brought to an ED after a head or spinal cord injury, the emergency nurse should explain and answer any questions about the child's condition. When possible, the family or caregivers should be allowed to see, talk to, and touch the child.

A child who is discharged home with a mild head injury needs to be continuously observed for about

48 hours. The child's family needs to be given instructions (see Appendix A) that include how to perform a brief neurologic assessment, including observation for behavioral changes, pupillary inequality, and changes in gait. The emergency nurse should be sure that the parent or caretaker has a thorough understanding of what to watch for and to either call for assistance or bring the child back to ED. The child may be treated with acetaminophen for analgesia (Dolan, 1992).

REFERENCES

Allison M (1992). The effects of neurologic injury on the maturing brain. *Headlines* 3:2–10

Bernardo L, Bove M (1993). *Pediatric procedures.* Boston: Bartlett & Jones, pp 143–152

Bohn D, Armstrong D, Becker L, Humphreys R (1990). Cervical injuries in children. *Journal of Trauma* 30:463–469

Bruce D (1993). Head trauma. In Eichelberger M (ed), *Pediatric trauma.* St. Louis: Mosby Year Book, pp 353–361

Bucklew P, Osler T, Eidson J, Clevenger F, Olson S, DeMarest G (1992). Falls and ejections from pickup trucks. *Journal of Trauma* 32:468–472

Cardona V, Hurn P, Mason P, Scanlon A, Veise-Berry S (1994). *Trauma nursing: From resuscitation through rehabilitation.* Philadelphia: Saunders, pp 693–720

Dickman C, Rekate H (1993). Spinal trauma. In Eichelberger M (ed), *Pediatric trauma.* St. Louis: Mosby Year Book, pp 362–377

Dolan M (1992). Head trauma. In Barkin R (ed), *Pediatric emergency medicine.* St. Louis: Mosby Year Book, pp 184–198

Duhaime A, Alario A, Lewander W, et al (1992). Head injury in very young children: Mechanisms, injury types, and ophthalmologic findings in 100 hospitalized patients younger than 2 years of age. *Pediatrics* 90:179–185

Evans T, Billittier A (1990). Rationale for burr hole decompression in the emergency management of head injuries. *Topics in Emergency Medicine* 11:64–68

Gerhart K (1991). Spinal cord injury outcomes in population-based sample. *Journal of Trauma* 31:1529–1535

Haley K, Baker P (1993). *Emergency nursing pediatric course.* Park Ridge, Il: Emergency Nurses Association, pp 109–152

Jaimovich D, Blostein P, Rose W, Stewart D, Shabino C, Buechler M (1991). Functional outcome of pediatric trauma patients identified as "non-salvageable survivors." *Journal of Trauma* 31:196–199

Johnson D (1988). Head injury. In Eichelberger M, Pratsch G (eds), *Pediatric trauma care.* Rockville, Md: Aspen, pp 87–99

Lower J (1992). Rapid neuro assessment. *American Journal of Nursing* 92:38–45

Luerssen T (1993). General characteristics of neurologic injury. In Eichelberger M (ed), *Pediatric trauma.* St. Louis: Mosby Year Book, pp 345–352

Massagli T, Jaffe K (1990). Pediatric spinal cord injury: Treatment and outcome. *Pediatrician* 17:244–254

Mayer T (1985). *Emergency management of pediatric trauma.* Philadelphia: Saunders

McKenna P, Welsh D, Martin L (1991). Pediatric bicycle trauma. *Journal of Trauma*, 31:392–394

Medina F (1992). Neck and spinal cord trauma. In Barkin R (ed), *Pediatric emergency medicine.* St. Louis: Mosby Year Book, pp 230–260

Mitchell P, Ackerman L (1992). Secondary brain injury reduction. In Bulechek G, McCloskey J (eds), *Nursing interventions.* Philadelphia: Saunders, pp 558–573

Paul M, Fahner T (1991). Closed depressed skull fracture in childhood reduced with suction cup method: Case report. *Journal of Trauma* 31:1551–1552

Peclet M, Newman K, et al (1990). Patterns of injury in children. 1(25):85–91

Pediatric Alert (1993). Epidural hematomas in children. 18:37–38

Reynolds E (1992). Controversies in caring for the child with a head injury. *American Journal of Maternal/Child Nursing* 17:246–251

Schafermeyer R, Ribbeck B, Gaskins J, Thomason S, Harlan M, Attkisson A (1991). Respiratory effects of spinal immobilization in children. *Annals of Emergency Medicine* 20:1017–1019

Semonin-Holleran R (1991). Pediatric trauma patients: Differences and implications for emergency nurses. *Journal of Emergency Nursing* 17:24–33

Shapiro K (1990). Emergency care of the head injured child. *Topics in Emergency Medicine* 11:36–42

Soud T (1992). Airway, breathing, circulation, and disability: What is different about kids. *Journal of Emergency Nursing* 18:107–116

Spaite D, Murphey M, Criss E, Valenzuela J, Meislin H (1991). A prospective analysis of injury severity among helmeted and nonhelmeted bicyclists involved in collisions with motor vehicles. *Journal of Trauma* 31:1510–1516

Stein S, Ross S (1992). Mild head injury: A plea for early routine CT scanning. *Journal of Trauma* 33:11–13

Sternbach G (1992). The great mutilator of American youth. *Journal of Emergency Medicine* 10:201–202

Steuland D, Layde P, Lee B (1991). Agricultural injuries in children in central Wisconsin. *Journal of Trauma* 31:1503–1509

Tepas J, DiScala C, Ramenofsky M, Barlow B (1990). Mortality and head injury: The pediatric perspective. *Journal of Pediatric Surgery* 25:92–96

Thompson R, Thompson D, Rivara F, Salazar A (1993). Cost effectiveness of bicycle helmet subsidies in a defined population. *Pediatrics* 91:902–907

Wagner M (1992a). Neurologic emergencies in the young: Evaluation and stabilization. *Emergency Medicine* 6:204–213

Wagner M (1992b). Neurologic emergencies in the young: Infection and injury. *Emergency Medicine* 6:214–224

Wesson D, Scorpio R, Spencer L, et al (1992). The physical, psychological, and socioeconomic costs of pediatric trauma. *Journal of Trauma* 33:252–257

Widner-Kolberg M, Maloney-Harmon P (1988). Pediatric trauma. In Cardona V, Hurn P, Mason P, Scanlon-Schilpp A, Veise-Berry S (eds), *Trauma nursing.* Philadelphia: Saunders, pp 664–691

SUGGESTED READING

Barkin R (1992). *Pediatric emergency medicine.* St. Louis: Mosby Year Book

Eichelberger M (1993). *Pediatric trauma.* St. Louis: Mosby Year Book

Haley K (ed) (1993). *Pediatric nursing core course.* Chicago: Emergency Nurses Association

Neff J, Kidd P (1993). *Trauma nursing: The art and science.* St. Louis: Mosby Year Book

Seidel J, Henderson D (1991). *Emergency medical services for children: A report to the nation.* Washington: National Center for Education in Maternal and Child Health

Thomas D (1991). *Pediatric emergency nursing.* Rockville, Md: Aspen

CHAPTER 19

Musculoskeletal Trauma

ANNE PHELAN

INTRODUCTION

When children suffer injury to the musculoskeletal system, the concerns of the emergency department (ED) nurse are twofold. The first priority is to minimize the discomfort through immobilization, elevation, and application of ice when appropriate. The second priority is to preserve the best possible level of function of the injured part by assessment of distal pulses, sensation, color, temperature, motion, and capillary refill both before and after any splinting or immobilization is performed.

There are two important differences between the skeletal systems of children and adults. The first is that children have an epiphyseal plate or growth cartilage at the ends of all long articulating bones. Fractures that disrupt or transect the epiphyseal plate may interfere with the growth of the bone, leading to a limb length discrepancy. The second difference is that the bones of children are more porous than those of adults, which increases the likelihood of fractures. Children also have a thicker periosteal covering, however, which enables them to produce more periosteal recalcification to smooth out and remodel the bone after a fracture is sustained. Figure 19–1 illustrates and Table 19–1 describes fracture patterns of the long bones.

As with any injury to a child, the emergency nurse must be aware of the possibility of inflicted injury. In collaboration with the physician, assessment should be made regarding the consistency of the his-

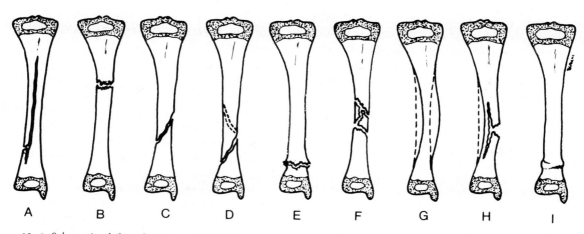

Figure 19–1. Schematic of tibia of a 3-year-old child showing types of fractures. **A.** Longitudinal. **B.** Transverse. **C.** Oblique. **D.** Spiral. **E.** Impacted. **F.** Comminuted. **G.** Bending, bowing. **H.** Greenstick. **I.** Cortical, torus. (From Ogden JA [1990]. *Sketetal injury in the child* [2nd ed] Philadelphia: Saunders, p 7)

TABLE 19–1. FRACTURE PATTERNS OF LONG BONES

Type	Pattern
Longitudinal	The fracture occurs lengthwise on a long bone.
Transverse	The fracture occurs crosswise on a long bone.
Oblique	The fracture transsects the long bone at an angle.
Spiral	The fracture line curves up a length of long bone.
Impacted	Crush injury; the fracture line is often indistinct.
Comminuted	The fractured bone is in more than two fragments.
Bowing	Bending causes deformity without an actual fracture.
Greenstick	The fracture may be oblique, transverse, or longitudinal without angulation; a portion of the periosteum is intact.
Torus	The bone buckles and may have some bowing without distinct fragments.

(Adapted from Ogden JA [1991]. Skeletal trauma. In Grossmman M, Dieckmann R.A (eds), Emergency medicine. Philadelphia: Lippincott, p 289)

tory with the injury sustained to determine the need for further investigation or protective intervention. Table 19–2 lists fractures suggestive of child abuse (see Chapter 8).

It is important to remember that for a patient with multiple system trauma, fractures are rarely life-threatening injuries. Although fractures may be readily apparent, the ABCs (airway-breathing-circulation) of trauma resuscitation take priority.

The nurse's approach to a child with musculoskeletal injuries varies with the developmental level of the child and the child's ability to cooperate. Whenever possible the child should be asked about the events leading up to the injury and to pinpoint the area of pain. Active range of motion is preferable to passive and may be accomplished by having the child reach for or grasp an interesting object.

The initial assessment of the neurovascular status of an injured extremity involves the suspected fracture site and the body parts distal to it. It is important to document the evaluation of the distal color, sensation, motion, temperature, capillary refilling, and degree of swelling. This assessment is repeated after immobilization and at regular intervals to detect any changes that require intervention.

EPIPHYSEAL INJURIES

The epiphyseal plate or growth cartilage is located between the metaphysis and the epiphysis at the articulating ends of long bones. Injury to the epiphyseal plate may cause a growth disturbance in that bone, producing a length discrepancy as the child matures.

For this reason careful assessment and management are essential.

Etiology and Pathophysiology

The epiphyseal plate may be more vulnerable to injury because it has partial ligamentous attachments, which can cause disruption from avulsion, shearing, or compression forces. The five types of epiphyseal fractures are classified by Salter and Harris (Figure 19–2). The potential for alteration in growth patterns increases from a Type I to a Type V fracture (Mayeda, 1990).

Type I injury is the result of a shearing or avulsion force that results in the separation of the epiphysis from the metaphysis without disruption of the epiphyseal plate. This injury may not be evident on x rays. It is characterized by pain, tenderness, and soft tissue swelling directly over the growth plate. Evidence of healing—periosteal recalcification—is usually present after about 7 days.

Type II is the most common type of epiphyseal fracture. It involves the slipping of an epiphyseal plate with fracture through the metaphysis. It is visible on x ray as a triangular metaphyseal fragment.

Type III is an intra-articular fracture of the epiphysis with slippage of a growth plate. This type of fracture is most commonly seen at the distal tibial epiphysis and the lateral condyle of the distal humerus.

Type IV is an intra-articular fracture that extends through the epiphysis, epiphyseal plate, and metaphysis. This fracture is commonly seen at the lateral condyle of the humerus.

Type V is a rare injury in which an axial compression causes a crush injury to the epiphyseal plate. Growth arrest is common and this injury is difficult to see on initial x rays.

TABLE 19–2. FRACTURES STRONGLY SUGGESTIVE OF CHILD ABUSE

Fractures inconsistent with history
Fractures inconsistent with developmental stage of child
Fractures with associated injuries suggestive of abuse
Multiple fractures, particularly in various stages of healing
Multiple, complex, or depressed skull fractures
Epiphyseal-metaphyseal rib fractures
Spiral fractures of the femur or tibia in preambulating children
Spiral fractures of the humerus
Metaphyseal chip (corner) fractures
Avulsion fractures of clavicle and acromion process

(Reproduced with permission from Bachman D, Santora S [1993]. Orthopedic trauma. In Fleisher G, Ludwig S [eds], Textbook pediatric emergency medicine [3rd ed]. Baltimore: Williams & Wilkins Publishers, p 1244.)

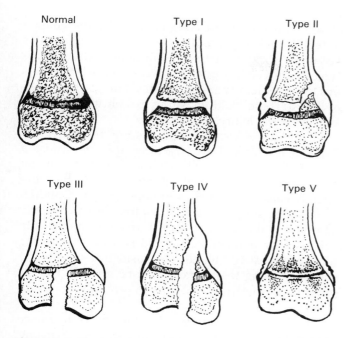

Normal   Type I   Type II

Type III   Type IV   Type V

Figure 19–2. The Salter–Harris classification system used in epiphyseal injuries. (From Simon RR, Koenigsknecht SJ [1989]. *Emergency orthopedics: The extremities* [2nd ed]. Norwalk, Conn: Appleton & Lange p 19)

History

The triage nurse obtains a history of the events leading to the injury and any measures taken to treat it before arrival at the ED.

Physical Assessment

Initial assessment involves documenting the location of point tenderness, any evidence of soft tissue swelling or discoloration, any limitation in range of motion or loss of function, alterations in sensation perception, and changes in pulses, temperature, or capillary refill distal to the injury site. Immobilization must be provided utilizing appropriate splints or a sling and documenting reassessment of the distal pulses, color, temperature, sensation, and capillary refill after splinting.

Diagnostic and Laboratory Tests

In many EDs the triage nurse orders the initial x rays. It is best to include the joint above and the joint below the suspected fracture site. Both the child and the parents should be made aware that the patient should take nothing by mouth in case sedation or operative fixation is necessary to reduce the suspected fracture.

TRIAGE
Epiphyseal Trauma

Emergent —
A child with an open fracture with exposed bone or suspected distal femoral fractures; marked swelling. A child with pulselessness, cool color, and delayed capillary refill distal to the injury.

Urgent —
A child with closed skin but an obvious bony deformity; intact pulses; color, sensation, motion, and capillary refill distal to the injury.

Non-urgent —
A child with closed skin; no obvious bony deformity; good range of motion of the injured part; no alteration in color, sensation temperature, motion, or capillary refill distally.

Nursing Diagnosis
High Risk for Infection:

Defining Characteristics
- Inadequate primary defenses (broken skin)
- Traumatized tissues
- Tissue destruction and increased environmental exposure

Nursing Interventions
- Irrigate open fracture sites in a sterile manner
- Initiate intravenous access and draw baseline blood tests
- Administer antibiotics as ordered

Expected Outcomes
- Body temperature remains normal
- Wound shows no evidence of purulent drainage or surrounding erythema
- White blood cell count and erythrocyte sedimentation rate remain within normal limits

Nursing Diagnosis
Pain

Defining Characteristics
- Verbal communication of pain
- Nonverbal indicators of pain (facial expression, protective of injury site, crying)

- Autonomic responses to pain (changes in blood pressure, heart rate and respiratory rate, diaphoresis)

Nursing Interventions

- Provide a calm, soothing environment
- Provide simple and clear explanations of all procedures before carrying them out
- Immobilize the injured part and provide elevation and ice whenever possible
- Administer medication as ordered

Expected Outcomes

- Vital signs return to normal
- The child appears comfortable when the injured part is not being actively manipulated
- The child states that the level of pain has improved
- The child appears to have decreased anxiety

Nursing Diagnosis
Bathing/Hygiene, Toileting, Feeding Self Care Deficit

Defining Characteristics

- Inability to complete self feeding, bathing, toileting
- Requires help from another person

Nursing Interventions

- Include family members in discharge teaching
- Assure that the home environment is amenable to the level of increased assistance that will be required
- Make appropriate referrals to community agencies for assistance with home management

Expected Outcomes

- The family verbalizes their understanding of the child's increased need for assistance with activities of daily living
- The family verbalizes their initial plans for home management (taking turns staying home with child or availability of a relative or caretaker until child returns to school)

Management
Once the presence of an epiphyseal fracture is confirmed, the child is referred for orthopedic evaluation. Type I injuries are usually immobilized with a cast or splint for about 3 weeks; bone growth problems are rare. Type II fractures are usually manipulated with closed reduction. These children may require sedation in the ED for this procedure (see section on Conscious Sedation). Type II fractures of an upper extremity are typically placed in a cast for 3 weeks; Type II fractures of a lower extremity are immobilized in a cast for up to 6 weeks. These children rarely exhibit growth problems after the injury.

Surgical reduction is frequently necessary for Type III fractures. These fractures also may cause a growth disturbance. Type IV fractures typically require open reduction and internal fixation; they frequently cause disturbances in bone growth. Children who require surgical reduction of fractures are usually admitted to the hospital. Type V fractures are usually managed by immobilization and non-weight-bearing for approximately 3 weeks. They usually disrupt blood supply, leading to an arrest in bone growth. Parents should be forewarned that growth problems are likely to occur.

In addition to documenting the child's tolerance of procedures and responses to and recovery from any medications, it is important to document the status of distal circulation, sensation, and motion after any manipulation and immobilization.

UPPER EXTREMITY TRAUMA

Fractures of the upper extremities are common in children and may occur as a result of falls on an outstretched hand (Figure 19–3), direct blows, or sports injuries.

Etiology and Pathophysiology

Clavicular Fractures. Proceeding from proximal to distal, clavicular fractures usually result from a direct blow or a fall in which the child lands on the shoulder. A fractured clavicle also may be caused by a fall on an outstretched hand. There is decreased range of motion on the affected side and tenderness on palpation. There is frequently a palpable bony deformity.

Acromioclavicular Separations. Separations of the acromioclavicular (AC) joint usually occur in older children. These injuries frequently are caused by a direct blow to the shoulder or a fall in which the child lands on the shoulder. They are characterized by point tenderness and soft tissue swelling over the AC joint.

Anterior Shoulder Dislocations. Anterior shoulder dislocation usually results from a fall on an extended arm causing the head of the humerus to slide forward. This is the most common shoulder dislocation in child-

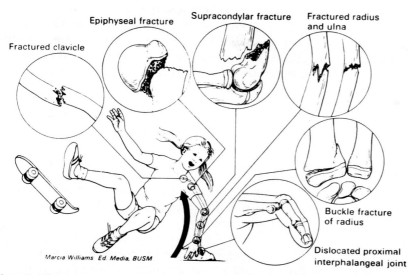

Figure 19–3. Trauma resulting from progression of force in a fall on an outstretched hand. (From Segal D [1979]. Pediatric orthopedic emergencies. *Pediatric Clinics of North America* 26:794)

hood. The humeral head is usually palpable anterior to the distal clavicle, and the deltoid musculature has markedly decreased tone. This injury is likely to cause alterations in sensation and circulation.

Scapular Fractures. Fractures of the scapula rarely occur in children; they usually are the result of severe blunt trauma. These fractures may be seen in association with other injuries. When a scapular fracture is seen as an isolated injury in the absence of a history of force, the possibility of nonaccidental trauma should be investigated.

Humeral Fractures. Fractures of the proximal epiphysis of the humerus are more common in adolescents and older children than in infants and young children and are usually the result of a backward fall on an extended arm or of a direct blow. These injuries may present without bony deformity because the fragments are minimally displaced. Fractures of the shaft of the humerus are less common in children than in adults and may result from a twist, a fall, or a direct blow.

Elbow Fractures and Dislocations. Supracondylar fractures of the humerus are the most common elbow fracture in children. This fracture usually results from a fall and can be differentiated from a subluxation of the head of the radius, or "nursemaid's elbow," by the presence of marked soft tissue swelling. Fractures of the lateral epicondyle of the humerus (capitellum) usually result from a fall on an extended arm. This fracture typically has a Salter Type IV configuration. Medial epicondylar fractures of the humerus are rare in children but may cause complications because of their proximity to the ulnar nerve.

Posterior dislocation of the elbow usually results

from a fall on a hyperextended arm. This is a common dislocation among children and may be seen in association with a supracondylar fracture of a flexed elbow. Subluxation of the head of the radius is one of the most common injuries among toddlers and preschoolers. It usually results from a sudden pull on a pronated forearm. The history is usually that an adult tried to pick up a child or to stop him or her from running. Afterward the child refused to use the grabbed arm and complained during any attempt at passive motion. There is usually an absence of swelling and the child typically holds the arm in pronation. Fractures of the neck of the radius usually result from a fall on an outstretched hand and may require surgical reduction if angulation is severe.

Forearm Fractures. Fractures of the forearm usually are caused by a fall in which the child lands on the palm of the hand; they also may be the result of a direct blow. The child usually presents with localized pain, soft tissue swelling, and bony deformity. There are seven common forearm fractures (Mayeda, 1990).

Common Forearm Fractures

1. Monteggia fracture—a single bone fracture with overriding fragment associated with a dislocation of the head of the radius
2. Torus fracture—a buckle fracture that may involve both bones. There usually is no displacement, but there is a disruption of the cortex, common in children, usually at the metaphyseal area.
3. Colles fracture—transection of the distal radius with dorsal angulation associated with a Salter Type II epiphyseal fracture of the ulnar styloid
4. Smith fracture—reverse of a Colles fracture. Fracture of distal radius with volar angulation, usually caused by direct blow to a pronated forearm.

5. Greenstick fracture—a longitudinal fracture involving one side of the cortex of one bone
6. Barton fracture—a radial fracture, marginal, of the volar or dorsal surface associated with dislocation of the carpal bones and hand
7. Galeazzi fracture—fracture of the middle to distal third of the radius associated with radio-ulnar subluxation

Hand Injuries. Hand injuries are common in children. Fractures of the navicular bone are common in older children; they may result from a fall on a dorsiflexed hand. The child presents with local tenderness, possibly with swelling and discoloration, and usually has reduced grasp strength. These fractures are rarely seen on initial x rays. Metacarpal fractures usually occur as a result of a crush injury or direct blow. The child presents with marked swelling, tenderness, and deformity. Finger fractures are common among children and often result when a hand is crushed in a closing door. A finger fracture associated with a skin laceration is managed as an open fracture. Mallet finger deformity is a fracture at the base of a distal phalanx with disruption of the extensor tendons of the distal interphalangeal (DIP) joint. The child presents with an obvious deformity, tenderness and swelling of the DIP joint, and an inability to extend the finger. Amputation of fingers usually results from entrapment in machinery, such as threshers, lawn mowers, and snow blowers. Though dramatic in presentation, an amputation is rarely life-threatening. Degloving injuries are frequently the result of an attempt to pull the hand out of machinery once trapped. This crushing injury may result in extensive soft tissue injury and dislocations.

History
The history should include the mechanism of injury, treatment measures taken before arrival at the ED and initial vital signs. The presence of any concomitant injuries, such as head trauma or loss of consciousness, at the scene should be ascertained. It is also beneficial to document any known allergies, immunization status, and last food and fluids ingested.

Physical Assessment
Documentation of current neurovascular status, any obvious deformity, areas of point tenderness, limitations in range of motion, breaks in skin or areas of ecchymosis should be noted. Immobilization of the suspected fracture increases comfort by preventing the grating of fragments on motion. For most upper extremity fractures, a sling or sling and swathe is adequate. For suspected hand and distal forearm fractures, splinting is necessary. Neurovascular status should be assessed and documented after immobilization.

Laboratory and Diagnostic Tests
The x rays should include at least two views, including the joint above and the joint below the suspected fracture site. Application of ice helps control swelling and minimize discomfort.

TRIAGE
Upper Extremity Trauma

Emergent
A child with an open fracture and exposed bone; amputation or degloving injury; evidence of neurovascular compromise.

Urgent
A child with a bony deformity; intact skin; no evidence of neurovascular compromise.

Non-urgent
A child with no obvious deformity; mild soft tissue swelling; no evidence of neurovascular compromise.

Nursing Diagnosis
High Risk for Infection

Defining Characteristics
- Inadequate primary defenses (broken skin, traumatized tissues)
- Tissue destruction and increased environmental exposure

Nursing Interventions
- Irrigate open fracture sites in a sterile manner
- Initiate intravenous access
- Administer antibiotics as ordered

Expected Outcomes
- Body temperature remains normal
- Wound shows no evidence of purulent drainage or surrounding erythema

Nursing Diagnosis
Pain

Defining Characteristics
- Verbal communication of pain
- Nonverbal indicators of pain (facial expression, protection of injury site, crying)
- Autonomic responses to pain (changes in blood

pressure, heart rate and respiratory rate, diaphoresis)

Nursing Interventions

- Provide a calm, soothing environment
- Provide simple and clear explanations of all procedures before carrying them out
- Immobilize the injured part and provide elevation and ice whenever possible
- Administer medication as ordered

Expected Outcomes

- Vital signs return to normal
- The child appears comfortable when the injured part is not being actively manipulated
- The child states that the level of pain has improved

Nursing Diagnosis

Bathing/Hygiene, Toileting, Feeding, Self-Care Deficit

Defining Characteristics

- Inability to complete self feeding, bathing, toileting
- Requires help from another person

Nursing Interventions

- Include family members in discharge teaching
- Assure that the home environment is amenable to the level of increased assistance that will be required
- Make appropriate referrals to community agencies for assistance with home management

Expected Outcomes

- The family verbalizes their understanding of the child's increased need for assistance with activities of daily living
- The family verbalizes their initial plans for home management (taking turns staying home with child or availability of a relative or caretaker until child returns to school)

Management

Shoulder Injuries. *Clavicular fractures* rarely require manipulation. Immobilization with a padded figure-of-eight strap or harness or sling and swathe is usually necessary for 3 weeks. Powdered pads in the axilla help prevent chafing. *Acromioclavicular separation* also is managed with a sling and swathe or figure-of-eight

splint. Separation of the AC joint with more than 1 cm of upward displacement of the distal clavicle may require surgical intervention. *Anterior shoulder dislocations* must be manipulated into place. These children usually require intravenous muscle relaxants and analgesics (see section on Conscious Sedation). There are several positions for and methods of applying traction and manipulation to relocate the humeral head. Post-reduction x rays are usually obtained to assure adequate relocation and reveal any concurrent fractures. These children's arms are usually immobilized with a sling and swathe for approximately 4 weeks to allow the joint capsule to heal. *Scapular fractures* are usually managed with sling and swathe immobilization when this injury occurs by itself.

Humeral Fractures. Fractures of the proximal epiphysis of the humerus with less than 1 cm of separation and less than 40° of angulation and no malrotation are treated by sling and swathe or a shoulder immobilizer. Surgical intervention is needed in the presence of greater angulation or fractures with three or more fragments. Fractures of the shaft of the humerus without severe angulation or displacement may be immobilized in a sugar-tong splint applied from wrist to axilla with the arm in 90° of flexion. Supracondylar fractures of the distal humerus and lateral epicondyle (capitellum) require immediate reduction and immobilization with the elbow flexed at 90°. Reduction is often performed in the operating room. These children are usually admitted to the hospital for monitoring of their neurovascular status. Fractures of the medial epicondyle of the humerus with less than 1 cm of displacement are typically managed by splinting. Indications for open reduction and admission to the hospital include ulnar nerve compression and more than 1 cm of displacement. Children with fractures of the medial epicondyle are usually admitted to monitor their neurovascular status carefully because of the possibility of compartment syndrome.

Elbow Injuries. Posterior elbow dislocation requires manipulation. These children typically receive intravenous muscle relaxants and analgesics prior to reduction. Gentle traction is used to relocate the elbow. Post-reduction x rays are usually obtained to assure good results and to uncover associated fractures. The arm is splinted at 90° of flexion, usually for 2–3 weeks. Subluxation of the head of the radius does not require orthopedic evaluation. The ED physician reduces the subluxation by using one hand to supinate the forearm while flexing the elbow with the other hand over the head of the radius. A palpable click on completion of this maneuver indicates success. The child usually begins to use the affected arm within a brief period.

Forearm Fractures. Fractures of the neck of the radius, when nondisplaced or having less than 20° of angulation, do not require reduction. They are immobilized in a long arm splint that includes the wrist. Greater degrees of angulation may require open reduction. Forearm fractures that are not rotated and have less than 15° of angulation are immobilized for 4–6 weeks. For greater degrees of angulation and when both bones are fractured, reduction, possibly open reduction, is necessary.

Hand Injuries. Fractures of the navicular (scaphoid) bone are usually immobilized with a long arm cast to include the thumb, metacarpohalangeal (MCP) and elbow. The cast remains in place for 7–8 weeks. The hands of children with metacarpal fractures are usually immobilized in a cast in flexion from the distal phalanges to the middle of the forearm once reduced. Fractures of the distal phalanx or middle phalanx are usually immobilized by finger splints. Epiphyseal injuries, rotational or angulated deformities, and open fractures may require internal fixation to assure proper alignment. Mallet finger deformities with less than 25% of subluxation are usually splinted in hyperextension. Greater degrees of displacement require internal fixation.

Avulsion injuries and digital amputation are irrigated and treated as open fractures. Antibiotic prophylaxis is indicated. If the digit is to be reimplanted, care must be taken to wrap the finger in sterile gauze that has been moistened with Ringer lactate. The wrapped finger is placed in a sealed plastic bag, and the bag is placed in ice. This system prevents tissue masceration. X rays of the hand and the amputated part are needed to assess viability and associated fractures. The child's hand should be wrapped in a dry, sterile dressing. Children with degloving injuries require aggressive pain management. Thorough irrigation and debridement are usually performed in the operating room. A sterile occlusive dressing is applied after cleansing. Antibiotic prophylaxis may be necessary. The child's hand is assessed for the need for skin grafting.

In addition to documenting the child's responses to procedures and tolerance to and recovery from any medications, it is important for the ED nurse to reassess and document neurovascular status after any manipulation, reduction, or application of immobilization device such as a splint or cast.

LOWER EXTREMITY TRAUMA

Motor vehicle crashes, bicycle injuries, contact sports, and recreational activities account for most lower extremity trauma among children.

Etiology and Pathophysiology

Pelvic Fractures. Pelvic fractures usually result from motor vehicle crashes in which the child was a pedestrian or passenger. These fractures generally result from direct blunt trauma; they are more common among older children. The child usually complains of localized pain and has asymmetric movement or crepitus on rocking the pelvis. Pelvic fractures often occur at multiple sites around the pelvic girdle. These children require careful evaluation for the possibility of blood loss and damage to underlying intra-abdominal structures such as the bladder and urethra.

Femoral Fractures. Femoral fractures are common in childhood. The femur is the primary weight-bearing bone. When the femur is broken, there may be considerable swelling due to blood loss into surrounding tissues. These children may present with pain, swelling, refusal to move the affected leg, or refusal to bear weight.

Knee Injuries. Patellar dislocations are most common among teenaged girls. They usually occur as a result of a direct blow or internal rotation. The patellar dislocation is usually palpable, and a knee effusion may be present. Patellar fractures are usually caused by direct blunt trauma. The patient may be unable to fully extend the knee.

Osgood–Schlatter disease is common in athletic and active preteens and adolescents. Patients with this disease often present with a history of intermittent painful swelling over the tibial tuberosity noted after periods of physical activity; the swelling usually resolves with rest. The activity causes the patellar tendon to pull on the tibial tuberosity, causing a partial avulsion.

Lower Leg Fractures. Fractures of the tibial shaft are common in children. Fractures of the fibula may occur in conjunction with a tibial fracture or may occur alone. The child presents with difficulty in weight bearing and localized tenderness and swelling; a deformity may not be present.

Ankle and Foot Injuries. Ankle sprains are common in all age groups of ambulatory children. An inversion twist is the most common cause, leading to swelling over the lateral malleolus and tenderness over the ligaments. Eversion twists are more likely to be associated with a fracture. The most common ankle fracture occurs at the lateral malleolus and is usually the result of a twisting injury. In addition to local pain and swelling, the child has pain on dorsiflexion of the foot.

Fractures of the midshaft of the metatarsals usually result from direct blunt trauma, and fractures at the base of the fifth metatarsal from inversion. The child usually exhibits local pain, swelling, and difficulty with weight bearing.

Assessment

In addition to documenting the mechanism of injury, the nurse must assess the injured extremity for the quality of distal pulses, color, sensation, temperature, and capillary refill. Any gait disturbance or inability to bear weight should be noted along with limitations in range of motion. The injured extremity should be elevated in a wheelchair and ice should be applied while the child goes for x rays. As with application of any immobilization device, neurovascular status should be reassessed after application of the splint.

T R I A G E
Lower Extremity Trauma

Emergent

A child with an open fracture with exposed bone; amputation or degloving injury of foot; evidence of neurovascular compromise.

Urgent

A child with a bony deformity; intact skin; no evidence of neurovascular compromise.

Non-urgent

A child with no marked deformity; mild soft tissue swelling; able to bear weight partially; no evidence of neurovascular compromise.

Nursing Diagnosis
High Risk for Infection

Defining Characteristics

- Inadequate primary defenses (broken skin, traumatized tissues
- Tissue destruction and increased environmental exposure

Nursing Interventions

- Irrigate open fracture sites in a sterile manner
- Initiate intravenous access
- Administer antibiotics as ordered

Expected Outcomes

- Body temperature remains normal
- Wound shows no evidence of purulent drainage or surrounding erythema

Nursing Diagnosis
Pain

Defining Characteristics

- Verbal communication of pain
- Nonverbal indicators of pain (facial expression, protection of injury site, crying)
- Autonomic responses to pain (changes in blood pressure, heart rate, respiratory rate; diaphoresis)

Nursing Interventions

- Provide a calm, soothing environment
- Provide simple and clear explanations of all procedures before carrying them out
- Immobilize the injured part and provide elevation and ice whenever possible
- Administer medication as ordered

Expected Outcomes

- Vital signs return to normal
- The child appears comfortable when the injured part is not being actively manipulated
- The child states that the level of pain has improved

Nursing Diagnosis
Bathing/Hygiene, Toileting, Feeding, Self Care Deficit

Defining Characteristics

- Inability to complete self bathing or toileting; lack of mobility
- Requires help from another person

Nursing Interventions

- Include family members in discharge teaching.
- Assure that the home environment is amenable to the level of increased assistance that will be required
- Make appropriate referrals to community agencies for assistance with home management

Expected Outcomes

- The family verbalizes their understanding of the child's increased need for assistance with activities of daily living
- The family members verbalize their initial plans for home management (taking turns staying home with child or availability of a relative or caretaker until child returns to school)

Management

Pelvic Fractures. Uncomplicated pelvic fractures may be managed with bedrest for a period of 2–4 weeks, with gradual resumption of ambulation. Crush injuries to the pelvis warrant close assessment and intervention to preserve the function of the internal organs and prevent or treat hemorrhage. A pneumatic anti-shock garment (PASG) may be of benefit.

Femoral Fractures. Fractures of the femur may be immobilized with a Hare or Thomas traction splint before definitive care is undertaken. Care usually involves operative reduction or placement in traction. Careful evaluation of neurovascular status after splinting is always a priority.

Knee Injuries. Patellar dislocations are usually managed by gentle closed manipulation in the ED. Both the patellar dislocations and fractures may be immobilized in extension with a knee immobilizer and crutch walking to avoid weight bearing. Osgood–Schlatter disease is managed with the knee immobilizer in extension for 2–4 weeks, with gradual return to the child's activities. Children with an avulsed tibial tubercle may require surgical intervention to prevent nonunion or avascular necrosis.

Lower Leg Fractures. Fractures of the fibula alone can be treated with a short-leg walking cast. Nondisplaced tibial-fibular fractures are usually treated with a long-leg cast. Children with displaced tibial fractures are usually admitted to the hospital after reduction to monitor neurovascular status.

Ankle and Foot Injuries. Ankle sprains vary in degree of severity and may be treated by immobilization using an elastic bandage or posterior splint. Weight bearing may resume as the child becomes comfortable. Ankle fractures may require reduction to return fragments to their functional position and immobilization with casting and crutch walking to restrict weight bearing. Some ankle fractures may require open reduction and internal fixation. Metatarsal fractures may require a short-leg walking cast for 5–6 weeks to promote healing. Displaced metatarsal fractures may require surgical reduction.

Patient and Family Teaching and Psychosocial Support

Parents and children should receive oral and written instructions about restrictions in weight bearing. They should be well informed on how to check the neurovascular status distal to the injury site, especially when a cast has been applied. The importance of any recommended orthopedic follow-up care should be emphasized to promote adequate healing and return to function. Children with casts may require assistance with bathing, at least initially. The importance of keeping the cast dry is emphasized. The parents should be given the phone number to contact the ED or the orthopedist in case difficulties arise.

CONSCIOUS SEDATION

Although controversy exists surrounding the use of conscious sedation for pediatric ED procedures, it is becoming more common in practice. For painful, brief emergency procedures such as repair of a laceration or fracture reduction, the use of rapid-acting agents with a short half life can greatly reduce the discomfort and anxiety of a child. Policies and procedures governing the use of these medications must be in place and well understood by the ED staff.

During triage the emergency nurse can identify children likely to require sedation. In addition to the typical history of the event, physical assessment, initial vital signs (with weight in kg), allergy and immunization history, the triage nurse should instruct the patient to take nothing by mouth and should document the last oral intake of food and fluids (Hammer, 1990).

The type and route of conscious sedation may vary with the age of the child and type of procedure. The drugs are typically determined and administered by the ED attending physician. As with other narcotics, the ED nurse is responsible for double checking calculation and assuring an appropriate dosage.

The nurse also has an integral role in the monitoring of the child. In addition to frequent (every 5–15 minutes) monitoring of apical pulse rate and respiratory rate, a cardiorespiratory monitor and transcutaneous pulse oximeter should be used. Constant nursing observation may be necessary during most of the procedure and recovery period.

The following drugs (Miller and Leno, 1991) may be used alone or in combination to produce conscious sedation. The appropriate reversal agents (flumazenil and naloxone) should be readily available, as should oxygen and suction equipment. Table 19–3 contains dosages and nursing considerations.

Fentanyl. A synthetic narcotic with few hemodynamic effects, fentanyl has a rapid onset with effects lasting 30–40 minutes. The effect of fentanyl is reversible with naloxone. Patient may require supplemental oxygen. Fentanyl may be given intravenously. The nasal and oral mucosal routes are being studied for efficacy.

TABLE 19–3. DRUGS COMMONLY USED IN CONSCIOUS SEDATION

Drug	Dosage and Route	Nursing Considerations
Fentanyl	1–5 μg/kg/dose IV	Rapid onset. Effects last 30–40 minutes. Monitor VS, esp. resp. status frequently; include pulse oximetry when possible. Reversible with naloxone.
Ketamine	1–2 mg/kg/dose IV	Rapid onset. Effects last less than 2 hours. Side effects: vomiting, ataxia, laryngospasm, and hallucinations. Monitor VS and oxygen saturation during sedation.
Merperidine, promethazine, and chlorpromaxine cocktail	Dose not to exceed 2 mg/kg: 1 mg/kg and 1 mg/kg IV	Longer onset of action (30–40 minutes) Longer duration of action (usually more than 2 hours) Monitor for signs of respiratory depression.
Midazolam	0.05–2 mg/kg IV slowly or intra-nasally	Rapid onset of effect. Short duration (30–40 minutes) Monitor for resp. depression, hypotension, and bradycardia.
Nitrous oxide	Administered by inhalation in combination with oxygen	Rapid onset of action. Short duration of effect on withdrawal (less than 5 minutes) May cause nausea and vomiting. Monitor oxygenation status and assure continued consciousness by talking with the child. Usually used in children older than 5 years.
TAC	Tetracaine 0.5% Adrenaline 0.05% Cocaine 11.8% topical solution	Applied directly to wound by liquid compress (held in place with parent's gloved hand for 20–30 minutes). Should see some blanching of surrounding skin. Not to be used on cuts involving mucous membranes, genitalia, or fingers or toes because of increased absorption of cocaine and potential for cocaine toxicity.

Vs, vital signs.

Ketamine. Ketamine is a sedative agent with rapid onset of action. The duration of action is usually less than 2 hours. The most common side effects are vomiting, ataxia, laryngospasm, and hallucinations.

Meperidine, Promethazine and Chlorpromazine Cocktail. This combination of drugs has a long onset of action, 30–40 minutes and a longer duration of action, about 2 hours. The patient must be monitored for respiratory depression. This medication is given intramuscularly.

Midazolam. A benzodiazepine, midazolam has a rapid onset of action and a short duration of effect. It reduces anxiety and causes sedation and amnesia. Midazolam may be used in lower dosages in combination with fentanyl.

Nitrous Oxide. An analgesic agent administered by inhalation, nitrous oxide has a rapid onset of action, usually less than 5 minutes, and a short duration of effect on withdrawal, usually less than 5 minutes. Side effects may include nausea and vomiting. The nurse monitors oxygenation status by pulse oximetry and assures continued consciousness, usually by having the child hold the mask in place.

TAC. Tetracaine 0.5%, adrenaline 0.05%, and cocaine 11.8% are combined to form a local anesthetic agent that is applied directly to the wound by liquid compress. The compress should not be applied to lacerations involving mucous membranes, genitalia, or fingers or toes because of the high vascularization of these areas and the potential for cocaine toxicity. The drugs are placed on an appropriate-sized gauze pad and usually held in place by a parent's gloved hand for 20–30 minutes. There should be some blanching of the skin immediately around the laceration.

Patient and Family Teaching and Psychosocial Support

Parents and the child should receive oral and written instructions for cast care. They should also be made aware of signs of swelling under the cast, such as local pain, distal swelling, decreased temperature, color changes, delayed capillary refill, altered sensation or motion. They should be instructed to return to the ED or to contact their orthopedist if these signs develop.

Parents and caretakers also need to be aware that activities of daily living may require varying amounts of assistance depending on the age of the child and the limb that is placed in a cast. Diversional activities, especially for a younger child, may require some creativity. For example a child who is unable to draw or paint or play computer games may be entertained by a modification of the game of 20 questions, such as "I'm thinking of a word that begins with B." These are the times when all of a parent's talents are required.

Follow-up care with an orthopedic specialist is necessary to assure optimal healing and return of function. A cast check may be necessary in 24 hours. The parents should be given the phone number of the ED or orthopedist.

REFERENCES

Hammer SJ (1992). Conscious sedation for infants and children in the emergency department. *Journal of Emergency Nursing* 18:165–167

Mayeda DV (1990). Orthopedic injuries. In Barkin RM, Rosen P (eds), *Emergency pediatrics: A guide to ambulatory care.* St. Louis: Mosby, pp 418–449

Miller R, Leno T (1991). Advances in pediatric emergency department procedures. *Emergency Medicine Clinics of North America* 9:639–653

SUGGESTED READING

Altieri M, Bogema S, Schwartz RH (1990). TAC topical anesthesia produces positive urine tests for cocaine. *Annals of Emergency Medicine* 19:577–579

Bachman D, Santora S (1993). Orthopedic trauma. In Fleisher G, Ludwig S (eds), *Textbook of emergency medicine.* Baltimore: Williams & Wilkins, pp 1236–1287

Fitzmaurice LS, Wasserman GS, Knapp JF, Roberts DK, Waecherie JF, Fox M (1990). TAC use and absorption of cocaine in a pediatric emergency department. *Annals of Emergency Medicine* 19:515–518

Gahagan S, Rimsza ME (1991). Child abuse or osteogenesis imperfecta: How can we tell? *Pediatrics* 88:987–992

Gamis AS, Knapp JF, Glenski JA (1989). Nitrous oxide analgesia in a pediatric emergency department. *Annals of Emergency Medicine* 18:177–181

Hennes HM, Wagner V, Bonadio V, et al (1990). The effect of oral midazolam on anxiety of preschool children during laceration repair. *Annals of Emergency Medicine* 19:1006–1009

Mellick L, Ressor K (1990). Spiral tibial fractures of children: A commonly accidental spiral long bone fracture. *American Journal of Emergency Medicine* 8:234–237

Ogden JA (1991). Skeletal trauma. In Grossman M, Dieckmann RA (eds), *Emergency medicine.* Philadelphia: Lippincott, p 289

Ramoska EA, Linkenheimer R, Glasgow C (1991). Midazolam use in the emergency department. *Journal of Emergency Medicine* 9:247–251

Terndrup TE, Dire DJ, Madden CM, Davis H, Cantor RM, Gavula DP (1991). A prospective analysis of intramuscular meperidine, promethazine, and chlorpromazine in pediatric emergency department patients. *Annals of Emergency Medicine* 20:31–35

Thomas SA, Rosenfield NS, Leventhal JM, Markowitz RI (1991). Long-bone fractures in young children: Distinguishing accidental injuries from child abuse. *Pediatrics* 88:471–476

Wright SW (1992). Conscious sedation in the emergency department: The value of capnography and pulse oximetry. *Annals of Emergency Medicine* 21:551–555

CHAPTER 20

Ophthalmic Emergencies

BETH S. NACHTSHEIM

INTRODUCTION

Seventy thousand children younger than 15 years are treated annually in the United States for ophthalmic injuries (Levin, 1991). When other children with eye-related complaints are added to this group, it becomes apparent that pediatric ophthalmic problems are commonly seen in emergency departments (EDs). Staff in these departments are typically not ophthalmologists; thus initial assessment and intervention depend on pediatricians and emergency physicians. It is imperative, therefore, that ED staff be trained to care for common pediatric eye problems and know when referral to an ophthalmologist is warranted.

GENERAL HISTORY

Chemical injuries to the eye are usually considered to be the only truly emergent ophthalmic problems requiring immediate intervention. With most other problems, there is time for a thorough history and physical examination. In many instances, the child's eye problem may be concurrent with other systemic or traumatic processes; consequently, the importance of a thorough assessment cannot be minimized. When other systems have been affected, as in central nervous system trauma, eye problems are usually evaluated only after life-saving measures have been instituted.

The history should be complete and should include chronic illnesses, previous ocular problems, allergies, immunization status, and recent medications. When applicable, the child's normal visual acuity should be noted. Although it is not common, some

small children do wear corrective lenses. The mechanism of injury in traumatic insults should be evaluated. The nurse should keep a high level of suspicion because not all injuries are readily apparent.

GENERAL ASSESSMENT

Ophthalmic problems may produce tremendous anxiety, not only for the child but also for the caretakers. If possible, parents should be encouraged to assist with the examination. To minimize stress, all equipment and personnel needed should be assembled before the examination is begun. Table 20–1 lists supplies frequently stocked in EDs for this purpose.

The initial assessment may be done with the child in the caretaker's lap. This offers the child support and security. If the child remains fearful, toys can be used to provide distraction. Initially it is best to assess children without touching them. The external ocular area

TABLE 20–1. SUGGESTED EMERGENCY DEPARTMENT OPHTHALMIC SUPPLIES

Eye pads	Artificial tears
Protective metal eye shields	Topical anesthetic agents
Morgan therapeutic eye lens	Tetracaine 0.5%, 1%
Eye charts	Proparacaine 0.5%
Wood lamp	Mydriatic agents
Slit lamp	Phenylephrine 2.5%
Nonsterile examination gloves	Tropicamide 1%
Protective eye wear	Cycloplegic agents
Nitrazine paper	Cyclopentolate 0.5, 1%
Fluorescein	

is examined first. The lid margins, lashes, and symmetry are evaluated. If lacerations are present, their location is noted for the presence of canalicular involvement (Figure 20–1). The conjunctiva is inspected and the presence and character of any drainage are noted. Ocular motility should be described. Toys may prove useful in measuring the child's ability to follow objects.

The second part of the ocular assessment is to examine the child's level of vision. If the child has corrective lenses, they should be worn during the visual examination. If the lenses are not available, several holes can be placed closely together in a piece of cardboard with an 18-gauge needle. Visual acuity is then measured as the child looks through these holes. If the child's visual level is improved with the piece of cardboard, visual impairment is most likely due to a refractive error (Levin, 1991).

Each eye should be examined separately. Vision in the opposite eye is completely occluded with an eye patch and tape. There are several different eye charts available for young children (Figure 20–2). The tumbling E chart can be used successfully with children about 5 years of age. Charts with toys and figures may be used for those who are younger or developmentally delayed. It can be helpful to have the child identify the toys and figures on the chart (Figure 20–3) in advance so he or she is not confused naming the pictures during the examination. Identification starts at the bottom of the chart. Most children have short attention spans, so it is best not to waste time having them identify the largest lines. If the use of any chart is precluded by the child's condition, fingers or other objects may be used instead to test vision. Documentation of the findings

should be specific, for example, "the child read one inch lettering at 18 inches," or "the child recognized 2 fingers at 2 feet." Acceptable vision in children varies with age, ranging from 20/40–50 for a 3-year-old to 20/20–30 for a 5-year-old (Sprague, 1990).

Next, pupillary responses are tested. Pupillary size should be the same in each eye despite the level of ambient light. Twenty-five percent of the population has anisocoria (unequal pupils); therefore, unless the pupillary response is more pronounced in dim, rather than bright light, the inequality can be considered a normal physiologic variation (Nelson, 1984). The pupillary reactions are documented in millimeters so that other staff will have objective numbers with which to compare future responses.

For a physician to examine the internal globe, pupillary dilation is usually required. Mydriatic or cycloplegic agents may be used for this purpose. The lowest strength solution available should be used because excessive doses may cause central nervous system stimulation (Sprague, 1990). Mydriatic agents may cause hypertension in low-birth-weight infants (Nelson, 1984); consequently, cycloplegic agents are recommended for this group. Dark brown irises may require two doses or a greater strength solution to produce dilation. Longer-acting dilating agents, such as atropine, usually have no use in the ED. Two drops of the dilating solution are placed in the lower conjunctival pocket. Universal precautions should be followed when the mucous membranes are touched. Twenty to thirty minutes should elapse for the best results before the examination is continued.

The final part of a thorough examination is to palpate the orbital rim. This step is performed last

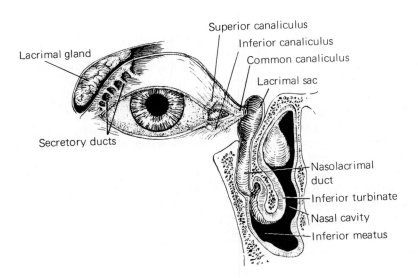

Figure 20–1. The lacrimal system.

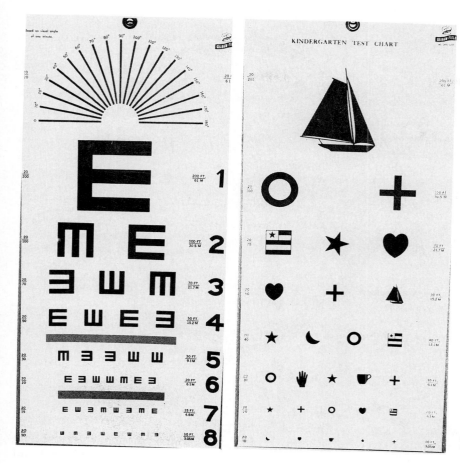

Figure 20–2. Sample eye charts. **A.** Tumbling E eye chart. **B.** Toys and figures chart. (Kindergarten Test Chart by Graham-Field, New York, NY)

because it may be upsetting or painful for the child. Any bony abnormalities are documented.

Some EDs have slit lamps. Trained physicians use these to perform thorough examinations of the cornea in cooperative children.

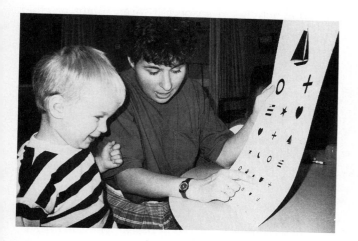

Figure 20–3. Child identifying toys and figures on chart before visual examination.

CONJUNCTIVITIS

Conjunctivitis is the most common ophthalmic problem in children and frequently requires treatment in the ED.

Etiology and Pathophysiology

The conjunctiva is a mucous membrane composed of a thin transparent layer of epithelial cells (Figure 20–4). It lines the inner eyelid and covers the entire eyeball except the cornea. Conjunctivitis is an inflammatory process that affects the conjunctiva; it may be caused by toxins, allergens, viruses, or bacteria. The problem is usually self-limiting and is easily treated.

Exposure of the conjunctiva to chemical irritants may result in the development of a toxic conjunctivitis. Allergic reactions frequently occur during the spring and summer from environmental agents such as molds and pollens. The most common viral conjunctivitis is caused by the adenovirus and usually follows an upper respiratory infection. In a neonate, bacteria, such as *Chlamydia* and *Neisseria gonorrhoeae*, may cause conjunctivitis as well as concurrent severe systemic dis-

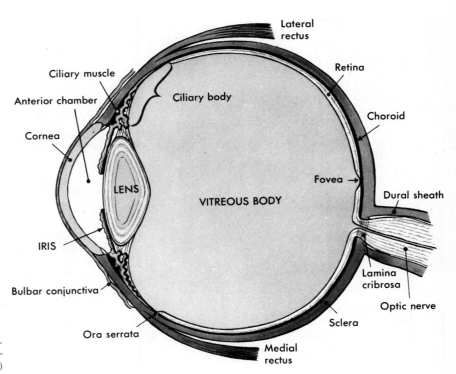

Figure 20–4. The eye cut in horizontal section. (From Stein HA, Slatt BJ, Stein RM [1987]. *Ophthalmic terminology* [2nd ed] St Louis: Mosby.)

ease. Organisms that cause conjunctivitis in older children include *Haemophilus influenzae, Staphylococcus aureus,* and *Streptococcus pneumoniae;* they usually produce only localized infections (Good, 1991).

Nonbacterial conjunctivitis can become superinfected at any time, particularly if frequent eye rubbing occurs.

History

Toxic conjunctivitis should be suspected anytime a child has watery eye drainage and there has been chemical irritation of the eye. It may be seen in a 2-day old infant after the instillation of silver nitrate eye drops. Allergic reactions may present similarly to toxic conjunctivitis, although a history of chemical exposure is lacking. Viral conjunctivitis is very contagious; hence, a history that reveals several affected family members or an upper respiratory infection is helpful in establishing the diagnosis.

As previously stated, the bacterial infections in older children are frequently localized. The history usually includes awakening with the eyelids of one or both eyes adhered with dried grainy crusts. However, when these symptoms first appear on the third day of life, the more serious infections of *N. gonorrhoeae* and *Chlamydia* are part of the differential diagnosis. Family members may deny, or be unaware of, any history of sexually transmitted diseases.

Physical Assessment

Either toxic or allergic conjunctivitis may present with a watery discharge. The conjunctiva is inflamed and chemotic. Viral and bacterial infections usually manifest a more purulent yellow drainage. If the infection is systemic, as in *N. gonorrhoeae,* other symptoms may be present, such as temperature instability, irritability, and altered feeding behavior.

Laboratory and Diagnostic Tests

Cultures of eye drainage may be acquired when bacterial conjunctivitis is suspected in an infant or child; they are mandatory for neonates. Because the conjunctivitis may represent only one part of a systemic infection, newborn infants usually require further diagnostic procedures such as a lumbar puncture, a complete blood count (CBC), and blood cultures to determine the extent of the disease process.

T R I A G E
Conjunctivitis

Urgent ─────────────────────
A newborn with *N. gonorrhoeae* or *Chlamydia* infection.

Nursing Diagnosis
Impaired Tissue Integrity

Defining Characteristics

- Disruption of mucous membrane tissue
- Erythema
- Edema

Nursing Interventions

- Administer medication as ordered
- Apply dressing as ordered
- Use good hand-washing technique

Expected Outcomes

- Infection is eliminated
- Erythema and edema are reduced
- Nosocomial transmission of infection is prevented

Nursing Diagnosis
Knowledge Deficit (Conjunctivitis)

Defining Characteristics

- Verbalization of a deficiency in knowledge related to management of conjunctivitis
- Incorrect administration of ophthalmic medication

Nursing Interventions

- Assist family in understanding their child's type of conjunctivitis and mode of transmission
- Explain proper administration and schedule for medication

Expected Outcomes

- Parents verbalize methods to prevent transmission of conjunctivitis to other family members
- Parents demonstrate proper administration of medication and verbalize accurate schedule for medications (Carpenito, 1991)

Management
Children with toxic, allergic, or viral conjunctivitis may benefit initially from cold compresses on their eyes to reduce edema. Warm compresses may be soothing after 24 hours. Universal precautions should be followed when touching the mucous membranes. Treatment of bacterial conjunctivitis varies according to the causative organism. Infants with chlamydial or gonorrheal infections may require hospitalization and intravenous antibiotics. Deutsch (1990) suggests erythromycin ointment for general use on bacterial conjunctivitis because as many as one-third of children are sensitive to neomycin. Corticosteroids should be avoided for all types of conjunctivitis because they retard healing (Levin, 1991). An eye patch is applied if ordered. If there has been no improvement after 36–48 hours a consultation with an ophthalmologist is warranted.

Patient and Family Teaching and Psychosocial Support
Parents should be reminded that conjunctivitis is usually a self-limited and easily treated infection and that good hand washing is mandatory to prevent infection of the entire household if the conjunctivitis is viral or bacterial.

PERIORBITAL AND ORBITAL CELLULITIS

Periorbital cellulitis is more common and usually less serious than orbital cellulitis (Grossman, 1991). It is very important to determine which form of cellulitis the child has because management and patient outcome may differ.

Etiology and Pathophysiology
Periorbital cellulitis involves the facial tissues anterior to the orbital septum. The most common causes of either infection are a penetrating injury to the facial soft tissues, sinus infection, or dental disease (Deutsch, 1990). Factors influencing these causes are the proximity of the paranasal sinuses to the orbit, absence of a lymphatic drainage system, profuse venous connections, and relatively thin skin that surrounds the eye. A systemic or intracranial infection can occur with either type of cellulitis. These children can appear quite ill. *H. influenzae* is responsible for many non-traumatic infections in nonimmunized children younger than 5 years. When the infection follows an injury, *S. aureus* is frequently the causative agent.

History
Periorbital infections are often unilateral. When the orbit is the site of infection, however, there may be pain and loss of vision. Fever usually presents with either infection.

Physical Assessment

Periorbital infections can present with considerable lid and facial swelling. There may be chemosis and purulent drainage. In addition, orbital infections often cause decreased ocular motility, proptosis, and an abnormal pupil response.

Laboratory and Diagnostic Tests

To determine the level of systemic or intracranial involvement, tests such as a CBC, blood culture, computed tomography (CT), and lumbar puncture may be performed.

T R I A G E
Periorbital and Orbital Cellulitis

Urgent
An infant or child with appreciable lid and facial swelling.

Nursing Diagnosis

Sensory/Perceptual Attentions (Visual)

Defining Characteristics

- Negative change in amount or pattern of incoming stimuli
- Disorientation about people
- Fear

Nursing Interventions

- Attempt to reduce fears and concerns by explaining equipment, its purpose, and noises
- Allow family to provide comfort and support throughout examinations and procedures

Expected Outcomes

- Child verbalizes understanding of surroundings.
- Child remains calm

Nursing Diagnosis

Pain

Defining Characteristics

- Report or demonstration of discomfort
- Crying, moaning
- Facial mask of pain

Nursing Interventions

- Discuss with the child and family the therapeutic uses of distraction
- Teach noninvasive pain relief measures such as relaxation
- Administer medications as ordered

Expected Outcomes

- Child verbalizes elimination of discomfort
- Child is quiet, relaxed
- Facial grimacing stops (Carpenito, 1991)

Management

The treatment of periorbital cellulitis with IV antibiotic therapy is controversial (Levin, 1991). Oral antibiotics may be given to children who do not appear to have systemic disease; however, these children should be re-evaluated in 24 hours. If the infection has not subsided, the child should be hospitalized and given intravenous antibiotics. Ill-appearing children, and all infants, with periorbital or orbital infections require hospitalization. A consultation with an ophthalmologist is suggested for any child whose orbital infection is not responsive to intravenous antibiotics.

Patient and Family Teaching and Psychosocial Support

Facial swelling, proptosis, and irritability from pain can be very distressing for the family. In addition, they may have concerns regarding disfiguration and permanency of vision loss. The nurse should review the etiology, nursing interventions, and expected outcomes of the care with the family. Offering comfort and support, and encouraging the family to do the same for the child, may ease the family's distress. The nurse assists the family in providing pain relief and teaches them relaxation and distraction techniques to use with the child.

CORNEAL ABRASIONS

A corneal abrasion occurs when the top epithelial layer of the cornea is abraded or eroded. It is frequently associated with blurred vision and pain, causing a great deal of anxiety for children and families when they appear in the ED.

Etiology and Pathophysiology

The most common causes of corneal abrasions are fingernail scratches, playground dirt, sticks, sharp toys, and cigarette burns. Contact lenses produce fewer abrasions in children than they do in adults, because children are less likely to wear them. The cornea is covered by a thin, transparent layer of epithelial cells. This tissue has a very rich sensory nerve supply. When the cornea is damaged, pain, photophobia, and production of tears are common. Ciliary spasm (see Figure 20–4) may contribute to the photophobia and pain the child experiences.

History

Because so many corneal abrasions are caused by foreign bodies, any such history should be documented. It should be noted if the foreign body is made of wood, because unremoved wooden objects are associated with the development of fungal infections (Deutsch, 1990).

Physical Assessment

Children with corneal abrasions may present with excessive production of tears, blepharospasm, photophobia, pain, and blurred vision. Application of a topical anesthetic usually provides immediate pain relief and allows for a thorough examination. When ciliary spasm is the cause of the child's pain, topical anesthetic agents do not provide relief, and the affected pupil may react to light sluggishly (Nelson, 1985).

If a foreign body is suspected, the physician carefully searches the child's eye. Frequently, foreign bodies are found under the upper eyelid. Eversion of the lid is easily accomplished by the ED physician (Figure 20–5).

Laboratory and Diagnostic Tests

The eye should be examined with fluorescein and a cobalt blue light or Wood lamp. Fluorescein dye is applied from an impregnated strip that has been moistened with a sterile eye-wetting solution. Several drops of the dye should be allowed to accumulate in the lower conjunctival pocket, then the child is allowed to blink. The epithelium is hydrophilic and repels the fluorescein. Exposed subepithelial tissue stains a brilliant green. Visibility of the defect caused by an abrasion is enhanced with the use of a Wood lamp.

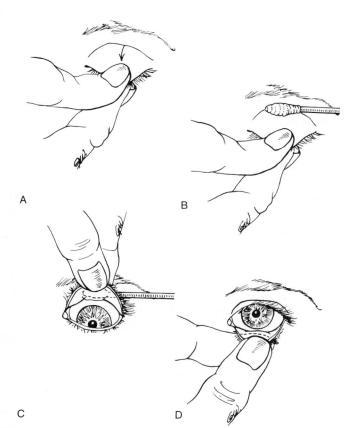

Figure 20–5. Four steps to eyelid eversion. **A.** Draw eyelid down. **B.** Place a clean cotton swab across the superior tarsal margin. **C.** In one motion, pull the swab slightly downward and pull the eyelid slightly upward. **D.** Place finger at base of lower lid and gently retract it in a caudal and posterior direction while the child looks up.

T R I A G E
Corneal Abrasions

Emergent
A child with severe pain; blurred vision; foreign body.

Urgent
A child with mild to moderate pain; intact vision; no history of foreign body.

Nursing Diagnosis
Impaired Tissue Integrity

Defining Characteristic

* Disruption of corneal tissue

Nursing Interventions

* Administer medications as ordered
* Apply eye pads as ordered
* Provide family information and support to reduce anxiety

Expected Outcomes

* Abrasion resolves

- There is no delayed wound healing from bacterial super-infections or repetitive blinking
- Family remains calm

Nursing Diagnosis
Pain

Defining Characteristics
- Report or demonstration of discomfort
- Crying, moaning
- Facial mask of pain

Nursing Interventions
- Administer medications as ordered
- Teach noninvasive pain relief measures such as relaxation
- Discuss with the child and family the therapeutic uses of distraction

Expected Outcomes
- Child verbalizes elimination of discomfort
- Child is quiet, relaxed
- Facial grimacing stops (Carpenito, 1991)

Management
The epithelial tissue of the cornea heals very rapidly, usually within 2–3 days. Although topical anesthetic agents are helpful during the examination, their continued use at home to reduce pain is not advised because they may retard re-epithelialization (Nelson, 1985). As in conjunctivitis, antibiotic ointment or drops are frequently prescribed. They provide lubrication and a prophylaxis for bacterial infection. When a painful ciliary spasm is present, a cycloplegic agent may be ordered.

A pressure eye patch should be applied for at least the first 24 hours to prevent repeated blinking, which delays wound healing. One or two eye pads are folded and placed over the closed affected eye. A third pad is then placed over the eye and two pieces of tape are applied (Figure 20–6). Children younger than 1 year are prone to amblyopia from prolonged eye patching; therefore, pads should be removed within 24 hours (Levin, 1991). An ophthalmologist is consulted whenever the corneal abrasion is extensive, caused by contact lenses, or not improving within 24 hours (Levin, 1991).

Patient and Family Teaching and Psychosocial Support
Corneal abrasions are easily treated and heal quickly; however, families can become very distressed when their children complain of blurred vision or pain. The nurse provides information and support, assists the

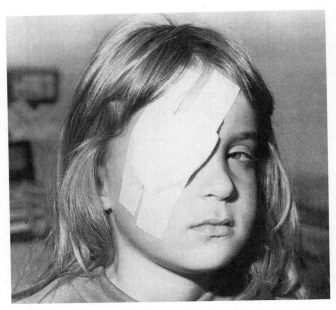

Figure 20–6. Proper eye patching technique.

family with pain relief, and teaches the family relaxation and distraction techniques to use with the child. The family is allowed to view the fluorescin-stained abrasion because this helps them to better understand the child's condition and care. The family is taught how to administer any ordered ophthalmic medications and to apply eye patches.

CHEMICAL INJURIES

Chemical injuries to the eye are usually considered to be the only truly emergent ophthalmic injuries; they require immediate intervention.

Etiology and Pathophysiology
Alkali solutions quickly penetrate ophthalmic tissues and can produce severe burns. Acidic solutions, although caustic to epithelial tissues, usually do not produce such severe burns. Household cleaning solutions, automotive lubricants, and house and garden products are among the most common caustic agents causing ophthalmic injuries in children.

History
Parents usually have a high index of suspicion regarding what chemical their child has been exposed to and may bring the agent with them to the ED.

Physical Assessment
Children may present with blepharospasm, tearing, chemosis, and pain.

Laboratory and Diagnostic Tests

Irrigation of the affected eye must not be delayed. Vision tests and pH testing of ophthalmic secretions should be performed after the irrigation.

TRIAGE
Chemical Injuries

Emergent —————————————————
An infant or child with ophthalmic chemical exposure.

Nursing Diagnosis
Sensory/Perceptual Alterations (Visual)

Defining Characteristics

- Negative change in amount or pattern of incoming stimuli.
- Disorientation about people
- Fear

Nursing Interventions

- Attempt to reduce fears and concerns by explaining equipment, its purpose, and noises
- Allow family to provide comfort and support throughout examinations and procedures

Expected Outcomes

- Child verbalizes understanding of surroundings
- Child remains calm

Nursing Diagnosis
Pain

Defining Characteristics

- Report or demonstration of discomfort
- Crying, moaning
- Facial mask of pain

Nursing Interventions

- Administer medications as ordered
- Discuss the therapeutic uses of distraction

Expected Outcomes

- Child is quiet, relaxed
- Child verbalizes elimination of discomfort
- Facial grimacing stops (Carpenito, 1991)

Management

Irrigation of the affected eye should be performed immediately, and both eyes should be flushed if there is any doubt regarding the extent of the exposure. Irrigation should be attempted before arrival at the ED. A child can be placed in the bathtub or sink; tepid tap water should then be run over the eyes for 10–15 minutes. Ideally the water should contact the medial portion of the eye and run out the lateral side so that the caustic agent is flushed away; this can be difficult to accomplish with a writhing toddler.

Once the child is in the ED a more thorough irrigation can be performed with a Morgan Therapeutic Eye Lens (Figure 20–7). Universal precautions are followed. This device allows for thorough flushing of the conjunctival pockets and fits most children, although open-ended macrodrip IV tubing may be used. It is often helpful to administer a topical anesthetic agent before inserting the eye lens. Each eye needs to be flushed with at least 2 L of normal saline solution over 20 minutes. After irrigation, ophthalmic secretions are tested with nitrazine paper. The ophthalmic pH should be between 6.5 and 7.5 (Levin, 1991), and irrigations should be continued until this range has been reached. An ophthalmologist should always examine a patient who has had an ophthalmic chemical exposure.

Patient and Family Teaching and Psychosocial Support

Permanent eye damage is every parent's worst fear after chemical exposure, and ophthalmic irrigations are initiated quickly, often before any explanation can be offered to the family. During the eye flush, however, time can be taken to discuss with family members the equipment used and the plan for care of chemical injuries. Caregivers may need to be taught about administration of medication and eye patching. The nurse assists the family in providing pain relief. The family is taught relaxation and distraction techniques to use with the child. Safety and accident prevention information is offered as well.

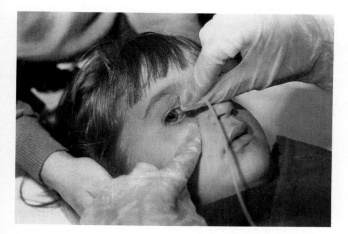

Figure 20–7. Insertion of a Morgan therapeutic eye lens.

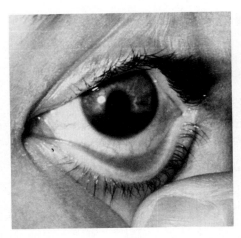

Figure 20–8. Hyphema. Note the presence of blood in the anterior chamber.

HYPHEMA

A hyphema is caused by bleeding that has taken place in the anterior chamber of the eye (see Figure 20–4). The size of the hyphema may range from large and grossly obvious (Figure 20–8) to microscopic, requiring a slit lamp for visualization.

Etiology and Pathophysiology
Most hyphemas are caused by blunt trauma to the eye. Less commonly, they follow a penetrating eye injury. There may be concurrent facial, ophthalmic, or head injuries. Secondary damage from rebleeding 3–5 days after the initial injury may worsen the visual prognosis. The actual bleeding occurs from a torn iris root or ciliary body. When blood accumulates in the anterior chamber, intraocular pressure increases, which may impede the drainage of normal aqueous fluid.

History
The history should include the circumstances surrounding the injury and if there was a loss of consciousness or vision. Head injuries are frequently associated with hyphemas. Suspicions may arise regarding child abuse. Decreased ocular motility may indicate an orbital fracture. Pre-existing hemoglobinopathies or bleeding disorders can impede a full visual recovery.

Physical Assessment
The child may have mild pain, tearing, lid swelling, ecchymosis, headache, vomiting, or decreased visual acuity.

Laboratory and Diagnostic Tests
A thorough examination, including a vision test, should be performed by an ophthalmologist. If the hyphema is suspected, but not obvious, the use of a slit lamp is required. The internal globe is examined for any signs of injury. X rays and CT may be helpful in determining the extent of the injury.

T R I A G E
Hyphema

Emergent —————————————————
An infant or child with signs of blunt trauma to eye.

Nursing Diagnosis
Pain

Defining Characteristics
- Report or demonstration of discomfort
- Crying, moaning

Nursing Interventions
- Administer medication as ordered
- Teach noninvasive pain relief measures such as relaxation
- Discuss with family the therapeutic uses of nonvisual distraction, such as music

Expected Outcomes
- Child verbalizes elimination of discomfort
- Child is quiet, relaxed

Nursing Diagnosis
Fear

Defining Characteristic
- Feelings of dread, fright, apprehension related to risk for loss of vision

Nursing Interventions
- Accept child's and family's fear; provide explanations; share with child and family that it is acceptable to have these fears
- Speak slowly and calmly when discussing care outcomes with the child and family
- Provide an emotionally nonthreatening atmosphere

Expected Outcomes
- Child and family discuss fears
- Child is quiet, relaxed (Carpenito, 1991)

Management

All patients with hyphemas (known or suspected) should be examined by an ophthalmologist. Management, however, is controversial. Levin (1991) supports rest and avoidance of valsalva maneuvers for 3–5 days even if sedation is required. Deutsch (1990) reports that quiet activity should be allowed with a protective eye shield in place and that bilateral eye patching and sedation are unnecessary. Cyclopegic agents may be prescribed to relieve ciliary spasm. To reduce intraocular pressure, the head of the child's bed should be elevated. The nurse should speak slowly and provide a calm, relaxing environment.

Patient and Family Teaching and Psychosocial Support

Providing information and support to the family is imperative because the visual prognosis is uncertain at the time of the injury. The child and family should be allowed to voice concerns regarding reduced activity and eye patching. The family should be assisted in distracting and entertaining the child while in the ED.

FRACTURES OF THE ORBITAL WALL

Orbital fractures occur when a blunt force to the eye produces increased intraorbital pressure (Figure 20–9) with resultant damage to the bony structures. The medial wall and orbital floor are the weakest bones and are most easily damaged (Nelson, 1985). Close by are nerves and the vascular supply. Concurrent globe and head injuries are common and must not be overlooked.

History

As with hyphemas, the history should include the circumstances surrounding the injury. Concurrent head trauma is not uncommon.

Physical Assessment

Soft tissue damage may present as lid swelling or ecchymosis. Subcutaneous emphysema may occur. Because orbital contents, especially inferior rectus muscle and fat, may become entrapped in the fractured bone, extraocular motility should be assessed (Figure 20–10).

Laboratory and Diagnostic Tests

X rays and CT may be helpful in determining the extent of the injury.

TRIAGE
Fractures of the Orbital Wall

Emergent ————————————————————
A child with severe pain, blurred vision, foreign body, or blunt eye trauma.

Nursing Diagnosis
Pain

Defining Characteristics

- Report or demonstration of discomfort
- Crying, moaning
- Facial mask of pain

Nursing Interventions

- Discuss with the child and family the therapeutic uses of distraction
- Teach noninvasive pain relief measures such as relaxation
- Administer medications as ordered

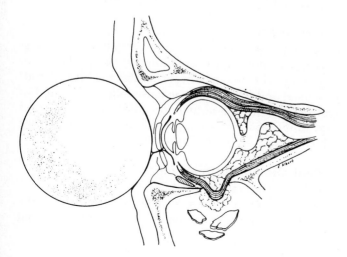

Figure 20–9. Fracture of the orbital floor with incarceration of inferior rectus muscle. (From Mayer T [1985]. *Emergency management of pediatric trauma.* Philadelphia: Saunders, p 304.)

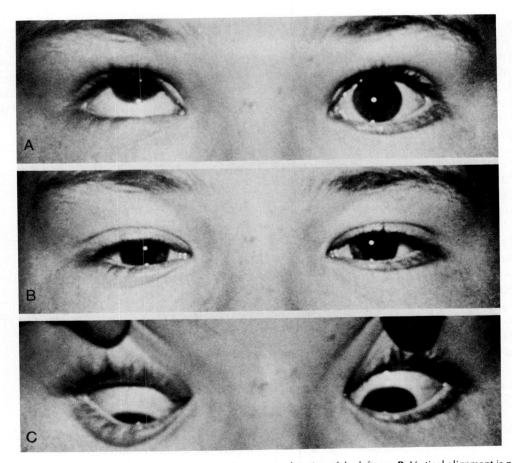

Figure 20–10. A. Entrapment of the inferior rectus muscle prevents elevation of the left eye. **B.** Vertical alignment is normal in primary gaze. **C.** Contusion injury to the inferior rectus muscle also prevents full depression of the left eye. (From Mayer T [1985]. *Emergency management of pediatric trauma.* Philadelphia: Saunders, p 350.)

Expected Outcomes

- Child verbalizes elimination of discomfort
- Child is quiet, relaxed
- Facial grimacing stops

Nursing Diagnosis
Body Image Disturbance

Defining Characteristic

- Verbal or nonverbal negative response to actual or perceived change in structure or function

Nursing Interventions

- Encourage child to express feelings, especially about the way he or she feels, thinks, or views self
- Encourage child and family to ask questions about health problems, treatment, progress, prognosis

Expected Outcomes

- Child verbalizes feelings about self
- Child asks questions and shows interest in plan of care and progress (Carpenito, 1991)

Management
All children who sustain blunt trauma to the eye must undergo a thorough evaluation by an ophthalmologist. Surgical management for orbital fractures is controversial and if necessary usually follows a period of rest that allows for reduction of edema. This period may range from 7 to 10 days if there are no concurrent injuries requiring more aggressive care.

Patient and Family Teaching and Psychosocial Support
When the inferior rectus muscle is entrapped by the orbital floor, families can become very disturbed that

their child will have a permanent facial deformity. The nurse provides support and comfort to the family. They should be allowed to voice their concerns. The nurse discusses with the family the plan of care and how the family can assist in keeping the child calm.

EYELID LACERATIONS

Minor lacerations of the eyelids usually do not require consultation with an ophthalmologist unless there is involvement of the canalicular system (see Figure 20–1). Concurrent injuries such as global penetration may be present and must not be overlooked.

Etiology and Pathophysiology
The eyelids provide protection to the globe by lubricating it and serving as a barrier to foreign substances. The lacrimal glands located under the upper lateral lids provide the lubrication for the eyelids to spread during blinking. Injury to any part of this system may affect the globe; small puncture wounds may even extend to the cranial vault.

History
The history should include a description of the mechanism of injury. The potential for penetrating trauma or foreign bodies should be noted.

Physical Assessment
Bleeding may need to be controlled, however, judicial use of direct pressure is recommended until the extent of the injury is known. Sedation or restraint may be required to complete a thorough examination. For puncture wounds to the eyelids, eversion of the lid should be performed (see Figure 20–5) to determine wound depth. The internal globe should be examined if the lid has been penetrated.

Laboratory and Diagnostic Tests
For lacerations in the area of the canalicular system, probing of the wound by an ophthalmologist is usually necessary to assure ductal integrity.

TRIAGE
Eyelid Lacerations

Emergent ─────────────────────────
An infant or child with significant eyelid lacerations or puncture wounds of the surrounding area.

Urgent ─────────────────────────
An infant or child with minor, superficial lacerations to outer eyelids or surrounding area. No history of penetrating object or foreign body.

Nursing Diagnosis
Body Image Disturbance

Defining Characteristic
- Verbal or nonverbal negative response to actual or perceived change in structure or function

Nursing Interventions
- Encourage child to express feelings, especially about the way he or she feels, thinks, or views self
- Encourage child and family to ask questions about health problems, treatment, progress, prognosis

Expected Outcomes
- Child verbalizes feelings about self
- Child asks questions, shows interest in plan of care and progress

Nursing Diagnosis
Fear

Defining Characteristic
- Feelings of dread, fright, apprehension related to risk for disfigurement

Nursing Interventions
- Accept child's and family's fear; provide explanations; share with child and family that it is acceptable to have these fears
- Speak slowly and calmly when discussing care outcomes with child and family

Expected Outcomes
- Child and family discuss fears
- Child is quiet, relaxed (Carpenito, 1991)

Management
Small, superficial lacerations can usually be treated readily by ED personnel. Canalicular trauma, puncture wounds, and lacerations involving the lid margin should be evaluated by an ophthalmologist. Lacerations of the lid margin require meticulous attention for adequate repair to the gray line, where conjunctiva

and skin meet, in order to prevent disfigurement (Nelson, 1985). Canalicular trauma may require surgical repair if the integrity of the system has been compromised.

Patient and Family Teaching and Psychosocial Support

Families find even minor lacerations near the eye to be very distressing—they worry about the risk for visual damage and disfigurement. Parents should be reminded that most of these lacerations are repaired easily by ED staff. When injuries are severe, the family is offered information as it becomes available regarding the ophthalmologic evaluation and planned interventions. They should be allowed to express their feelings. The nurse provides the family with comfort and support and encourages them to do the same for the child.

PENETRATING EYE INJURIES

Penetrating eye injuries may occur from relatively small projectiles that enter the globe with great velocity or by larger objects such as pencils, knives, car antennae, and sticks.

Etiology and Pathophysiology

Unless the foreign object is large and protruding from the eye, as with a pencil, it may not be readily apparent that the child has a penetrating eye injury. The epithelial tissues of the cornea repair themselves quickly and can make small puncture wounds to the globe appear nearly invisible. Metal pieces may leave a small rust ring that becomes visible over time at the entry site, and wooden objects may cause fungal infections. Most foreign bodies, however, are inert and may display no telltale signs of their presence (Nelson, 1985).

History

As previously stated, global penetration is obvious when objects protrude from the eye; however, the ED staff must seriously consider that ophthalmic disruption may have occurred after contact with any foreign body. There may be concurrent corneal abrasions, lid lacerations, or head injuries, which must be evaluated and treated.

Physical Assessment

Children can present with pain, tearing, conjunctival inflammation, and visual loss. At times, the foreign body is easily visualized or even protrudes from the eye; however, it may be imbedded in the cornea or located intraocularly.

Laboratory and Diagnostic Tests

A history of penetration requires a consultation with an ophthalmologist, even if no visible signs are present. Topical anesthetic agents may ease the examination, as may pupil dilation. X rays and CT may be helpful in determining the extent of the injury.

T R I A G E
Penetrating Eye Trauma

Emergent ————————————————————————
A child with penetrating eye trauma.

Nursing Diagnosis
Sensory / Perceptual Alteration (Visual)

Defining Characteristics

- Negative change in amount or pattern of incoming stimuli
- Disorientation about people
- Fear

Nursing Interventions

- Attempt to reduce fears and concerns by explaining equipment, its purpose, and noises
- Allow family to provide comfort and support throughout examinations and procedures

Expected Outcomes

- Child verbalizes understanding of surroundings
- Child remains calm

Nursing Diagnosis
Pain

Defining Characteristics

- Report or demonstration of discomfort
- Crying, moaning

Nursing Interventions

- Administer medications as ordered
- Teach noninvasive pain relief measures such as relaxation

Expected Outcomes

- Child verbalizes elimination of discomfort
- Child is quiet, relaxed (Carpenito, 1991)

Management

Once a penetrating eye injury is suspected, the child's head should be kept elevated at least 30°. The child should take nothing by mouth. The child should be protected from dislodging large foreign objects, such as a radio antenna, him- or herself—by immobilization if necessary. Emergency department personnel must never remove imbedded or protruding objects themselves. An ophthalmologist may use x rays, ultrasonography, and CT in addition to direct visualization to determine the extent of injury (Nelson, 1985; Sears, 1990). The visual prognosis may be uncertain while the patient is in the ED. Surgical intervention can be hazardous, but it may be required.

Patient and Family Teaching and Psychosocial Support

Families usually panic at the sight of an object imbedded in their child's eye. They are justifiably worried about permanent loss of vision. They should be allowed to express their fears. Offering comfort and support and encouraging the family to do the same for the child may ease distress. The nurse teaches the family nonpharmacologic pain relief measures and how to administer ordered medications.

REFERENCES

Carpenito L (1991). *Handbook of nursing diagnosis.* Philadelphia: Lippincott

Deutsch T (1990). Ocular emergencies in childhood. *Pediatrician* 17:173–176

Good W (1991). Eye trauma. In Grossman M, Dieckmann R (eds), *Pediatric emergency medicine.* Philadelphia: Lippincott, pp 256–261

Grossman M (1991). Sinusitis and periorbital cellulitis. In Grossman M, Dieckmann R (eds), *Pediatric emergency medicine.* Philadelphia: Lippincott, pp 541–544

Levin A (1991). Eye emergencies: Acute management in the pediatric ambulatory care setting. *Pediatric Emergency Care* 7:367–377

Nelson L (1984). *Pediatric ophthalmology.* Philadelphia: Saunders, pp 42; 231; 236

Nelson L (1985). Eye injuries. In Mayer T (ed), *Emergency management of pediatric trauma.* Philadelphia: Saunders, pp 301–315

Sears M (1990). Eye injuries. In Touloukian R (ed), *Pediatric trauma.* St. Louis: Mosby, pp 246–265

Sprague J (1990). Eye trauma. In Barkin R, Rosen P (eds). *Emergency pediatrics: A guide to ambulatory care.* St. Louis: Mosby, pp 355–360

SUGGESTED READING

Bernardo L, Bove M (1993). *Pediatric emergency procedures.* Boston: Jones and Bartlett

Clark R, Farber J, Sher N (1989). Eye emergencies and urgencies. *Patient Care* 23:24–34

Diamond G (1988). Ophthalmic emergencies. In Fleisher G, Ludwig S (eds), *Textbook of pediatric emergency medicine.* Baltimore: Williams & Wilkins, pp 995–1007

Diamond G (1988). Red eye. In Fleisher G, Ludwig S (eds). *Textbook of pediatric emergency medicine.* Baltimore: Williams & Wilkins, pp 268–271

Poe C (1990). Eye irrigating lens more effective if applied seconds after accident. *Occupational Health and Safety* 59:43–47

Rahman W, O'Connor T (1992). Facial trauma. In Barkin R (eds). *Pediatric emergency medicine.* St. Louis: Mosby Year Book, pp 199–220

Thompson S (1990). Eye injuries. *Emergency care of children.* Boston: Jones and Bartlett

Chapter 21

Burns

WENDY L. DALY
JOAN MEUNIER-SHAM

INTRODUCTION

Approximately 385,000 children 18 years of age and younger sustain burn injuries in the United States each year (Hall, 1992). Thermal injuries have potential life-altering effects related to disfigurement and severe functional disability. Burns of children are most often thermal, such as scalds, contact with a hot object, or exposure to flame. Chemical and electrical injuries occur less often among children, but they are associated with greater morbidity.

Most pediatric burns are minor injuries requiring basic wound care, often on an outpatient basis. Many moderate pediatric burns can be effectively managed in a community hospital, but patients with large or complex injuries require transfer to a specialized burn center. The survival of these patients depends on proper initial management and resuscitation by a coordinated trauma team of emergency care professionals.

THE EPIDEMIOLOGY OF PEDIATRIC BURNS

Burn injuries to children often follow predictive patterns related to the child's developmental level. Most of these injuries occur in or near the home, are unintentional, and are related to lapses in adult attention or supervision (Lindblad and Terkelsen, 1990). However, the emergency department (ED) nurse must be alert to the fact that as many as 10% of child abuse cases involve burns (Bernardo and Sullivan, 1991). Physical findings that are inconsistent with the reported history, delays in seeking medical assistance, and con-

flicting histories should alert the ED staff to the possibility of an inflicted injury (see Chapter 8).

Scalds are the leading cause of burns of infants and young children. Hot liquids that are accidentally spilled on a child are a common cause of burn injury. Microwave preparation of foods has added to the risk of oral scald burns because actual temperature is difficult to judge (Powell and Tanz, 1993). Hot tap water in the bathtub is also a frequent cause of scald burns in infancy and early childhood. Household hot water heaters are often set above the recommended 130°F. At a temperature of 130°F it takes only 10 seconds to cause a full-thickness injury to a young child's skin (Nebraska Burn Institute, 1987).

As children become more mobile and curious, their exposure to household burn hazards expands. Electrical burns can occur by chewing on electrical wires or inserting objects into electric sockets. Contact burns from ovens, hot irons, and radiators become more common.

School-aged children are attracted to match and fire play. Some lighters can be manipulated by children as young as 2 years. Flame burns associated with clothing ignition are often complicated by the melting of synthetic fabrics. Participation in risk-taking behaviors such as cigarette smoking and the handling of flammable liquids contributes to the burn problem for older children. These injuries can have a chemical or inhalation component when gasoline or explosives are involved.

In addition to the child's developmental level, a child's socioeconomic status may place him or her at increased risk for thermal injury. Substandard housing units often lack functioning smoke detectors and escape ladders. Lack of finances to afford heat has caused families to resort to unsafe heat sources such as space heaters, kerosene, and charcoal (Locke et al, 1990).

Burns, like all pediatric injuries, are largely preventable. Emergency department nurses can play an important role in developing educational strategies aimed at children and parents and advocate environmental controls (Erdmann et al, 1991).

GENERAL PATHOPHYSIOLOGY

Burn injuries are caused by the effects of heat on skin. As the largest organ of the body, the skin provides many vital functions, including protection from infection and fluid loss. It has a role in the regulation of body temperature, the sensation of pleasure and pain, and perception of body image. Damage or loss of skin influences each of these functions.

The skin is composed of two layers: the epidermis and the dermis. The outer epidermal layer serves as a barrier to fluids and microorganisms, continually

sloughing its outer layer of dead cells. The epidermal cells are generated here in the stratum germinativum. The inner dermal layer is composed of collagen and fibrous connective tissue, which provides the skin with strength and durability. The dermis contains hair follicles and sweat and sebaceous glands. These appendages are lined with epithelial cells, which can become the source of epithelial regeneration if the entire epidermis is destroyed (Figure 21–1).

Severity and Characteristics of Burn Wound

The severity of a burn injury depends on both the intensity of the heat and the duration of its contact with the skin. The effects of this damage vary with age and the location on the body. That the skin of children is delicate and thin makes children very susceptible to the effects of thermal injury. A large or deep burn is considered multisystem trauma with consequences that extend well beyond the actual burn site.

Deep thermal damage to skin is not uniform. These wounds have three zones, each with unique tissue effects. The surface area, the zone of hyperemia, appears warm and red. The adjacent zone of stasis contains damaged capillaries, which allow fluid to leak

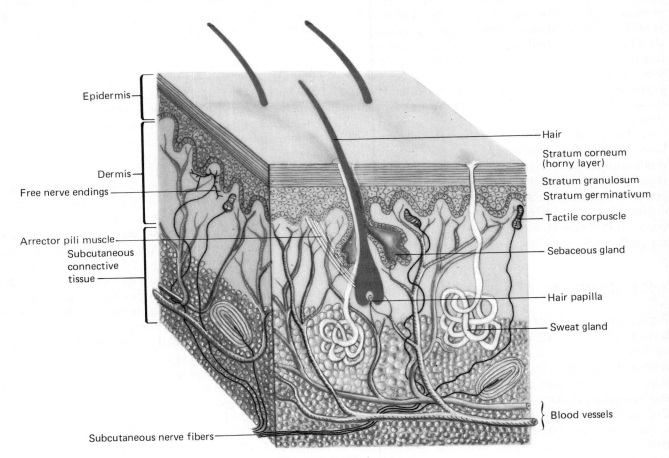

Figure 21–1. Skin layers.

from the vascular system into the interstitial space. There is a resultant local edema and associated burn shock in a large burn injury. The deepest area is the zone of coagulation, where heat-damaged cells occlude the blood vessels. As a result, oxygen, nutrients and the protective components of the immune response are unable to reach the injured tissue.

Depth and Extent of Burn

The depth of a burn wound in skin is described as partial thickness or full thickness. A superficial partial-thickness burn involves only the epidermis. Deep partial-thickness burns involve epidermis and only part of the dermis; there are enough remaining epidermal cells in the lining of the appendages to allow regeneration. In full-thickness burns, the entire epidermis and dermis are destroyed, sometimes extending into the subcutaneous tissues of fat, muscle, and bone. A partial-thickness wound can be converted to a deeper thickness if there is additional tissue destruction from infection, hypoxia, or direct mechanical damage (Table 21–1).

The actual depth of a burn injury can be difficult to determine from inspection of the skin surface alone. Wound appearance, pain, and tissue pliability are used to assess the extent of damage. A thorough injury history, establishing the nature of the burning agent and the extent of exposure, provides additional information on which to base the plan of care. It may take several days for even a skilled clinician to accurately assess burn depth.

The extent of these injuries is also described as the percent of the body surface area (BSA) burned. The Lund and Browder (Figure 21–2) or Berkow chart is used to calculate BSA in children, taking into account the proportional changes that occur during growth. Deep partial- and full-thickness burns are measured as a percent of the whole, and these areas are then com-

bined to determine the total body surface area (TBSA) affected (Table 21–2). This calculation provides a consistent reference for communication among the burn care team. It is important in the calculation of fluid resuscitation needs.

Accurate assessment of the depth and extent of the burn is pivotal in the selection of a treatment plan. The effects of thermal injury may be limited to the local area only and may heal spontaneously with minimal intervention. Patients with large burns, those with a respiratory component, or with burns involving the face, hands, feet, or perineum require ongoing assessment and specialized burn care.

Local and Systemic Effects of Burn Injury

The impact of a burn injury can range from a minor local injury to multisystem involvement in the case of moderate or major burns. Systemic responses are often seen in burns greater than 20% of the TBSA.

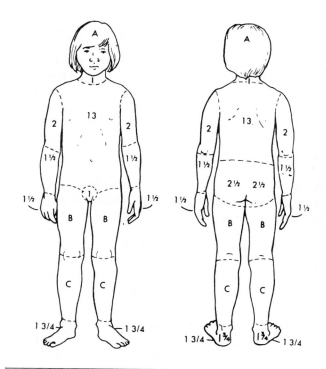

	<1 yr	1 yr	5 yr	10 yr	15 yr	Adult
A: half of head	9½	8½	6½	5½	4½	3½
B: half of thigh	2¾	3¼	4	4¼	4½	4¾
C: half of leg	2½	2½	2¾	3	3¼	3½

Figure 21–2. Calculation of burn surface area, after Lund and Browder. (From Barkin RM, Rosen P [1990]. *Emergency pediatrics* [3rd ed] St Louis: Mosby.)

TABLE 21–1. BURN DEPTH CATEGORY AND APPEARANCE

Surface Appearance	Superficial Partial Thickness	Deep Partial Thickness	Full Thickness
Color	Pink or red	Mottled, red or mixed pink and white	White, or sclerosed blood vessels with mahogany or blackened areas
Capillary refill	Excellent	Adequate, uneven	None
Condition	Dry, no blisters	Moist, intact or broken blisters	Dry, leathery or waxy
Edema	Minimal or none	Surface	In underlying tissues

TABLE 21–2. LUND AND BROWDER CHART FOR ESTIMATING PERCENTAGE OF BURNS ACCORDING TO BODY AREA

Area	Birth–1 year	1–4 years	5–9 years	10–14 years	15 years	Adult	Partial Thickness 2°	Full Thickness 3°	Total
Head	19	17	13	11	9	7	_____	_____	_____
Neck	2	2	2	2	2	2	_____	_____	_____
Anterior trunk	13	13	13	13	13	13	_____	_____	_____
Posterior trunk	13	13	13	13	13	13	_____	_____	_____
Right buttock	2½	2½	2½	2½	2½	2½	_____	_____	_____
Left buttock	2½	2½	2½	2½	2½	2½	_____	_____	_____
Genitalia	1	1	1	1	1	1	_____	_____	_____
Right upper arm	4	4	4	4	4	4	_____	_____	_____
Left upper arm	4	4	4	4	4	4	_____	_____	_____
Right lower arm	3	3	3	3	3	3	_____	_____	_____
Left lower arm	3	3	3	3	3	3	_____	_____	_____
Right hand	2½	2½	2½	2½	2½	2½	_____	_____	_____
Left hand	2½	2½	2½	2½	2½	2½	_____	_____	_____
Right thigh	5½	6½	8	8½	9	9½	_____	_____	_____
Left thigh	5½	6½	8	8½	9	9½	_____	_____	_____
Right leg	5	5	5½	6	6½	7	_____	_____	_____
Left leg	5	5	5½	6	6½	8	_____	_____	_____
Right foot	3½	3½	3½	3½	3½	3½	_____	_____	_____
Left foot	3½	3½	3½	3½	3½	3½	_____	_____	_____
						Total	_____	_____	_____

Cardiovascular. The increased vascular permeability that occurs with a major burn causes a major shift of fluid from the vascular to the interstitial spaces and a loss of protein through the wound itself. These fluid and protein shifts become most pronounced in the first 4–24 hours after the burn. If not properly anticipated and treated, they cause a burn shock that presents as hypovolemia, hypoproteinemia, and decreased oxygen tension (Demling and LaLonde, 1989).

Renal. As essential proteins and electrolytes also pass through the damaged capillaries, alterations in sodium and potassium metabolism contribute to the overall acid-base imbalance. There is often a compensatory renal response to the fluid and electrolyte imbalance. Antidiuretic hormone and aldosterone are secreted to conserve water and sodium. The breakdown of blood and muscle cells in a severe burn releases hemoglobin and myoglobin into the bloodstream. These substances are filtered through the kidney, turning urine a deep red-brown (hemoglobinuria). Adequate urine output is necessary to prevent these hemochromogens from clogging the renal tubules.

Altered Thermoregulation. The ability to control body temperature is impaired. Tissue deficits and persistent evaporative water losses lead to ongoing loss of body heat. Large injuries are followed by a hypermetabolic state, and the body compensates by mobilizing energy stores to meet increased metabolic needs.

Infection. The primary cause of morbidity for patients who survive the initial postburn phase is systemic infection. A burn patient's susceptibility to infections increases if wounds remain open, metabolic demands exceed nutritional intake, protein losses continue, and the host defense mechanism is suppressed. Survival is not assured until all wounds are covered with the patient's own skin. This may involve spontaneous healing, skin grafting, or the application of cultured epithelial cells.

PATHOPHYSIOLOGY OF SPECIFIC INJURIES

Electrical Injuries

Electrical burns are caused by heat that is generated from the resistance of tissues to the flow of electrical current. Higher resistance results in higher heat. Body tissues have varying resistance characteristics. Skin acts as an insulator to the flow of electricity, but this resistance can be easily overcome in the presence of moisture or strong electrical current. Dense tissues such as bone and fat are the most resistant, and blood vessels and nerves are the least resistant. The severity of tissue damage in an electrical burn depends on the path of the electrical current, the voltage of the electrical current, and the amount of time that the body was exposed to the electrical charge.

Electrical burns in children often result from contact with low-voltage current from household appliances. These injuries often occur when children chew on electrical cords or place objects in electrical sockets. Damage from such injuries causes local tissue destruction without systemic effects. The focus of treatment should be on local wound treatment and careful follow-up care (Monafo and Freedman, 1987).

High-voltage or amperage injuries are seen occasionally in adolescents and older children and usually involve contact with high tension wires. The severity of a high voltage or amperage injury is not always apparent from an inspection of the body surface. Therefore, clinicians must maintain a high index of suspicion for systemic damage, which may not be evident for several days.

Patients should be carefully assessed for the identification of an entrance and an exit wound, which often provide information about the path of the electrical current. Patients require careful observation for signs of deep damage such as myoglobinuria and compartment syndrome. The patient must also be carefully assessed for electrocardiographic changes because the electrical pathway may interrupt the normal cardiac cycle.

Chemical Burns

Tissue damage caused by contact with chemicals leads to a localized tissue necrosis that continues to progress even after the caustic agent has been removed. The severity of these injuries is related to the nature of the chemical, its concentration, and the duration of contact. Most pediatric chemical burns are caused by household cleaners containing strong alkalis and acids. These injuries in older children are most often associated with school laboratory environments and the handling of flammable liquids and explosives. First aid treatment of chemical burns consists of wound irrigation with copious amounts of water until a neutral ph is reached. Such irrigation always takes precedence over determination of the exact caustic agent (Doyle and Guzzardia, 1992).

Inhalation Injuries and Carbon Monoxide Poisoning

Inhalation injury includes but is not limited to damage caused by the breathing of heat, smoke, and toxic fumes. Thermal injury caused by exposure to high environmental temperatures and hot gases and liquids affects the upper airways. The mouth, nasopharynx and oropharynx, and larynx rapidly become edematous. Internal narrowing of the airway occurs that can quickly progress to total obstruction of the small upper airways of a child.

Lower airway damage is primarily related to the chemicals found in smoke. It is currently implicated in 30–80% of burn-related deaths (Herndon et al, 1988). Symptoms of lower airway injury are generally not apparent until 24 hours after the inhalation injury. Therefore, patients with a potential inhalation injury must be carefully monitored for signs of increasing respiratory distress.

Carbon monoxide poisoning often occurs in conjunction with an inhalation injury. It is the result of the inhalation of the products of the incomplete combustion of organic materials such as wood, paper, and cotton. The carbon monoxide molecule combines with the hemoglobin molecule, thereby reducing the ability of the blood to carry oxygen to tissues. The physical signs and symptoms of carbon monoxide poisoning include the presence of cherry-red mucous membranes, dizziness, nausea and vomiting, and alterations in consciousness ranging from stupor to coma.

Blood measurement of carboxyhemoglobin is helpful in diagnosing carbon monoxide poisoning, although prehospital oxygen administration often decreases the measurable levels on admission. Untreated, severe carbon monoxide poisoning leads to tissue hypoxia, altered cerebral functioning, coma, and death.

The identification of a child with an inhalation injury can be challenging; it is often determined on the basis of injury history and surface signs. Actual respiratory or ventilatory changes may occur immediately or take several hours to develop. Direct bronchoscopic inspection may be useful but is not always readily available in the ED. An inhalation injury should be suspected in patients with any of the following signs.

Signs of Inhalation Injury

- A history of being burned in an enclosed space
- Ignition of clothing of the upper body
- A burn of the face or neck, including a scald
- Singed facial, nasal, or scalp hairs
- Soot in nose, mouth, or sputum
- Hoarseness, brassy cough, or stridor
- Elevated carboxyhemoglobin level

Children with any of the findings in the list should be monitored extremely closely and intubated electively before airway edema occurs.

ASSESSMENT

History

The importance of obtaining a thorough history of the burn injury cannot be overemphasized. Small burns, although not a threat to survival, may have a clinical, functional or social significance that is not readily apparent. The details of how and where the injury occurred, the nature and extent of exposure to the burning agent, and first aid measures taken should be ascertained. Age, weight, allergies, relevant medical history, and current medications should be documented. Immunization status, especially tetanus prophylaxis, must be clarified.

Clinicians must be alert to the possibility of burns resulting from abuse or neglect. Inconsistencies between history and physical findings, delays in seeking treatment and conflicting histories necessitate further follow-up care and social service referral.

The management of moderate or major burn requires a co-ordinated trauma team effort to maximize the child's chances of recovery and rehabilitation (Locke et al, 1990). Although the physical manifestations of a major burn may be overwhelming, clinicians must first look past the burn to ensure that the child's ventilation, oxygenation, and perfusion are optimized. This is accomplished by a rapid primary survey focused on airway, breathing and circulation (ABCs) and the institution of emergency measures to support these vital functions (American College of Surgeons, 1980).

Primary Survey

Airway. The airway should be carefully assessed for patency and maintained by the use of positioning and establishment of adjunct naso- and oropharyngeal airways. Cervical spinal protection should be instituted and maintained if there is risk for a cervical spinal injury. One hundred percent warm humidified oxygen should be administered by a non-rebreather mask and titrated according to arterial blood gas (ABG) results. A child with upper body burns, facial burns, or possible smoke inhalation is at risk for airway obstruction from mucosal edema and airway narrowing. Clinical findings such as face and neck edema; soot in the mouth, nose or sputum; or singed nasal hairs merit early intubation to ensure a patent airway as airway swelling increases.

Breathing. Effective breathing and ventilation may be impaired after a moderate or major burn, even in the absence of an inhalation injury. An altered mental status, circumferential burns of the chest, and carbon monoxide poisoning can limit effective ventilation. Assessment of ventilation should include respiratory rate, respiratory effort, and auscultation of breath sounds. Breath sounds should be evaluated for the presence of rales, rhonchi, or wheezes. Absent or ineffective ventilations should be supported with a bag-mask-valve device until intubation is accomplished.

Circulation. Moderate and major burns cause fluid losses from the intravascular space and burn wound that may lead to cardiovascular collapse. Perfusion should be assessed by the simultaneous palpation of proximal and distal pulses, capillary filling time (not less than 2 seconds), and heart rate. Diminished peripheral pulses, tachycardia, and a prolonged capillary filling time are often signs of early shock in a pediatric patient. Hypotension is a late sign of shock in children and should not be relied upon as the only indicator of impaired perfusion. Vascular access with two large-bore intravenous or intraosseous lines should be promptly established and fluid resuscitation initiated (see the section on Management).

Disability. A child's neurologic status may be impaired from a variety of causes, including smoke inhalation, carbon monoxide poisoning, shock, or associated head injuries. The child's level of consciousness should be rapidly assessed using the Glasgow Coma Scale (GCS) modified as appropriate to the child's developmental level. Pupillary responses should be evaluated.

Exposure. The child's large surface-to-volume ratio places him or her at greater risk than an adult for hypothermia after a burn injury. Ambient room temperature should be increased as much as possible. Wet or smoldering clothing should be immediately removed, and the child should be fully examined for the extent of burn and other existing injuries. Jewelry and other restricting items should be removed. The child should then be covered with dry sterile sheets to decrease the evaporative losses.

Losses of moderate to large surfaces of skin covering also place the child at increased risk for the development of infection. Emergency department nurses can play an important role in reducing the risk of infection by ensuring that personnel caring for the patient don appropriate protective clothing. Masks, gowns, caps, and gloves should be worn by anyone having direct contact with the burn injury. Sterile bed linens and gowns should be used. These items are often kept in a readily accessible burn pack in most EDs.

Secondary Survey

The secondary survey consists of a comprehensive head-to-toe examination and continuing reassessment of the ABCs (Table 21–3). Depth and extent of the burn injury should be carefully mapped using a Lund and Browder or Berkow chart. Thorough examination is important, because burns of the scalp, eyes, back, and inner ears are easily overlooked.

TABLE 21–3. SECONDARY SURVEY

Area	Assessment
Head and neck	Examine for entrance and exit wounds; soot in mouth, nose, or sputum; singed eyebrows, eyelashes, or hair; circumferential neck burns; presence of other injuries, such as lacerations, contusions, or hematomas
Eyes	Assess for pupillary response, extraocular movements (EOM), corneal opacity
Chest	Observe for chest expansion, retractions, circumferential burns; signs of possible abuse, such as hematomas, bruises, or scars; auscultate for rhonchi, wheezes, and rales
Abdomen	Observe for abdominal distention, rigidity; signs of trauma, such as bruising, old scars; auscultate bowel sounds
Back	Look for evidence of old injuries, such as scars or bruises
Extremities	Assess for circumferential burns; evaluate for compartment syndrome by palpation of pulses

LABORATORY AND DIAGNOSTIC TESTS

Laboratory tests obtained in the ED can provide important baseline and diagnostic information in the management of thermal, electrical, or inhalation injury. Such tests routinely include a complete blood count (CBC) with differential, hemoglobin and hematocrit, determination of electrolyte levels, and renal function tests (blood urea nitrogen [BUN] and creatinine concentration). Frequent bedside monitoring of glucose levels is important in young children and infants.

Arterial blood gases and carboxyhemoglobin levels should be drawn if inhalation injury or respiratory compromise is suspected. Liver function—serum glutamic-oxaloacetic transaminase (SGOT), serum glutamic pyruvate transaminase (SGPT), and amylase—and cardiac enzymes—creatine phosphokinase (CPK)—should be measured if there is any risk of high-voltage electrical injury.

Urinalysis should be done to evaluate for the presence of myoglobin. Myoglobin often results from muscle breakdown associated with burns of more than 30% of the TBSA and electrical injuries.

The selection and timing of other diagnostic efforts are related to specific injuries and relative risks. An ECG and cardiac monitoring are necessary for a large or electrical burn. Bronchoscopy can clarify the extent of a respiratory injury. Chest and other x ray examinations are performed as needed for endotracheal tube (ET) and line placement.

MANAGEMENT

ABCs

Management of the patient's ABCs should proceed as outlined in the primary survey. The focus is on continual re-evaluation of the patient's ventilation and oxygenation. Supplemental oxygen (100%) should be administered and titrated with the use of pulse oximetry and ABGs. Intubation should be considered early if there is a facial burn, upper airway edema, or suspected inhalation injury. Ventilatory support should be provided as needed. Nasogastric tubes should be inserted to decompress the stomach in children who are mechanically ventilated or who have a severe burn injury.

Vital signs and peripheral perfusion are monitored to assess adequacy of circulation. Electrocardiographic monitoring should be instituted and a 12-lead electrocardiogram (ECG) performed for all patients with a high-voltage electrical injury. Peripheral circulation requires careful monitoring in extremities with electrical or circumferential burns because local tissue edema can cause obstruction of arterial flow resulting in compartment syndrome.

Noninvasive blood pressure values should be trended over time. Two large-bore peripheral lines or intraosseous lines should be placed for fluid resuscitation (see section on Fluid Resuscitation). Adequacy of fluid resuscitation and perfusion should be monitored through an indwelling Foley catheter. Hourly urine output should be maintained at 1.5 mL/kg/hour during the first 24 hours.

Hypothermia can place further demands on the body's vital functions. Therefore, the child's temperature should be carefully monitored with a tympanic or rectal thermometer. Environmental temperature should be increased and the child's body covered as much as possible.

Fluid Resuscitation

Fluid resuscitation is a major focus of care of seriously burned patients during the emergent phase. The goal of such treatment is to compensate for intravascular fluid losses related to increased vascular permeability and protein loss. Several pediatric fluid resuscitation formulas are available for reference. Physician preference varies, but each formula is based on the relation between body weight and burn size (Table 21–4).

The fluid formula requirements are generally 2–4 mL/kg of body weight times the TBSA burned (Demling, 1990). These rates should be used only as guidelines; actual prescribed fluids and rates are adjusted according to the patient's response. For children the goal is to maintain urine output of 1.5 mL/kg/hour, with stable vital signs and appropriate mental status

TABLE 21–4. FLUID RESUSCITATION FORMULAS

	Evans	Brooke	Parkland	Modified Brooke
■ DAY 1				
Colloid	1 ml/kg/% burn	0.5 ml/kg/% burn	None	None
Crystalloid	Lactated Ringer solution: 1 mL/kg/% burn	Lactated Ringer solution: 1.5 mL/kg/% burn	Lactated Ringer solution: 4 mL/kg/% burn	Lactated Ringer solution: 2 mL/kg/% burn (adult) 3 mL/kg/% burn (child)
D_5W	2000 mL/m²	2000 mL/m²	None	Same as Brooke
Rate	½ total in first 8 hours ¼ total in next 8 hours ¼ total in next 8 hours	½ total in first 8 hours ¼ total in next 8 hours ¼ total in next 8 hours	½ total in first 8 hours ¼ total in next 8 hours ¼ total in next 8 hours	
Volume calculation	Use burn area up to a total of 50 TBSA; if greater than 50%, calculate as a 50% burn	Same as Evans	Use total burn area regardless of size	Same as Parkland
■ DAY 2				
Colloid	0.5 mL/kg/% burn	0.25 mL/kg/% burn	Only if needed to maintain plasma volume	0.3–0.5 mL/kg/% burn
Crystalloid	Lactated Ringer 0.5 mL/kg/% burn	Lactated Ringer 0.75 mL/kg/% burn	None	None
D_5W	1500–2000 mL	1500–2000 mL	Sufficient to maintain urine output	Sufficient to maintain urine output

TSBA, total body surface area; D_5W, 5% dextrose in water.

(Herrin, 1990). The quantity, color, and specific gravity of urine may provide clues to the existence of damaged blood vessels and muscles from an electrical injury. Reddish brown urine often signifies myoglobinuria from deep injuries. Careful monitoring of the child's blood glucose is imperative because small children and infants have limited glycogen stores which are easily depleted. Dextrose is generally administered in boluses of 25% dextrose or 10% dextrose during the acute resuscitative stage.

Pain Management

Pain management involves more than administration of analgesics. The pain following a burn injury can range from mild to severe. Feelings of fear and anxiety can heighten the perception of pain. This can be complicated by the experience of the hospital setting and the awareness of parental emotions. Wound pain is compounded by invasive procedures such as laboratory tests and placement of intravenous lines. Vital signs and body language may provide the best clues to level of comfort and anxiety.

Intravenous narcotics are indicated for the pain associated with burns. Morphine sulfate or fentanyl, often in combination with a short acting anxiolytic agent, is used during the emergent phase. All medications should be given intravenously because of the

incomplete and unpredictable absorption from body tissues after a burn. These drugs should be given in small increments and titrated to patient response.

Patient comfort interventions may involve maintaining a calm supportive environment, explaining procedures, and allowing the parents to be present as much as possible. Increasing the room temperature, adding warm blankets, and limiting exposure of body parts to the air further decrease discomfort from shivering or air currents passing over burns.

Wound Care

Wound care should be instituted only after the child's condition is adequately stabilized, and adequate analgesia is achieved. Assessment of the burn wound should be performed in a clean, warm environment after all clothing is removed. Treatment of the burn wound during the emergent phase is focused on accurate assessment, basic cleansing and debridement, and prevention of complications. Assessment of burn depth may be difficult in the emergent phase, yet estimation of extent of TBSA burned should be as accurate as possible. Burn charts such as the Lund and Browder and Berkow can facilitate this process.

Burn wounds are washed with a warm solution of mild soap and sterile saline solution. Loose tissue should be debrided, although removal of intact blisters is controversial. Dressings are applied using aseptic technique. Burn wound dressings should be loosely applied to allow for the anticipated swelling. Access to peripheral pulses and sites of intravenous (IV) lines should be anticipated. Dressings should be bulky to absorb drainage. Topical agents may be prescribed for wound treatment; the agent used varies with physician preference. Silver sulfadiazine is commonly used because of its broad-spectrum bacteriocidal action. Table 21–5 describes the advantages and disadvantages of the topical agents used in burn care. Unless recommended, no topical agents should be applied if a patient is to be transferred to a burn center.

Tetanus Prophylaxis

Tetanus prophylaxis should be administered to children who have not completed their immunization course or who have received a tetanus immunization more than 5 years before the injury. Tetanus prophylaxis in the form of tetanus-diphtheria (TD) should be administered to children older than 7 years. Children younger than 7 years should receive tetanus prophylaxis in the form of diphtheria-pertussis-tetanus (DPT) unless they have (1) had an adverse reaction to DPT; (2) have had pertussis, or (3) have a chronic seizure disorder. Children in these three categories should receive tetanus prophylaxis in the form of TD (Committee on Infectious Diseases, 1991).

MINOR BURNS

Most burns treated in the ED are minor. Once the ABCs are ensured, the focus of intervention is on wound care, pain management, and patient and family education. Wound care focuses on gentle cleansing with a mild soap and sterile saline solution. Small burns are generally treated with silver sulfadiazine or bacitracin on an outpatient basis. To decrease the discomfort of application, the ointment should be spread aseptically on open unfolded sterile gauze. The gauze can then be cut to the proper size and placed directly on the burn. The wound is then gently wrapped with a bulky bandage to provide protection and accommodate swelling.

Facial burns of older children are often treated open with a thin layer of bacitracin covering the burns. The wound is cleansed twice a day, and a new layer of bacitracin is applied. This method is often not practical in small children and infants because of their limited cognitive ability.

Mild pain and discomfort can generally be treated by acetaminophen administered 30–40 minutes before wound care. Anxiety regarding wound care often can be lessened with the use of distraction techniques. Most children also cope better if allowed to play an active role in the procedure.

Patient and parent teaching should focus on the care of the wound as outlined earlier and signs and

TABLE 21–5. ADVANTAGES AND DISADVANTAGES OF THE TOPICAL AGENTS USED IN BURN CARE

Topical Agent	Advantages	Disadvantages
Silver sulfadiazine	Can be used with or without dressings Is painless Can be applied to wound directly Broad-spectrum Effective against yeast	Does not penetrate into eschar
Silver nitrate	Broad-spectrum Nonallergenic Dressing application is painless	Poor penetration Discolors, making assessment difficult Can cause severe electrolyte imbalances Removal of dressings is painful
Povidone-iodine	Broad-spectrum Antifungal Easily removed with water	Not effective against *Pseudomonas* May impair thyroid function Painful application
Mafenide acetate	Broad-spectrum Penetrates burn eschar May be used with or without occlusive dressings	May cause metabolic acidosis May compromise respiratory function May inhibit epithelialization Painful application
Gentamicin	Broad-spectrum May be covered or left open to air	Has caused resistant strains Ototoxic Nephrotoxic
Nitrofurazone	Bactericidal Broad-spectrum	May lead to overgrowth of fungus and *Pseudomonas* Painful application

(From Tofrin RB [ed] [1991]. Nursing care of the burn-injured patient. Philadelphia: Davis, p 46)

symptoms of wound infection. Parents should be encouraged to increase the child's fluid intake to decrease the chance of dehydration. Mild temperature elevations up to 38°C (101°F) are to be expected and can be treated by appropriate doses of acetaminophen. Higher temperature elevations may be indicative of wound infection and may merit medical intervention. Most minor burns should be re-examined within 24–48 hours of initial presentation because the appearance of the burn may change considerably.

TRIAGE

Triage decisions related to an initial transport destination for a burn patient may be made in the field based on the criteria of the local emergency response system. Arrival of a patient in the ED may be anticipated and well coordinated with appropriate personnel on hand. In many cases, however, a child with a burn injury is carried into the ED by a family member. The challenge for the ED nurse is to quickly assess the type, extent, and severity of the burn to assign a triage rating and provide appropriate treatment.

The American Burn Association (ABA) has developed criteria for the classification of the severity of burn injury. These criteria can be used to assist with triage decisions. The categories can be further described as follows.

Criteria for Classification of Severity of Burn Injury

- Minor burn injury
    Partial-thickness burns less than 10% of TBSA on children
    Full-thickness burns less than 2% of TBSA that do not involve face, hands, eyes, ears, or genitalia
- Moderate burn injury
    Partial-thickness burns; 10–20% of TBSA on children
    Full-thickness burns less than 10% of TBSA that do not involve face, hands, feet, eyes, ears, or genitalia
- Major burn injury
    Partial-thickness burns greater than 20% of TBSA on children
    Full-thickness burns, 10% of TBSA or greater
    All burns involving face, hands, eyes, feet, ears, or genitalia
    All burn injuries complicated by inhalation injury or major trauma
    Electrical burns

These classifications may be helpful in performing accurate triage of a child with a burn injury, yet each patient must be evaluated individually. Rapid assessment of the ABCs, neurologic status, pain status, and emotional state of child and family are intrinsic components of the triage assessment.

TRIAGE
Burns

Emergent
A child with major burns as classified by the ABA; respiratory distress; altered level of consciousness.

Urgent
A child with moderate burns as classified by the ABA; severe pain or discomfort; severe emotional distress; burns from possible abuse or neglect; burns more than 24 hours old.

Non-urgent
A child with minor burn injury as classified by the ABA if child is awake, alert, and in little or no pain.

NURSING DIAGNOSES

The possible nursing diagnoses for a burn patient vary with the nature and the extent of injury. Nursing care of a burned child involves the family, both in planning and in psychosocial support. Patient and family teaching and appropriate referrals may be the focus of care of a minor burn. Life-saving priorities are the needs in a moderate or major injury. Burns are considered a surgical problem; therefore, many of the nursing interventions are collaborative.

Nursing Diagnosis
Ineffective Airway Clearance

Defining Characteristics

- Facial or upper body burns, swollen mucous membranes
- Singed nasal or scalp hairs, carbonaceous sputum
- Hoarseness, cough, dyspnea
- Facial, nasal, oral, neck, or chest edema

Nursing Interventions

- Monitor quality of respirations and observe for signs of impaired airway; prepare appropriate equipment for intubation

- Elevate head of bed
- Administer humidified oxygen as ordered
- Perform suction as necessary
- Establish naso- or oropharyngeal airway

Expected Outcome

- Patent airway maintained

Nursing Diagnosis
Impaired Gas Exchange

Defining Characteristics

- Labored breathing, dyspnea, cough with increasing sputum
- Decreased lung sounds, rales, rhonchi, or wheezing
- Decreased pO_2, restlessness

Nursing Interventions

- Monitor breath sounds, effectiveness of cough.
- Assess amount and quality of pulmonary secretions
- Administer humidified oxygen and medications as ordered
- Monitor blood gases, oxygen saturation
- Assist in and maintain endotracheal intubation and mechanical ventilation as appropriate

Expected Outcomes

- Breath sounds are clear; mobilization of secretions is effective
- Arterial blood gases are normal
- Respiratory pattern is regular and unlabored

Nursing Diagnosis
Fluid Volume Deficit

Defining Characteristics

- Decreased blood pressure, capillary refill, and urinary output
- Increased pulse rate
- Altered mental status, thirst, dry mucous membranes, edema

Nursing Interventions

- Weigh patient
- Monitor vital signs, monitor hourly urine output, report trends
- Administer IV crystalloids as ordered
- Maintain position and patency of IV line

Expected Outcomes

- Adequate fluid and electrolyte balance are maintained
- Tissue perfusion maintained
- Vital signs and mental status are appropriate for age

Nursing Diagnosis
Altered Tissue Perfusion (Cardiopulmonary, Renal, Peripheral, Cerebral)

Defining Characteristics

- Increased heart rate, decreased urine output
- Metabolic acidosis with increased respiratory rate
- Diminished or absent peripheral pulses
- Altered mental status, restlessness, lethargy, or coma

Nursing Interventions

- Assess peripheral perfusion frequently
- Monitor vital signs, oxygen saturation, mental status, and laboratory data

Expected Outcomes

- Adequate cardiac output and tissue perfusion are maintained
- Peripheral pulses are present and equal
- Unburned skin color and temperature are normal

Nursing Diagnosis
Impaired Skin Integrity

Defining Characteristics

- Disruption of skin surface
- Destruction of skin layers

Nursing Interventions

- Assess skin, body temperature
- Estimate size of burn using Lund and Browder chart
- Apply loose, clean dry dressings and warm blankets
- Increase environmental temperature

Expected Outcomes

- Normal body temperature is maintained
- Integrity of intact skin and remaining tissues is protected

Nursing Diagnosis
Pain

Defining Characteristics

- Verbalization of pain, crying, screaming
- Clenched teeth, tight lips, facial grimaces, withdrawal or resistance to moving the affected area
- Increased heart rate, blood pressure, respiratory rate

Nursing Interventions

- Assess level of pain with verbal reports, age-appropriate pain rating scale, or observed signs
- Provide calm environment, reassure child and family
- Administer IV analgesics as ordered
- Evaluate effectiveness of analgesics

Expected Outcomes

- Patient shows evidence of pain control with verbal reports, nonverbal cues, and vital signs
- Patient is able to cooperate with care as appropriate for age

Nursing Diagnosis

High Risk for Infection

Defining Characteristics

- Loss of skin barrier related to burn injury
- Immunosuppression related to burn injury

Nursing Interventions

- Institute infection control measures (mask, gown, and gloves) for all in contact with burn injury
- Obtain culture of burn wound
- Use aseptic technique when cleansing wound and applying dressings
- Apply topical antimicrobial agents to burn as ordered

Expected Outcome

- Patient remains free from infection

PATIENT AND FAMILY TEACHING AND PSYCHOSOCIAL SUPPORT

The emotional state of the child and family after a moderate or major burn injury can be extremely variable. A child with a severe burn injury is often in pain and extremely anxious about what is happening. Older children may be concerned about whether they will die. The emergency nurse caring for a child with a serious burn must juggle the need to provide expedient care while maintaining a calm demeanor. Nursing interventions should focus on providing the child with developmentally appropriate explanations and reassurance as appropriate to the situation.

During the acute resuscitative stage a consistent clinician or staff member should be available to the parents to provide frequent updated information regarding the child's condition and progression of care. Parents should be allowed to visit with the child as soon as possible. It is extremely important that the parents be prepared for what to expect before seeing the child. Parents are often overwhelmed by the burn dressings and indwelling tubes. As appropriate, parents should be informed that burn dressings are often much larger than the involved area. Parents should be informed of what to expect if paralytic agents are used or if the child is extremely sedated.

Parents often experience a variety of feelings including shock, disbelief, anger, and guilt. Being available to listen and provide understanding is an important aspect of emergency nursing care. Parents are always concerned about the child's chances of survival and the extent of possible disfigurement. Parents should be informed that everything possible is being done for the child. They should be told that the extent of scarring is difficult to predict during the emergency period.

TABLE 21–6. ADMISSION GUIDELINES FOR BURNED CHILDREN

More than 10% of total body surface area
More than 5% full-thickness burns
Location
Face
Neck
Both hands
Both feet
Perineum
Burn types
Inhalation
Electrical
Chemical
Circumferential
Associated injuries
Disabling soft tissue trauma
Fractures
Head injury
Complicating medical conditions
Diabetes
Heart disease
Pulmonary disease
Social problems
Child abuse
Neglect
Homelessness

(Reproduced with permission from Salivanov V [1991]. Thermal injury. In Grossman M, and Dieckmann R A (eds), Pediatric Emergency Medicine. Philidelphia: Lippincott, p 319)

TABLE 21–7. AMERICAN BURN ASSOCIATION CRITERIA FOR PATIENT REFERRAL TO BURN CENTER

Second- and third-degree burns over more than 10% of the total body surface area (TBSA) of patients less than 10 or more than 50 years of age

Second- and third-degree burns of more than 20% of TBSA in other age groups

Second- and third-degree burns with a serious threat of functional or cosmetic impairment that involve face, hands, feet, genitalia, perineum, and major joints

Third-degree burns of more than 5% TBSA in any age group

Electrical burns including lightning injury

Chemical burns with serious threat of functional or cosmetic impairment

Inhalation injury with burn injury

Circumferential burns of the extremity and chest

Burns of patients with pre-existing medical disorders that could complicate management, prolong recovery, or affect mortality

Concomitant trauma, in which the burn injury poses the greater risk of morbidity or mortality

Burns of children when local facility is unable to provide specialized pediatric care

(Adapted from The American Burn Association's Guide to development and operation of burn centers [1993] American Burn Association: New York, NY)

DISPOSITION

As previously discussed, children with minor burns are usually discharged home if a reliable caretaker is available to provide wound care and observe for signs and symptoms of infection. Follow-up visits should be arranged with the child's pediatrician or nurse practitioner because small burns on children often may be deeper than initially assessed.

Many moderate burns can be successfully treated in non-burn-center hospitals. The guidelines for hospital admission are found in Table 21–6. The ABA has established criteria (Table 21–7) for the type of injuries that require referral to a specialized burn center. These type of injuries require the acute burn and rehabilitation expertise available in a specialized burn center.

The process of transfer should be well coordinated with the receiving facility. An adequate airway must be assured. Intravenous lines must be patent and well secured. Patients should be transferred in dry dressings with warm blankets. Transfer plans should be made with the physician at the burn center. The patient and family need support and information about the benefits of transfer to a specialized burn center.

REFERENCES

American College of Surgeons Committee on Trauma (1980). *Advanced trauma life support course providers manual.* Chicago: American College of Surgeons, pp 159–170

Bernardo LM, Sullivan K (1991). Care of the pediatric patient with burns. In Tofrino RB (ed), *Nursing care of the burn-injured patient.* Philadelphia: Davis, p 250

Committee on Infectious Diseases American Academy of Pediatrics (1991). *Report of the committee on infectious diseases.* Elk Grove Village, Il: American Academy of Pediatrics

Demling RH (1990). Pathophysiologic changes after acute burns and approach to initial resuscitation. In Martyn JA (ed), *Acute management of the burned patient.* Philadelphia: Saunders, p 21

Demling RH, LaLonde C (1989). *Burn trauma.* New York: Theime, p 27

Doyle CJ, Guzzardia LJ (1992). Chemical burns. *Patient Care* 2:232–248

Erdmann TC, Feldman KW, Rivara FP, Heimbach DM, Wall HA (1991). Tap water burn prevention: The effects of legislation. *Pediatrics* 88:572–577

Hall JR (1992). *Burn injuries.* Quincy, MA: National Fire Protection Association, p 3

Herndon DN, Barrow RE, Linares HA, et al (1988). Inhalation injury in burned patients: Effects and treatment. *Burns* 14:349–356

Herrin JT (1990). Renal function in burns. In Martyn JA (ed), *Acute management of the burned patient.* Philadelphia: Saunders, p 244

Lindblad BE, Terkelsen CJ (1990). Domestic burns in children. *Burns* 16:254–256

Locke JA, Rossignol AM, Burke JF (1990). Socioeconomic factors and the incidence of hospitalized burn injuries in New England counties, USA. *Burns* 16:273–277

Monafo WW, Freedman BM (1987). Electrical and lightning injury. In Boswick JA (ed). *The art and science of burn care.* Rockville, Md: Aspen, p 247

Nebraska Burn Institute (1987). Pediatric burn temperature sensitivity. *Advanced burn life support course: Providers manual.* Lincoln, Neb: Nebraska Burn Institute

Powell EC, Tanz, RR (1993). Comparison of childhood burns associated with use of microwave ovens and conventional stoves. *Pediatrics* 91:344–349

SUGGESTED READING

Atchison NE (1991). Pain during burn dressing change in children: Relationship to burn area, depth and analgesic regimens. *Pain* 47:41–45

Bernstein NC, Robson MC (1983). *Comprehensive approaches to the burned person.* New York: Medical Examination

Burke JF (1990). From desperation to skin regeneration: Progress in burn treatment. *J Trauma* 30:36–40

Kinner MA, Daly WL (1992). Skin transplantation. *Critical Care Nursing Clinics of North America* 4:173–178

McLaughlin EG (ed) (1990). *Critical care of the burn patient: A case study approach.* Rockville, Md: Aspen

Tompkins RG, Burke JF (1990). Progress in burn treatment and the use of artificial skin. *World J Surg* 14:819–824

CHAPTER 22

Ingestions and Poisoning

BONNIE S. DEAN

INTRODUCTION

Accidental childhood poisoning occurs in seconds. The few seconds it takes to answer the telephone or to put dinner into the oven is enough time for a young child to grab a bottle and take a few mouthfuls of a red liquid that has the same appeal as cherry soda. A child's senses of smell and taste are not fully developed, therefore he or she cannot differentiate cherry soda from an aromatic cherry-scented lamp oil. Tragically, five young children have died during the past 8 years because they ingested lamp oil.

Accidental childhood poisoning continues to be a major health care problem in the United States. Although 75% of all reported pediatric poisonings can be successfully managed in the home, the other 25% mandate referral to a health care facility for medical intervention. The field of toxicology is constantly expanding and changing. In the past decade many important advances have contributed to the recognition, assessment, diagnosis, and treatment of poisoning in children. It is vitally important for the emergency nurse to be aware of the most current toxicology treatment protocols, the most appropriate methods of gastric decontamination, the existence of and the need for antidotal therapy, and the initiation of extracorporeal elimination procedures so as to improve the quality of care and increase the child's chance for survival.

EPIDEMIOLOGY OF PEDIATRIC POISONING

During years 1985 through 1989, 3,810,405 poisonings involving children younger than 6 years were reported to the American Association of Poison Control Centers (Litovitz and Manoguerra, 1992). Of this number, 2,117 children experienced a life-threatening effect or residual disability and an additional 111 children died as a direct result of unintentional poisoning (Litovitz and Manoguerra, 1992). The three most commonly implicated substance categories, resulting in 30.4% of the reported poisonings among young children, included cosmetics and personal care products, cleaning substances, and plants (Litovitz and Manoguerra, 1992). Although these categories contain a multitude of substances or products that are frequently implicated in pediatric poisoning, their toxicity hazard is considered to be quite low. Conversely, iron supplements, antidepressants, cardiovascular medications, methyl salicylate, hydrocarbons (including lamp oil), pesticides and selenious acid-containing gun bluing were substances or products responsible for the deaths of children by poisoning during this time period.

ETIOLOGY OF PEDIATRIC POISONING

Children are naturally curious. Their immediate environment includes areas around the home that afford easy access to a wide variety of toxins. A closed cabinet door, or even a high shelf, becomes a challenge to a child to discover what treasures lie there. Many household products are marketed in attractive packages that are intended to catch the eye of potential buyers. However, an array of colorful attractive containers also challenges the inquisitiveness of a young child. Young children have increased hand-to-mouth activity. During this developmental period a child places anything

365

and everything into his or her mouth, and toxins are no exception. Because the greatest numbers of accidental childhood poisonings occur around mealtimes, a child's hunger and thirst must be considered to be causal factors. Children love to copy and imitate behaviors of their caregivers. A child might accidentally ingest as many as 58 extra-strength acetaminophen caplets after watching his or her mother take two for a headache. These are but a few of the many factors that contribute to accidental childhood poisoning. Additional vigilance and education and prevention efforts on the part of consumers, parents, health care providers, poison centers, manufacturers, and regulatory governmental agencies must continue in an attempt to eradicate the morbidity and mortality associated with pediatric poisoning.

INITIAL ASSESSMENT AND STABILIZATION

Successful management of poisoning can generally be accomplished as outlined in Figure 22–1. Overriding all other considerations must be that the care of the child is the first priority. The familiar adage, "Treat the patient, not the poison," is appropriate. It is of no value for a nurse to make heroic attempts at gastric emptying if a child is not breathing or if the blood pressure is dangerously low. The first step is to assess the patient's condition and to stabilize it.

History

A history may not always be easy to obtain and may be inaccurate, especially if the patient is a young child and the ingestion was not witnessed by an adult caretaker. In addition, patients' accounts of events are confused and often unreliable. Therefore, the nurse must always correlate the history with the physical examination. The child or the family should be asked to describe the exposure. Where, when, why, how much, and who else witnessed the event are specific questions an emergency nurse can ask.

Also important is to discern what if any symptoms occurred between the ingestion and the emergency department (ED) presentation (eg, vomiting, ataxia, tremors, or a change in the level of consciousness).

Were there coingestants? Pediatric poisoning fre-

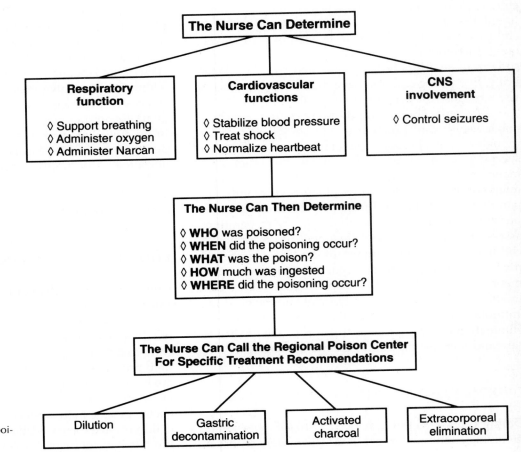

Figure 22–1. Assessment of a poisoned child.

quently occurs when children ingest drugs that have been mixed into one container to facilitate storage in a purse or pants pocket. Children have ingested mixtures of solvents that were stored in a glass jar in the garage (Litovitz and Manoguerra, 1992).

Has any therapy been done before presentation in the ED? If the caretaker placed a telephone call to the regional poison center, treatment may already have begun. A regional poison center gathers historical data, fully and accurately documents the history, formulates and documents a treatment plan specific to the toxin and the child, and relays this information to the treating ED while the child is en route.

Poisoning ingestions in infants are largely a result of therapeutic overdosing (Atwood, 1980). Ingestions are most often accidental in children 1–5 years of age. A child older than 6–7 years at the time of the overdose should be evaluated for psychological dysfunction, because in this age group poisoning is rarely an accident (Atwood, 1980).

Physical Assessment and Stabilization

The clinical presentation of acute poisoning may vary from no symptoms and normal vital signs to coma. Children with no symptoms or mild symptoms should not be dismissed as insignificantly intoxicated because depending on the substance ingested, they are at risk for rapid deterioration in both mental status and vital signs. The nurse must assess by evaluating the patient's breathing. Oxygen may need to be administered or mechanical ventilation started. Is the patient's blood pressure stabilized? Shock is best treated with a fluid challenge and, if necessary, vasopressor agents. Is there normal sinus rhythm? Is the patient experiencing seizures, tremors, or is he or she comatose?

Initial Therapy. Intravenous access should be established and the appropriate solution administered. Naloxone hydrochloride, 0.1 mg/kg, should be administered intravenously (or endotracheally or intramuscularly if intravenous access is compromised or delayed) to children with a decreased level of consciousness (Krenzelok and Dunmire, 1992).

If a rapid dipstick method of determining serum glucose level is available, it should be used because hypoglycemia is a frequent manifestation of acute poisoning. If the level cannot be measured or if it measures less than 80 mg/dL, the child may need an intravenous bolus of 50% glucose solution or the intramuscular administration of glucagon (Krenzelok and Dunmire, 1992).

Airway Management. Maintenance of the airway should always take priority in management of an

TABLE 22–1. INDICATIONS FOR INTUBATION OF A POISONED CHILD

Respiratory insufficiency

Decreased level of consciousness with accompanying danger of aspiration

Combativeness to degree that performance of therapeutic measures is inhibited

Intoxication with a substance that results in rapid clinical deterioration, eg, cyclic antidepressants, calcium channel blockers, clonidine

acutely poisoned child. Although the decision to intubate is not difficult in the case of comatose patients, it does become a dilemma in combative or moderately lethargic patients. Indications for intubation are listed in Table 22–1. Children who have ingested a large amount of a rapidly acting agent, such as cyclic antidepressants or calcium channel blockers, might need to be intubated on arrival in the ED, even if mental status has not yet deteriorated (Krenzelok and Dunmire, 1992).

Management of Hypotension. Some of the drugs most commonly involved in severe acute poisoning (opiates, cyclic antidepressants, sedatives, cardiovascular drugs) can cause vascular dilatation and relative hypovolemia, leading to hypotension. The initial approach to hypotension in acutely poisoned children should always include aggressive administration of fluids. When adequate blood volume adjustment fails to raise blood pressure, use of vasodepressor agents may be necessary (Krenzelok and Dunmire, 1992).

After cardiorespiratory functions are supported, the next step is to obtain a history of the poisoning incident.

Laboratory and Diagnostic Tests

During the initial evaluation, measurement of the serum glucose level and collection of a serum or urine specimen for a toxicology screen may prove beneficial. A high index of suspicion about the specific toxin ingested by the child may make the toxicology screen unnecessary. In such a case, a specific request for laboratory confirmation of the suspected toxin is sufficient. Qualitative analysis, which merely indicates the presence or absence of a substance, is acceptable unless quantitation of the toxin is essential to treatment or diagnosis. It is important for the nurse to remember that toxicology screens are not universally identical and are usually not totally inclusive. Therefore, if results of a urine or blood screen are negative, it is important to know what toxins were included in the assay.

The following questions should be asked to validate the need for toxicologic laboratory analysis: Will

TABLE 22–2. POISON TREATMENT

Substance	Code
Acetominophen	2, 7
Acetone	9
Acids	
Ingestion	1
Eye Contamination	4
Topical	6
Inhalation if mixed with bleach	5
Aerosols	
Eye Contamination	6
Inhalation	8
After Shave Lotions	
Less than 15 ml	1
More than 15 ml	2
Airplane Glue	9
Alcohol	
Ingestion	4
Eye Contamination	6
Alkali	
Ingestion	4
Eye Contamination	6
Topical	5
Inhalation	8
Ammonia	
Ingestion	4
Eye Contamination	6
Inhalation	8
Amphetamines	2
Analgesics	See Specific Type
Antacids	1
Antibiotics	9
Antidepressants	
Tricyclic	2
Others	2
Antidiarrheal Agents	
Prescription	2
Non-Prescription	9
Antifreeze (Ethylene Glycol)	
Ingestion	2, 7
Eye Contamination	6
Antihistamines	2
Batteries	
Dry Cell (Flashlight)	1
Button (Hearing Aid, Calculator)	9
Wet Cell (Automobile)	4
Benzene	
Ingestion	9
Inhalation	8
Topical	5
Benzodiazepines	2
Birth Control Pills	1
Bleaches	
Liquid Ingestion	1
Solid Ingestion	4
Eye Contamination	6
Inhalation when mixed with acids or ammonia	5
Boric Acid	4
Bromides	6
Bubble Bath	8
Caffeine	2
Camphor	6
Camphorated Oil	8
Candles	2
Caps	See Specific Type
Carbon Monoxide	9
Chalk	2
Chlorine Bleach	
Liquid Ingestion	1
Solid Ingestion	4
Eye Contamination	6
Inhalation if mixed with acids or ammonia	8
Cigarettes	
Less than one	1
One or More	2
Dehumidifying Packets	1
Denture Adhesives	1
Denture Cleansers	4
Deodorants, Personal	
Ingestion	1
Eye	6
Deodorizer Cakes	2
Deodorizers, Room	9
Desiccants	1
Detergents	
Liquid Dishwashing	1
Electric Dishwasher	4
Laundry Detergent	9
Dextromethorphan	2, 7
Diaper Rash Ointment	1
Diet Aids	2
Digitalis Glycosides	2
Dishwasher Detergents	2
Disinfectants	1
Drain Cleaners	
Ingestion	4
Eye Contamination	6
Topical	5
Inhalation if mixed with bleach	8
Dyes	1
Electric Dishwasher Detergent	4
Epoxy glue	
Catalyst	1
Resin or When Mixed	2
Epson Salts	4
Ethyl Alcohol	
Ingestion	4
Eye Contamination	6
Ethylene Glycol	
Ingestion	2, 7
Eye Contamination	6
Hallucinogens	9
Hand Cream	1
Hand Lotions	1
Herbicides	9
Heroin	7
Hydrochloric Acid	
Ingestion	4
Eye Contamination	6
Topical	5
Inhalation if mixed with bleach	8
Inks	
Ballpoint Pen	1
Laundry Marking	9
Printer's	2, 7
Insecticides	
Ingestion	1
Topical	2
Iron	2, 7
Isopropyl Alcohol	
Ingestion	4
Eye Contamination	6
Kerosene	9
Laundry Marking Ink	9
Laundry Pre-washes	9
Laxatives	9
Lead	9
Lighter Fluid	9
Liniments	9
Lipstick	1
LSD (Lysergic Acid Diethylamide)	9
Lye	
Ingestion	4
Eye Contamination	6
Topical	5
Magic Markers	1
Make-up	1
Marijuana	9
Model Cement	9
Modeling Clay	1
Morphine	7
Moth Balls	2
Mushrooms	9
Nail Polish	2
Nail Polish Remover	9
Narcotics	7
Natural Gas	9
Nicotine	2
Oil of Wintergreen	2
Opium	7
Oven Cleaner	
Ingestion	4
Eye Contamination	6
Topical	5
Inhalation if mixed with bleach	8
Paint	
Acrylic	1
Latex	1
Lead Base	2, 7
Oil Base	2
Paint Chips	2, 7
Paint Thinner	9
PCP (Phencyclidine)	2
Pencils	1
Perfume	1
Permanent Wave Solution	
Ingestion	4
Eye Contamination	6
Peroxide (Hydrogen 3%)	1
Pesticides	
Ingestion	9
Topical	5
Petroleum Distillates	9
Phencyclidine	2
Phenothiazines	2
Pine Oil	9
Plants	1
Polishes	2
Pre-washes	9
Silica Gel	1
Sleep Aids	9
Snake Bite	9
Soaps	9
Soldering Flux	4
Spider Bite	9
Starch, Washing	1
Street Speed	2
Strychnine	9
Sulfuric Acid	
Ingestion	4
Eye Contamination	6
Topical	5
Inhalation if mixed with bleach	8
Sun Tan Preparation	9
Swimming Pool Chemicals	4
Talc	
Ingestion	1
Inhalation	9
Tear Gas	8
Teething Rings	1
Thyroid Preparations	9
Thermometers (All types)	1
Theophylline	2
Toilet Bowl Cleaner	
Ingestion	4
Eye Contamination	6
Toilet Water	
Less than 15 ml	1
More than 15 ml	2
Toothpaste	1
Toys, Fluid Filled	9
Tranquilizers	2
Tricyclic Antidepressants	2

Poisoning Substance Index and Treatment Codes

Substance	Treatment
Antiseptics	9
Appetite Suppressants	2
Aquarium Products	9
Arsenic	2, 7
Aspirin	2
Baby Oil	1
Ball Point Ink	1
Barbiturates	2
Bar Soap	1
Bathroom Bowl Cleaner	
Ingestion	4
Eye Contamination	6
Inhalation if mixed with bleach	8
Topical	5
Clay	1
Cleaning Fluids	9
Cleanser (household)	1
Cocaine	9
Codeine	2, 7
Cold Remedies	9
Cologne	
Less than 15 ml	1
More than 15 ml	2
Contraceptive Pills	1
Corn-Wart Removers	4
Cosmetics	See Specific Type
Cough Medicines	9
Crayons	
Children's	8
Others	5
Cyanide	7
Eye Make-up	1
Fabric Softeners	9
Fertilizers	9
Fish Bowl Additives	9
Fluoride, Sodium	1
Food Poisoning	3
Furniture Polish	9
Gas (Natural)	8
Gasoline	9
Glue	9
Gun Products	9
Hair Dyes	
Ingestion	9
Eye Contamination	6
Topical	5
Markers	
Indelible	2
Water Soluble	1
Matches	
Less than 12 wood or 20 paper	1
More than the above	2
Mercurochrome	9
Mercury	
Metallic (Thermometer)	8
Salts	2, 7
Metal Cleaners	9
Methadone	7
Merthiolate	9
Methyl Alcohol	2, 7
Methyl Salicylate	2
Mineral Oil	1
Printer's Ink	9
Putty	1
Rodenticides	9
Rubbing Alcohol	
Ingestion	1
Eye Contamination	6
Sachet	1
Sedatives	9
Shampoo	
Ingestion	1
Eye Contamination	6
Shaving Cream	1
Shaving Lotion	
Less than 15 ml	1
More than 15 ml	2
Shoe Dyes	9
Shoe Polish	1
Tub and Tile Cleaner	1
Turpentine	9
Typewriter Cleaners	9
Varnish	9
Vitamins	
Water Soluble	1
Fat Soluble	2
With Iron	2, 7
With Other Minerals	9
With Sodium Fluoride	9
Wart Removers	4
Weed Killers	9
Window Cleaner	9
Windshield Washer Fluid	2, 7
Wood Preservatives	4

Suggested General Treatment for Poisoning Management

1. Dilute with water. (Call Poison Center for further information.)

2. Prevent absorption of the substance. The method used to prevent the absorption of a substance is dependent upon . . . the clinical condition of the patient . . . pre-existing medical problems . . . amount and substance ingested . . . and the time since ingestion.

   The treatment modalities listed below can be used alone or in combination depending upon the Poison Center's recommendation.

   Induce Vomiting: Give Syrup of Ipecac in the following dosages:

   Under Five Years of age:
   One measuring tablespoonful (15 ml) followed by a minimum of 5 to 10 ounces of clear liquid, preferably water. (Avoid milk.)

   Over Five Years of Age:
   Two measuring tablespoonfuls (30 ml) followed by a minimum of 8 to 16 ounces of clear liquid, preferably water. (Avoid Milk.)

   DO NOT INDUCE VOMITING IF THE PATIENT HAS A DECREASED LEVEL OF CONSCIOUSNESS, IS COMATOSE, OR IS CONVULSING.

   Gastric Lavage may be indicated for the comatose patient or if Syrup of Ipecac fails to induce vomiting.

   THE POISON CENTER may recommend that the adsorbent, ACTIVATED CHARCOAL, be administered after vomiting has been induced. (DO NOT give prior to the use of Syrup of Ipecac.)

   The following doses are recommended:
   Children: 25–50 grams
   Adults: 50–100 grams

   To prepare an activated charcoal slurry from powder, add 30 ml of tap water for every 10 grams of activated charcoal into a jar, cover tightly, and shake the jar vigorously for at least 30 seconds. There are premixed activated charcoal slurries available commercially. Call Poison Center for specific information.

3. Treat symptomatically unless botulism is suspected. Call Poison Center for specific information.

4. Dilute with water, DO NOT INDUCE VOMITING. Gastric lavage should be avoided. This substance may cause burns of the mucous membranes. Call Poison Center for specific information. Consult ENT specialist following emergency treatment.

5. Immediately wash skin thoroughly with a gentle stream of running water. Call Poison Center for further treatment.

6. Immediately wash eyes with a gentle stream of tepid running water. Continue for 15 minutes. Call Poison Center for further treatment.

7. Specific antagonist may be indicated. Call Poison Center for specific information.

8. Remove to fresh air. Support respirations. Call Poison Center for further treatment.

9. Call Poison Center for specific instructions.

Most important in the management of all poisoning emergencies is to support the patient's vital functions. After the patient is stabilized, the Poison Center should be consulted immediately. The treatment chart was designed to provide guidelines and recommendations when an emergent situation necessitates initial treatment be given before a Poison Center can be contacted. The chart obviously addresses acute poisonings only, and recommendations listed are not absolute.

the test influence the child's treatment? Will the test affect the child's disposition or prognosis? Are there impending medico-legal consequences? Is academic interest the only motivating factor for the assay?

A representative, but certainly not inclusive, list of toxins that require a specific quantified level include acetaminophen, carbon monoxide, digoxin, ethylene glycol, iron, lithium, methanol, methemoglobin, and theophylline.

TRIAGE
Poisoning

Emergent
A child with known or suspected ingestion with altered level of consciousness; unstable vital signs; or respiratory difficulty. A child who has ingested a potentially toxic amount of a potent drug. A child who has ingested an unknown substance.

Nonurgent
A child who has ingested a nontoxic substance.

Nursing Diagnosis
Ineffective Airway Clearance

Defining Characteristics

- Change in rate or depth of respiration
- Abnormal breath sounds

Nursing Interventions

- Assess and support airway continually
- Insert oropharyngeal airway in unconscious patient.
- Perform oropharyngeal suctioning as necessary
- Assist in endotracheal intubation if indicated

Expected Outcomes

- Airway remains patent
- Respiratory rate and pattern are normal

Nursing Diagnosis
Ineffective Breathing Pattern

Defining Characteristics

- Abnormal blood gas values
- Tachypnea

- Dyspnea
- Pallor or cyanosis

Nursing Interventions

- Assess and support breathing continually
- Artificially ventilate patient as needed
- Monitor arterial blood gas values
- Interrupt absorption of toxic substance
- Administer antidote
- Carefully monitor vital signs

Expected Outcomes

- Respirations are adequate to provide oxygenation
- Blood gas values are normal
- Color is pink
- Toxic substance is removed or absorption is slowed
- Vital signs are stable

Nursing Diagnosis
Knowledge Deficit (Child Safety)

Defining Characteristics

- Failure to provide child safe environment
- Verbalization of lack of knowledge related to child safety

Nursing Interventions

- Teach parents ways to provide a safe environment for the child
- Encourage practices that decrease the chances of accidental poisoning
- Instruct parents to notify their poison control center when ingestions occur
- Instruct parents to keep ipecac syrup in home but use only when instructed

Expected Outcomes

- Parents provide a safe environment for the child
- The child does not have exposure to poisonous substances in future
- Parents keep phone number of poison control center at ready access

MANAGEMENT

Approximately 80% of all poisonings result from ingestions. Table 22–2 provides the suggested general treatment for management of a poisoning. After the patient's condition is stabilized, the next step is to determine if gastric decontamination is necessary and, if so, what technique should be used to prevent further absorption of the ingested toxin (Krenzelok and Dunmire, 1992).

Gastric Decontamination Procedures

There is no one right method or combination of methods for decreasing systemic absorption of ingested poisons for all patients. Each child must be considered individually in terms of the ingestant, the clinical presentation, and available resources to determine the optimal treatment regimen. It is important for the nurse to use the consultation resources of a clinical toxicologist and the staff of certified specialists at a regional poison center. These professionals help clarify difficult or questionable cases and assist with treatment recommendations.

Syrup of Ipecac. Emesis induced by syrup of ipecac is the most frequently used method of gastric emptying in poisoning emergencies (Krenzelok, 1988). Ipecac is safe, is effective, acts rapidly, is inexpensive, and is readily available as an over-the-counter medication. It is frequently recommended by the professional poison center staff to facilitate gastric emptying in children who have ingested toxins of mild to moderate toxic potential. It is most frequently used in the home a short time after a poisoning incident.

The emetic action of syrup of ipecac is produced by the alkaloids emetine and cephaline, which are derived plants (Abdallah and Tye, 1967). Ipecac produces emesis primarily through a peripheral gastric irritant mechanism and secondarily through central stimulation of the medullary chemoreceptor trigger zone (Boxer et al, 1969).

Syrup of ipecac is an extremely effective emetic. If ipecac is used properly, emesis should occur within 15–20 minutes (Dean and Krenzelok, 1985). Ipecac is administered orally and followed by 6–12 ounces of clear fluids. The standard dose of 30 ml is recommended for children 12 months of age and older as well as for adolescents and adults (Dean and Krenzelok, 1985). For children younger than 1 year, ipecac should be administered cautiously. Ipecac syrup should not be given to children younger than 6 months because vomiting precludes the possiblity of sufficient airway protection and places the infant at great risk for aspiration (Krenzelok and Dean, 1985).

Absolute contraindications to the use of syrup of ipecac include (1) a decreased level of consciousness because of the risk of aspiration, (2) the ingestion of a corrosive substance such as an acid or an alkali that could result in oral, esophageal, or gastric erosion or perforation, and (3) the ingestion of drugs that result in rapid clinical deterioration in children (cyclic antidepressants, calcium channel blockers, clonidine HCl).

Gastric Lavage. Properly performed gastric lavage is superior to ipecac-induced emesis in poisonings with serious toxic potential, such as a rapid decrease in the level of consciousness, seizures, central nervous system depression, or respiratory depression. The child should be positioned in the left lateral recumbent position with the head lowered approximately 10° in the Trendelenburg position. A 16F–32F orogastric tube is used for children. Typically, a passive lavage system can be used. For pediatric patients, the 10 mL/kg of lavage solution is used (Rodgers and Matyunas, 1986). The lavage solution is retrieved either by suction or by lowering the tube to the floor and siphoning out the effluent (Rudolph, 1985). Warm lavage solution is recommended because it can increase the rate of dissolution of pills while decreasing gastric peristalsis, thereby decreasing the potential loss of medication through the pylorus (McDougal and Maclean, 1981). Lavage is performed until there is a clear return. Activated charcoal (1 g/kg in infants and 25–50 g in children older than 12 months) should be instilled in the orogastric tube after gastric lavage (Krenzelok and Dunmire, 1992).

Whole Bowel Irrigation. Whole bowel irrigation (WBI) is the latest technique proposed to decrease systemic absorption of some ingested poisons such as iron pills (Tenenbein, 1985). Whole bowel irrigation involves the administration through an oral or gastric tube of large volumes of a hypertonic, nonabsorbable polyethylene glycol electrolyte solution with the resultant induction of an osmotic catharsis (Postuma, 1988). Administration of 1–2 L of polyethylene glycol electrolyte solution per hour is recommended for children older than 5 years. Administration rates of 150–500 mL/hour have been used for children younger than 5 years. The highly osmotic solution is administered until the rectal discharge has the same appearance as the ingested fluid; this may take 6–10 hours. Adverse effects include abdominal cramping, vomiting, profuse diarrhea, and hyperchloremia (Burkhart et al, 1990; Mann et al, 1989; Postuma, 1988).

TABLE 22–3. RECOMMENDED ANTIDOTES

Drug/Toxin	Antidote
Acetaminophen	N-Acetylcysteine
Beta-adrenergic blockers	Glucagon
Carbon monoxide	Oxygen
Cardiac glycosides	Digoxin immune Fab
Ethylene glycol	Ethyl alcohol
Iron	Deferoxamine
Methyl alcohol	Ethyl alcohol
Methemoglobinemia	Methylene blue
Narcotics	Naloxone

Fab, fragment, antigen-binding

TABLE 22–4. AMERICAN ASSOCIATION OF POISON CONTROL CENTERS CERTIFIED REGIONAL POISON CENTERS, APRIL 1993

■ ALABAMA
Regional Poison Control Center
The Children's Hospital
   of Alabama
1600 7th Ave. South
Birmingham AL 35233-1711
Emergency Phone: (205) 939-9201,
   (800) 292-6678 (AL only) or
   (205) 933-4050

■ ARIZONA
Arizona Poison and Drug
   Information Center
Arizona Health and Sciences Center;
   Rm. #3204-K
1501 N. Campbell Ave.
Tucson AZ 85724
Emergency Phone: (800) 362-0101,
   (AZ only) (602) 626-6016

Samaritan Regional Poison Center
Good Samaritan Regional
   Medical Center
1130 E. McDowell,
Suite A-5
Phoenix AZ 85006
Emergency Phone: (602) 253-3334

■ CALIFORNIA
Fresno Regional Poison Control Center
   of Fresno Community Hospital
   and Medical Center
2823 Fresno Street
Fresno CA 93721
Emergency Phone: (800) 346-5922 or
   (209) 445-1222

San Diego Regional Poison Center
UCSD Medical Center; 8925
225 Dickinson St.
San Diego CA 92103-8925
Emergency Phone: (619) 543-6000,
   (800) 876-4766 (in 619 area code only)

San Francisco Bay Area
   Regional Poison Control Center
San Francisco General Hospital
1001 Potrero Ave., Building 80,
   Room 230
San Francisco CA 94122
Emergency Phone: (415) 476-6600

Santa Clara Valley Medical Center
   Regional Poison Center
751 South Bascom Ave.
San Jose CA 95128
Emergency Phone: (408) 299-5112,
   (800) 662-9886 (CA only)

■ CALIFORNIA (*continued*)
University of California, Davis,
   Medical Center Regional Poison
   Control Center
2315 Stockton Blvd
Sacramento CA 95817
Emergency Phone: (916) 734-3692;
   (800) 342-9293 (Northern
   California only)

■ COLORADO
Rocky Mountain Poison and
   Drug Center
645 Bannock St.
Denver CO 80204
Emergency Phone: (303) 629-1123

■ WASHINGTON DC
National Capital Poison Center
Georgetown University Hospital
3800 Reservoir Rd., NW
Washington, DC 20007
Emergency Numbers: (202) 625-3333,
   (202) 784-4660 (TTY)

■ FLORIDA
The Florida Poison Information
   Center at Tampa
   General Hospital
Post Office Box 1289
Tampa FL 33601
Emergency Phone: (813) 253-4444
   (Tampa), (800) 282-3171 (Florida)

■ GEORGIA
Georgia Poison Center
Grady Memorial Hospital
80 Butler Street S.E.
P.O. Box 26066
Atlanta GA 30335-3801
Emergency Phone: (800) 282-5846
   GA only, (404) 589-4400

■ INDIANA
Indiana Poison Center
Methodist Hospital of Indiana
1701 N. Senate Boulevard
P.O. Box 1367
Indianapolis IN 46206-1367
Emergency Phone: (800) 382-9097
   (IN only), (317) 929-2323

■ MARYLAND
Maryland Poison Center
20 N. Pine St.
Baltimore MD 21201
Emergency Phone: (410) 528-7701,
   (800) 492-2414 (MD only)

National Capital Poison Center
   (D.C. suburbs only)
Georgetown University Hospital
3800 Reservoir Rd., NW
Washington, DC 20007
Emergency Numbers: (202) 625-3333,
   (202) 784-4660 (TTY)

■ MASSACHUSETTS
Massachusetts Poison Control System
300 Longwood Ave.
Boston MA 02115
Emergency Phone: (617) 232-2120,
   (800) 682-9211

■ MICHIGAN
Blodgett Regional Poison Center
1840 Wealthy S.E.
Grand Rapids MI 49506-2968
Emergency Phone: (800) 632-2727
   (Michigan only), TTY (800) 356-3232

Poison Control Center
Children's Hospital of Michigan
3901 Beaubien Blvd.
Detroit MI 48201
Emergency Phone: (313) 745-5711

■ MINNESOTA
Hennepin Regional Poison Center
Hennepin County Medical Center
701 Park Ave.
Minneapolis MN 55415
Emergency Phone: (612) 347-3141,
Petline: (612) 337-7387,
TDD (612) 337-7474

Minnesota Regional Poison Center
St. Paul-Ramsey Medical Center
640 Jackson St.
St. Paul MN 55101
Emergency Phone: (612) 221-2113

■ MISSOURI
Cardinal Glennon Children's Hospital
   Regional Poison Center
1465 S. Grand Blvd.
St. Louis MO 63104
Emergency Phone: (314) 772-5200,
   (800) 366-8888

(*continued*)

TABLE 22–4. *(Continued)*

■ MONTANA
**Rocky Mountain Poison and
    Drug Center**
645 Bannock St.
Denver CO 80204
Emergency Phone: (303) 629-1123

■ NEBRASKA
The Poison Center
8301 Dodge St.
Omaha NE 68114
Emergency Phone: (402) 390-5555
    (Omaha), (800) 955-9119 (NE)

■ NEW JERSEY
**New Jersey Poison Information
    and Education System**
201 Lyons Ave.
Newark NJ 07112
Emergency Phone: (800) 962-1253

■ NEW MEXICO
**New Mexico Poison and Drug
    Information Center**
University of New Mexico
Albuquerque NM 87131-1076
Emergency Phone: (505) 843-2551,
    (800) 432-6866 (NM only)

■ NEW YORK
Hudson Valley Poison Center
Nyack Hospital
160 N. Midland Ave.
Nyack NY 10960
Emergency Phone: (800) 336-6997,
    (914) 353-1000
**Long Island Regional Poison
    Control Center**
Winthrop University Hospital
259 First Street
Mineola NY 11501
Emergency Phone: (516) 542-2323,
    2324, 2325, 3813
New York City Poison Control Center
N.Y.C. Department of Health
455 First Ave., Room 123
New York NY 10016
Emergency Phone: (212) 340-4494,
    (212) P-O-I-S-O-N-S,
    TDD (212) 689-9014

■ OHIO
Central Ohio Poison Center
700 Children's Drive
Columbus OH 43205-2696
Emergency Phone: (614) 228-1323,
    (800) 682-7625, (614) 228-2272
    (TTY), (614) 461-2012

**Cincinnati Drug & Poison
    Information Center and
    Regional Poison
    Control System**
231 Bethesda Avenue, M.L. 144
Cincinnati OH 45267-0144
Emergency Phone: (513) 558-5111,
    800-872-5111 (OH only)

■ OREGON
Oregon Poison Center
Oregon Health Sciences University
3183 S.W. Sam Jackson Park Road
Portland OR 97201
Emergency Phone: (503) 494-8968,
    (800) 452-7165 (OR only)

■ PENNSYLVANIA
**Central Pennsylvania Poison
    Center**
University Hospital
Milton S. Hershey Medical Center
Hershey PA 17033
Emergency Phone: (800) 521-6110

**The Poison Control Center serving
    the greater Philadelphia
    metropolitan area**
One Children's Center
Philadelphia PA 19104-4303
Emergency Phone: (215) 386-2100

Pittsburgh Poison Center
3705 Fifth Ave. @ DeSoto St.
Pittsburgh PA 15213
Emergency Phone: (412) 681-6669

■ RHODE ISLAND
Rhode Island Poison Center
593 Eddy St.
Providence RI 02903
Emergency Phone: (401) 277-5727

■ TEXAS
North Texas Poison Center
5201 Harry Hines Blvd.
P.O. Box 35926
Dallas TX 75235
Emergency Phone: (214) 590-5000,
    Texas Watts (800) 441-0040
Texas State Poison Center
The University of Texas Medical Branch
Galveston TX 77550-2780
Emergency Phone: (409) 765-1420,
    (Galveston), (713) 654-1702
    (Houston)

■ UTAH
**Intermountain Regional Poison
    Control Center**
50 North Medical Drive
Salt Lake City UT 84132
Emergency Phone: (801) 581-2151,
    (800) 456-7707 (UT only)

■ VIRGINIA
Blue Ridge Poison Center
Box 67
Blue Ridge Hospital
Charlottesville VA 22901
Emergency Phone: (804) 924-5543,
    (800) 451-1428

**National Capital Poison Center
    (Northern VA only)**
Georgetown University Hospital
3800 Reservoir Rd., NW
Washington, DC 20007
Emergency Numbers: (202) 625-3333,
    (202) 784-4660 (TTY)

■ WEST VIRGINIA
West Virginia Poison Center
3110 MacCorkle Ave. S.E.
Charleston WV 25304
Emergency Phone: (800) 642-3625
    (WV only), (304) 348-4211

■ WYOMING
The Poison Center
8301 Dodge St.
Omaha NE 68114
Emergency Phone: (402) 390-5555
    (Omaha), (800) 955-9119 (NE)

Activated Charcoal. Because gastric emptying techniques do not completely evacuate the stomach, other measures must be undertaken to prevent absorption of the remaining toxin. Activated charcoal is an excellent adsorbent and is customarily used for this purpose. Activated charcoal is the residue remaining after the pyrolysis of a variety of organic materials, such as wood pulp. The activation process cleans and fragments the charcoal by exposing it to an oxidizing gas of steam, oxygen, and acids at temperatures exceeding 500°F. The process not only cleans the charcoal but also increases its surface area by creating a network of external and internal pores that serve as reservoirs for the adsorption of ingested toxins (Neuvonen et al, 1983).

Activated charcoal is used alone or as an adjunct in the management of many types of oral poisoning. Inorganic and organic substances with a molecular weight of 100–1000 are most effectively adsorbed by activated charcoal (Cooney, 1980).

Activated charcoal should be administered as soon as possible. Adsorption or binding of a toxin to activated charcoal can occur anywhere in the gastrointestinal (GI) tract. The longer the delay between ingestion of the poison and administration of the activated charcoal, the less effective the charcoal is in binding the toxin. If gastric lavage is the method of gastric decontamination, activated charcoal can be administered before and after the lavage procedure.

An infant dose of 1 mg/kg has been established. Children should receive 25–50 g. The charcoal is prepared as an aqueous slurry. Many commercial products are available that contain 25–50 g of activated charcoal and require only that the nurse vigorously shake the container before administering the charcoal. These prepared activated charcoal products are also available with sorbitol. The addition of sorbitol gives the product a sweet taste and a smooth texture. Sorbitol also serves as a cathartic to assist in the passage of the toxin-activated charcoal complex. Commercial products must be cautiously used in young children because the amount of sorbitol is fixed and may produce severe diarrhea (Krenzelok and Dunmire, 1992).

Although activated charcoal has traditionally been used in a single dose to manage acute poisoning ingestions, multiple-dose activated charcoal is now being used in some overdoses. The primary application is in patients who have ingested toxins that are enterohepatically circulated. Repetitive doses of charcoal bind toxin that is being secreted in biliary secretions and prevent reabsorption of the toxin.

Although still controversial, the use of activated charcoal without concurrent gastric emptying may be indicated (Albertson et al, 1989; Kulig et al, 1985; Neuvonen et al, 1983). Research has shown that the administration of activated charcoal is as effective as gastric emptying in certain toxic situations (Albertson et al, 1989; Kulig et al, 1985).

Because activated charcoal does not bind toxins irreversibly, it is important to hasten the elimination of the toxin-charcoal complex through the GI tract with an osmotic cathartic (Krenzelok and Dunmire, 1992). Sorbitol produces the most rapid cathartic effect; however, it should be used cautiously in children because it can produce considerable fluid and electrolyte losses (Krenzelok and Dunmire, 1992).

Methods of Enhancing Drug Excretion

The elimination of certain drugs from the body can be aided by certain pharmacokinetic agents that effect drug excretion (Arena, 1970). The action of high-molecular weight polar compounds can be diminished because these drugs are reabsorbed into the stomach or intestine through the biliary system. Interruption of this pathway facilitates fecal elimination of the toxin. Activated charcoal binds drugs in the GI tract that are "enterohepatically recycled" (Park et al, 1986). Nonionizing drugs and poisons dissolved in the blood are able to diffuse across GI membranes by passive diffusion and are effectively removed by multiple doses of activated charcoal. A toxin whose excretion may be enhanced by multiple-dose activated charcoal must have a small volume of distribution, must be extensively bound to plasma proteins or other blood components, must be lipophilic, or must undergo enterohepatic circulation (Park et al, 1986).

Hemodialysis and hemoperfusion are extracorporeal methods of enhancing elimination of toxins in certain cases of severe poisoning. These procedures require an extracorporeal chamber through which blood is passed over a membrane dialyzer, a bed of charcoal, or a synthetic resin (Park et al, 1986). The advantages and disadvantages of extracorporeal means of toxin removal are related not to technology but to the chemical and pharmocologic characteristics of the poison that limit the role of these procedures. Specific toxins for which hemodialysis may be extremely efficacious include methanol, ethylene glycol, salicylates, phenobarbital, lithium, and isopropanol. Hemoperfusion can achieve increased clearance with substances such as amanita mushrooms, digitoxin and digoxin, gyromitra mushrooms, ethchlorvynol, paraquat, and theophylline.

Administration of an Antidote

The purpose of antidotal therapy is to reduce toxicity by either inhibiting the translocation of the toxin to the effector site or reducing toxin concentration or action at the effector site (Loomis, 1973). Use of an antidote is rarely the essence of the treatment of a poisoned child.

Although a number of specific antidotes are available, their use should not take the place of good general supportive measures. Consulting the local regional poison center can provide contemporary toxicologic information and management advice about when and how to use specific pharmacologic antidotes. A list of available antidotes is given in Table 22–3.

As in all medical emergencies, good supportive care is the cornerstone of managing an acute pediatric poisoning. Aggressive support of the cardiovascular, respiratory, and central nervous systems, along with appropriate gastric decontamination, greatly reduces morbidity and mortality and improves the child's ultimate outcome.

PATIENT AND FAMILY TEACHING AND PSYCHOSOCIAL SUPPORT

Nurses and other health educators can provide an adult caregiver with the following suggestions aimed at reducing the incidence of childhood poisoning.

Prevention of Childhood Poisoning

- Store all medications in a locked cabinet, out of a child's reach. Use child-resistant containers for all prescription and over-the-counter drugs. Never introduce medications to a child by comparing them to candy.
- Discard household cleaning products that are no longer used by wrapping them completely before placing them in the garbage.
- Keep all items in their original containers. Return all containers to their locked cabinet after use.
- Never mix chemicals such as household bleaches with toilet bowel cleaners or ammonia.
- Have the telephone number of the local regional poison center posted on the telephone (Table 22–4). Call this number immediately if you believe a poisoning has occurred.

REFERENCES

Abdallah AH, Tye A (1967). A comparison of the efficacy of emetic drugs and stomach lavage. *American Journal of Diseases of Children* 113:571–575

Albertson TE, Derlet RW, Goulke GE, et al (1989). Superiority of activated charcoal alone compared with ipecac and activated charcoal in the treatment of acute toxic ingestions. *Annals of Emergency Medicine* 18:56–59

Arena J (1970). The clinical diagnosis of poisoning. *Pediatric Clinics of North America* 17:477–494

Atwood S (1980). The laboratory in the diagnosis and management of acetaminophen and salicylate intoxications. *Pediatric Clinics of North America* 27:871–879

Boxer L, Anderson FP, Rowe DS (1969). Comparison of ipecac-induced emesis with gastric lavage in the treatment of acute salicylate ingestion. *Journal of Pediatrics* 74:800–803

Burkhart KK, Kulig KW, Rumack B (1990). Whole-bowel irrigation as treatment for zinc sulfate overdose. *Annals of Emergency Medicine* 19:1167

Cooney DO (1980). *Activated charcoal.* New York: Marcel Dekker

Dean BS, Krenzelok EP (1985). Syrup of ipecac: 15 vs 30 ml in pediatric poisonings. *Clinical Toxicology* 23:165–170

Krenzelok EP (1988). Ipecac vs lavage: Pros and cons. *Critical Decisions in Emergency Medicine* 3:1–8

Krenzelok EP, Dean BS (1985). Syrup of ipecac in children less than one year of age. *Clinical Toxicology* 23:171–176

Krenzelok EP, Dunmire SM (1992). Acute poisoning emergencies: Resolving the gastric decontamination controversy. *Postgraduate Medicine* 91:179–186

Kulig K, Bar-Or D, Cantrill SV, et al (1985). Management of acutely poisoned patients without gastric emptying. *Annals of Emergency Medicine* 14:562–567

Litovitz TL, Manoguerra AS (1992). Comparison of pediatric poisoning hazards: An analysis of 3.8 million exposure incidents. *Pediatrics* 89:999–1006

Loomis TA (1973). *Essentials of toxicology* (3rd ed). Philadelphia: Lea and Febiger

Mann KV, Picciotti MA, Spevack TA, et al (1989). Management of acute iron overdose. *Clinical Pharmacy* 8:428

McDougal C, Maclean M (1981). Modification in the technique of gastric lavage. *Annals of Emergency Medicine* 10:514–517

Neuvonen P, Vartiainen M, Tokola O (1983). Comparison of activated charcoal and ipecac syrup in prevention of drug absorption. *European Journal of Clinical Pharmacology* 24: 557–562

Park G, Spector R, Goldberg M, et al (1986). Expanded role of charcoal therapy in the poisoned and overdosed patient. *Archives of Internal Medicine* 146:969–973

Postuma R (1988). Whole bowel irrigation in pediatric patients: A comparison of irrigating solutions. *Journal of Pediatric Surgery* 23:769

Rodgers G, Matyunas N (1986). Gastrointestinal decontamination for acute poisoning. *Pediatric Clinics of North America* 33:261–285

Rudolph J (1985). Automated gastric lavage and a comparison of 0.9% normal saline solution and tap water irrigant. *Annals of Emergency Medicine* 14:1156–1159

Tenenbein M (1985). Inefficacy of gastric emptying procedures. *Journal of Emergency Medicine* 3:133–136

PART 5

Medical Emergencies

CHAPTER 23

Ear, Nose, and Throat Disorders

PATRICIA KRAEPELIEN-BARTELS

INTRODUCTION

Ear, nose, and throat (ENT) complaints account for frequent visits to pediatric emergency departments (EDs). Complaints of fever, earache, upper respiratory infection (URI), or sore throat accounted for 25% of visits to both general and pediatric tertiary care EDs in two studies. Minor trauma, including ENT trauma, accounted for 22% of total diagnoses in a tertiary pediatric ED and 42% in a general ED (Krauss et al, 1991; Nelson et al, 1992).

OTITIS

Otitis is inflammation of the structures of the ear (Figure 23–1). It is usually associated with pain. Acute otitis media, one of the most common illnesses in infants and toddlers, affects almost all children during the first years of life; the peak incidence is 7–9 months of age (Teele, 1992). Ear pain may be caused by a bacterial infection in the middle ear (otitis media), by infection of the tympanic membrane (TM) itself (bullous myringitis), or by pressure and bleeding within the middle ear space (aerotitis media).

Etiology and Pathophysiology

Otitis media is inflammation of the middle ear. It is usually associated with antecedent events, such as an URI or respiratory allergy. The mucous membranes of the middle ear and mastoid process are continuous with those of the nasopharynx via the eustachian tube. Congestion of the mucous membranes causes obstruction of the narrowest portion of the eustachian tube,

and secretions of the middle ear have no egress and accumulate. This effusion may be serous, mucoid, or purulent. Microbial pathogens may be present in this effusion, or may come from reflux or aspiration from the nasopharynx up the eustachian tube and into the middle ear. The usual pathogens in otitis media are *Streptococcus pneumoniae, Moraxella catarrhalis,* and *Haemophilus influenzae;* there also has been a rise in beta-lactamase-producing strains of influenza (Bluestone et al, 1992).

Anatomic or physiologic abnormalities of the eustachian tube are important factors in otitis media. Inflammation due to an allergy may cause intrinsic mechanical obstruction of the eustachian tube. In infants, the eustachian tube is shorter and more horizontal than in older children, increasing the likelihood of

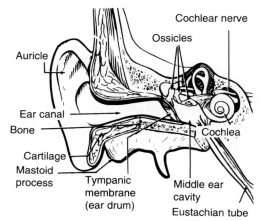

Figure 23–1. Ear canal, middle ear, and inner ear. (From Rudy EB, Gray VR [1986]. *Handbook of health assessment* (2nd ed). Norwalk, Conn: Appleton & Lange, p 79)

otitis media secondary to URI. Other factors in eustachian tube dysfunction include ciliary dyskinesia, immunologic syndromes, and mucous membrane irritation from environmental pollutants such as woodstoves and cigarette smoke. Otitis media with effusion is almost always present in unrepaired cleft palate (Bluestone and Klein, 1988). Otitis occurs more often in winter than in summer. The hematologic spread of bacteria to the middle ear may cause otitis media, but this is uncommon (Schutzman et al, 1991).

For children infected with the human immunodeficiency virus (HIV), the causative agents are similar to those for children without the virus. In recurrent otitis media, the presence of a nasopharyngeal mass should be suspected (Lucente, 1991).

Bullous myringitis is believed to be a viral infection of the TM. It causes swelling and vesiculation. As secondary bacterial infection often results, an antibiotic treatment is usually prescribed.

Aerotitis media occurs with sudden pressure changes, as in scuba diving and airplane descents, that cause the TM to stretch. Capillaries rupture within the middle ear space, causing painful hematotympanum and hearing loss due to a decrease in sound conduction.

In *perforation of the TM*, there is usually unilateral otorrhea. After carefully wicking or suctioning drainage from the external canal, one may see the perforation of the TM. Perforation of the TM and drainage of serous or purulent material may be associated with an acute otitis. The perforation releases pressure and pain, and drainage through the eustachian tube may improve. Perforation usually heals within 1 week, and cultures usually show the same pathogens as acute otitis media. Spontaneous perforation occurs with almost every case of otitis media in native Alaskan and American Indian infants and children (Bluestone and Klein, 1988). A draining ear may signal otitis externa. However, otitis externa usually does not have an antecedent URI and fever.

History

The history includes antecedent URI with fever, or allergic disease. Symptoms of otalgia and hearing loss are usually elicited. The patient and family should be asked about previous ear infections. Infants may have a fever, be fussy, pull at or slap their ears and head, and have loose stools.

Physical Assessment

The physical findings include reduced mobility and dull erythema or injection of the TM, which may be bulging (obscuring bony landmarks) or severely retracted. Tympanometry reveals decreased impedance. If perforation has occurred, ear drainage may be seen.

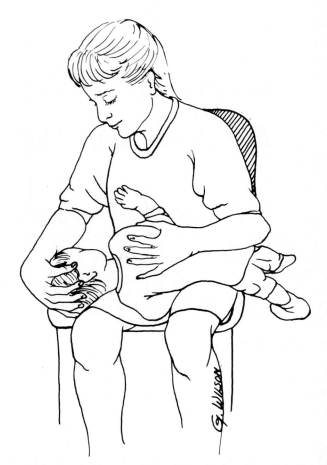

Figure 23–2. Mother using lap position of infant for examination of the infant's ear.

The infant or child should be assessed for signs of respiratory infection and sepsis, and the child's level of activity should be noted.

Figure 23–2 indicates how the caretaker should hold an infant during an otoscopic examination. Figure 23–3 illustrates how a toddler can be held.

In *bullous myringitis*, the history includes sudden onset of intense otalgia with a mild hearing loss. Physical assessment shows small, amber-colored bullous lesions of the TM.

In *aerotitis*, there is a history of recent barotrauma to the ear with sudden onset of pain and hearing loss. Physical assessment reveals the TM to be hemorrhagic and purple, dark blue, or almost black. Tympanometry shows marked impedance.

Laboratory and Diagnostic Tests

If the temperature is higher than 38.4°C and the child is younger than 1 year, a complete blood count (CBC) and blood culture should be ordered for evaluation of sepsis.

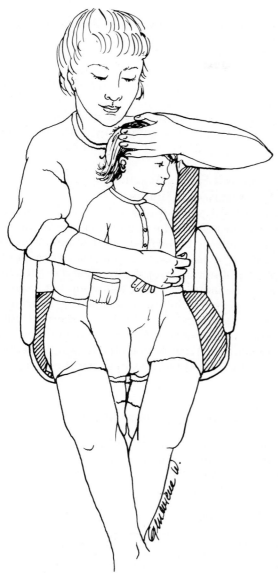

Figure 23–3. Mother assisting in restraining a toddler for examination of the ear.

TRIAGE
Otitis

Emergent ────────────────────
A neonate with fever > 40°C; toxic appearance with meningeal signs (see Chapter 26).

Urgent ─────────────────────
An infant with fever > 39.5°C; otalgia; expiratory wheezing.

Non-urgent ──────────────────
An infant or child with otalgia; fever; antecedent URI or respiratory allergy; ear drainage; history of recent barotrauma.

Nursing Diagnosis
High Risk for Altered Body Temperature

Defining Characteristics

- Body temperature greater than 37.8°C orally or 38.8°C rectally
- Flushed skin
- Warm skin
- Increased pulse and respirations

Nursing Interventions

- Monitor temperature
- Administer antipyretic as needed
- Assess for signs of dehydration
- Educate parent about temperature taking and temperature control measures

Expected Outcomes

- Patient's temperature is normal
- Parent can explain temperature taking techniques and control measures

Nursing Diagnosis
Pain

Defining Characteristics

- Communication verbal or coded for pain
- Distraction behavior (crying, restlessness, rocking)
- Autonomic response (diaphoresis, blood pressure and pulse change, increased respiratory rate)

Nursing Interventions

- Educate parent about pain management techniques
- Administer analgesics
- Monitor effectiveness of analgesics

Expected Outcomes

- Child exhibits signs of pain relief with interventions
- Parent describes methods of pain management

Nursing Diagnosis
Altered Family Processes

Defining Characteristics

- Verbalization of inability to care for ill child
- Disruption of normal family routines

Nursing Interventions

- Educate parent about illness and therapy

- Assess parental ability to provide therapy
- Provide support services as needed to assist family in providing therapy
- Provide parent with emotional support

Expected Outcomes

- Parent describes therapy.
- Parent vocalizes comfort caring for ill child.
- Parent identifies support services needed to assist family in providing therapy.

Management

Table 23–1 describes the antibiotic medication regimen for otitis media and bullous otitis. If a child has head congestion and a cough, an oral decongestant may be suggested. If the child has known or suspected allergy, an antihistamine may be suggested. However, the efficacy of decongestants or antihistamines in the treatment of otitis itself has not been shown (Mandel et al, 1987; Woolbert, 1990). Analgesic and antipyretic agents are used for a minimum of 48 hours. Local heat to the affected ear may be helpful.

Neonates with *sepsis and otitis* may be hospitalized for parenteral administration of antibiotics. In other types of otitis, they are sent home. The parents are instructed to make an appointment for an ear examination by their primary care provider in 2–3 weeks.

In *perforation*, a combination of antibiotic and steroid otic drops (Table 23–1) may be prescribed. Strict water precautions (no water in the ear or swimming) for 4 weeks must be followed.

In *aerotitis*, all interventions are aimed at improving eustachian tube function to decrease pressure in the middle ear. Decongestant-antihistamine combinations are prescribed. The use of a humidifier is suggested. Aerotitis is prevented by frequent yawning, swallowing, chewing gum, or by pinching the nostrils and gently exhaling into the nasopharynx.

Patient and Family Teaching and Psychosocial Support

Symptoms should subside in 2–3 days. If not, the family should contact the primary care provider or ED. Signs of allergy to the medication should be reviewed. The use of antipyretic and analgesic agents (acetaminophen or ibuprofen) for the first few days of treatment should be emphasized. A follow-up ear examination in 2–3 weeks, including assessment of hearing, is important (Jones et al, 1989). With recurrent otitis, the nurse must acknowledge the patient's and parents' frustration and fear of potential hearing loss or speech delay; they must be reassured that these sequelae are rare.

MASTOIDITIS AND PERIOSTEITIS

Acute mastoiditis occurs in almost every child with acute otitis media because mastoid air cells also are inflamed. Periosteitis occurs when the infection progresses.

TABLE 23–1. EAR, NOSE, AND THROAT ANTIBIOTICS

Medication	Dosage/24 Hours and Frequency	Indications
Amoxicillin	40 mg/kg/day in 3 divided doses	Otitis, rhinitis, sinusitis
Trimethoprim/sulfamethoxazole	8 mg/kg TMP/40 mg SMZ/kg/day in 2 divided doses	Otitis, rhinitis, sinusitis
Erythromycin	40 mg/kg/day in 3 divided doses	Streptococcal infection, bullous myringitis
Erythromycin 200 mg/sulfisoxazole 600 mg/5cc	40 mg/120 mg/kg/day in 3 divided doses	Otitis, rhinitis sinusitis
Amoxicillin-clavulanate	40 mg/kg/day in 3 divided doses	Resistant or recurrent otitis, rhinitis, sinusitis
Cephalexin	500 mg tid	Adolescent sinusitis
Cefixime	8 mg/kg/day once daily	Resistant or recurrent otitis
Cefprozil	30 mg/kg bid	Otitis, streptococcal infection
Penicillin V	50 mg/kg/day in 3 divided doses	Streptococcal infection, bullous myringitis Otitis in children older than 6 years
Doxycycline	100 mg bid on day 1, then once a day	Adolescent sinusitis
Otic drops (Cortisporin[a] Otic Suspension) (Cortisporin[a] Otic Solution)	3 drops tid 3 drops tid	Otitis externa (perforation) Otitis externa

[a]Polymyxin B sulfate–neomycin sulfate–hydrocortisone.
(Information from Bluestone, et al, 1992; Durbin, 1992; Jacobs, 1992; Josephson, 1991; Kaban and Jacobs, 1992; Zenk and Ma, 1990)
TMP, trimethoprim; SMZ, sulfamethoxazole.

Etiology and Pathophysiology
Infection in the mastoid air cells spreads to the periosteum covering the mastoid process; the bony trabeculae are destroyed; and an empyema forms.

History
The history includes antecedent otalgia and fever.

Physical Assessment
A physical examination shows signs of otitis media. In addition there is postauricular erythema, tenderness, and slight swelling. There may be swelling or sagging of the posteriorsuperior wall of the ear canal. There also may be purulent otorrhea. The pinna may be displaced inferiorly and anteriorly. There may be fluctuant subperiosteal abscess or a draining fistula from mastoid to postauricular area. The postauricular crease may be lost.

Laboratory and Diagnostic Tests
Computed tomographic findings are abnormal in the area of bony destruction. There are no laboratory tests specific for mastoiditis.

TRIAGE
Mastoiditis and Periosteitis

Urgent —
An infant or child with otitis; evidence of postauricular erythema and pain in the bone.

Non-urgent —
A child with otitis; slight fever; no wheezing.

Nursing Diagnosis
Fear

Defining Characteristics
- Verbalization or demonstration of feelings of apprehension
- Autonomic responses indicative of fear

Nursing Interventions
- Explain admitting procedures to child and parent
- Assess for presence of visceral-somatic activity
- Provide for child's support (parents, special toys from home)

Expected Outcomes
- Child's responses stabilize

- Child and parent explain admitting procedures
- Child exhibits an increase in psychological comfort

Nursing Diagnosis
Pain

The nursing diagnosis for pain in mastoiditis is the same as that for otitis

Nursing Diagnosis
High Risk for Altered Body Temperature

The nursing diagnosis for high risk for altered body temperature in mastoiditis is the same as that for otitis.

Nursing Diagnosis
Parental Role Conflict

Defining Characteristics
- Verbalization of concerns about changes in parenting role
- Verbalization of feelings of anxiety or guilt

Nursing Interventions
- Explain parental visitation policies
- Acknowledge parental role in decision-making during hospitalization

Expected Outcomes
- Parent verbalizes feelings about child's illness and hospitalization
- Parent identifies and uses available support systems

Management
Management of mastoiditis in the ED includes administration of antipyretics and analgesics. Intravenous administration of antibiotics may be initiated in the ED. All children with mastoiditis are admitted to the hospital for myringotomy and parenteral administration of antibiotics.

Patient and Family Teaching and Psychosocial Support
The child and family need to be prepared for hospitalization. They should be informed that hearing returns with proper treatment.

OTITIS EXTERNA

Otitis externa, an inflammation of the lining of the external ear canal, is a common problem in children.

Etiology and Pathophysiology

Otitis externa occurs after prolonged exposure to heat and moisture (eg, swimming, using ear phones), exposure to irritant chemicals, or traumatic injury such as scratches by cotton-tip applicator, bobby pin, or other object. Inflammation and swelling cause pain. *Pseudomonas* is the usual bacterial pathogen (Marcy, 1987). In children who have had positive HIV tests, the usual bacterial or fungal pathogens are suspected. The external canal should be subsequently inspected for masses (Kaposi sarcoma) in adolescent patients. The possibility of pneumocystic infection or severe otomycosis should be considered, and intense, systemic therapy may be necessary (Lucente, 1990).

History

The history usually includes onset of pain with movement of the pinna or tragus and an odorous discharge from the ear. There is often a recent history of swimming or of traumatic injury. There may be hearing loss due to a decrease in sound conduction on the affected side.

Physical Assessment

A physical examination shows an occluded external canal with pain on movement of the tragus and purulent discharge. At times visualization of the TM is not possible.

Laboratory and Diagnostic Tests

A culture of the exudate is not usually obtained.

TRIAGE
Otitis Externa

Urgent

An infant with a temperature higher than 38.4°C; draining ear.

Non-urgent

An infant or child with draining ear; mild fever.

Nursing Diagnosis

Impaired Tissue Integrity

Defining Characteristics

- Disruption of lining of external ear canal
- Erythema
- Pain

Nursing Interventions

- Educate parent about precautions and treatment
- Administer analgesics
- Monitor drainage from ear

Expected Outcomes

- Parent can describe precautions and therapy
- Child does not show characteristics of pain
- Discharge from ear is controlled

Nursing Diagnosis

The nursing diagnosis for pain in otitis externa is the same as that for pain in otitis.

Management

A combination antibiotic-steroid ear drops is prescribed (Table 23–1). If canal lumen has narrowed by 50% or more, rolled cylinder of cotton is inserted to a depth of 1 cm. This aids in penetration of topical medicine; it should be removed 48 hours after insertion. If the lumen is occluded, and if cervical adenopathy is present, the wick also is used for 48 hours. Treatment also includes a 10-day course of systemic antibiotics (eg, penicillin or erythromycin) (Jacobs, 1992). Analgesia should be administered in the ED.

Patient and Family Teaching and Psychosocial Support

Analgesia is used for a minimum of 48 hours. Water precautions (no water in the ears or swimming) are followed for 4 weeks. The parents are taught the proper way to instill ear drops: The child lies on his or her side with the affected ear facing up. The drops are instilled during gentle movement of the pinna. The child then lies still for 2–3 minutes to ensure penetration of the medication into the ear canal.

Prophylactic treatment for swimmers should be taught: Instill 1:1 vinegar-water or 1:1 vinegar-alcohol tid after swimming to decrease the recurrence of swimmer's ear (Marcy, 1987). A hair dryer can be used to dry the inside of the ears.

EAR TRAUMA

Trauma to the ear may occur in a variety of ways—by compression injury, explosion, rupture of the TM causing ossicular discontinuity with sudden sensorineural hearing loss, abrasions, contusions, or lacerations to the pinnae, and head injury with basilar or temporal bone skull fracture.

History

A careful history of the mechanism of injury should be elicited. A history of loss of consciousness or bleeding should be noted. The possibility of child abuse (intentional injury) should be considered during this assessment.

Physical Assessment

Minor Trauma

Minor Blunt Trauma. A hematoma is present on the auricle or pinna. The shearing forces of injury may have separated the auricle from its cartilage. The nurse should inspect for lacerations.

Tympanic Membrane Trauma. Because of blows, blasts, barotrauma, foreign body, or careless attempt at removal of a foreign object, the TM has a defect that is slit-shaped and irregular.

Laceration. The external ear is a delicate skin-cartilage structure due to poor circulation. A laceration that is penetrating or deep may be slow to heal.

Major Trauma

Ossicular Chain Injury. This injury is caused by penetrating trauma, a temporal bone fracture, or a blast. It is characterized by an overly compliant TM on tympanometry and considerable conductive hearing loss. There may be rupture of the TM.

Temporal Bone Fracture. Penetrating or blunt trauma may cause a longitudinal fracture with bleeding from the external canal, conductive hearing loss (TM damage, ossicular disruption, hematotympanum), loss of consciousness, or cerebrospinal fluid (CSF) otorrhea (fluid should be tested for pH and glucose). Post-auricular ecchymosis (Battle sign) may be seen 2–3 days after the fracture. Less often, there is sensorineural hearing loss or dizziness, which is temporary and delayed in onset (Finklestein et al, 1991). Transverse fractures, occurring in 20% of temporal bone fractures, are usually caused by an occipital insult that is much more intense than the cause of a longitudinal fracture. Severe and immediate sensorineural hearing loss occurs with hematotympanum, CSF otorrhea, and total vestibular functional loss. Immediate facial paralysis occurs 50% of the time (Finklestein et al, 1991).

Laboratory and Diagnostic Tests

Hearing acuity and tympanometry may be ordered. For major head and ear trauma computed tomography (CT) and a serum B-2 transferrin level are ordered (McGuirt and Stool, 1992). Blood is differentiated from CSF fluid by observing drop of bloody fluid on filter or tissue paper: spinal fluid has a more rapid diffusion pattern than blood, and concentric rings may be seen (double ring or halo sign).

TRIAGE
Ear Trauma

Emergent ———————————————
An infant or child with skull fracture; loss of consciousness; ecchymosis over mastoid; ear bleeding.

Urgent ———————————————
Infant or child with acute ear trauma, unilateral ear bleeding, unilateral hearing loss, ear laceration.

Nursing Diagnosis
Impaired Tissue Integrity

Defining Characteristics

- Disruption of tympanic membrane
- Pain
- Ear discharge

Nursing Interventions

- Administer analgesics as needed
- Educate parent and child about therapy

Expected Outcomes

- Parent and child identify causes of ear trauma
- Parent describes therapy measures

Nursing Diagnosis
Altered Parenting

Defining Characteristics

- Unrealistic expectation of child by parent
- Inappropriate parenting behaviors

Nursing Interventions

- Help parent identify factors with potential for injury
- Help parent identify factors resulting in this injury

Expected Outcomes

- Parent demonstrates positive parent-child interactions
- Parent can describe safety precautions appropriate to age of child

Nursing Diagnosis
Pain

The nursing diagnosis for pain in trauma is the same as that for pain in otitis.

Management

Minor Ear Trauma. Lacerations are sutured if appropriate. A plastic surgeon may be consulted to repair delicate skin and cartilage and because of the poor circulation. Ice packs are placed on the external ear if ecchymosis is present. The patient is discharged home, with a follow-up appointment in 1 week to assess healing and one in 2–3 weeks to assess hearing.

Blunt Trauma. Surgical evaluation with firm repositioning is the treatment.

Laceration. A multilayered closure is performed by microsurgical techniques for complete avulsion.

Tympanic Membrane Trauma. Irrigation is avoided. Sufficient analgesia is provided, and antibiotics are prescribed (see Table 23–1). Follow-up care is in 1–2 days with an otolaryngologist to assess membrane edges.

Major Trauma. The initial treatment is stabilization of respiratory, cardiovascular, and neurologic systems.

Facial Nerve Function. If the patient is in a state of depressed consciousness, painful stimuli may be necessary to assess nerve function.

Patient and Family Teaching and Psychosocial Support

The patient and family are told to expect return of hearing acuity as healing occurs. The parents are taught about injury prevention according to child's developmental level.

FOREIGN BODY: NOSE OR EAR

Small children are inquisitive and manipulative with food and toys. Among 2–3-year-old children, one-third of foreign body diagnoses in the ED pertain to the ear and nose (Baker, 1992). Common objects include beads, small parts of toys, stones, peanuts, and other vegetable matter. Animals, most commonly insects, worms, and larvae, can enter as mobile adults or be deposited as eggs (Santamaria and Abrunzo, 1992).

History

There may be a history of insertion of a foreign object, or no known history. There may be a history of recurrent epistaxis, foul smell, pain, drainage, or fever.

Physical Assessment

A foreign body in the ear produces pain and decreased hearing; those in the nose may produce pain, an odorous discharge, and occasionally bleeding (Baker, 1992). It is important to examine both sides of the nose and both ears, even when only one foreign object is suspected.

Laboratory and Diagnostic Tests

X rays may be ordered, although foreign objects are often non-radiopaque. Computed tomography may be performed to identify a foreign object in the posterior aspect of the nose.

TRIAGE
Foreign Body in the Nose or Ear

Urgent ————————————————————
A child with suspected foreign body in nose or ear; pain; bleeding; fever.

Non-urgent ————————————————
A child with suspected foreign body in nose or ear.

Nursing Diagnosis
Ineffective Family Coping: Disabling

Defining Characteristics
- Unrealistic expectations of child by parent
- Inappropriate child care provisions

Nursing Interventions
- Assess parental understanding of child's developmental level
- Assess parental understanding of safety issues

Expected Outcomes
- Parents seek assistance in child-proofing home
- Parents can describe safety precautions appropriate to child's developmental level

Management
Most foreign bodies in the nose and ear can be removed in the ED under direct visualization and with proper restraint of the child. All procedures should be carefully explained to parents and child. Careful restraint of the child is essential to prevent further injury during removal. If the parent or child has tried to remove the object and failed, the child should be referred to an otolaryngologist for retrieval of the object.

Ear. The first attempt should be a forceps grasp of the foreign body or scooping with a cerumen spoon. If the foreign object is not vegetable matter or paper, an attempt should be made to irrigate the area with a WaterPik or butterfly tubing attached to a syringe; to perform suction with a small-gauge plastic catheter; or to make the object adhere to cyanoacrylate placed on the tip of a straightened paper clip. Topical application of a small amount of lidocaine to the external ear canal may expedite exit of live insects, such as roaches. Alcohol may be instilled to kill the insect before removal.

Nose. Some authors advocate blowing into the child's mouth to dislodge a nasal foreign body (Baker, 1992). Nasal secretions may be aspirated by using a Frazier suction catheter. Two to three drops of 4% cocaine solution, 1% epinephrine, or 2% pontacaine can be used for anesthesia, vasoconstriction, and shrinkage of the mucous membrane. The object is removed with a bayonet forceps, a tiny long forceps, or a "snatcher instrument" under direct visualization. Prophylactic treatment with oral antibiotics (see Table 23–1) may be given for 10 days after removal.

Patient and Family Teaching and Psychosocial Support
Prevention of recurrence by surveillance of the environment for small parts should be emphasized. Behavioral modification techniques may be used to decrease this activity by the child.

EPISTAXIS

Epistaxis, or nosebleeds, is a common occurrence in childhood. Bleeding beyond a few minutes often is cause for an ED visit.

Etiology and Pathophysiology
Ninety percent of nosebleeds are from a localized, single-artery bleeding site on one side of the nasal septum and within 2 cm of the nasal tip. The artery may be damaged by picking the anterior septum, insertion of a foreign body, forceful sneezing or nose blowing, or facial or nasal injury. There may be overdrying of the mucous membrane from overheating in winter or overuse of topical nasal sprays. Hypervascularity associated with rhinitis or sinusitis may increase the chance of arterial damage. Idiopathic epistaxis occurs in children 5–12 years of age. Other sources of epistaxis are rare in pediatrics, including arterial hypertension, and side effects from medications such as warfarin, aspirin, phenothiazines, and nonsteroidal anti-inflammatory agents.

Nosebleeds may originate from a more active, posterior site. Such nosebleeds are rare in children; they are usually associated with specific conditions such as recovery from an adenoidectomy, nasal trauma, polyps,

nasopharyngeal angiofibroma, and blood dyscrasias due to leukemia, drug ingestion, thrombocytopenia, and hepatic or renal disease (Jacobs, 1992).

History
The history-taking includes determining the duration and volume of the bleeding and whether it is unilateral or bilateral. Questions are asked about concurrent illnesses or allergies and about the use of aspirin. The precipitating event, if any, must be determined. The child and family often arrive extremely fearful, with active bleeding occurring through partial clots in both nares. The initial determination of anterior or posterior and unilateral or bilateral bleeding site may be difficult. The child may be nauseated from swallowing blood.

Physical Assessment
The physical assessment includes a rapid scan of the skin and mucous membranes for ecchymosis and petechiae. Blood pressure and pulse should be obtained. Epistaxis due to a nasal fracture usually stops spontaneously within an hour of injury. Continued bleeding may require reduction of the nasal fracture.

Laboratory and Diagnostic Tests
In a hypovolemic child, a hemoglobin level and blood type and cross match should be obtained. If anemia or coagulopathy is suspected, a CBC, partial thromboplastin time (PTT), platelet count, and bleeding time should be obtained.

TRIAGE
Epistaxis

Emergent
A child with epistaxis with prolonged or rapidly flowing blood loss; decreasing blood pressure; evidence of coagulopathy on skin or other mucous membrane.

Urgent
A child with active epistaxis from suspected anterior site.

Non-urgent
A child with repeated short nose bleeds; chronic septal mucosa injury; flecks of blood in nasal secretions.

Nursing Diagnosis
Impaired Tissue Integrity

Defining Characteristic

- Bloody nasal drainage

Nursing Interventions

- Monitor nasal discharge
- Provide bleeding control
- Educate child and parent on bleeding control
- Educate child and parent on prescribed treatment

Expected Outcomes

- Child has no bloody nasal discharge
- Child and parent describe bleeding control
- Child and parent describe prescribed treatment

Nursing Diagnosis
Parental Role Conflict

Defining Characteristics

- Verbalization of concerns about changes in parenting role
- Disruption in family routines
- Verbalization of feelings of inadequacy in providing for child's needs

Nursing Interventions

- Acknowledge parent's apparent discomfort with blood
- Educate parent and child about bleeding control
- Educate parent and child about treatment

Expected Outcomes

- Parent and child describe bleeding control
- Parent and child describe treatment

Management

Initial Stabilization. The nurse must try to help the patient to remain calm by giving continued reassurance. The skin and mucous membranes are inspected for ecchymosis or petechiae. The patient and examiner are covered with blood barrier gowns. The examiner should wear gloves and protective eye gear. The patient should sit upright with his or her head tilted slightly forward. This inclines the floor of the nose slightly anteriorly and may prevent further passage of blood posteriorly. Blood should be spit out, not swallowed. The clinician should observe for rate of blood loss and unilateral or bilateral flow. Patient should be encouraged to gently blow out any clots. For examination, the patient should clench 4×4-inch gauze pads rolled between the front teeth and breathe through the mouth with open lips. Figure 23–4 pro-

vides an overview of the evaluation and management of epistaxis.

Intervention

Localization of Bleeding Site. Table 23–2 lists examination and treatment equipment. The nares are inspected with a headlight and nasal speculum after clots are cleared. Usually the arterial bleeder is seen within 2 cm on the anterior nasal septum. The area may need to be rubbed with a cotton-tip applicator to reinstitute active bleeding. If no active bleeder is seen, no cauterization is needed. Preventive teaching is accomplished with this visit; the child can return to the ED if there are future signs of epistaxis.

Initial Control of Bleeding. Bleeding is usually controlled by packing the nasal cavity tightly with cotton dampened with 4% cocaine or tetracaine-phenylephedrine mixture. Epinephrine 1% or pontacaine 2% may be used if the other agents are unavailable. The mucosa becomes anesthetized with adequate vasoconstriction. The pack is left in place for 10 minutes. If bleeding recurs, the pack is reapplied for 10 more minutes. Blood pressure and pulse are reassessed. When cocaine solution is used, the total amount should not exceed 200 mg, or 3 ml of 4% cocaine solution. Cardiopulmonary resuscitation (CPR) equipment should be readily available if an adverse cardiopulmonary reaction to the cocaine or tetracaine-phenylephedrine mixture occurs.

Definitive Control of Bleeding. Cautery with silver nitrate is usually the first method of choice for control of a small bleeding vessel in the anterior nasal septum. Silver nitrate is less effective when applied to vessels that are actively bleeding. Its use is contraindicated if diffuse mucosal hemorrhage is occurring, such as in blood dyscrasias (Josephson et al, 1991).

Anterior Nasal Packing by a Physician. If cautery is unsuccessful, or if an obscure bleeding site is located in the first 5 cm of the nasal tip, a physician is called for anterior packing. Anterior packing is contraindicated in nasal trauma or if a CSF leak is suspected. Packing may increase the chance of cribriform plate injury or infection.

Anteroposterior Packing by an Otorhinolaryngologist. If the bleeding site is posterior the child is admitted to the hospital for posterior packing, observation, and antibiotics are prescribed.

Patient and Family Teaching and Psychosocial Support
Prevention of recurrences by humidification, use of saline nose drops or spray, gentle nose blowing, and by decreasing nose-picking habits is emphasized. The

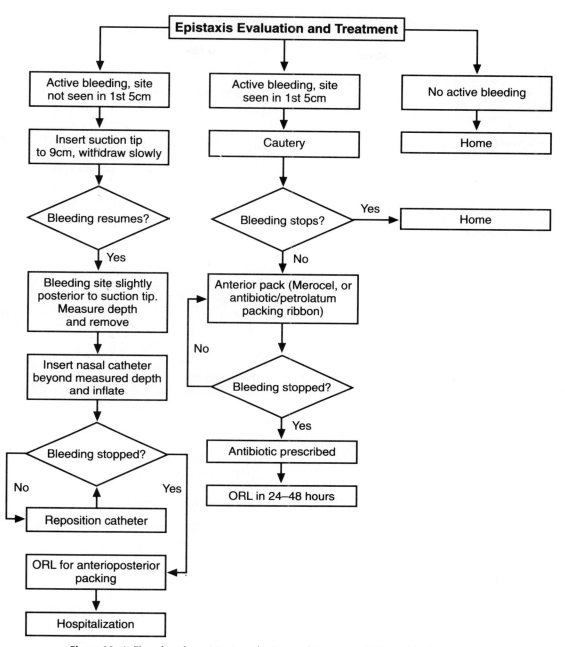

Figure 23–4. Flowchart for epistaxis evaluation and treatment. ORL, otorhinolaryngologist.

first aid for simple epistaxis is having the child sit up. This lowers blood pressure and decreases the likelihood that the child will swallow blood. As the child leans forward slightly, the caregiver pinches the entire soft portion of nose firmly for 10–15 minutes. The child should then rest quietly for 30 minutes. If there is anterior packing, the importance of follow-up care with an otolaryngologist within 48–72 hours should be emphasized.

NASAL OBSTRUCTION

Partial nasal obstruction is a common pediatric event because of the obligate nose breathing of infants until they are 3 months of age and because of the small caliber of the nasal passages of small children. Noisy, labored breathing in small children can sometimes be traced to obstruction of the nasal passages.

The upper one-third of the nose has bony sup-

TABLE 23–2. EPISTAXIS EXAMINATION AND TREATMENT EQUIPMENT

Coaxial headlight
Topical anesthetic
   2–4% pontocaine or 2–4% lidocaine
Topical decongestant solution
   0.25% phenylephrine or 4–10% cocaine solution
     (for vasoconstriction and anesthesia)
   or 1% epinephrine
Short and long nasal specula
Bayonet forceps
Silver nitrate sticks
4 x 4-inch gauze pads
No. 7, No. 9 Frazier suction tips
Yankauer suction tips
Source of suction
1/2" petrolatum gauze or petrolatum-antibiotic ointment gauze ribbon
   or prefabricated compressed sponge packs
No. 16–18 Foley catheters with 30-ml balloon, tip cut off or
   specifically designed nasal balloon

port, and the lower two-thirds has cartilage support. The nasal septum forms the medial wall of each nasal cavity; it is supported by both bone and cartilage. The septum is covered by a mucous membrane, which is richly supplied by blood. The nasal turbinate bones (the superior, medial, and inferior) are three shelf-like structures protruding from the lateral nasal wall into the nasal cavity. The mucous membranes of these bones have a rich blood supply. Sinuses drain through these turbinate bones at the meatus. The functions of the mucous membranes of the nasal cavities are cleansing, humidification, and temperature control of inspired air.

Etiology and Pathophysiology

In acute rhinitis, the mucosa is erythematous and swollen, with a thin, watery or thick, purulent bilateral discharge. In allergic rhinitis the mucosa is swollen and boggy, with a pale bluish hue. Furuncles, bacterial invasion of the hair follicles that line the nasal passages anteriorly, may cause erythema and pustules, which are swollen and tender. Polyps, glistening pedunculated growths that may be smooth or grapelike, are often associated with atopy or recurrent infection. They are unusual before 10 years of age unless associated with cystic fibrosis. Foreign bodies in the nose often do not cause nasal obstruction initially, but by 24–48 hours after insertion there is a unilateral nasal discharge. Nasal trauma may cause obstruction from a blood clot in the nasal cavity, an acutely displaced nasal septum, fracture displacement of the nasal pyramid, or reactive mucosal edema (Jacobs, 1992).

History

The history includes antecedent events such as an URI or allergy, nasal trauma, and the possibility of the presence of a foreign body.

Physical Assessment

The physical assessment includes inspection of the nasal mucosa for color, swelling, exudate, and bleeding site. The nasal septum is inspected for deviation, bleeding site, and perforation. The nasal turbinate bones are inspected for exudate, swelling, and polyps. Respiratory rate, breath sounds, color, and the presence of retractions are continually assessed.

T R I A G E
Nasal Obstruction

Emergent

An infant younger than 3 months with cyanosis; decreased breath sounds; tachypnea. A child with nasal injury and bleeding.

Non-urgent

An infant or child with nasal obstruction; without signs of respiratory distress.

Nursing Diagnosis
Impaired Tissue Integrity

Defining Characteristics
- Nasal discharge
- Nasal obstruction

Nursing Interventions
- Monitor nasal discharge
- Educate child and parent about therapy such as bulb suctioning, saline nose drops

Expected Outcome
- Child and parent describe therapy

Nursing Diagnosis
Ineffective Airway Clearance

Defining Characteristic
- Inability to remove airway secretions

Nursing Interventions
- Provide humidified air

- Perform suction of nasal secretions as needed
- Provide teaching about therapy measures

Expected Outcomes

- Child clears airway
- Parent describes therapy
- Airway remains clear

Nursing Diagnosis
Ineffective Breathing Pattern

Defining Characteristics

- Inability to move airway secretions
- Increased respiratory distress in environment containing allergens

Nursing Interventions

- Provide health teaching about known causative factors
- Teach therapy

Expected Outcomes

- Parent and child state causative factors, if known
- Parent and child describe methods to avoid known allergens
- Parent and child describe therapy

Management

Acute Viral Rhinitis. Humidified air is provided. Nasal decongestant, oral medication, or nose drops are administered as directed.

Allergic Rhinitis. Humidified air is provided. An antihistamine or other allergy medication is administered as directed. A steroid nasal spray may be given to school-aged or adolescent patients.

Bacterial Rhinitis. Humidified air is provided, and a decongestant is administered. Antibiotics are prescribed (see Table 23–1).

HIV Infection. The usual causative agents of rhinitis are similar to those in children without HIV infection. Treatment is standard. Recurrent bacterial rhinitis is a part of the syndrome. If there are giant herpetic ulcers on the nares and facial skin, treatment with oral acyclovir is in order. Consideration should be given to infection with other, less routine agents, such as cytomegalovirus, *Legionella, Acanthamoeba, Candida, Pseudallescheria, Alternaria,* and *Cryptococcus* (Lucente, 1991).

Patient and Family Teaching and Psychosocial Support

Safety teaching may be appropriate. The child may need to avoid allergens. Humidification of air in the environment is important. Parents should be taught bulb suctioning and use of saline nose drops.

NASAL FRACTURE

Injury to the face may result in a fracture of the nose.

History

There is history of injury to the face and nose. The possibility of child abuse (intentional injury) should be considered when obtaining the history.

Physical Assessment

Physical assessment shows widening of the dorsum of the nose, with loss of dorsal height. There may be swelling, epistaxis, or external deformity. On palpation there is tenderness and bony crepitus. Telescoping or foreshortening indicates more complex injury. The nurse should look for widening of the intercanthal distance, periorbital emphysema, and CSF rhinorrhea (Barot, 1991). Assessment for additional injury to facial bones, the skull, and the spinal column should be accomplished. The child's vital signs and neurologic status should be assessed continually.

Laboratory and Diagnostic Tests

For a hypovolemic child, a hemoglobin concentration and blood type and crossmatch should be obtained.

TRIAGE
Nasal Fracture

Emergent ————————————————
A child with facial injuries; evidence of airway compromise; loss of consciousness.

Urgent ————————————————————
A child with nasal swelling; tenderness; epistaxis.

Nursing Diagnosis
Pain

The nursing diagnosis for the pain of a nasal fracture is the same as that for pain in otitis.

Nursing Diagnosis
Body Image Disturbance

Defining Characteristics

- Negative response to a change in structure and function of nose
- Avoidance of looking at face and nose

Nursing Interventions

- Provide support for child and parent's understanding of healing process
- Provide support regarding feelings

Expected Outcomes

- Child and parent can describe healing process
- Child and parent articulate feelings about injury

Management

Ice is applied to the nose to decrease swelling. If there is a simple fracture, the physician may reduce the bone to position with a nasal elevator or Walsham forceps. If there is considerable deformity, surgical reduction may be performed using general anesthesia in 3–7 days, when swelling has subsided. The nose is immobilized by nasal packing for 3–4 days and by external splint for 7–10 days. Ice is applied intermittently to reduce swelling and pain. Pain relief is usually accomplished by acetaminophen. Decongestants should not be used because of their effect on blood supply to healing areas. Parents should be instructed to telephone their primary care provider or return to the ED if the child becomes lethargic or has persistent vomiting due to head trauma.

SINUSITIS

Acute sinusitis is a bacterial inflammation of the paranasal sinuses; it is common in children.

Etiology and Pathophysiology

The sinuses are invaginations of the mucous membranes of the nasal cavity. They lie within the maxilla and frontal bones of the skull. The mucosa is lined with ciliated, columnar epithelium, which both produces and transports secretions. The ethmoid and maxillary sinuses develop by 3–5 months of gestational age. The frontal sinuses, developed in the first year of life, are radiologically apparent by the age of 3–4 years. The sphenoid sinuses, developed by the age of 4–5 years, are radiologically apparent by the age of 9 years. The sinus functions include olfaction, mucous production, voice resonance, decrease in skull weight and density, and defense against infection.

Inflammation of the sinuses may be caused by an URI or allergy. There is mucosal swelling and vascular congestion. With absence of pulsatile movement of the cilia of the mucosa, there is stagnation of secretions and proliferation of pathogens. The pathogens may be viral or bacterial, but sinusitis is usually treated as a bacterial infection because of the high percentage of secondary bacterial invasion with *S. pneumoniae, H. influenzae,* or *M. catarrhalis* (Josephson, 1991).

There may be host variations in anatomy and physiology, such as midface anomalies or immunodeficiencies. Predisposing conditions include dental disease, adenotonsilitis, a foreign body in nares, adenoid hyperplasia, nasal polyps, deviated septum, tumor, and trauma (Kaban and Jacobs, 1992).

History

The history usually shows a recent URI, allergy, or barotrauma. Symptoms are prolonged, without amelioration by usual treatment. There may be a cough, with persistent postnasal discharge. Children often have a night cough as secretions drain during position changes. There may be frequent sniffing, snorting, or throat clearing. There may be halitosis, fever, malaise, dizziness, and headache; there is facial discomfort when the head drops forward.

Physical Assessment

Physical assessment includes examination of the nares for discharge and erythema. There may be tenderness to palpation over the sinuses, which is aggravated by sudden head movements. Less common is periorbital swelling, which is most obvious upon waking.

Laboratory and Diagnostic Tests

Sinusitis is generally confirmed by sinus x rays. These x rays show opacification of sinus cavities and the presence of air-fluid levels in the sinus cavities, which are pathognomonic of sinusitis. There is an underreporting of ethmoid sinus disease (Josephson, 1991).

T R I A G E
Sinusitis

Emergent ————————————
A neonate with a fever.

Urgent ————————————
An infant or child with fever; rhinitis; facial pain.

Non-urgent ————————————
An infant or child with rhinitis; cough; no wheezing.

Nursing Diagnosis

The nursing diagnosis for pain and high risk for altered body temperature in sinusitis are the same as those for these two problems in otitis. The nursing diagnosis for impaired tissue integrity is the same as that in nasal obstruction.

Management

Humidification by cool mist and adequate hydration is essential. Analgesic and antipyretic agents are used for a minimum of 48 hours. Decongestants are used only if they provide symptomatic relief. The therapeutic effects are controversial in sinusitis. Antibiotics are prescribed (see Table 23–1).

The patient usually goes home after the ED visit. A follow-up visit to the primary care provider is made 3 weeks after the ED visit. Hospitalization may be required if sinusitis is associated with periorbital cellulitis or an abscess, osteomyelitis, or meningitis.

Patient and Family Teaching and Psychosocial Support

The importance of completing the 2–3 week antibiotic treatment to completely eradicate the infection should be emphasized. Follow-up care is needed if sinus infections are recurring to assess the underlying cause (eg, polyps or a deviated septum).

OROPHARYNGEAL BLEEDING AND INJURY

Bleeding from the oropharyngeal area may be a serious situation, warranting immediate action.

Etiology and Pathophysiology

Intraoral bleeding is usually associated with trauma to the teeth, tongue, or pharyngeal area. Injury may be minor, such as a laceration with a popsicle or lollipop stick, or major, such as a penetrating injury with a knife or sharp-edged toy. Post-tonsillectomy bleeding is usually intermittent and mild for 7–10 days postoperatively. Catgut sutures used to control surgical bleeding usually dissolve about 1 week after the operation. Postsurgical hemorrhage may occur.

History

A history of antecedent events is elicited. Blood loss is estimated.

Physical Assessment

The physical examination is specific for the site of bleeding. Vital signs are assessed frequently. If an *injury* is suspected, the intraoral hard and soft tissues are inspected for laceration, bleeding, ecchymosis, and mobility. The mandible and maxilla are assessed for fractures. The dental arches are assessed for alveolar fracture, tooth trauma, and mobility. Occlusion and tooth alignment and number are assessed. Avulsed teeth must be accounted for. If teeth are found at the scene of the accident, they should not be wiped; they should simply be rinsed of dirt or debris. The teeth are placed in milk- or saline-moistened gauze for transport and storage. If partially avulsed, the teeth are left in the mouth unless they pose a threat for airway aspiration. If a hemorrhage has occurred after an extraction, the site of bleeding must be identified.

Laboratory and Diagnostic Tests

If inspection of the skin and mucous membranes shows evidence of coagulopathy, a CBC, PTT, and bleeding time may be considered.

TRIAGE
Oropharyngeal Bleeding and Injury

Emergent
An infant or child with pharyngeal hemorrhaging; unstable blood pressure; serious injury; uncontrolled blood loss after extraction or injury; evidence of coagulopathy.

Non-urgent
An infant or child with no active bleeding; history of minor mouth or oropharyngeal injury.

Nursing Diagnosis
Fluid Volume Deficit

Defining Characteristics
- Decreased fluid volume from bleeding
- Blood pressure and pulse instability

Nursing Interventions
- Monitor for signs and symptoms of shock
- Collaborate with physician to replace fluid losses at a rate to maintain urine output >0.5 mL/kg/hour
- Provide support to reduce anxiety and fear
- Educate child and parent about therapy

Expected Outcomes
- Child maintains a urine output of 30 mL/hour
- Vital signs remain stable
- Child shows no signs of anxiety and fear
- Child and parent can describe therapy

Nursing Diagnosis
High Risk for Injury

Defining Characteristics
- Lack of knowledge of environmental hazards
- History of injury in home or other environment
- Lack of clear history of event by responsible adult

Nursing Interventions
- Educate parent about safety issues
- Assist in identifying community resources to help with safety in the home environment

Expected Outcomes
- Parent describes plans for increasing safety in the home for child
- Parent identifies potential hazards in the home

Management

Initial Stabilization. Personnel should use blood-barrier gowns, eye gear, and gloves during the procedure. The patient should be lying down with the head slightly dependent.

Minor Injury. If the bleeding site can be seen, the function of the soft palate, tongue, and pharynx are assessed. The patient is discharged home.

Active Bleeding. An intravenous line should be established, and intravenous volume replacement is begun, if necessary. The site of bleeding is determined. To do this, the physician uses a headlamp light source, freeing both hands for treatment. A tongue blade is inserted followed by a tonsil suction tip to the back of the pharynx. Clots and blood are suctioned out. If the bleeding site is seen, the suction tip can be placed directly over it and kept there until definitive tamponade can be performed (Jacobs, 1992). Tamponade using a 4×4-inch gauze sponge held by a hemostat clamp (Kelly) may be accomplished. This maneuver is more effective if counterpressure is applied against the tonsillar fossa externally by placing fingers posterior to the ramus of the mandible. This maneuver should be effective in controlling massive bleeding in a patient recovering from a tonsillectomy until the patient can be removed to the operating room for definitive treatment.

After Tonsillectomy. In a patient recovering from a tonsillectomy, if the bleeding site cannot be determined, it is probably the inferior pole of one of the tonsillar fossae, near the base of the tongue. The physi-

cian places the suction tip blindly to one side of the pharynx to assess if bleeding ceases. If it does not, the same maneuver is attempted on the other side.

Hemorrhage After Tooth Extraction. A moist gauze sponge is placed over the site of extraction. The patient compresses the area by biting down for 30 minutes. If bleeding resumes, this is evidence of a small bone bleeder. Local anesthetic (eg, lidocaine 2% with epinephrine 1:100,000) is infiltrated into the maxillary or buccal and palatal side of the extraction socket. A 000 catgut suture may be placed, or gelatin foam sponge may be placed and packed into the socket. If the extraction occurred in the mandible, an inferior alveolar nerve block is performed. Follow-up care is with an oral surgeon.

Dental Injury. The airway is assessed. Intraoral debris is removed and noted. An oral surgeon is called for stabilization of teeth and for treatment. Tetanus toxoid is administered. Antibiotics are prescribed for 5–7 days (see Table 23–1).

Patient and Family Teaching and Psychosocial Support
In minor trauma, with cessation of bleeding and normal function, education centers on prevention and safety teaching. The patient and family are prepared for operative assessment and treatment. Hospitalization is necessary if there is considerable hemorrhaging.

STOMATITIS AND PHARYNGITIS

Infection of the mucous membranes of the mouth and throat are common in children. Dysphagia may be severe; it usually leads to anorexia and sleep disturbances.

Etiology and Pathophysiology
Stomatitis and pharyngitis are inflammations of the mucous membranes of the mouth and throat. They may be caused by an allergy or an infection by a fungus, virus, or bacteria.

Peritonsillar abscess, although rare, is serious; it occurs in association with infection by *Streptococcus* or *Staphylococcus.* The abscess occurs between the pseudocapsule of the tonsil and the muscles of the pharyngeal wall. It usually develops as a complication of simple bacterial tonsillitis and may occur during the antibiotic treatment itself (Dudley, 1989).

In children with HIV infection the oropharynx is a common site of infection. Candidiasis may have erythematous, hyperplastic, or atrophic forms (Lucente,

1991). Herpes is often more severe and widespread than in children without HIV. The ulcers may be 1–3 mm in diameter. Aphthous ulcers may be seen in giant forms.

History

A history of fever and of contact with other people with contagious disease should be elicited. There may be history of dysphagia and decreased appetite.

Physical Assessment

A physical examination may lead to a differential diagnosis of the infection.

Peritonsillar Abscess. The patient has a sudden onset of high fever with severe unilateral throat pain radiating to the ipsilateral ear. There is medial displacement of the tonsil toward the middle. The uvula may be edematous. A fluctuant tender mass is palpable in the soft palate near the superior pole of the involved tonsil. The child is quite febrile, and there is enlargement of the ipsilateral tonsilar lymph nodes. The child has localized pain, which becomes progressively severe. Dysphagia and trismus may be present. There is exquisite tenderness in the neck, with torticollis to minimize the pressure of the sternocleidomastoid over the inflamed lymph nodes. Speech is thickened or muffled, giving the characteristic "hot potato" voice caused by poor palatine movement. Serious airway problems usually do not develop (Dudley, 1989).

Gingivostomatitis. Erythema and vesicles are found.

Herpes. There are vesicles and generalized erythema of the gingival mucosa. A very painful initial infection occurs with fever and adenopathy. Recurrences involve vesicles on the lip.

Coxsackie. The lesions are yellow ulcerations with red halos. Painful erythematous vesicles develop on the tonsilar pillars, soft palate, palms, and the plantar surface of the foot. Fever and adenopathy are present.

Aphthous Ulcers. One to several shallow, painful ulcers with erythematous halos appear; there is no adenopathy. Aphthous ulcers are often related to trauma, stress, or allergies.

Candida. Erythema with white plaques occurs on the buccal mucosa, tongue, and palate. There is no adenopathy.

Viral Pharyngitis or Tonsillitis. Erythema and dysphagia are found.

Group A Beta Hemolytic Streptococcus. Fever, bright red tonsils which may have white exudate, halitosis, and palatal petechiae may be found with anterior lymphadenopathy, which is tender. Some children have abdominal pain. There may be an erythematous, pinpoint papular rash on the body. A carefully conducted rapid test for latex agglutination enzymes is positive, or a culture is positive for bacteria (Turnik et al, 1990).

Epstein-Barr Virus (Mononucleosis). Marked malaise and anorexia, a white exudate on the tonsils, halitosis, fever, and generalized lymphadenopathy are found, and the child may have splenomegaly. A CBC shows increased atypical lymphocytes. A heterophile test for Epstein-Barr virus becomes positive during the course of disease. Epstein-Barr virus is frequently associated with a secondary bacterial tonsillitis (Jacobs, 1991).

Adenovirus. Conjunctivitis and a nonexudative tonsillar inflammation are found; cervical adenopathy is present.

TRIAGE
Stomatitis and Pharyngitis

Emergent ————————————————
A child with sudden-onset fever and severe unilateral dysphagia radiating to ipsilateral ear.

Urgent ————————————————
A child with mouth or throat pain; mild to moderate fever; no respiratory distress.

Nursing Diagnosis

The nursing diagnosis for high risk for altered body temperature and pain in stomatitis and pharyngitis are the same as those in otitis.

Nursing Diagnosis

Altered Oral Mucous Membrane

Defining Characteristics

- Oral burning or pain
- Change in tolerance of food of extreme temperatures and of acidic or highly spiced foods
- Ulcerations in oral mucosa

Nursing Interventions

- Provide adequate oral hydration and hygiene

- Educate parent and child about hydration and nutrition
- Reduce pain by analgesia as needed

Expected Outcomes

- Child and parent can describe oral hygiene measures
- Child and parent can describe hydration and nutrition plan
- Child shows no signs of pain

Nursing Diagnosis
Impaired Swallowing

Defining Characteristics

- Difficulty swallowing
- Coughing

Nursing Interventions

- Assess level of difficulty swallowing
- Educate child and parent on measures to promote ability to swallow
- Assess adequate hydration

Expected Outcomes

- Child and parent can describe measures to promote ability to swallow
- Child has adequate hydration

Management

Peritonsillar Abscess. The child is admitted to the hospital for parenteral administration of antibiotics and surgical incision and drainage. Intravenous access is established in the ED.

Viral Stomatitis and Pharyngitis. The child is hydrated with small, frequent sips of water or licks on popsicles. Analgesic and antipyretic agents are given; they should be continued as needed at home. The judicious use of a topical anesthetic, such as viscous lidocaine 1% solution mixed with 5 mL mouthwash and used to rinse the mouth 5 minutes before meals, may be considered for severely painful vesicles (Jacobs, 1992). Cardiac arrhythmias may occur with frequent, large doses of this solution.

Viral Stomatitis in a Child with HIV Infection. Treatment is more aggressive. Oral acyclovir is prescribed for herpes simplex. For giant aphthous ulcers, oral or topical dexamethasone is prescribed to decrease inflammation and relieve pain (Lucente, 1991).

Candida Stomatitis. Adequate hydration and feeding are important. The nurse teaches the parents about decontamination of fomites, such as nipples and pacifiers. Treatment is nystatin oral drops, 1 mL, each side qid for 10 days.

Group A Beta Hemolytic Streptococcus. Adequate hydration and feeding are important. Antibiotics are given (see Table 23–1).

Patient and Family Teaching and Psychosocial Support
The parents are taught the importance of completing antibiotic treatment, if prescribed, to completely eradicate streptococcal bacterial infection and to prevent sequelae, such as pyogenic complications of cervical adenitis and peritonsillar or retropharyngeal abscess, and nonpyogenic complications such as rheumatic fever. The parent's role in supporting hydration and providing analgesia with viral stomatitis is emphasized.

KAWASAKI DISEASE

Early recognition of acute Kawasaki disease, with its classic oropharyngeal signs, may be life saving. An acute febrile multisystem vasculitis, Kawasaki disease usually occurs in children younger than 4 years with a peak incidence at the age of 1 year (Murrant, 1990). The etiology is unknown. Asian American children have a threefold higher yearly incidence than other ethnic groups (Terndrup, 1990). A 1–2% mortality from the development of coronary and arterial aneurysms, myocarditis, pericarditis, or acute vascular insufficiency may occur. Echocardiography demonstrates a coronary artery aneurysm in 20–30% of patients with Kawasaki disease. This is the most important form of acquired heart disease among children (Terndrup, 1990).

History
The history reveals a sudden onset of fever that has been unresponsive to antibiotics for 5 days or more.

Physical Assessment

Acute Phase (Weeks 1–2). Fever and irritability occur with conjunctival erythema, cracked, red lips, and erythema of the oral mucosa and tongue. There is unilateral cervical adenitis. Anterior uveitis may be apparent during a slit-lamp examination. Erythema and edema of the hands and feet occur. A truncal rash, polymorphous in type, may be present. An electrocardiogram (ECG) may show sinus tachycardia, PR interval prolongation, or nonspecific ST and T wave changes. The child may be profoundly ill with arthritis or myocarditis or may have aseptic meningitis with CSF pleocytosis (10–15 white blood cells/mm³, predominance of mononuclear cells).

Subacute Phase (Weeks 2–3). The fever resolves, and there is desquamation of the fingers and toes. Thrombocytopenia and an elevated erythrocyte sedimentation rate (ESR) may be seen. The child may have urethritis with sterile pyuria, obstructive jaundice with diarrhea, and abdominal pain. Echocardiography may show coronary arterial aneurysms, or the child may have palpable arterial aneurysms.

Convalescent Phase (Weeks 3–4). The clinical stigmata have resolved. At this time the cardiovascular changes become overt in 20–30% of untreated children. The greatest peak of sudden death occurs during convalescence.

TRIAGE
Kawasaki Disease

Emergent
Infant or child with fever over 40°C, erythematous oral and eye mucosa, tachypnea, and signs of meningitis.

Urgent
Infant or child with fever over 40°C and erythematous eye and oral mucosa.

Nursing Diagnoses
The nursing diagnoses for high risk for altered body temperature and pain are the same as those in otitis. The nursing diagnosis for fear related to hospitalization is the same as that for mastoiditis.

Management
Hospitalization is required for supervised bedrest and cardiac monitoring. Intravenous gamma globulin and oral aspirin are administered within 10 days of the onset of the disease. This treatment results in a threefold reduction in the frequency of coronary artery aneurysms (Terndrup, 1990).

Patient and Family Teaching and Psychosocial Support
The importance of long-term follow-up by a cardiologist should be emphasized. Because of the sudden and severe nature of this illness, the patient and parents need a great deal of support.

FOREIGN BODY IN THROAT

Foreign bodies in the throat usually lodge in the hypopharynx or cervical esophagus. They cause pain and anxiety in the child. Chicken or fish bones, toy parts, coins, nuts, hot dog pieces, or candy may be found (May, 1992).

History
A history of suspected ingestion of foreign body is elicited.

Physical Assessment
The child should be carefully assessed for any respiratory distress, drooling, or dysphagia. A physical examination may reveal the foreign object.

Laboratory and Diagnostic Tests
A plain x ray is useful for radiopaque objects such as a bone, but it is not useful for vegetable matter or meat. The x ray should be carefully evaluated for air in the area of the cervical esophagus because this represents air in the postcricoid region.

TRIAGE
Foreign Body in Throat

Emergent
An infant or child with respiratory distress; pharyngeal bleeding; history of foreign body ingestion.

Urgent
An infant or child with blood-tinged secretions; history of foreign body ingestion.

Nursing Diagnosis
Ineffective Airway Clearance

Defining Characteristics
- Ineffective cough
- Inability to remove airway secretions

Nursing Interventions
- Assess respiratory functioning
- Provide measures to promote optimum respiratory functioning
- Educate child and parent about therapy
- Provide support to reduce anxiety and fear

Expected Outcomes
- Child maintains optimum respiratory functioning

- Child demonstrates effective coughing and increased air exchange in lungs
- Child and parent can describe therapy
- Child shows no signs of anxiety or fear

Nursing Diagnosis

Altered Nutrition: Less than body requirements

Defining Characteristics

- Inadequate food intake
- Metabolic needs in excess of intake

Nursing Interventions

- Assess needs and ability for intake
- Educate child and parent about methods to facilitate intake

Expected Outcomes

- Child and parent can describe nutritional requirements and methods to facilitate intake
- Oral intake is adequate to meet child's needs
- Child and parent can describe causative factors for swallowing difficulties

Nursing Diagnosis

Altered Family Processes

Defining Characteristics

- Verbalization of stress regarding injury
- Verbalization of guilt regarding injury
- Disruption in normal family routines

Nursing Interventions

- Encourage verbalization of guilt or anger by parents
- Facilitate communication within family to identify safety issues in the home
- Reinforce parental role to set priorities regarding safety in the home

Expected Outcomes

- Parent can explain modifications to be made in the home environment that will improve safety
- Parent can identify external resources available to increase safety in the home
- Parent can resume system of mutual support of each family member

Management

An otolaryngologist removes the object. The parents are instructed regarding prevention of further epi-sodes of foreign objects in the throat. The child and parents need a great deal of reassurance.

REFERENCES

Baker MD (1992). Foreign bodies of childhood. In May HL, Aghababian RV, Fleisher GR (eds), *Emergency medicine.* Boston: Little, Brown, pp 1892–1893

Barot L (1991). Maxillofacial trauma. *Topics in Emergency Medicine* 13:17–26

Bluestone CD, Klein JO (1988). *Otitis media in infants and children.* Philadelphia: Saunders, pp 55; 123–124

Bluestone CD, Stephenson JS, Martin L (1992). Ten-year review of otitis pathogens. *Pediatric Infectious Diseases* 11:87–811

Dudley JP (1989). Ear, nose, throat, sinus infections. *Topics in Emergency Medicine* 10:43–51

Durbin W (1992). Otitis media. In May HL, Aghababian RV, Fleisher GR (eds), *Emergency medicine.* Boston: Little, Brown, pp 1839–1842

Finklestein JM, Schaffer SR, Drezner DA (1991). Otologic injuries. *Topics in Emergency Medicine* 13:17–26

Jacobs EE (1992). Acute nasal problems, acute ear problems, acute oral and pharyngeal problems. In May HL, Aghababian RV, Fleisher GR (eds), *Emergency medicine.* Boston: Little, Brown, pp 1383–1404

Josephson GD, Godley FA, Stierna P (1991). Practical management of epistaxis. *Medical Clinics of North America* 75:1311–1320

Josephson JS (1991). Update on diagnosis and treatment of sinus disease: The functional endoscopic sinus surgery approach. *Medical Clinics of North America* 75:1293–1309

Jones SL, Jones PK, Katz J (1989). A nursing intervention to increase compliance in otitis media patients. *Applied Nursing Research* 2:68–73

Kaban LB, Jacobs EE (1992). Facial pain and swelling. In May HL, Aghababian RV, Fleisher GR (eds), *Emergency medicine.* Boston: Little, Brown, pp 1377–1380

Krauss B, Harakal T, Fleisher G (1991). The spectrum and frequency of illness presenting to a pediatric emergency room. *Pediatric Emergency Care* 7:67–71

Lucente FE (1991). Otolaryngologic aspects of acquired immunodeficiency syndrome. *Medical Clinics of North America* 75:1389–1398

Mandel EM, Rockette HE, Bluestone CD, Paradise JL, Nozza RJ (1987). Efficacy of amoxicillin with and without decongestant-antihistamine for otitis media with effusion in children. *New England Journal of Medicine* 316:432

Marcy SM (1987). Swimmer's ear: Timely management tips. *Patient Care* 21:28–43

May HL, Aghababian RV, Fleisher GR (eds) (1992). *Emergency medicine Volume II.* Boston: Little, Brown

McGuirt WF, Stool S (1992). Temporal bone fractures in children: A review with emphasis on long-term sequelae. *Clinical Pediatrics* 31:12–18

Murrant NJ, Cook, JA, Murch SH (1990). Acute admission in Kawasaki disease. *The Journal of Laryngology and Otology* 104:581–584

Nelson DS, Walsh K, Fleisher GR (1992). Spectrum and frequency of pediatric illness presenting to a general community hospital emergency department. *Pediatrics* 90:5–10

Santamaria JP, Abrunzo TJ (1992) Ear, nose, and throat. In Barkin RM (ed), *Pediatric emergency medicine.* St. Louis: Mosby, pp 642–687

Schutzman SA, Petrycki S, Fleisher GR (1991). Bacteremia with otitis media. *Pediatrics* 87:48

Teaching rounds (1992). Air travel and barotitis. *Hospital Medicine* 28:52–57

Teele DW (1992). Otitis media. In Reece RM (ed), *Manual of emergency pediatrics* (4th ed). Philadelphia: Saunders, pp 363–364

Terndrup TE (1990). Kawasaki disease. *Topics in Emergency Medicine* 12:23–29

Tunik MG, Fierman AH, Dreyer BP, Kraskinski K, Hanna B, Rosenberg C (1990). Latex agglutination for the rapid diagnosis of streptococcal pharyngitis: Use by house staff in a pediatric emergency service. *Pediatric Emergency Care* 6:93–95

Woolbert LF (1990). Do antihistamines and decongestants prevent otitis media? *Pediatric Nursing* 16:365–367

Zenk KE, Ma H (1990). Pharmacologic treatment of otitis media and sinusitis in pediatrics. *Journal of Pediatric Health Care* 4:297–303

SUGGESTED READING

Carpenito LJ (1992). *Nursing diagnosis: Application to clinical practice.* Philadelphia: Lippincott

CHAPTER 24

Diabetic Emergencies

BARBARA WOODRING
LAURETTE QUINN

INTRODUCTION

The hormones and glucocorticosteroid secretions of the endocrine system influence almost every type of emergency situation. However, neither infection of, trauma to, nor tumors of endocrine organs produce as many emergent problems in children as does a disorder of carbohydrate metabolism known as diabetes mellitus.

Diabetes mellitus is a result of faulty pancreatic function, the absolute cause of which is still unknown. Most authorities, however, acknowledge strong viral, immunologic, or genetic links among people with Type 1 insulin-dependent diabetes mellitus (IDDM) (Barkin and Rosen, 1990; Davidson, 1991; Kitabachi and Goodman, 1987). The dysfunction can be divided into four major categories, all having glucose intolerance in common: insulin-dependent (Type 1), non-insulin-dependent (Type 2), gestational, and malnutrition-related. Type 1 diabetes, which most commonly affects children and young adults, is the focus of this chapter. The onset of IDDM frequently occurs after an infection or during the growth spurts of childhood and adolescence (Davidson, 1991).

In the United States there are approximately 14 million people with diabetes (7 million cases diagnosed, 7 million cases undiagnosed), about 10% of whom have Type 1 IDDM (American Diabetes Association, 1991). On the basis of previous trends and current US Bureau of Census data, it is projected that the prevalence of diabetes in the younger population will remain at about 1 million through 2050 (Helms, 1992).

Therefore, one can project that the number of children experiencing diabetic emergencies will remain fairly consistent in the years ahead.

Before they have completed their basic nursing education, nurses have mastered the common warning symptoms, major methods of treatment, and anticipated complications of diabetes in adults. Conceptually the pathophysiology and management of diabetes in children and adults is similar. However, psychosocial, emotional and developmental factors make the care divergent. The most notable differences are (1) the length of the disease process; (2) the fact that a child is dependent on insulin and will remain so for the rest of his or her life unless she or he has an islet cell or pancreatic transplant; and (3) the frequency with which a child experiences hypo- or hyperglycemic episodes.

ETIOLOGY AND PATHOPHYSIOLOGY

Because the emergency department (ED) nurse generally sees a child with diabetes mellitus during some type of crisis, the emphasis in this chapter is placed on the most frequently encountered crises: loss of glucose homeostasis resulting in (1) hypoglycemia or (2) hyperglycemia, referred to as diabetic ketoacidosis (DKA). These emergencies represent opposite extremes of glucose regulation. Hypoglycemic crises arise from high levels of exogenous insulin and counterregulatory deficiencies. Conversely, hyperglycemic crises arise from insulin depletion and heightened counterregulation.

Emergency treatment is aimed at identification and reversal of the imbalance (Kitabachi and Rumbak, 1989).

Hyperglycemia–Diabetic Ketoacidosis

In spite of advances in the understanding and treatment of DKA, it is still responsible for 41% of all diabetes-related deaths among people younger than 24 years (American Diabetes Association, 1991). Most of these deaths could be prevented through early recognition and intervention. Diabetic ketoacidosis is an acute complication characterized by an elevated serum glucose level, acidosis, and ketosis; it closely resembles a fasting state. Diabetic ketoacidosis results from a relative or absolute lack of insulin, accompanied by a concomitant increase in counterregulatory hormones such as glucagon, catecholamine, cortisol, or growth hormone. An absolute insulin deficiency exists when a child with diagnosed IDDM omits an insulin dose. A relative insulin deficiency exists when a child's insulin dose is not increased in spite of worsening hyperglycemia. The counterregulatory hormones, secreted during times of physiologic or emotional stress, oppose the effects of insulin, and worsen this absolute or relative lack of insulin (Kitabchi and Murphy, 1988).

Insulin is the primary anabolic hormone of the feed state. The major fuels for energy metabolism are carbohydrates, fats, and proteins. After a meal, these fuels are converted to glucose, amino acids, and free fatty acids. Insulin is released from the beta cells of the pancreas primarily in response to glucose, amino acids, and a number of gastrointestinal hormones. In the liver, insulin promotes glycogen synthesis while at the same time inhibiting glycogen breakdown. In addition, insulin enhances glucose transport to sensitive tissue, such as muscle (Karam et al, 1991).

Pathophysiology of Diabetic Ketoacidosis

Glucagon is the most important catabolic hormone of the fasting state. The major role of glucagon is to ensure normal blood glucose levels during a fast by stimulating the breakdown of hepatic glycogen thereby protecting the brain from hypoglycemic injury (Kitabchi and Murphy, 1988). During DKA there is an increase in the glucagon-to-insulin ratio, resulting in an accelerated rate of hepatic glucose production and ketogenesis. Because of the lack of insulin, there is an overproduction of glucose and a decrease in glucose utilization that potentiate hyperglycemia. The levels of counterregulatory hormones are increased. Catecholamine stimulates glycogenolysis and lipolysis, resulting in the release of free fatty acids and glycerol, which are subsequently converted to glucose and ketone bodies in the liver. Cortisol increases hepatic gluconeogenesis and proteolysis (Kreisberg, 1990). The release of

growth hormone results in an increase in hepatic glucose production, a decrease in peripheral glucose uptake, and an increase in lipolysis; thus ketogenesis is enhanced. The hyperglycemia of DKA, therefore, results from an interplay of insulin, glucagon, and counterregulatory hormones.

Hyperglycemia causes an osmotic diuresis, which leads to dehydration, electrolyte depletion, and hypertonicity. When hyperglycemia exceeds the renal threshold, glucose spills into the urine (glycosuria) and acts as an osmotic diuretic, pulling water from the vascular space and causing polyuria and polydipsia. An older child with an intact thirst mechanism and normal renal function may become moderately hyperglycemic during DKA because the kidneys are able to adequately excrete some of the increased glucose load. However, a small child who relies on caregivers to satisfy thirst-needs may be unable to meet the demands of the diuresis, and volume depletion occurs rapidly (Krane, 1987). Continued hyperglycemia produces dehydration, volume depletion, and reduced glomerular filtration rates (GFRs). Reduction of the GFR causes decreased renal excretion of glucose, thereby intensifying the hyperglycemia (Krane, 1987).

Osmotic diuresis also causes passive loss of electrolytes and free water. The free water loss depends on the severity and the length of the episode. Considerable sodium loss occurs in DKA, although the serum sodium level often appears decreased on initial presentation. The serum hypertonicity draws water from the intercellular to the extracellular space, diluting the sodium (Krane, 1987). Each 100 mg/dL elevation of glucose lowers the serum sodium concentration by 1.6 mEq/L (Katz, 1973). As treatment causes a decrease in the blood glucose level, water moves intercellularly, and there is a subsequent rise in serum sodium concentration.

The net effect of increased lipolysis (caused by increases in glucagon and the counterregulatory hormones) is metabolic acidosis, as explained in Figure 24–1. Kussmaul (deep, rapid) respirations develop as the body attempts to reduce CO_2 levels through respiratory compensation. The characteristic fruity odor of the breath is from the acetone. Severe metabolic acidosis can result in depression of the respiratory vasomotor center, compromised cardiovascular output, and reduced vascular tone. The result may be cardiovascular collapse with generation of lactic acid, which adds to the already existing acidosis (Karam et al, 1991).

Total body potassium stores are depleted because of an intracellular-to-extracellular shift during both metabolic acidosis and protein catabolism. There is further loss of potassium through solute diuresis. Initial potassium levels are normal or increased in early

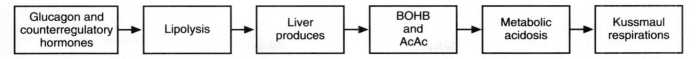

Figure 24–1. Physiologic development of Kussmaul respirations. BOHB, ketone bodies; AcAc, Acetone.

DKA because of intracellular-to-extracellular shifts and decreased glomerular filtration. As fluid and insulin therapy progresses, and dehydration and acidosis are corrected, hypokalemia can be present. Hypokalemia, if it occurs, is caused by an extracellular-to-intracellular shift of potassium, resulting in the reduction of circulating potassium (Krane, 1987). An overview of the symptoms produced by the inadequate supply of insulin is illustrated in Figure 24–2.

Hypoglycemia

Hypoglycemia is defined as a blood glucose level less than 50 mg/dL as evidenced by serum analysis or by amelioration of symptoms by administration of glucose (DDCT, 1991). Hypoglycemia has always been a part of the life of a child with IDDM. The severity of the episode may range from mild irritability to seizure and coma. With the development of more intensive insulin regimens, the risk of hypoglycemia is even greater, because the major cause of these episodes in children is inappropriate insulin regulation (Alberti, 1988). It is difficult to mimic normal physiologic insulin release. For example, an attempt to decrease morning hyperglycemia by increasing the evening dose of intermediate-acting insulin can cause nocturnal hypoglycemia. In addition, there is always the risk of administering the incorrect amount or type of insulin, using an inappropriate site, or reducing caloric intake

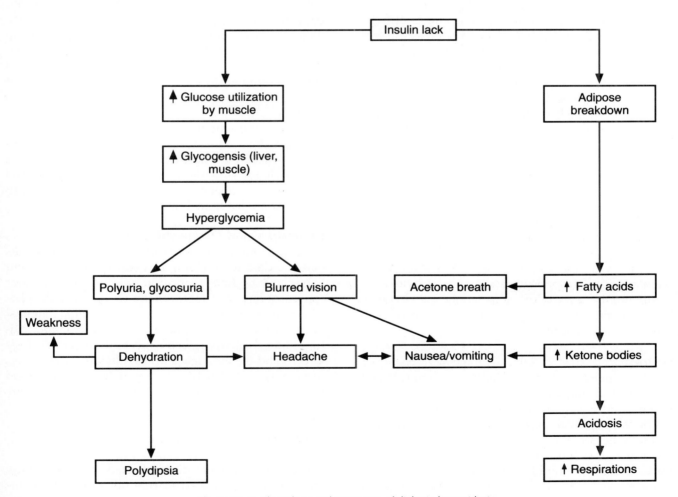

Figure 24–2. Physiology and symptoms of diabetic ketoacidosis.

or delaying or omitting meals, each of which may cause hypoglycemia. Exercise-induced hypoglycemia also may result from increased fuel utilization without a concomitant decrease in insulin levels.

Pathophysiology of Hypoglycemia

Glucose is an obligate fuel for the brain and the central nervous system (CNS) and an alternative fuel for many other organ systems. The brain is unable to synthesize or to store glucose and must rely on circulating blood glucose levels for survival. In children without IDDM, normal glucose levels are maintained through the complex interrelationship between the insulin, glucagon, and counterregulatory mechanisms described earlier. In children with IDDM, this fine metabolic tuning is deranged. The signs and symptoms of hypoglycemia result from both neuroglycopenia (when there is insufficient glucose to meet the needs of the CNS) and activation of the sympathetic nervous system. The symptoms related to neuroglycopenia can include cognitive impairment, fatigue, dizziness, tremors, anxiety, pallor, seizures, loss of consciousness, and death (Cryer and Gerich, 1990). Most children with IDDM exhibit no obvious effects of hypoglycemia, yet neurologic dysfunction may result from recurrent episodes. Children who have once experienced the confusion or seizures of hypoglycemia live in constant fear of repeated episodes in which they are unable to command the control of their bodies.

In summary, loss of glucose hemostasis carries the risk of emergencies at opposite extremes of dysregulation: hyper- or hypoglycemia.

ASSESSMENT

The depth of assessment depends on the condition of the child upon initial encounter. Evaluation of airway, breathing, circulation, and level of consciousness always assume first priority. The child's level of consciousness and responsiveness may vary widely according to the severity of the metabolic imbalance, the length of time it has existed, and the efforts of the body to rectify the imbalance.

History

Insulin-dependent diabetes mellitus is commonly first diagnosed during early school age. Therefore, a conscious child is capable of providing a fairly accurate historical portrayal of the experience. For younger children the parent or caregiver has to give the history. The onset of describable symptoms in children is reported to be quite rapid. Often the child or parent can report the exact day or time they began noticing symptoms. The classic symptoms of polydipsia, polyphagia, and polyuria are usually present. In addition, the parent may recall the incongruity of increased appetite accompanied by weight loss, a sticky substance on the floor around the toilet (from glycosuria), or urinary accidents or reversion to bedwetting (from polyuria). The child may also complain of nausea, vomiting, fatigue and abdominal pain. The complaint of vomiting must be evaluated carefully: nausea accompanied by vomiting may indicate the presence of a dehydration state, which can rapidly escalate into a state of shock if untreated in diabetic children. An allergy history should be obtained, and evidence of recent viral or bacterial infections should be elicited. If the child is known to have diabetes, the nurse should determine the time, type, and amount of last food ingested as well as the time, type, and amount of insulin (and any other medication) last administered.

Of importance for a child with previously undiagnosed diabetes is the assessment of (1) a familial linkage to diabetes mellitus; (2) the existence of gestational diabetes during the mother's pregnancy; and (3) the birth weight of the child, since mothers with gestational diabetes frequently give birth to infants who are large for their gestational age. Additional historical data would be important in developing a complete nursing care plan, but eliciting this data can be delayed until the child's condition is stabilized and the child is admitted to the hospital or begins outpatient care.

Physical Assessment

A systematic head-to-toe assessment produces data on which to accurately base a nursing diagnosis. Findings from each assessment category that could indicate the presence of diabetic complications, DKA, or hypoglycemia are listed in Table 24-1.

Laboratory and Diagnostic Tests

Diagnostic information obtained in the ED serves as baseline data for ongoing assessment and treatment. Laboratory findings that could indicate the two major complications of diabetes mellitus—DKA and hypoglycemia—are presented in Table 24-2. Initial diagnostic studies should include a urinalysis (routine, culture and sensitivity, glucose, acetone, and toxicology screen) and hematologic studies (glucose, electrolytes, osmolality, complete blood count (CBC), arterial blood gases, culture and sensitivity, and toxicology screen).

DIFFERENTIAL DIAGNOSIS

All of the assessment data collected must be rapidly and carefully evaluated to rule out causative agents other than diabetes. Many of the symptoms presented,

TABLE 24–1. PHYSICAL ASSESSMENT FINDINGS

System	Diabetic Ketoacidosis	Hypoglycemia
Skin	Face flushed Skin dry, warm	Pale, circumoral pallor Cold, clammy, heavy sweating
Cardiovascular	Pulse normal to slightly rapid BP decreased	Tachycardia, strong pulse Bradycardia in deep coma BP normal to slightly elevated
Respiratory	Initial: deep, rapid Late: dyspnea, Kussmaul respirations Breath: fruity odor	Initial: normal to increased rate Shallow in coma Normal breath odor
Musculoskeletal	Muscle weakness, fatigue	Normal muscle strength
Eyes	Double or blurred vision Eyeballs soft (dehydration)	Dazed Pupils dilated (late)
Gastrointestinal	Thirst, anorexia, nausea, vomiting, abdominal cramping and tenderness, weight loss, dry mucous membranes	Hunger (delayed or missed meals) Stable weight Numb mouth and tongue
Neurologic	Irritability-to-lethargy Initial: dull, confused, normal to diminished reflexes, headache Late: signs of cerebral edema, coma	Irritability, anxiety-to-delirium Initial: hand tremors, difficulty concentrating, speaking, coordinating, headache Late: staggering gait, hyperreflexia (Babinski reflex inappropriately present), seizure, coma
Genitourinary	Polyuria (initial) to oliguria (late) Urine positive for sugar and acetone	Normal urine output Urine negative for sugar by second voiding

BP, blood pressure.

TABLE 24–2. LABORATORY ANALYSIS[a]

■ HEMATOLOGY	Normal 1–13 years	DKA	Hypoglycemia
Glucose (mg/dL)	60–105	250–1500	<50
pH (arterial)	7.3–7.45	<7.25 (acidic)	WNL
Bicarbonate (mEq/L)	21–29	<15	WNL
BUN (mEq/L)	6–20	Elevated	WNL
Creatinine (mg/dL)	0.3–1.0	Elevated	WNL
Hemoglobin (g/dL)	10–16	Elevated, related to level	WNL
Hematocrit (g/dL)	35–50	of dehydration	WNL
Osmolality (mOsm/L)	280–300	300–325	WNL
Glycosylated hemoglobin	Varies but provides insight into blood sugar levels maintained in past several months		
Potassium (mEq/L)	3.5–5	May be normal, increased or decreased and fluctuating continually	
Sodium (mEq/L)	134–146		
WBC (cells/mm³)	5–15,000	>20,000: related to dehydration >30,000: may indicate infection	

■ URINE			
Glucose	Not present	Present	None by second voiding
Ketone	Not present	Present	None by second voiding

[a]Values may vary with laboratory methods used.
DKA, diabetic ketoacidosis; BUN, blood urea nitrogen; WNL, within normal limits; WBC, white blood cells.

TABLE 24–3. DIFFERENTIAL DIAGNOSIS

Presenting Symptom	Possible Diagnosis
Hyperglycemia	Salicylate poisoning
Ketonuria	Fasting or starvation state
	Gastroenteritis with vomiting
	Anorexia
	Salicylate poisoning
Polyuria (enuresis)	Urinary tract infection
Acidosis	Severe gastroenteritis
	Ingestions of salicylates, iron, alcohol, or methanol
Coma	Hypoglycemia
	Medication overdose (sedative, hypnotic, narcotic)
	CNS trauma or infection

CNS, central nervous system.

especially by DKA, could indicate other disorders such as ingestions (eg, medication, ethanol) fasting or starving states, or CNS compromise. Other diagnoses that need to be considered are listed in Table 24–3.

T R I A G E
Diabetic Crisis

Emergent
A child with severe dehydration; cool extremities (indicating poor perfusion); profound Kussmaul respirations; tachycardia; a lethargic-to-comatose state.

Urgent
A child with abdominal pain accompanied by abdominal tenderness, nausea and vomiting or with signs of early dehydration; elevated pulse rate that is diminished in quality; respirations that are labored and rapid; a fruity odor to breath.

Non-urgent
A child with polydipsia; polyphagia; polyuria (in absence of signs of dehydration); irritability; weight loss; minimal distress.

Nursing Diagnosis

There are ten North American Nursing Diagnosis Association diagnostic categories that can be used in planning the care of a diabetic child.

Nursing Diagnoses for Diabetes in a Child

- High risk for fluid volume deficit related to increased urine excretion and osmotic diuresis
- High risk for injury related to hypoglycemic seizures and coma
- Altered comfort related to insulin injections and blood glucose testing
- Fear related to diagnosis of diabetes and potential complications and long-term outcome
- High risk for altered nutrition related to decreased ability to utilize glucose, lack of knowledge, or ineffective coping with diagnosis
- Social isolation related to fear of embarrassment (food restriction, insulin injections, blood glucose monitoring) before peers
- High risk for noncompliance related to complexity and chronicity of treatment regimen and peer interaction
- High risk for altered health maintenance related to insufficient understanding of disease, glucose self-monitoring, diet and exercise balance, medication administration, or hypo- or hyperglycemic reactions
- Knowledge deficit related to inappropriate explanation of treatment and long-term care requirements presented at developmental level of child or caregiver
- Altered family process related to child's chronic illness.

Each of these diagnoses may be appropriate at varying stages of the disease. However, one is especially important to consider during emergency care and is given here as an example.

Nursing Diagnosis
Fluid Volume Deficit

Defining Characteristics

- Output greater than intake
- Dry skin and mucous membranes
- Thirst, anorexia
- Decreased skin turgor
- Decreased blood pressure and pulse
- Urinary frequency, dilute urine
- Weakness
- Altered mental status

Nursing Interventions

- Assess physical condition and mental status
- Establish parenteral fluid access route
- Evaluate degree of fluid deficit
- Monitor and evaluate vital signs

- Evaluate mucous membranes, skin turgor, and capillary refill
- Observe amount, color, and specific gravity of urine
- Obtain and evaluate hematologic data.
- Correct fluid deficit
- Initiate IV therapy with isotonic saline solution
- Monitor and record urinary output and fluid intake
- Adjust IV glucose, electrolytes and total fluid volume based on repeated hematologic measures
- When appropriate, provide liquids in a form acceptable to the child—popscicles, gelatin dessert, soft drinks
- Reassure the child and parent that symptoms will subside as deficits are corrected

Expected Outcomes

- Fluid and electrolyte balance return to normal
- Serum glucose level is within normal range for age
- Child is alert, responsive, and taking oral fluids
- Child and parent verbalize understanding of the cause of DKA

MANAGEMENT

When a child is admitted to the ED exhibiting seizure activity, extreme lethargy, or coma, the initial management is always the same, regardless of precipitating cause: assure the *airway;* assess *breathing* and other vital signs; assess *circulation* and provide venous access; prevent *damage;* and protect from further injury.

A comatose child, with a compromised respiratory status, should have an endotracheal tube inserted to secure the airway. Aspiration pneumonia is a major cause of respiratory failure in this population; therefore, gastric decompression by a nasogastric tube and suctioning should be initiated for any comatose, lethargic, or obtunded child who has abdominal distention, pain, or absence of bowel sounds. The search for the cause of the problem is rapidly initiated. An intravenous (IV) access route must be established to allow rapid access for hematologic sampling and for fluid replacement. A venous or capillary glucose measurement using a glucose meter or glucose-reagent strip and a ketone measure with a ketone-reagent strip may be time efficient while the laboratory results are awaited. It must be noted that commercial products for measuring ketones cause a nitroprusside reaction that measures acetone not ketone bodies. Because the ketone-to-acetone ratio is increased in DKA, the amount of ketone bodies can be severely underestimated in DKA (Krane, 1987).

Emergency management depends on which of the diabetic crises the child is facing. Because the management of DKA and that of hypoglycemia are so divergent, they are covered separately. The physical findings for each of these complications are presented in Table 24–1.

Hypoglycemia

If the initial assessment reveals a blood glucose level of 50 mg/dL or less, the child is considered to have hypoglycemia. If the child is unconscious or having a seizure, immediate glucose therapy is required. Into the existing peripheral IV access line, 25% dextrose is administered as a bolus at the dose of 1–2 mg/kg of the child's body weight (Walker, 1991). This dose may be repeated in 10 minutes if the child remains unconscious. This administration of glucose should resolve several of the hypoglycemia-related symptoms rather rapidly, but the time required for complete resolution of the symptoms depends on the duration of hypoglycemia before arrival in the ED and the severity of the hypoglycemia. The adrenergic symptoms generally dissipate rapidly, but the CNS symptoms may take longer to resolve. A continuous infusion of 10% dextrose, accompanied by an intermittent bolus of 25–50% dextrose, may be necessary after the initial resolution of hypoglycemia to maintain levels within a normal range (Kitabachi and Rumbak, 1989; Yealy and Wolfson, 1989). This is especially important if the child is still lethargic and unable to take food orally.

An alternative treatment for an unconscious child or a child younger than 6 years, when venous access is unavailable, is 0.25–1.0 mg of glucagon (based on the child's weight) given intramuscularly or subcutaneously (Chase, 1992). This therapy mobilizes hepatic glycogen stores and raises blood glucose levels. After injection of glucagon, the patient should be positioned on his or her side, because glucagon may cause nausea and it is important to avoid aspiration.

When caring for any child, the developmental levels and abilities must be considered. Nursing care should be individualized according to the child's ability to cope and respond. A summary of developmental characteristics that influence management is given in Table 24–4.

The child should be monitored closely in the ED for any change in symptoms. Vital signs should be taken at least every half hour. Capillary blood glucose testing should be done hourly. It is extremely important to monitor the child's level of consciousness throughout the ED stay. A decreased level of consciousness in a child who had previously shown im-

TABLE 24–4. DEVELOPMENTAL CHARACTERISTICS AND ASSOCIATED MANAGEMENT ISSUES

Age Group	Characteristic	Management Issue
Toddler	Independence Temper tantrums Frightened of pain Mimics actions Picky eater	Cannot be relied upon to remain still for injection Mimics parental attitudes and facial expressions related to injections
Preschool-aged	Energetic Sense of pride in accomplishments Magical thinking Short attention span Needs reassurance Needs limit-setting	Can assist in food selections Able to gather supplies for blood and urine test Able to select injection sites Can distinguish colors on test strips; may be able to read numbers on glucose monitor Able to activate spring for finger sticks
School-aged	Excited about trying new things Longer attention span Able to think and reason General muscle coordination	Able to identify foods having varying amounts of sugar Progressively able to push plunger of syringe, draw up correct insulin dosage (not mix), administer own injections, differentiate between feelings of hypo- and hyperglycemia
Pre-adolescent		Can select foods based on exchanges and own diet plan Can do own glucose monitoring Can independently rotate injection sites Capable of wearing insulin pump
Adolescent	Independent, easily embarrassed, confrontational, weight-conscious Well-developed musculoskeletal system Capable of critical thinking Wants peer acceptance Fantasy: nothing-can-happen-to-me	Able to plan meals and snacks (may select junk food) Capable of monitoring insulin pump Can mix two insulins in one syringe Suggests insulin adjustments based on planned activities

provement may indicate continued hypoglycemia or a coexisting problem with neurologic manifestations.

A hypoglycemic child who is alert and able to swallow should be given a fast-acting source of carbohydrate, such as apple juice concentrate, orange juice, a regular (not diet) soft drink, or some form (tablet, liquid, or gel) of concentrated glucose product. A capillary blood glucose level should be checked before the child ingests the carbohydrate and periodically until values normalize. Hospital admission is indicated for any hypoglycemic child who exhibits hemodynamic instability. No child should leave the ED until after eating a substantial meal (peanut butter or grilled cheese sandwich, fresh fruit, and milk).

The nurse should explore with the child and the family the possible reasons for the hypoglycemic reaction. A detailed history as described earlier should be obtained. If known to have diabetes, the child should be encouraged to carry a carbohydrate source at all times and to wear medical-alert identification. The frequency of these reactions should be noted. If there is an increased frequency of hypoglycemic reactions, or if the child exhibits hypoglycemic unawareness, he or she must be referred to a physician or diabetes educator for educational follow-up care.

Hyperglycemia–Diabetic Ketoacidosis

The successful management of hyperglycemia involves prompt recognition of the DKA and institution of emergency measures. These measures include insulin therapy, fluid and electrolyte maintenance, appropriate bicarbonate management, monitoring, and treatment of complications, and detection of the precipitating cause.

Prompt Recognition. The clinical appearance of a child with DKA depends on a variety of factors, including the degree of dehydration and acidosis. Seldom does one see a child in the ED unless the hyperglycemia is so severe that DKA and lethargy or a coma occurs. Approximately 29% of patients with DKA present in a comatose or stuporous state (Kitabachi and Murphy, 1988). In DKA the child may exhibit Kussmaul respirations with a corresponding acetone odor to the breath. The child's face may be flushed because high levels of carbon dioxide in the blood cause vasodilatation. The respiratory response is ineffective as the acidosis becomes more severe; increasing acidosis depresses the respiratory centers.

Immediate IV access must be established to initiate fluid therapy. Dehydration of varying degrees based on the fluid loss is present. A child with DKA may exhibit typical signs and symptoms of dehydration: dry skin, dry mucous membranes, sunken eyeballs, hypotension, and a weak, thready pulse. If a previous weight is known, a fairly accurate percentage of fluid loss can be calculated. It can be assumed that children with DKA have lost approximately 10% of their body weight (Barkin and Rosen, 1990; Sperling, 1990). Treatment with 0.9% normal saline solution should be initiated in the first hour. Sperling (1990) recommends 500 ml of normal saline solution for a child weighing 30 kg.

Attachment of a cardiac monitor provides information related to cardiac rate and rhythm and to the presence of electrolyte abnormalities (tall, peaked T waves may reflect hyperkalemia). It is advisable to continue cardiac monitoring of the child because of the dynamic nature of fluid and electrolyte shifts that may occur during treatment.

After confirmation of the DKA state, treatment is focused on three major factors: insulin therapy; replacement of fluid loss; and maintenance of fluid, electrolyte, and bicarbonate balance.

Insulin Therapy. Initiation of insulin therapy to a child with DKA results in not only a reduction in hyperglycemia but also correction of acidosis. Because there are fewer long-term side effects, the insulin of choice in treating children is the genetically manufactured human insulin. Although there are several traditional modes of insulin therapy that include combinations of intravenous, subcutaneous, and intramuscular U100 insulin, the preferred method is a low-dose continuous insulin infusion (Kitabachi and Rumbak, 1989; Sperling, 1990). This method uses a priming dose (bolus) of 0.1 U/kg of regular insulin intravenously followed by a continuous intravenous infusion of regular insulin at 0.075–0.1 U/kg/hour beginning in the second hour (Walker, 1991). When the blood glucose concentration reaches 300 mg/dL and the acidosis is resolved, the insulin infusion should be discontinued. If the acidotic state has not been corrected by the time the child's glu-

ose level reaches 300 mg/dL, the insulin infusion is continued at a rate of 0.5–1.0 U/kg/hour while 5–10% dextrose is added to the IV infusion to maintain blood glucose levels at 200–300 mg/dL. This dosage allows for correction of acidosis while avoiding hypoglycemia and prevents too great a fall in plasma osmolality.

Subcutaneous injection of 0.2–0.4 U/kg of regular insulin should be initiated 30 minutes before the continuous insulin–IV infusion is discontinued. Subcutaneous insulin *cannot* be administered until dehydration has been corrected. If dehydration exists, insulin is not transported, remains in the subcutaneous tissue, then enters the system as a bolus.

Fluid, Electrolyte and Bicarbonate Balance. Ideally fluid and electrolyte replacement is carried out over a 36-hour period, but it is initiated in the ED. The 36-hour replacement process is used to prevent too rapid a fall in plasma osmolality, which may predispose a child to cerebral edema. The volume of fluid used is based on the child's weight and electrolyte levels. The child is given 10–20 ml/kg of 0.9% normal saline solution intravenously in the first hour, followed by 10–20 ml/kg of 0.45% normal saline solution with appropriate amounts of potassium added in the second hour. From hours 3–12, the 0.45% normal saline plus potassium infusion should be maintained. Over the next 24 hours 5% dextrose in 0.2 normal saline solution with potassium is infused (Aoki and Hanson, 1991; Sperling, 1990). Of course, the fluid rate and volume and the dosage of potassium must be adjusted according to the child's weight and hemodynamic response. A summary of these guidelines is found in Table 24–5.

TABLE 24–5. INTRAVENOUS FLUID REPLACEMENT IN DIABETIC KETOACIDOSIS

Intervention	Immediate	First hour	Hours 2–4	
Type of fluid	0.9% NSS	0.9% NSS	0.45% NSS	
Insulin		Regular 0.75–0.1 U/kg (bolus)	Regular 0.75–0.1 U/kg/hour by IV infusion	
Rate of infusion	20 ml/kg/hour	20 mL/kg/hr	■ CHILD'S WEIGHT[a]	■ FLUID RATE
			<10 kg	7 ml/kg/hour
			<10–20 kg	6 ml/kg/hour
			<20–40 kg	5 ml/kg/hour
			>40 kg	4.5 ml/kg/hour
Bicarbonate		Use only if pH is <7.0 Give NaHCO$_3$ 1–2 mEq/kg IV over 1–2 hours		
Potassium			■ SERUM K$^+$ (mEq/L)[b]	■ INFUSE K$^+$ (mEq/L)
			<3	40–60
			3–4	30
			4–5	20
			5–6	10

[a]Wexler I (1992). Diabetic ketoacidosis. In Reece R (ed), *Manual of emergency pediatrics*. Philadelphia: Saunders, pp 174–176
[b]Salatino R (1992). Endocrine and metabolic disorders. In Barkin R (ed), *Pediatric emergency medicine*. St. Louis: Mosby, pp 688–704
NSS, normal saline solution.

Rapid correction of acidosis using bicarbonate is generally not recommended for three reasons: (1) an abrupt correction can result in a shift of the oxyhemoglobin curve, decreasing oxygen delivery to the tissue and producing tissue anoxia (Krane, 1987); (2) bicarbonate infusions may lead to a worsening in cerebral acidosis (Sperling, 1990); and (3) rapid correction of acidosis may cause hypokalemia from the rapid shift of potassium into the cells (Karam et al, 1991). The potential benefits and risks of bicarbonate therapy must be weighed against the other potential risks associated with acidosis, such as impending cardiac decompensation. Therefore, the use of bicarbonate may be indicated in certain situations. If the blood pH is 7.1 or less, 40 mEq/m^2 may be infused over several hours (Sperling, 1990). Bicarbonate should never be given as a bolus except in cardiopulmonary resuscitation.

Assessment of Complications of DKA Therapy. The child must be monitored closely to assess for any complication of therapy. Any changes in mental status must be evaluated carefully because they may represent a worsening of metabolic control, development of cerebral edema, the onset of hypoglycemia, or a manifestation of a precipitating illness. The major concern in treating a child with DKA is the development of cerebral edema. The onset of cerebral edema usually occurs 6–10 hours after the initiation of therapy (Israel, 1989); therefore, is not usually seen in the ED. The nurse should keep in mind when monitoring children being treated for DKA that cerebral edema may have an iatrogenic component. Cerebral edema can occur unpredictably in a child who appears to be responding well to treatment. Therefore, any complaints of headache during treatment should be evaluated immediately. The possibility of cerebral edema should be considered until proven otherwise. Hypoglycemia also can result from overzealous insulin therapy. Children who have experienced DKA are admitted for monitoring, regulation, and education once their condition has stabilized.

Recognition of Precipitating Factors. It is important that the precipitating factors in the cause of DKA be detected as quickly as possible. Infection and omission of, or inappropriately low, doses of insulin are the major causes of DKA in children with IDDM. Children who are seen in the ED with frequent bouts of DKA should be referred to a Certified Diabetes Educator (CDE). Inadequate or inaccurate knowledge may be a problem that the CDE can remedy.

PATIENT AND FAMILY TEACHING AND PSYCHOSOCIAL SUPPORT

Although the time available for teaching during an ED visit is limited, several key factors must be empha-

sized. If the child and caregivers are learning for the first time that diabetes mellitus is suspected or confirmed, teaching must be limited to a brief description of the disease itself. That IDDM is a treatable, but not curable, disease is all that can be comprehended at the time. The child is admitted for additional diagnostic work and regulation. A complete teaching plan is developed during the hospitalization.

The major difference in treating Type 1 and Type 2 diabetes relates to administration of insulin. Type 1 diabetes is always insulin-dependent; therefore, any teaching opportunity must reinforce insulin administration techniques and positive health practices. At this time few children use insulin pumps, but the nurse should be certain to verify whether or not the patient uses this equipment. Teaching efforts are always influenced by the developmental level of the child and should include the parent and caregiver, but they should not be geared toward the parent while coincidentally including the child. An example of material appropriate for school-aged children is presented in Figure 24–3. Children are able to assume aspects of managing their diabetes as cognitive and musculoskeletal development progress. Table 24–4 re-

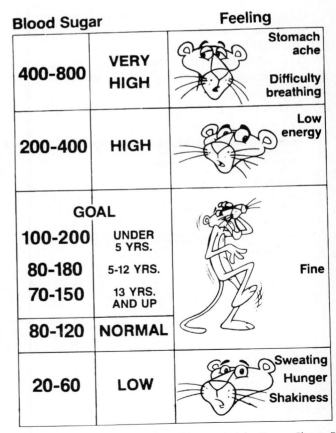

Figure 24–3. Age-appropriate teaching material. (From Chase P [1992]. *Understanding insulin dependent diabetes* [7th ed]. Denver: University of Colorado Health Science Center, p 28)

TABLE 24–6. SUGGESTED EDUCATIONAL MATERIALS

Diabetes '92, '93 Subscription Department American Diabetes Association 1660 Duke Street Alexandria, VA 22314	*Diabetes Self Management* P.O. Box 51125 Boulder, CO 80321
Diabetes Forecast American Diabetes Association Membership Center P.O. Box 2055 Harlan, IA 51593	*The Diabetic's Book* by T. B. Beirman Los Angeles: J. Tarcher, Inc. 1990.
Diabetes in the News Ames Center for Diabetes Education Miles Incorporated P.O. Box 3105 Elkhart, IN 46515	*Health-O-Gram* SugarFree Center 13725 Burbank Blvd Van Nuys, CA 91401 *Understanding Insulin Dependent Diabetes* (7th ed) by H. Peter Chase Children's Diabetes Foundation 700 Delaware Street Denver, CO 80204

flects some of the major developmental characteristics and associated management issues to be kept in mind.

In addition to insulin administration skills, the nurse should review and reinforce the needs for: consistent and appropriate dietary intake; accurate monitoring of blood glucose level; adequate exercise and rest; rapid recognition of signs of hypo- or hyperglycemia; wearing medical alert identification; carrying a rapid source of glucose (sugar cubes, tube of cake icing, not candy because candy is too tempting to eat at any time); and consistent follow-up health care. A number of excellent teaching materials and resources are available; examples of these are included in Table 24–6. The child and caregiver should be given some type of educational material to use as a reference during or after the teaching session.

CONCLUSION

The emergency nursing care of a child experiencing altered insulin or glucose metabolism should focus on rapid assessment of airway, breathing, circulation, and level of consciousness; prompt recognition of the differential diagnosis; immediate initiation of fluid resuscitation; administration of insulin as indicated; ongoing evaluation; patient and family teaching; and discharge planning and follow-up care.

REFERENCES

Alberti K (1988). Diabetic emergencies. In Galloway J, Potvin J, Shuman C (eds), *Diabetes mellitus* (9th ed). Indianapolis: Eli Lilly, pp 254–274

American Diabetes Association (1991). *Diabetes: 1991 vital statistics.* Alexandria, Va: ADA

Aoki B, Hanson, J (1991). Diabetic ketoacidosis. In Grossman M, Dieckman R (eds), *Pediatric emergency medicine: A clinician's reference.* Philadelphia: Lippincott, pp 133–137

Barkin R, Rosen P (eds) (1990). *Emergency pediatrics: A guide to ambulatory care* (3rd ed). St. Louis: Mosby, pp 502–506

Bubb J, Pontious S (1991). Weight loss from inappropriate insulin manipulation: An eating disorder variant in an adolescent with insulin dependent diabetes mellitus. *Diabetes Educator* 17:29–32

Chase HP (1992). *Understanding insulin dependent diabetes* (7th ed). Denver: University of Colorado Health Science Center, p 2

Cryer P, Gerich J (1990). Hypoglycemia in insulin dependent diabetes mellitus: Insulin excess and defective glucose counterregulation. In Rafkin H, Porte D (eds), *Diabetes mellitus: Theory and practice* (4th ed). New York: Elsevier, pp 526–546

Davidson M (1991). *Diabetes mellitus: Diagnosis and treatment* (3rd ed). New York: Churchill-Livingston, pp 243–255

DCCT Research Group (1991). Diabetes control and complications trials (DDCT): Results of feasibility study. *Diabetes Care* 10:1–19

Helms R (1992). Implications of population growth on prevalence of diabetes. *Diabetes Care* 15:6–9

Israel R (1989). Diabetic ketoacidosis. *Emergency Medicine Clinics of North America* 7:859–869

Karam J, Salber P, Forsham P (1991). Pancreatic hormones and diabetes mellitus. In Greenspan F (ed), *Basic and clinical endocrinology* (3rd ed). East Norwalk, Conn: Appleton & Lange, pp 592–650

Katz M (1973). Hyperglycemia induced hyponatremia: Calculation of expected serum sodium depression. *New England Journal of Medicine* 289:843–844

Kelley S, Roberts C (1988). Endocrine emergencies. In Kelley SJ (ed), *Pediatric emergency nursing.* East Norwalk, Conn: Appleton & Lange, pp 389–399

Kitabachi A, Goodman R (1987). Hypoglycemia: Pathophysiology and diagnosis. *Hospital Practice* 22:45–60

Kitabachi A, Murphy M (1988). Diabetic ketoacidosis and hyperosmolar hyperglycemic nonketonic coma. *Medical Clinics of North America* 72:1545–1563

Kitabachi A, Rumbak M (1989). The management of diabetic emergencies. *Hospital Practice* 24:129–160

Krane E (1987). Diabetic ketoacidosis. *Pediatric Clinics of North America* 34:935–960

Kreisberg R (1990). Diabetic ketoacidosis. In Rifkin H, Porte D (eds), *Diabetes mellitus: Theory and practice* (4th ed). New York: Elsevier

Sperling M (1990). Diabetes mellitus. In Kaplan S (ed), *Clinical pediatric endocrinology.* Philadelphia: Saunders, pp 127–164

Salatino R (1992). Endocrine and metabolic disorders. In Barkin RM (ed), *Pediatric emergency medicine.* St. Louis: Mosby, p 142

Walker J (1991). Diabetic emergencies. In Thomas D (ed), *Quick reference to pediatric emergency nursing.* Gaithersburg, MD: Aspen, pp 141–150

Wexler I (1992). Diabetic ketoacidosis. In Reece R (ed), *Manual of emergency pediatrics.* Philadelphia: Saunders, pp 174–176

Yealy D, Wolfson A (1989). Hypoglycemia. *Emergency Medicine Clinics of North America* 7:837

SUGGESTED READING

Allen C, Duck S, Sufit R, Swick H, D'Alessio D (1992). Glycemic control and peripheral nerve conduction in children and young adults. *Diabetes Care* 15:502–506

Bledsoe B (1991). Dealing with diabetic emergencies. *Journal of Emergency Medical Services* 16:40–44; 46–47

Clark L, Plotnick L (1990). Insulin pumps in children with diabetes. *Journal of Pediatric Health Care* 4:3–10

Gray D, Golden M (1991). Diabetes care in schools: Benefits and pitfalls of Public Law 94-142. *Diabetes Educator* 17:33–36

Litman T, Difazio D, Meers R, Thompson R (1989). A developmental approach to diabetes in children: Birth through preschool. *The American Journal of Maternal/Child Nursing* 14:255–259

Litman T, Difazio D, Meers R, Thompson R (1989). A developmental approach to diabetes in children: School age–adolescence. *The American Journal of Maternal/Child Nursing* 14:330–332

Littlefield C, Cravens J, Rodin G, Daneman D, Murray M, Rydall A (1992). Relationship of self-efficacy and beginning adherence to diabetes regimen among adolescents. *Diabetes Care* 15:90–94

McCrea D, McCrea C (1991). Emergency department care of the patient with an insulin pump. *Journal of Emergency Nursing* 17:220–224

Pastors J (1992). Alternative to exchange system. *Diabetes Educator* 18:57–63

Puczynski S, Puczynski M, Ryan C (1992). Hypoglycemia in children with insulin-dependent diabetes mellitus. *Diabetes Educator* 18:151–153

Singer D, Nathan D, Fogel H, Schachat A (1992). Screening for diabetic retinopathy. *Annals of Internal Medicine* 116:660–661

Wheeler M, Warren-Boulton E (1992). Diabetes patient education programs: Quality & reimbursement. *Diabetes Care* 15:36–40

CHAPTER 25

Hematologic Emergencies

SUSAN J. KELLEY

SICKLE CELL DISEASE

Sickle cell disease (SCD) is an autosomal recessive hereditary disorder characterized by the presence of an abnormal type of hemoglobin (hemoglobin S) in the red blood cell. Hemoglobin S may be manifested as active sickle cell disease or as the sickle cell trait. Approximately one out of every 500 African American children has sickle cell disease; 8% have sickle cell trait. Sickle cell disease is found predominantly in people from Africa, the Mediterranean, the Middle East, and parts of India. As of 1990, 36 states included a newborn screening for sickle cell disease (Day et al, 1992).

People with sickle cell trait usually are not as severely affected as those with sickle cell disease. Those with sickle cell trait, however, may be affected by a decreased ability to tolerate extreme physical activity. These people are often unable to withstand atmospheric conditions of low oxygen and may have difficulty during pregnancy.

The prognosis for children with SCD is grave, although advances have been made in the treatment of SCD. Infection is the leading cause of death among young children with SCD. Prophylactic treatment with penicillin begins at 2–4 months of age and continues for at least 5 years. Preventive treatment with penicillin has dramatically decreased the occurrence of serious infection. In older children or young adults death is usually the result of the long-term effects of repeated infarcts and complications. In a sample of 310 children with SCD followed since birth, 7.8% had one or more strokes by the age of 14 years (Balkaran et al, 1992).

Etiology

The basic defect in sickle cell disease is the substitution of valine for glutamic acid in the sixth position of the beta polypeptide chain of the hemoglobin molecule. This structural change facilitates the sickling phenomenon.

Children with SCD are at increased risk for subtle neuropsychological deficits and for behavioral and psychological problems (Iloeje, 1992).

Pathophysiology

In the presence of deoxygenation, a stacking of sickle hemoglobin molecules occurs, and the cell assumes an irregular shape. The abnormally shaped cells increase blood viscosity, which causes stasis and sludging of the cells and further deoxygenation. This leads to further sickling, eventual occlusion of small vessels, and tissue ischemia with infarction and necrosis (Figure 25–1). Before the age of 10 years, the spleen in children with sickle cell anemia may become completely infarcted, often referred to as autosplenectomy. This loss of splenic function makes these children susceptible to life-threatening infections.

Sickle Cell Crisis

Episodes of sickling with localized or generalized pain, profound anemia, debilitation, and weakness are referred to as sickle cell crises. The sickling phenomenon takes place when the oxygen tension in the blood is lowered. This condition may be precipitated by infection, dehydration, exposure to cold, and physical or emotional stress.

There are three primary types of sickle cell crises: vaso-occlusive, aplastic, and sequestration. Vaso-

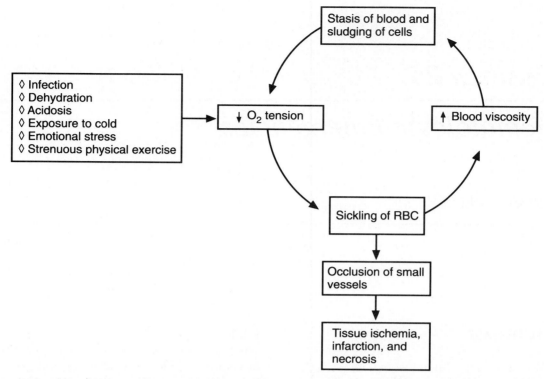

Figure 25–1. The sickling phenomenon. (Redrawn from Thompson SW [1990]. *Emergency care of children.* Bostone:Jones and Bartlett, p 149)

occlusive crisis is the most common. It is caused by intravascular sickling, stasis, and occlusion of the vessels. The most common sites for a vaso-occlusive crisis include the bones, abdominal viscera, liver, spleen, lungs, and central nervous system.

A carefully taken history may reveal a recent infection, physical exertion, exposure to cold, or emotional stress. In some instances no precipitating event is identified. The pain is usually intense in the organ where vascular occlusion is occurring. These children may complain of painful and swollen joints, severe abdominal pain, back pain, and severe headache. The hemoglobin and hematocrit values may be unchanged or slightly elevated because of hemoconcentration.

An aplastic crisis often occurs in association with an upper respiratory infection, gastroenteritis, or viral syndrome. In an aplastic crisis, erythropoiesis ceases or drastically decreases while hemolysis continues. This can result in a life-threatening anemia. Congestive heart failure may occur. The hemoglobin level is low compared with the patient's baseline hemoglobin count, and no reticulocytosis is seen.

In the more uncommon and rapidly fatal sequestration crisis, the blood pools in the spleen and other visceral organs, resulting in severe anemia and hypovolemic shock. This occurs most often in young children. The child may initially appear pale and lethargic, with left-sided abdominal pain, a rapidly en-

larging spleen, chills, fever, and jaundice. Hypovolemic shock rapidly ensues, and death can occur (Powell et al, 1992).

History

A patient with SCD may arrive at the emergency department (ED) in a variety of physical states. Even when newborn screening has been done, many parents do not know the results (Losek, 1991). A family history of SCD or trait should be carefully elicited. An infant with undiagnosed SCD may have a history of frequent infections, failure to thrive, jaundice, or anemia. Manifestation of SCD rarely occurs before the age of 6 months because of the presence of fetal hemoglobin. Between the ages of 6 months and 2 years, dactylitis (hand-foot syndrome) (Figure 25–2) is commonly observed in children with sickle cell anemia. It is characterized by soft tissue swelling and tenderness over the affected appendages. Older children may have a history of joint pain, chest pain, frequent infection, abdominal pain, headache, nausea, and vomiting. The diagnosis of SCD should be considered in any young African American or other black child with a history of fever, unexplained joint pain or swelling, chest pain, pneumonia, meningitis, sepsis, neurologic abnormality, splenomegaly, or anemia.

It is important to identify any medications or analgesics taken on a regular basis or within the past 24

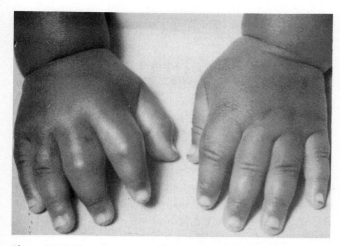

Figure 25–2. Dactylitis occurs when a clot forms on the hands or feet. (Reproduced from *Sickle Cell Anemia.* NIH Publication No 90-3058, 1990, p 8)

TABLE 25–1. HEMATOLOGIC VALUES IN SICKLE CELL DISEASE

Hematologic Parameter	Normal Value	Value in Sickle Cell Disease
Hemoglobin (g/dL)	12	5.5–9.5
Hematocrit (%)	36	17–29
Reticulocyte count (%)	1.5	5–25
WBC count (cells/mm³)	7500	12,000–35,000

hours. Infants and children with SCD usually are receiving penicillin prophylaxis. A history of recent fever, illnesses, pain, or any past hospitalizations or operations, such as a splenectomy, should be noted. Patients with SCD often have glucose-6-phosphate dehydrogenase (G6PD) deficiency, which is an inherited enzyme deficiency related to hemolytic anemia. It is critical to know the child's immunization status, because children with SCD are highly susceptible to infection.

Physical Assessment

The nursing assessment includes an initial evaluation of airway, breathing, and circulation (ABCs). The vital signs, including temperature, should be monitored continually, with special attention to any signs of hypovolemic shock or sepsis.

Location, type, and intensity of pain should be assessed carefully. Painful or swollen joints should be examined for redness, degree of warmth, and range of motion. Sickling in the mesenteric vessels may cause a complaint of abdominal pain. There may be tenderness upon palpation—guarding and rebound. The liver and spleen may be enlarged. Priapism may be present.

Hydration status should be assessed continually and fluid intake and output carefully recorded. Respiratory status should be assessed, because these children are susceptible to bacterial pneumonias. Any sign of cyanosis should be noted. Fast or difficult breathing may indicate an acute chest syndrome (ACS), that is, pulmonary involvement secondary to lung infarction or infection, or a combination of both (SCD Guideline Panel, 1993).

Scleral icterus is typically present in children with

SCD, but any increase in icterus should be noted. Parents may be helpful in observing any increase in scleral icterus because they are familiar with the child's baseline level of scleral icterus. A neurologic assessment should be conducted because a central nervous system infarction can occur with severe sequelae. Limping or paresis could indicate a stroke.

Laboratory and Diagnostic Tests

If prior sickle cell screening test results are not readily available, screening should be conducted in the ED (Losek, 1991). Blood sickling tests such as the Sickledex test and sickle cell slide preparation test are used to screen for the presence of hemoglobin S. If the screening test is positive, a stained blood smear or hemoglobin electrophoresis is used to diagnose SCD.

Hematologic values in SCD are outlined in Table 25–1. In addition to a complete blood count (CBC) with differential and reticulocyte count, it is necessary to obtain serum electrolyte levels, liver function tests, arterial blood gases, urine culture, urinalysis, and blood cultures. Chest, abdominal, and joint x rays should be obtained if indicated.

Early performance of computed tomography (CT) is useful in the diagnosis and rapid treatment of osteomyelitis (Stark et al, 1991). Magnetic resonance imaging (MRI) of the brain and transcranial ultrasonography are useful when there are neurologic signs. An electrocardiogram (ECG) should be obtained. Biventricular hypertrophy is common in children with SCD. Cor pulmonale may result from recurrent pulmonary infarctions.

T R I A G E
Sickle Cell Disease

Emergent ————————————————
A child with fever; severe pain, hypotension; tachycardia.

Urgent ————————————————
A child with a fever; hemodynamically stable condition; mild to moderate pain.

Nursing Diagnosis
Fluid Volume Deficit

Defining Characteristics

- Tachycardia
- Hemoconcentration

Nursing Interventions

- Administer humidified oxygen
- Administer intravenous fluids or blood products
- Carefully monitor vital signs

Expected Outcomes

- Vital signs return to normal
- Pain decreases

Nursing Diagnosis
Pain

Defining Characteristics

- Verbalization of pain
- Crying, irritability

Nursing Interventions

- Administer analgesics
- Administer fluids
- Immobilize painful joint

Expected Outcome

- Pain decreases

Nursing Diagnosis
Knowledge Deficit

Defining Characteristics

- Verbalization of lack of information
- Past treatment recommendations not followed

Nursing Interventions

- Teach importance and proper administration of medications
- Teach signs of sepsis, stroke, anemia emergency, osteomyelitis, acute chest syndrome
- Teach importance of maximum hydration
- Teach correlation of stress, coldness to sickle cell crisis
- Refer family to sickle cell disease treatment center

Expected Outcome

- Verbalization of knowledge of hydration, administration of medication, and signs of an emergency

Management

Impairment of circulation and oxygenation should be treated by administration of oxygen, hydration, and restoration of circulatory volume. Increased hydration by mouth or the intravenous route is critical. Fluids should be administered at 1.5–2.0 times maintenance. Dehydration causes decreased blood volume, sludging, increased blood viscosity, and further sickling. Fluid intake and output should be monitored strictly.

Administration of packed red blood cells at a rate of 5–10 ml/kg over 3–4 hours may be indicated during aplastic or hyperhemolytic crises. Close observation for signs of blood incompatibility is important. Raising the hemoglobin to high levels diminishes bone marrow production of additional sickle cells and dilutes the existing sickle cells with normal transfused erythrocytes. A high leukocyte count and an acute decrease in hemoglobin level are risk factors for stroke; therefore they need to be aggressively corrected (Balkaran et al, 1992).

Relief of pain in a child with SCD is essential. Mild pain can be treated with acetaminophen. The moderate to severe pain experienced by a child in sickle cell crisis usually requires administration of a strong analgesic such as codeine, meperidine, or morphine. Older children may use patient-controlled analgesia. Complications related to the use of parenteral narcotic analgesics include convulsions associated with meperidine and addiction (Pegelow, 1992). When dactylitis, or painful swelling of the hands or feet occurs, in addition to hydration and analgesics, applications of local warmth by compresses, massage, or warm baths may provide relief. The treatment of priapism is outlined in Table 25–2.

Antipyretic agents should be administered to febrile patients, because fever accelerates dehydration. The use of aspirin should be avoided if the patient also has G6PD deficiency. A cooling blanket may be needed. The child should have bedrest with the head of the bed elevated.

The risk for infection is markedly increased in

TABLE 25–2. MANAGEMENT OF PRIAPISM IN SICKLE CELL ANEMIA

Hospitalization if erection persists or if pain is severe.

Intravenous hydration with D5 1/4 NSS or D5 1/2 NSS at 1 1/2–2 × maintenance for 24–48 hours.

If swelling does not decrease, transfusion with red cells to raise hemoglobin level to 9–10 g/dL.

If no improvement after simple transfusion, exchange transfusion to reduce hemoglobins to less than 30% of total hemoglobin.

Aspiration and shunting procedures for patients in whom other forms of therapy have failed in the first 12–72 hours.

NSS, normal saline solution.
(*Reproduced with permission of Fleisher G, Ludwig S [eds], [1993]. Textbook of pediatric emergency medicine [3rd ed]. Baltimore: Williams & Wilkins, p 728*)

patients with SCD. They should be isolated from other children with infectious diseases. Intravenous antibiotics should be administered promptly in the ED.

At most sickle cell treatment centers, recent practice has been to admit to the hospital young children with SCD who are febrile pending blood culture results (Day et al, 1992).

Patient and Family Teaching and Psychosocial Support

A child in sickle cell crisis and the family members are often fearful and require extensive emotional support while in the ED. Children in sickle cell crisis fear painful procedures and repeat hospitalizations. Some children may express feelings of anger and frustration while in the ED.

In some cases the patient has known family members or friends who have died during a sickle cell crisis. The child therefore needs a great deal of reassurance from a calm, sensitive nurse. Younger children are fearful of separation from their parents and of painful procedures such as venipunctures and intramuscular injections. Parents should be permitted to remain close to their child while in the ED to alleviate the child's fears and anxiety. Children should be provided with age-appropriate toys that serve as a source of distraction from their pain while in the ED. Adolescents with SCD may need to discuss their concerns regarding feelings of frustration, social isolation, stigmatization, and loss of independence when hospitalized.

Children with SCD and their parents have many learning needs. For young children, the key to success is to avoid crisis situations through prevention. This includes maximum fluid intake to prevent stagnation and clogging of cells (Wright et al, 1992). Immunizations need to be kept current. It is important that children with SCD receive vaccination for *Haemophilus influenzae* type B (Rubin et al, 1992). The importance of compliance with prophylactic administration of penicillin cannot be over emphasized with patients and family members. Folic acid is also taken to stimulate blood cell production. The child and parents should carry a medical identification card that includes the child's diagnosis, medications, average hemoglobin level, blood type, allergies, and physician's name and telephone number. Parents should be instructed to protect their child from excessive cold and heat, dampness, and exposure to infections and to seek prompt medical attention for all injuries and febrile illnesses. Minor pain episodes may be managed at home with analgesics, rest, and hydration. Parents can be taught to palpate the spleen and to bring their child to the ED if the spleen enlarges (Powell et al, 1992).

The ED nurse should see to it that the family seeks not only episodic care during a crisis but is also closely followed at a SCD treatment center or hematology clinic, where the child can benefit from comprehensive, preventive, supportive, and educational measures.

Professionals and families can receive further information regarding SCD from either of the following agencies: National Sickle Disease Program, National Institutes of Health, Sickle Cell Disease Branch, National Heart, Lung & Blood Institute, Federal Building, Room 504D, 7550 Wisconsin Avenue, Bethesda, MD 20892-9905, (301) 496-6931; National Association for Sickle Cell Disease, 3345 Wilshire Boulevard, Suite 1106, Los Angeles, CA 90010-1880, (800) 421-8453.

HEMOPHILIA

Hemophilia refers to a group of inherited coagulation disorders in which there is a deficiency of one of the blood clotting factors. It affects males almost exclusively but is carried by females.

Etiology

The three most common forms of the disease are classic hemophilia (hemophilia A or factor VIII deficiency), Christmas disease (hemophilia B or factor IX deficiency), and von Willebrand disease. Seventy-five percent of people with hemophilia have classic hemophilia.

Pathophysiology

The prognosis varies greatly and can be predicted from the level of factor-coagulant activity. Patients with hemophilia are generally categorized into three groups according to the severity of the factor deficiency. Patients with severe hemophilia have less than 2% of the normal amount of factor involved. These children may bleed spontaneously or from mild injury. Those with moderate hemophilia have 2--5% of the normal amount of factor. This group does not usually bleed spontaneously but bleeds with only minimal trauma. Children with mild hemophilia have 5–25% of the normal amount of factor, and considerable trauma is needed to cause bleeding. These patients may have no symptoms for years until serious injury occurs or an operation is performed. Although very low factor VIII coagulant activity is associated with severe bleeding in von Willebrand disease, the relationship between laboratory findings and clinical course is less predictable than in other forms of hemophilia.

Patients with hemophilia in any of these three categories may seek emergency care. The classification of inherited bleeding disorders is very important in assessing these patients in the ED. For example, after mild head trauma a patient with severe hemophilia is at greater risk for intracranial bleeding than a patient with mild hemophilia. In a patient with mild hemophilia and extensive hemorrhage, severe trauma has probably occurred, and injury to internal organs should be suspected.

History

Children with hemophilia may have a history of traumatic or spontaneous bleeding. Prolonged bleeding may occur internally or externally. Subcutaneous and intramuscular hemorrhage and hemarthrosis, or bleeding into the joints, especially the ankles, knees, and elbows, is common. Prolonged bleeding may occur after circumcision or tooth extraction. A history of head trauma is very significant. Hematuria and epistaxis may result from spontaneous bleeding. A careful history of previous bleeding episodes, factor replacement therapy, and hospitalizations is important. A family history of hemophilia should be obtained. There may be a history of hepatitis or human immunodeficiency virus (HIV) infection acquired in transfusions with blood products.

Physical Assessment

Vital signs should be carefully monitored with close attention to heart rate and blood pressure. Tachycardia and hypotension may indicate impending shock. Careful assessment of cardiovascular, respiratory, central nervous, musculoskeletal, and gastrointestinal systems is important. Bleeding into the airway, neck, or chest is serious because of the risk of occluding the airway or respiratory tract. Emergency personnel should be alert to any unexplained or difficult-to-control bleeding in a patient with undiagnosed hemophilia.

Patients with hemophilia who have a history of headache, vomiting, altered mental status, or seizures may be experiencing an intracranial bleed. Paralysis, weakness, and asymmetric neurologic findings may signify a spinal cord hematoma. Bleeding into the central nervous system is often fatal.

Involvement of the elbows, knees, and ankles is common; joint tenderness, swelling, and limitation of range of motion are present (Barkin, 1992). Muscle bleeding is also common. Hematemesis and abdominal pain may signify bleeding in the gastrointestinal tract.

Laboratory and Diagnostic Tests

The following laboratory data should be obtained: CBC with hematocrit, blood coagulation studies including partial thromboplastin time (PTT), prothrombin time (PT), thrombin time (TT), bleeding time, urinalysis, and x rays as indicated by history and physical findings. Computed tomography is indicated if there has been head trauma.

TRIAGE
Hemophilia

Emergent
A child with serious hemorrhage; signs of hypovolemia; head injury; bleeding in airway.

Urgent
A child with moderate hemorrhage; bleeding into joint.

Non-urgent
A child with no sign of active bleeding; no complaint of pain.

Nursing Diagnosis
Fluid Volume Deficit

Defining Characteristics

- Tachycardia
- Hypotension

Nursing Interventions

- Administer intravenous fluids
- Control bleeding
- Monitor vital signs

Expected Outcomes

- Vital signs are normal
- Bleeding is controlled

Nursing Diagnosis
Activity Intolerance

Defining Characteristic

- Abnormal response to activity

Nursing Interventions

- Decrease child's level of activity while in ED
- Discuss child's toleration of physical activity with parents

Expected Outcomes

- Child rests while in ED
- Parents demonstrate an understanding of child's capacity for strenuous activity

Nursing Diagnosis
Pain

Defining Characteristics

- Verbalization of pain
- Demonstrates signs of pain such as irritability, tachycardia, facial grimacing by infant or nonverbal child

Nursing Interventions

- Administer analgesic as indicated
- Immobilize any joint that is painful and swollen

Expected Outcome

- Child describes a decrease in pain

Management

Emergency management is aimed at controlling bleeding, replacing fluid volume, administering the missing coagulation factor, and providing comfort. The type and amount of factor replacement depends on the factor deficiency and location and severity of hemorrhage. Fresh frozen plasma may be administered in the ED if the missing factor is not readily available.

If hemarthrosis is present, the joint should be immobilized. Analgesics may be necessary until the swelling subsides. Aspirin should never be used because its inhibitory effect on platelet function may aggravate the clotting disorder. Application of a cold pack to the affected joint may decrease pain and swelling. Arthrocentesis may be performed by a physician to remove blood from the joint to allow early mobilization and to increase range of motion. Aspiration of a joint is a frightening procedure for children; therefore, sedation may be given before the procedure. In addition, the nurse or parent may need to restrain the child during the procedure while providing reassurance and emotional support.

Muscle bleeding is usually superficial and easily controlled with a single dose of replacement therapy. Subcutaneous bleeding may occur but is rarely dangerous and rarely requires therapy. A subcutaneous bleed in the neck, however, may cause compression of the airway. Any bleeding in the neck muscles should be carefully monitored, and equipment to maintain a patent airway should be readily available, since airway obstruction could be sudden. Likewise, any bleeding in the oral cavity should be carefully monitored. Aminocaproic acid is given orally in conjunction with replacement therapy for any bleeding of the mouth, lip, or tongue.

Because of the numerous blood product transfusions that children with hemophilia receive, they are at an increased risk for acquired immune deficiency syndrome (AIDS) and hepatitis. All bodily secretions and blood specimens should therefore be handled with the appropriate precautions. As with all ED patients, universal precautions should be maintained.

Most children with hemophilia are treated and discharged home. Those with head trauma, retropharyngeal bleeding, or gastrointestinal bleeding usually are admitted for observation and further intervention.

Patient and Family Teaching and Psychosocial Support

Children with hemophilia need much support and reassurance while in the ED (Spitzer, 1992b). Research findings have indicated that children with hemophilia perceive illness and treatment-related experiences as threats. Children with hemophilia try to minimize their differences from other children and prefer not to be viewed as sick or different (Spitzer, 1992b). Children with hemophilia also have concerns regarding acquiring HIV infection through blood products, although this risk has been greatly reduced since screening of donated blood and blood products began in the early 1980s. Children with hemophilia who have acquired HIV through blood products and their families need to be supported as they cope with their grief and anger (Tsiantis et al, 1990).

The child and parents are usually frightened by the bleeding episode and need much reassurance and support from nursing personnel. All procedures and treatments should be carefully explained to the child and parents. The parents should be encouraged to remain at the child's bedside during the ED visit. Age-appropriate toys or reading materials should be provided to the child to keep the child calm and resting.

Research findings have indicated that children with hemophilia have major areas of knowledge deficiency, especially about how one contracts hemophilia and its treatment (Spitzer, 1992a). Parents of children with hemophilia also have many learning needs. Prevention of injury is very important. The nurse needs to teach parents how to protect the child from injury without becoming overprotective. Exercise should be encouraged to build strong muscles to help protect the joints from injury. All contact sports, however, should be avoided. A referral to a visiting nurse may be indicated to help the parents plan a safe home environment according to the child's developmental level. Children with hemophilia should wear a medical alert bracelet or carry a medical identification card.

The parents of a child with hemophilia should be referred to a parent support group. The National Hemophilia Foundation has more than 50 chapters across the United States to help families with financial, emotional, and medical needs. They can be contacted at: National Hemophilia Foundation, Soho Building, 110

Green St, Suite 303, New York, NY 10012, Telephone: (212) 219-8180.

IDIOPATHIC THROMBOCYTOPENIC PURPURA

Idiopathic thrombocytopenic purpura (ITP) is caused by a pronounced reduction in circulating platelets, causing purpura, or bleeding into the tissues. It is the most frequently encountered platelet disorder of childhood. Although ITP is usually an acute, self-limited disease, with most cases resolving within 6–12 months, it can be chronic, with numerous remissions. Serious bleeding is rare; it occurs in only 2% of patients.

Etiology

The thrombocytopenia is caused by an antiplatelet antibody produced in the spleen. It is associated with a spectrum of viral illnesses, including measles, rubella, mumps, chicken pox, infectious mononucleosis, and the common cold. Other causes include systemic lupus erythematosus, transfusions, and drug sensitivities. Possible complications, although rare, include intracranial hemorrhage, gastrointestinal bleeding, and hematuria (Barkin, 1992).

Pathophysiology

The acute form of ITP is preceded by a viral infection in 50% of patients. It can last anywhere from 3 weeks to several months. The chronic form of ITP is more indolent in its early stages but may recur over the years. Both forms are characterized by abrupt onset of petechiae, purpura, and ecchymoses over bony prominences and bleeding from the gastrointestinal tract, mouth, or gums, or epistaxis.

History

A history of a recent viral illness should be elicited. Any medications recently taken should be identified. Headaches or an altered level of consciousness may be related to an intracranial hemorrhage.

Physical Assessment

Airway, breathing, and circulation should be assessed continually. The skin should be carefully examined. The lesions of ITP are minute, flat, red hemorrhages in size from 0.5–3.0 or 4.0 mm; they often occur in association with petechiae. Bleeding from the mucous membranes of the mouth and nose should be noted. Hematuria and bloody stools may occur. A child with ITP who has sustained head trauma should be carefully evaluated for signs of increased intracranial pressure.

Laboratory and Diagnostic Tests

The platelet count is usually reduced to below 100,000 platelets/mm^3 (normal platelet count is 150,000 to 400,000/mm^3). If the count falls below 20,000 platelet/mm^3, the patient is at great risk for hemorrhage. A tourniquet test, bleeding time, and clot reaction are abnormal. Coagulation studies are normal. A bone marrow aspiration is performed to confirm the diagnosis and to rule out aplastic anemia or leukemia.

TRIAGE
Idiopathic Thrombocytopenic Purpura

Emergent
A child with severe hemorrhage; head trauma; acute onset.

Urgent
A child with mild hemorrhage; stable vital signs.

Nursing Diagnosis
Fluid Volume Deficit

Defining Characteristics

- Tachycardia
- Hypotension

Nursing Interventions

- Administer platelets as ordered
- Administer fresh frozen plasma as ordered
- Administer steroids as ordered
- Administer oxygen

Expected Outcomes

- Vital signs are stable
- Bleeding stops

Nursing Diagnosis
Fear

Defining Characteristic

- Verbalization of fear, anxiety

Nursing Interventions

- Keep child and family informed of all treatments
- Allow parents to remain at bedside while in ED

Expected Outcome

- Child and family express decrease in fear

Management

Emergency management focuses on controlling bleeding and preventing hemorrhage. The patient must be continually evaluated for shock and signs of increased intracranial bleeding. Transfusion with packed red blood cells may be necessary. Platelet transfusions may be administered during acute bleeding. Survival of the transfused platelets, however, is brief. Steroids such as oral prednisone 2 mg/kg/24 hours tid (maximum 60 mg/24 hours) are administered in severe or chronic cases. The effects of steroid therapy are usually apparent in 48–72 hours; more than 50% of children respond (Barkin, 1992). Splenectomy is reserved for children with thrombocytopenia that lasts more than 1 year or in the event of a life-threatening hemorrhage. Patients with platelet counts of less than 50,000 platelets/mm^3 should be admitted for evaluation and close monitoring.

Patient and Family Teaching and Psychosocial Support

In the initial phase of assessment, parents often fear that their child has a life-threatening illness, such as leukemia. They are also greatly disturbed by the changes in the appearance of their child caused by the purpura and petechiae. Parents and child need a great deal of emotional support and reassurance while in the ED.

If the child is discharged home, the parents need to be instructed to observe for any abnormalities. Accident prevention should be stressed, and the child should be instructed not to play any contact sports or rough games. The use of aspirin and aspirin products should be avoided. If steroids are prescribed, the parents should be instructed in their administration with special emphasis on not abruptly discontinuing them. The side effects of steroids, such as facial edema, weight gain, and increased appetite, should be explained.

DISSEMINATED INTRAVASCULAR COAGULATION

Disseminated intravascular coagulation (DIC) is an acquired disorder of hemostasis that occurs with the activation of clotting mechanisms and leads to a depression of clotting factors and intravascular formation of fibrin. The condition is manifested by diffuse hemorrhage and thrombosis.

Etiology

Disseminated intravascular coagulation is not a primary disease but is a secondary disorder that complicates a pathologic process such as hypovolemic shock; septic shock; viral, bacterial, rickettsial, or parasitic infections; multiple trauma; burns; respiratory distress syndrome; neoplasms; leukemia; intrauterine infections; severe birth asphyxia; snake bites; heat stroke; and intravascular hemolysis from an incompatible blood transfusion. Children with acute leukemia, especially acute promyelocytic leukemia (APML), are more prone to DIC than are children with other malignant diseases (Happ, 1987).

Pathophysiology

Disseminated intravascular coagulation occurs when the first stage of the coagulation process is abnormally stimulated. Thrombin is generated in larger amounts than can be neutralized by the body, and fibrinogen converts rapidly to fibrin with aggregation and destruction of platelets. In the second stage, the fibrinolytic mechanism is activated, causing extensive destruction of clotting factors. The child is then susceptible to uncontrollable hemorrhage and damage and hemolysis of red blood cells.

History

A history may reveal one of the secondary disorders described earlier. Careful attention should be given to the details of a history of a bacterial or viral illness. Disseminated intravascular coagulation most often is associated with bacterial septic shock.

Assessment

A child with DIC may present with petechiae, purpura, excessive bleeding from a venipuncture site, hypotension, acrocyanosis, ischemic necrosis of the skin and subcutaneous tissues, and dysfunction of organs from infarction and ischemia. Thrombosis in a blood vessel serving the central nervous system may cause changes in level of consciousness. Hematuria may indicate renal system involvement.

Laboratory and Diagnostic Tests

Hematologic abnormalities include anemia, thrombocytopenia, prolonged PT, prolonged PTT, prolonged TT, decreased platelet count, decreased fibrinogen level, decreased levels of factors V and VIII, and distortion of red blood cell structure. Blood and urine cultures, CBC, and arterial blood gases should also be obtained.

T R I A G E
Disseminated Intravascular Coagulation

Emergent ————————————————
A child with DIC.

Nursing Diagnoses

The nursing diagnoses for DIC are the same as those for ITP and its underlying conditions, such as septic shock.

Management

Initial attention should be directed toward stabilizing the patient's condition. Treatment involves correcting the underlying cause and supportive measures.

Fresh whole blood or packed red cells are administered if there is considerable hemorrhaging. Platelets and fresh frozen plasma may be administered to replace lost plasma components. Heparin may be given intravenously 50 U/kg, followed 4 hours later by 10–15 U/kg/hour by constant intravenous infusion.

Humidified 40% oxygen should be administered. Vital signs and temperature should be monitored carefully. Cardiac monitoring should be implemented. Continued assessment of neurologic, respiratory, and circulatory status is imperative during stabilization in the ED and subsequent transfer to an intensive care unit. The ED nurse should protect the child from any unnecessary bleeding episodes. The child's energy should be conserved in the ED by bedrest.

Patient and Family Teaching and Psychosocial Support

Parents are often frightened by the complication of DIC in an already stressful illness or injury in their child. Parents need to be informed of the child's progress and to be prepared for the child's admission to the hospital. Parents should be allowed to spend as much time as possible at the child's bedside while in the ED.

REFERENCES

Balkaran B, Char G, Morris JS, Thomas PW, Serjeant BE, Serjeant GR (1992). Stroke in a cohort of patients with homozygous sickle cell disease. *Journal of Pediatrics* 120:360–366

Barkin RM (1992). Hematologic and oncologic disorders. In Barkin RM (ed) *Pediatric emergency medicine.* St. Louis: Mosby, pp 828–844

Day S, Brunson G, Wang W (1992). A successful education program for parents of infants with newly diagnosed sickle cell disease. *Journal of Pediatric Nursing,* 7:52–57

Happ M (1987). Life threatening hemorrhage in children with cancer. *Journal of the Association of Pediatric Oncology Nurses,* 4:36–40

Iloeje SO (1991). Psychiatric morbidity among children with sickle cell disease. *Developmental Medicine and Child Neurology* 33:1087–1094

Losek JD (1991). Sickle cell screening practice in pediatric emergency departments. *Pediatric Emergency Care* 7:278–280

Pegelow CH (1992). Survey of pain management therapy provided for children with sickle cell disease. *Clinical Pediatrics* 31:211–214

Powell RW, Levine GL, Yang YM, Mankad VN (1992). Acute splenic sequestration crisis in sickle cell disease: Early detection and treatment. *Journal of Pediatric Surgery* 27:215–218

Rubin LG, Voulakas D, Carmody L (1992). Immunogenicity of Haemophilus influenzae type b conjugate vaccine in children with sickle cell disease. *American Journal of Diseases in Children* 146:340–342

Sickle Cell Disease Guideline Panel (1993). Sickle cell disease: Screening, diagnosis, management, and counseling. In: *Newborns and infants.* Rockville, MD: US Department of Health and Human Services. AHCPR Publication No. 93-0562

Spitzer A (1992a). Children's knowledge of illness and treatment experiences in hemophilia. *Journal of Pediatric Nursing,* 7:43–51

Spitzer A (1992b). Coping processes of school-age children with hemophilia. *Western Journal of Nursing Research* 14:157–169

Stark JE, Glasier CM, Blasier RD, Aronson J, Seibert JJ (1991). *Radiology* 179:731–733

Tsiantis J, Anastasopoulos D, Meyer M, et al (1990). A multilevel intervention approach for care of HIV-positive hemophiliac and thalassemic patients and their families. *AIDS Care* 2:253–266

Wright L, Brown A, Davidson-Mundt A (1992). Newborn screening: The miracle and the challenge. *Journal of Pediatric Nursing,* 7:26–42

CHAPTER 26

Infectious Disease Emergencies

ELLEN REYNOLDS
SUSAN J. KELLEY

INTRODUCTION

It is important for the emergency department (ED) nurse to be able to recognize infectious diseases and begin intervention. Many types of infectious disease present medical emergencies, and early identification and intervention may be essential in preventing morbidity and mortality. Also, since other ED patients may be immunocompromised or be susceptible to certain infectious diseases, the ED nurse may need to take special precautions to prevent the transmission of illness from one patient to another.

Some diseases, while not infectious in nature, may present with signs and symptoms similar to true infectious diseases. Because of this presentation and the need for differential diagnosis, some of these illnesses are discussed in this chapter.

ACQUIRED IMMUNE DEFICIENCY SYNDROME (AIDS)

Infection with the human immunodeficiency virus (HIV) is producing a new population of chronically and terminally ill children, many of whom may present to the ED with urgent or life-threatening conditions and complications. It is a challenge for the ED nurse to be prepared to treat not only the physical manifestations of these illnesses but also the long-term psychosocial implications for the child and family during the very brief ED contact.

AIDS was first reported in children younger than 13 years in 1983. As of April 1990, nearly 2200 cases of

pediatric AIDS had been reported to the Centers for Disease Control and Prevention (CDC) (Burroughs and Edelson, 1991), representing approximately 2% of the overall AIDS incidence (American Academy of Pediatrics, 1991). Children, like adults, manifest clinical signs and symptoms that range from mild general symptoms to a full-blown AIDS infection as defined by the CDC (Table 26–1). Most children with AIDS fail to thrive. They may have recurrent bacterial and fungal infections, chronic diarrhea, cardiomyopathy, neurologic deterioration, chronic anemia, or renal disease. Efforts can and should be made to focus the care of a child with AIDS in the home; hospital and community nursing support is given as needed.

Etiology and Pathophysiology

Children are infected with the HIV virus perinatally, through contaminated blood products, or through illicit sexual contact. Perinatal exposure is thought to be

---

TABLE 26–1. CENTERS FOR DISEASE CONTROL AND PREVENTION (CDC) DIAGNOSTIC CRITERIA FOR AIDS IN CHILDREN

- CHILDREN YOUNGER THAN 13 MONTHS HAVE ONE OF THE FOLLOWING:
  Confirmed human immunodeficiency virus (HIV) in blood or tissues
  Symptoms meeting CDC case definition
  HIV antibody and evidence of both cellular and humoral deficiency and symptoms

- OLDER CHILDREN HAVE ONE OF THE FOLLOWING:
  Confirmed HIV in blood or tissues
  HIV antibody
  Symptoms meeting CDC case definition

responsible for 80% of cases in infants and children (Thurber and Berry, 1990); 77% of mothers of children with HIV are themselves infected (Ward-Wimmer, 1988). The virus can be transmitted transplacentally, during the birth process, or more rarely through breast feeding. Perinatally acquired AIDS usually presents between 2 months and 2 years; transfusion-acquired AIDS can present from a few months to 5 years after the transfusion (Berry, 1988).

AIDS directly attacks the functioning B- and T-lymphocyte components of the immune system. B cells are mature lymphocytes that produce all antibodies and circulating immunoglobulins. T cells are responsible for cellular immunity and function to protect against most viruses, slow-growing intracellular bacteria, such as *Mycobacterium*, and fungi. They also mediate the hypersensitivity reaction. They are subdivided into T-helper lymphocytes, which support diverse immune functions, and T-suppressor cells, which function to shut down the immune response. Upon infection of a host, the HIV virus binds to a molecule known as the CD4 antigen, which is found on the surface of T-helper lymphocytes. The HIV virus then enters the T-helper cells and destroys them. As a result, cell-mediated immunity as well as T-cell support of antibody formation is compromised and the balance between immune suppression and activation is disrupted, leaving the child extremely vulnerable to infection (Thurber and Berry, 1990). Ordinary infections may become life-threatening, and opportunistic infections and cancers thrive. Infants who have not yet been able to develop immunity against common illnesses are especially vulnerable. Recurrence of infection is common, and gram-negative sepsis is the primary cause of death (Berry, 1988).

The ED nurse sees patients present for diagnosis of AIDS as well as patients in whom AIDS has already been diagnosed and who are being seen for an acute infection or complication. The remainder of this section applies to a child presenting for the first time with suspected AIDS.

History

An infant or young child with AIDS often presents with a history of failure to thrive. The parent may report a history of weight loss or failure to gain, chronic cough, diarrhea, and diaphoresis. The parent may also report a history of recurrent respiratory infections or thrush. Neurologic symptoms occur in 50% of affected children. These are usually manifested as progressive encephalopathy, characterized by developmental delay or loss of motor milestones after they have been mastered. Many of these infants are irritable and difficult to console.

A history of risk factors in both the child and mother needs to be elicited. Specifically, the mother should be asked about any history of blood transfusions, intravenous drug use, or sexual contact with intravenous drug users or bisexual men. She should be asked if the child has had any transfusions or blood products or if there has been any possibility of sexual contact or abuse.

Physical Assessment

Infection with HIV is multisystemic in nature, and presentation may vary greatly among patients. General characteristics should be carefully reviewed. Small size and the presence of dysmorphic features may be indicative of HIV infection in a young infant. Early findings during childhood may be nonspecific, but they tend to be persistent and more severe. Central nervous system (CNS) dysfunction accompanied by developmental delay is common.

Oral lesions indicating candidiasis may be noted. Generalized lymphadenopathy and signs of parotitis are common. Hepatomegaly may be present with or without splenomegaly.

The onset of *Pneumocystis carinii* pneumonia (PCP) may present with fever and tachypnea. Respiratory findings, including a cough, clubbing of the fingers, and lymphadenopathy, are associated with lymphoid interstitial pneumonitis (LIP), which is a criterion for a presumptive diagnosis of AIDS.

Laboratory and Diagnostic Tests

The primary and most successful diagnostic procedure is documentation of HIV by direct virus isolation. Serology tests are effective also, but because maternal antibodies are passively acquired by a newborn, testing by enzyme-linked immunosorbent assay (ELISA) with confirmation by Western blot is not diagnostic for infants and toddlers until approximately 15–18 months of age.

Infected infants and children often have increased immunoglobulin levels with decreased T4 cell counts and a decreased ratio of T4 (helper cells) to T8 (suppressor cells). Hypergammaglobulinemia may be present. A decreased lymphocyte response to mitogens and antigens also may be present. Viral culture, in vitro antibody production, and polymerase chain reaction (PCR) are other modalities of serodiagnosis that are not yet widely available.

General indices related to the presenting complaint should be examined. A complete blood count (CBC) may indicate anemia or the presence of infection as well as neutropenia, lymphopenia, and thrombocytopenia. Electrolytes may reveal hyponatremia or hypokalemia in the presence of diarrhea. Blood cultures may be warranted in acute infection.

TRIAGE
AIDS

Emergent

An HIV-infected child with symptoms of overwhelming infection; sepsis; hypovolemia; acute neurologic deterioration.

Urgent

A child with moderate respiratory distress; early dehydration; acute pain.

Non-emergent

A child with weight loss; mild diarrhea; infection but is awake and alert.

Nursing Diagnosis
Altered Nutrition: Less than body requirements

Defining Characteristics

- Less than 10th percentile for height and weight
- Thin, gaunt appearance
- Objective deficits based on 24-hour parent recall

Nursing Interventions

- Provide information on nutritional needs of child
- Assist with referral to nutritional services, such as the federally sponsored Women, Infants, and Children (WIC) program, as appropriate

Expected Outcome

- Weigh loss stabilizes, weight gain occurs

Nursing Diagnosis
Ineffective Breathing Pattern

Defining Characteristics

- Tachypnea
- Pallor, cyanosis

Nursing Interventions

- Administer oxygen
- Position with head of bed elevated to enhance respiratory effort
- Monitor vital signs

Expected Outcomes

- Respiratory rate normalizes
- Color normalizes

Nursing Diagnosis
Alterations in Cognitive Perception

Defining Characteristics

- Shrill cry
- Difficulty in being consoled
- Decreased responsiveness

Nursing Interventions

- Provide selective stimulation to child
- Teach parents techniques of calming, eg, swaddling infant
- Encourage respite care for parents

Expected Outcomes

- Amount of crying decreases
- Child is responsive

Management
There is no cure for AIDS. It is the ninth leading cause of death among children 1–4 years of age and the seventh leading cause of death among people 15–29 years of age (Novello et al, 1989). Management of AIDS involves a multidisciplinary effort aimed at prevention of infections and complications, support of optimal general health, and recognition and treatment of complications in their early stages.

The antiviral agent zidovudine (AZT) has been shown to be effective in delaying the progression of the disease in adults and is now used in children also. Weight gain, a decrease in liver and spleen size, an increased intelligence quotient, and increased immune function have been attributed to AZT (McKinney, 1991). The routine use of intravenous gamma (immune) globulin (IVIG) is controversial, but this drug has been used to provide passive immunity to children with recurrent infections. Trimethoprim-sulfamethoxazole (TMP-SMZ) prophylaxis against PCP is recommended for all children with the HIV who are younger than 1 year (American Academy of Pediatrics, 1991).

Children with AIDS should receive the usual childhood immunizations, inactivated polio vaccine (Salk) replacing oral polio vaccine. In addition, they should receive pneumococcal vaccine at 2 years and influenza vaccine annually. If they are exposed to measles or varicella, immunoglobulin or varicella-zoster immune globulin (VZIG), respectively, should be administered (Burroughs and Edelson, 1991).

Patient and Family Teaching and Psychosocial Support
Families of children with AIDS need constant support in dealing with the implications of a terminal illness

with many unknowns, with the stigma that society places on that illness, and with very complex physical care needs. The nurse can give such support by providing (1) information about the disease and treatment, (2) help to the family in talking with their children about the disease, (3) direct service, and (4) advocacy for the family and child.

The family's reaction to a diagnosis of AIDS may include shock, anger, guilt, and fear. These feelings may recur over and over again during various stages and exacerbations of the child's illness. Family members should be encouraged to express their feelings and concerns in times of crisis, which may often occur in the ED. As with other chronic illnesses, nurses and social workers who can provide continuity of care to the child and family during repeated visits should be identified early.

Extensive teaching needs to be done with the family, but the ED visit should focus on the teaching pertinent to the current presenting problem and resources should be identified for follow-up care. Families should be assured that casual contact does not result in transmission of the disease and that touching and cuddling are important for the child as well as the family. Parents should be taught basic principles of prevention of disease transmission to protect their immunocompromised child.

SEPSIS AND SEPTIC SHOCK

Sepsis, or septicemia, refers to a profound, life-threatening bacterial infection in the bloodstream. Bacteremia may progress to septicemia depending on clinical manifestations. Septicemia, however, can occur without bacteremia when endotoxemia is present (Behrman, 1992). Septic shock occurs in patients with septicemia when evidence of inadequate tissue perfusion is detected.

Neonates, especially those born prematurely, are highly susceptible to sepsis. Neonatal sepsis refers to the clinical syndrome of systemic illness associated with bacteremia during the first 4 weeks of life. All neonates evaluated in the ED with rectal temperatures 101°F or higher should be considered to have sepsis until proven otherwise, although many neonates with sepsis are afebrile and many neonates with fevers do not have sepsis.

The incidence of sepsis in the United States is estimated to be anywhere between 1 and 8 cases per 1000 live births. Boys are affected almost twice as often as girls and have a higher mortality. The overall mortality is 15–50%, depending on the infecting organism.

Etiology

In the neonatal period the pathogens most frequently responsible for sepsis are *Escherichia coli* and group B streptococcus. In infants and children older than 1 month, the organisms under suspicion are the same as those that produce meningitis in this age group. These organisms include *Hemophilus influenzae, Streptococcus pneumoniae,* and *Neisseria meningitidis.*

Pathophysiology

In contrast to bacteremia (bacteria in the blood), septicemia usually consists of bacteremia plus a constellation of signs and symptoms caused by microorganisms or their toxic products in the circulation (Behrman, 1992). Septic shock occurs when sepsis is accompanied by hypotension, signs of inadequate systemic perfusion, and metabolic acidosis.

Risk factors for neonates include low birth weight, prematurity, fetal distress, congenital anomalies, traumatic birth, and an Apgar score at 1 minute of 5 or less. Infants at high risk have a four-times greater risk of developing sepsis than healthy newborns. The source of infection for the neonate may be the umbilical stump; skin; mucous membranes of the eyes, nose, or pharynx; the ears; gastrointestinal (GI) tract; CNS; or urinary tract. While in the newborn nursery and neonatal intensive care unit (ICU), neonates are at risk for nosocomial infections, especially those on ventilators or with central lines.

Maternal risk factors for neonatal sepsis include endometritis, bacteremia, vaginal infection, premature rupture of the membranes, or a traumatic delivery.

Risk factors for older infants and children include sickle cell disease, HIV infection, immunocompromise, long-term use of antibiotics, recent surgical procedures or stays in ICUs, and burns or wounds.

History

A neonate may have a nonspecific history of "not doing well." A careful history may reveal poor feeding, vomiting, fever, diarrhea, abdominal distention, respiratory distress, apnea, lethargy, irritability, and seizures.

The history obtained for an infant or child older than 1 month may include fever, lethargy, irritability, vomiting, diarrhea, and poor feeding. A history of a localized infection, such as a respiratory tract infection, may be given. A history of a chronic or life-threatening disease such as sickle cell disease, HIV infection, or cancer should alert nurses to a child at increased risk for sepsis.

Physical Assessment

Airway, breathing, and circulation should be rapidly assessed and supported. The infant or child should immediately be assessed for symptoms of shock, including tachycardia, hypotension, tachypnea, decreased level of consciousness, and poor peripheral circulation. The examiner must keep in mind that hypotension is a late sign of shock in infants and young children; it indicates the shock is severe. The skin is often cool, especially at the extremities. Capillary refill time may be delayed (>2 seconds). Skin should be inspected for a petechial or purpuric rash, jaundice, pallor, cyanosis, or mottling. Neonatal body temperature should be carefully monitored and may fluctuate between hypothermia and hyperthermia. Older infants and children may have hyperthermia.

Vital signs should be carefully monitored. A cardiac monitor should be used in infants and children with indicators of septic shock. Fluid intake and output should be carefully monitored. Normal renal output is 2 mg/kg/hour in infants, 1 mg/kg/hour in children, and 0.5 mg/kg/hour in adolescents. Any decrease in urine output suggests that renal perfusion is compromised.

Ongoing neurologic assessment should include the patient's level of consciousness, lethargy, irritability, pupil reactivity, level of activity, seizure activity, and bulging fontanelles in infants. A decrease in response to painful procedures in infants and children is an ominous sign.

The liver should be inspected for hepatomegaly and the skin and sclerae for jaundice.

Laboratory and Diagnostic Tests

Blood Studies. Blood work includes a CBC with differential, platelet counts, prothrombin time (PT), partial thromboplastin time (PTT), and serum electrolyte with glucose levels. Arterial blood gas values may indicate metabolic acidosis in patients with shock.

Cultures. Two specimens for blood cultures from two different venipuncture sites should be obtained. A urine culture should be obtained by a suprapubic bladder tap or catheterization in infants and a clean voided or catheterized specimen in children. The nasopharynx, ear canals, and any skin lesion should be cultured in hopes of yielding the infective organism. In neonates the umbilical stump should be cultured.

Lumbar Puncture. A lumbar puncture is performed to rule out meningitis because 20–30% of neonates with septicemia also have bacterial meningitis.

X Rays. A chest x ray may be obtained to rule out the presence of pneumonia.

TRIAGE
Sepsis or Septic Shock

Emergent
An infant or child with sepsis or septic shock.

Nursing Diagnosis
Decreased Cardiac Output

Defining Characteristics

- Tachycardia
- Hypotension
- Poor capillary refill
- Cool extremities

Nursing Interventions

- Administer oxygen
- Administer medications
- Monitor fluid intake and output

Expected Outcomes

- Vital signs return to normal
- Capillary refill returns to normal
- Extremities are warm to touch

Nursing Diagnosis
Ineffective Thermoregulation

Defining Characteristics

- Increase or decrease in body temperature
- Tachycardia
- Tachypnea

Nursing Interventions

- Administer antipyretics for elevated body temperature
- Use warming or cooling blanket as indicated
- Administer antibiotics as ordered

Expected Outcomes

- Body temperature returns to normal
- Respiratory rate returns to normal
- Heart rate returns to normal

Nursing Diagnosis
Fluid Volume Deficit

Defining Characteristics

- Decreased urine output

- Decreased venous filling
- Decreased level of consciousness
- Hypotension

Nursing Interventions

- Administer intravenous fluids promptly
- Administer medications
- Monitor fluid intake and urinary output

Expected Outcomes

- Urine output increases
- Capillary filling returns to normal
- Blood pressure returns to normal
- Increased level of consciousness

Management

Early recognition and treatment of sepsis and septic shock are essential for increasing the chance of survival and decreasing long-term sequelae. Initial treatment includes support of airway, breathing, and circulation. The patient should be positioned to support maximal airway patency. Supplemental oxygen should be administered at 4–6 L/minute by mask. All necessary equipment for intubation should be available at the bedside in the event of rapid deterioration. Nursing interventions directed at decreasing oxygen demands should be instituted. These include thermoregulation, alleviation of pain, and reassurance of the child because emotional upset and fear increase oxygen consumption. A family member should be allowed to remain with the child as much as possible.

In patients with shock, systemic perfusion needs to be restored immediately. One or, preferably, two large-bore catheters should be inserted. If venous access cannot be achieved, an intraosseous needle should be inserted. A central venous pressure (CVP) line may be inserted for monitoring and fluid administration. Once the patient's condition is stabilized, an intra-arterial line may be inserted to monitor arterial blood pressure.

Isotonic crystalloids such as 0.9% normal saline solution or Ringer lactate are usually given. If the patient does not have signs of hypovolemia, an initial bolus of 20 mL/kg should be administered and repeated as needed until systemic perfusion improves. An indwelling urinary catheter should be inserted and fluid intake and output carefully monitored.

Patients with signs of septic shock may require a large volume of fluid to restore and maintain systemic perfusion. During the first hour of fluid resuscitation more than 40 mL/kg may be administered; 100–200 mL/kg or more may be required during the first several hours of therapy (Hazinski and Barkin, 1992).

Blood products may be given according to results of hematologic studies. When administration of blood or blood component therapy is necessary, 10 mL/kg boluses of type-specific packed red blood cells or 20 ml/kg of type-specific whole blood is given. Blood products should be warmed before administration.

Once the diagnosis of sepsis or septic shock is made, intravenous antibiotic therapy should be instituted immediately. The antibiotics administered vary according to the age of the patient and the presumed source of infection until culture results are available.

If present, metabolic acidosis should be corrected with sodium bicarbonate, 1 mg/kg/dose. Sympathomimetic and inotropic drugs such as epinephrine (0.05–0.15 μg/kg/minute titrated), norepinephrine 0.1 μg/kg/minute titrated), and dopamine (2–5 μg/kg/minute) may be used to increase heart rate and cardiac output in patients who continue to have poor myocardial function and poor systemic perfusion despite adequate oxygenation and fluid resuscitation.

Electrolyte imbalances are corrected according to laboratory results. Because infants are particularly vulnerable to hypoglycemia, glucose is often administered.

Ongoing assessment of the child's response to fluid resuscitation is essential. Indicators of a positive response include a decrease in heart rate, an increase in blood pressure, an increase in warmth of the extremities, improvement in color, an increase in urinary output, and an increase in level of consciousness.

Patient and Family Teaching and Psychosocial Support

Having an infant or child in the ED with sepsis or septic shock can be a very frightening experience for parents, who are often terrified by the suddenness and severity of the illness. Parents should be allowed to spend as much time as possible at the child's bedside while in the ED. They need to be prepared for the child's admission to the ICU or other in-patient setting.

■ INFECTIOUS DISEASES INVOLVING THE CENTRAL NERVOUS SYSTEM

Meningitis, encephalitis, and Reye syndrome are special challenges to the ED nurse. Early identification and intervention are essential in preventing morbidity and mortality. Although these CNS infections and postinfectious disease syndromes are critical illnesses, their initial presentations may resemble those of many minor pediatric illnesses, such as upper respiratory infections (URIs) and gastroenteritis. Infants and children with a CNS infection often present with such common pediatric complaints as fever, irritability, lethargy, vomiting, or headache. Therefore, the ED nurse must be knowledgeable in identifying and differentiating between the minor pediatric illnesses and the serious CNS diseases of meningitis, encephalitis, and Reye syndrome. These life-threatening diseases are amenable to treatment if they are diagnosed early in the ED.

MENINGITIS

The implementation of the *H. influenzae* type b (Hib) conjugate vaccine as a routine childhood immunization has resulted in a marked decrease in the incidence of meningitis in young children. *H. influenzae* type b conjugate vaccines were first licensed for use in the US in children at least 18 months of age in December 1987 and for infants at least 2 months of age in October 1990 (Adams, et al, 1993). As a result, the incidence of Hib disease among children younger than 5 years decreased 71% from 1989 to 1991 (Adams, et al, 1993). Currently immunization with Hib vaccine is routinely given to children at 2, 4, 6, and 15 months of age.

Meningitis carries a mortality of 20–50% among neonates and 1.5–5% among infants and children. If treated early, the prognosis is generally good. However, 20–40% of infants and children with meningitis suffer neurologic sequelae, loss of hearing being most common. Other long-term effects include delayed psychomotor development, seizure disorders, paraplegia, hydrocephalus, cranial nerve palsies, speech disorders, visual and hearing impairments, mental retardation, and changes in behavior. Early recognition and treatment are essential to decrease morbidity and mortality.

Etiology
Bacterial meningitis can be caused by a variety of bacterial agents, the most prevalent organisms varying by age of the child. Among neonates, group B streptococci, *E. coli*, and *Listeria monocytogenes* are the most frequent causative organisms. In infants and children younger than 5 years of age, *H. influenzae* type b, *S. pneumoniae*, and *N. meningitidis* (meningococcal) are the most frequent causative organisms. After the age of 9 years *S. pneumoniae* and *N. meningitidis* are the primary pathogens. The most common causative organisms in viral (aseptic) meningitis are the enteroviruses and echoviruses.

Pathophysiology
Meningitis, a potentially fatal infectious disease, is an inflammation of the meninges surrounding the brain caused by bacterial or viral infection. The meninges, the three membranes investing the spinal cord and brain are the dura mater (external); the arachnoid (middle); and the pia mater (internal).

In newborns, colonization by meningeal pathogens is usually acquired by vertical transmission from the maternal intestinal or genital tract or by horizontal transmission from newborn nursery staff. The pathogenesis of meningitis in older infants and children involves hematogenous dissemination of a causative organism that resides in the nasopharynx. The blood supply of the meninges lies adjacent to the venous system of the nasopharynx, mastoid process, and middle ear. This area provides an excellent environment for bacterial colonization because of the slower rate of venous circulation.

The invading organism enters the cerebrospinal fluid (CSF) and then spreads throughout the subarachnoid space. The infective process causes the brain to become hyperemic, edematous, and covered by a layer of purulent exudate. Intracranial sequelae may include hydrocephalus, ischemia, subdural effusions, venous sinus thrombosis, brain abscess, and temporary or permanent damage to the cranial nerves.

Although most children with meningitis have no predisposing factors, factors that predispose children to meningitis may include pre-existing CNS anomalies, neurosurgical procedures, severe head trauma, skull fractures with CSF leaks, sickle cell disease, immunoglobulin deficiencies, immunosuppressant drug therapy, cancer therapy, diabetes mellitus, cystic fibrosis, malnutrition, or primary infections elsewhere in the body. Maternal factors that increase the risk of meningitis in a neonate include premature rupture of the membranes, maternal infection during the last week of pregnancy, and prolonged labor.

History
A careful, detailed history should be obtained in all cases of suspected meningitis. The history obtained should include any recent febrile episodes; the child's recent level of activity, with special attention given to any history of irritability or lethargy; a decrease in appetite, total fluid intake in the last 24 hours; vomiting; diarrhea; seizures; or signs of respiratory distress. There may be a history of recent otitis media or an URI. A history of any underlying chronic illnesses or recent injuries should be elicited. The history may include an insidious onset of symptoms or a condition that has developed rapidly over a period of only hours.

The clinical presentation of meningitis varies with the age of the patient. The diagnosis of meningitis in neonates or infants is difficult because often the clinical sign in this age group is irritability. The irritability associated with meningitis often cannot be alleviated by any measure, even maternal comforting. A high-

TABLE 26–2. CLINICAL INDICATORS OF MENINGITIS IN INFANTS

Irritability
High-pitched cry
Lethargy
Bulging anterior fontanelle
Seizures
Apnea
Jitteriness
Fever
Hypothermia
Poor feeding
Vomiting
Petechiae
Purpura
General appearance of "sick infant"

pitched cry may be present. In any infant who presents with irritability or lethargy, the nurse must maintain a high index of suspicion for meningitis. A history of fever is variable in neonates but is almost always present beyond the neonatal period. There may or may or not be a history of fever in infants. Table 26–2 summarizes the clinical signs and symptoms of meningitis in infants.

In children older than 2 years, the history may contain some of the symptoms described for infants as well as symptoms more specific for CNS involvement. These patients may present with a history of the classic meningeal symptoms of headache, nuchal rigidity, vomiting, and fever. Table 26–3 summarizes the clinical presentation of meningitis in children older than 1 year. In either age group, meningitis may be abrupt in onset or insidious, often with a history of respiratory infection.

Physical Assessment

As with all critically ill patients, the first priority is assessment and support of airway, breathing, and circulation. Any respiratory distress should be noted. Apneic episodes are common in infants with meningitis. Tachypnea with or without other signs of respiratory distress may be present. Breath sounds should

TABLE 26–3. CLINICAL INDICATORS OF MENINGITIS IN CHILDREN

Headache
Vomiting
Fever
Nuchal rigidity
Positive Kernig sign
Positive Brudzinski sign
Altered mental status
Ataxia
Seizures
Petechiae
Purpura
Photophobia
Coma

be assessed for evidence of pneumonia, which may accompany meningitis. Skin should be assessed for petechial rash and purpura. The infant's color may be pale. Tachycardia may be present, and cardiac monitoring should be undertaken. Vital signs should be monitored every 15 minutes, more frequently if the patient's condition is unstable.

Five to ten percent of children with meningitis present with circulatory collapse marked by poor perfusion, mottling, delayed capillary refill, and altered mental status, which are due to vasoconstriction and increased venous pooling (Barkin, 1992). Therefore, children should be continually assessed for signs of septic shock. Signs of septic shock include fever, tachycardia, hypotension, decreased capillary filling, tachypnea or apnea, decreased level of consciousness, and decreased urinary output. Septic shock is often associated with meningococcemia and disseminated intravascular coagulation (DIC).

The child's temperature should be carefully monitored. A young infant with meningitis is often hypothermic; an older infant or child may be hyperthermic. The patient's neurologic status should be continually assessed for signs of increased intracranial pressure (ICP), which include a decrease in pulse and an increase in blood pressure. The child's level of consciousness, pupillary responses, cranial nerve assessment, and equality of movement and strength of extremities should be assessed continually.

In infants the anterior and posterior fontanelles should be observed and palpated while the infant is sitting. Normally the anterior fontanelle is soft and flat and may bulge slightly when the infant is crying. A bulging fontanelle may indicate increased ICP and is a late sign of meningitis. A depressed fontanelle may indicate dehydration.

Infants typically do not have nuchal rigidity. Older children may have nuchal rigidity, a Kernig sign (flexion of the hip 90° with subsequent pain on extension of the leg), a Brudzinski sign (involuntary flexion of the knees and hips after flexion of the neck while supine), and headaches.

Laboratory and Diagnostic Tests

Lumbar Puncture (Spinal Tap). A lumbar puncture should be performed immediately on all patients in whom meningitis is suspected. The CSF obtained is typically cloudy. The lumbar puncture should include measurement of opening and closing pressures and CSF leukocyte count with differential. In addition, a Gram stain and culture of the CSF should be performed to identify the particular bacterial organism causing the infection. Cerebrospinal fluid protein and glucose levels are obtained.

The child should be placed in the lateral decubitus

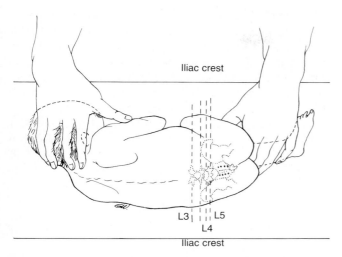

Figure 26–1. Position for lumbar puncture. The desired sites are the interspaces between L-3 and L-4 or between L-4 and L-5.

position, with the child's knees drawn up to the abdomen and the neck flexed forward (Figure 26–1) (Lang, 1993). The child should be secured in this position throughout the procedure, ensuring that the child's shoulders and hips are perpendicular to the examining table. One arm is placed over the child's neck and the other behind the child's knee (Lang, 1993). An alternative position for infants is upright. In the upright position, the infant is placed in a sitting position with his or her thighs against the abdomen and the neck flexed forward (Lang, 1993).

While the infant or child is held for the lumbar puncture, the child's respiratory and circulatory status must be assessed continually. An infant or child who has eaten just prior to the lumbar puncture is at risk for aspiration and respiratory arrest. Hyperflexion of the neck can lead to respiratory compromise. Holding the child too tightly can cause decreased venous return and lead to cardiopulmonary arrest. The infant or child needs much reassurance during the procedure. This involves talking softly and calmingly to the infant or child throughout the procedure.

Blood Studies. Serum electrolyte with glucose levels should be obtained. Decreased serum sodium level and serum osmolarity may indicate the syndrome of inappropriate antidiuretic hormone (SIADH). Most children with bacterial meningitis show evidence of SIADH. Therefore, careful monitoring of fluid and electrolytes is imperative.

A serum glucose level should be obtained before the lumbar puncture because the stress of the lumbar puncture may artificially raise the serum glucose level. The serum glucose level is compared with the CSF glucose level. In bacterial meningitis the CSF glucose level is less than one-half of the serum glucose level. It is important to note that infants are prone to becoming

hypoglycemic when critically ill, leading to seizures and respiratory arrest.

A CBC with differential may help differentiate between bacterial and viral meningitis. A platelet count should be obtained. One or more blood cultures should be obtained because of the high incidence of associated septicemia. The blood culture yields the infecting organism in 50% of cases of bacterial meningitis.

Urine Specimens. Urine electrolyte levels should include potassium, sodium, and urine osmolarity. These values assist in the diagnosis of the SIADH, which may develop within the first 72 hours of illness. A urine culture and urinalysis should be obtained, since there may be a concurrent urinary tract infection. The specific gravity of the urine is important in monitoring fluid and electrolyte balance.

Other Cultures. Cultures of purpuric lesions, abscesses, or middle ear infections should be obtained.

X Rays. A chest x ray should be obtained if pneumonia is suspected. Computed tomography (CT) may be performed if there are signs of increased ICP or cerebral edema.

TRIAGE
Meningitis

Emergent ─────────────────────────────
An infant or child with meningitis.

Nursing Diagnosis
Ineffective Breathing Pattern

Defining Characteristics

- Tachypnea
- Cyanosis

Nursing Interventions

- Administer oxygen
- Place patient in position to facilitate respiratory effort
- Monitor vital signs
- Administer medications as ordered

Expected Outcomes

- Respiratory rate improves
- Patient's color improves

Nursing Diagnosis
Ineffective Thermoregulation

Defining Characteristics

- Increase or decrease in body temperature
- Tachycardia
- Tachypnea

Nursing Interventions

- Administer antipyretics for elevated body temperature
- Use warming or cooling blanket as indicated
- Administer antibiotics as ordered

Expected Outcomes

- Body temperature begins to return to normal
- Respiratory rate improves
- Heart rate begins to return to normal

Nursing Diagnosis

Altered Tissue Perfusion (Cerebral)

Defining Characteristics

- Lethargy
- Irritability
- Bulging anterior fontanelle

Nursing Interventions

- Administer oxygen
- Elevate head of bed unless patient's condition is hemodynamically unstable
- Monitor vital signs
- Administer medications as ordered

Expected Outcomes

- Irritability decreases
- Level of consciousness improves
- Anterior fontanelle is soft and flat

Management. Meningitis is a true emergency that requires an immediate diagnosis and institution of therapy to prevent death and to avoid permanent neurologic impairment. Table 26–4 summarizes nursing intervention priorities for a child with meningitis. The child's airway, breathing, and circulation must be continually assessed and supported. Humidified oxygen

TABLE 26–4. PRIORITIES IN NURSING INTERVENTIONS FOR A CHILD WITH MENINGITIS

Assess and support airway, breathing, and circulation (ABCs).
Assess and prevent increase in intracranial pressure.
Administer steroids as soon as possible.
Administer antibiotics as soon as possible.
Monitor fluid intake and urine output.
Institute isolation and universal precautions.
Provide information and support to child and family members.

should be administered to all infants and children who are pale, cyanotic, or show sign of shock. Intubation and assisted ventilation are sometimes necessary. Intravenous access should be ensured. If the signs of septic shock previously described are present, shock may be corrected with rapid infusion of packed red blood cells or intravenous solutions.

If bacterial meningitis is identified or suspected, rapid administration of the appropriate antibiotics is essential. Antibiotics, selected by patient's age, CSF Gram stain results, and underlying disease are administered pending cultures results. Table 26–5 describes the appropriate antibiotic therapy. Antibiotics should be given immediately after the completion of the lumbar puncture. If intravenous access is not achieved, initial doses of antibiotics may be administered intramuscularly. If the child is in a state of shock, intraosseous administration of antibiotics and fluids may be appropriate (Barki, 1992).

Dexamethasone, 0.15 mg/kg every 6 hours intravenously, is sometimes administered before or immediately after administration of antibiotics and is continued for 4 days (16 doses) for meningitis caused by

TABLE 26–5. ANTIBIOTIC ADMINISTRATION IN BACTERIAL MENINGITIS

Age or organism	Drug/Dosage
■ INFANTS < 2 MONTHS	
Unknown etiology	Ampicillin 100–200 mg/kg/day q 4–6 hours IV *and*
	Cefotaxime 100–150 mg/kg/day q 8–12 hours IV
Group B streptococci	Penicillin G 150,000–250,000 U/kg/day q 4–6 hours IV *and*
	Gentamicin 5–7.5 mg/kg/day q 8–12 hours IV
E. Coli	Chloramphenicol 50–100 mg/kg/day q 6 hours IV *or*
	Cefotaxime 100–150 mg/kg/day q 8–12 hours IV
L. monocytogenes	Ampicillin 100–200 mg/kg/day q 4–6 hours IV
■ 2 MONTHS TO 10 YEARS	
Unknown etiology	Cefotaxime 200 mg/kg/day q 6 hours IV
H. influenzae	Cefotaxime 200 mg/kg/day q 6 hours IV
S. pneumoniae	Penicillin G 250,000 U/kg/day q 4 hours IV
N. meningitidis	Penicillin G 250,000 U/kg/day q 4 hours IV
■ OLDER THAN 10 YEARS	
Unknown etiology	Penicillin G 250,000 U/kg/day q 4 hours IV
S. pneumoniae	Penicillin G 250,000 U/kg/day q 4 hours IV
N. meningitidis	Penicillin G 250,000 U/kg/day q 4 hours IV

IV, intravenously.

H. influenzae. Dexamethasone is thought to have a beneficial effect on CNS inflammation and edema and reduces the likelihood of neurologic sequelae and hearing loss (Wendell and Harris, 1992). Recent investigations, however, have shown variable results when the results for patients treated by dexamethasone have been compared with those for patients receiving a placebo.

Increased ICP and cerebral edema may occur with meningitis; therefore, all measures should be taken to prevent, monitor, and treat cerebral edema and increased ICP. The patient's neurologic status should be assessed continually. Intravenous and oral fluid should be administered cautiously according to vital signs and hydration status. Initial fluid intake may be restricted to two-thirds maintenance to decrease the volume of fluid in the brain. Fluid and electrolyte balance needs to be carefully monitored. When necessary, the patient is hyperventilated to control pCO_2 levels between 25 and 30 mmHg. The head of the bed should be elevated to 30°; the patient's head should be maintained in a midline, neutral position to prevent obstruction of cranial venous return. If cerebral edema is evident, an osmotic diuretic such as mannitol 20% solution, 0.5 to 1.0 g/kg/dose every 4–6 hours intravenously, or glycerol (oral) may be administered.

Thermoregulation is essential because hyperthermia compounds cerebral edema by increasing the metabolic need for oxygen in the brain. Antipyretic agents should be administered orally if the patient is alert and rectally if the patient is unable to take medications by mouth. Acetaminophen, 15 mg/kg (maximum dose 650 mg), is administered every 4 hours for temperatures higher than 38.5°C (rectal). Ibuprofen 5–10 mg/kg may occasionally be alternated with acetaminophen. Tepid sponging or cooling blankets may be required. Rubbing alcohol should never be used because the alcohol may be absorbed through the skin and has been associated with acute toxicity and even death in some instances.

All necessary precautions should be taken in the ED to protect oneself and others from possible exposure to meningitis. All patients with suspected meningitis should be isolated upon arrival to the ED. Precautions include the wearing of masks, gowns, and gloves when having direct contact with the patient.

Children with meningitis are admitted for close observation, intravenous antibiotic therapy, and supportive measures.

Chemoprophylaxis for Contacts

Haemophilus Influenzae. The people at greatest risk for *H. influenzae* meningitis are young members of the household of the infected child, especially siblings younger than 6 years, and children attending the same day care center. Prophylaxis with rifampin is recommended. Infants younger than 1 month are treated with oral rifampin, 10 mg/kg every 24 hours for 4 days. Infants and children between 1 month and 12 years of age are treated with oral rifampin, 20 mg/kg every 24 hours for 4 days. Children older than 12 years and adults are treated with oral rifampin, 600 mg every 24 hours for 4 days.

Rifampin should not be administered to pregnant women. Others who are given rifampin should be warned that it reduces the efficacy of oral contraceptives and discolors urine, saliva, and tears. It can also permanently discolor contact lenses (Wendell and Harris, 1992).

Neisseria Meningitidis (Meningoccal Meningitis). Prophylaxis is recommended for all close contacts of a child with meningococcal meningitis. Infants younger than 1 month should be given oral rifampin, 5 mg/kg every 12 hours for 2 days. Infants and children 1 month to 12 years of age should receive oral rifampin, 10 mg/kg every 12 hours for 2 days. Children over 12 years and adult contacts should receive oral rifampin, 600 mg every 12 hours for 2 days.

Routine prophylaxis for hospital personnel who have come into contact with a patient with meningitis is usually not necessary. It is important to note that adults are not susceptible to infection with *H. influenzae* type b. Circumstances in which prophylaxis is indicated for health professionals include direct contact with the patient's saliva through mouth-to-mouth resuscitation or prolonged close contact with the patient before the institution of antibiotic therapy. Those at risk of infection should receive prophylaxis with oral rifampin 600 mg daily for 2 or 4 days, depending on the infective organism.

Current prophylactic agents do not reliably abort incipient meningitis. Therefore, close observation of those who have been exposed is extremely important. Contacts should be evaluated promptly with the first sign of fever, sore throat, otitis media, rash, or other sign of infection.

Viral Meningitis

Viral, or aseptic, meningitis is generally much milder in clinical presentation than bacterial meningitis. Usually it is self-limiting and does not require specific therapy. The presenting symptoms are similar to those seen in bacterial meningitis and include fever, nuchal rigidity, headache, malaise, photophobia, seizures, abdominal pain, sore throat, and generalized muscle aches. The onset of symptoms may be abrupt or insidious. Increased ICP is infrequent in viral meningitis. The assessment and management of viral meningitis are similar to those of bacterial meningitis, except that antibiotic therapy is of no value in the treatment of viral meningitis. However, antibiotic therapy may be administered and isolation enforced until a definitive diagnosis is made and the possibility of bacterial meningitis eliminated. Most patients with viral meningitis are admitted for close monitoring; however, older children in whom the diagnosis is solid may be followed on an outpatient basis.

Patient and Family Teaching and Psychosocial Support

The term meningitis still provokes thoughts of death or permanent disability in the minds and emotions of most people. Therefore, it is important to provide emotional support and accurate information to the child and parents. They need careful explanations of all procedures and treatments. Lumbar punctures are particularly frightening to children, as well as to their parents. Many parents cannot tolerate observing the lumbar puncture and should be encouraged to wait in another area of the ED until the procedure has been completed. Fears need to be allayed with information and reassurance. Some children and parents erroneously believe that during a lumbar puncture the needle goes through the spinal cord and can cause paralysis. Therefore, parents and older children need to be informed that the needle does not enter the spinal cord itself, but rather enters a space between two lumbar vertebrae, below the point where the spinal cord ends. Parents and the child also need to be prepared for the child's admission to the hospital.

ENCEPHALITIS

Encephalitis, an inflammation of the brain, has a wide range of severity of clinical manifestations. Because the diagnosis can be made with absolute certainty only by direct examination of brain tissue, the diagnosis is most often made on the basis of neurologic manifestations and history.

Etiology

Encephalitis is most often caused by the arboviruses (arthropod-borne viruses) acquired through an arthropod vector. The vector reservoir for these arboviruses is the mosquito, therefore the incidence is highest in the summer months. In the US four arboviruses are the major causes of viral encephalitis. Eastern equine encephalomyelitis (EEE) is found primarily in the eastern and north central US. It has a predilection for young infants and is associated with a high morbidity and mortality. St. Louis encephalitis (SLE), found in most sections of the US with the exception of the northeast, is more common in adolescents and adults than in children. Children infected with SLE often have no symptoms. Western equine encephalomyelitis (WEE) is found primarily in the western US and Can-

ada and scattered areas farther east. It is associated with severe sequelae, especially in infants. California encephalitis (CE) is found in rural areas throughout the US and primarily affects 5-to-9-year-olds. Severe illness, seizures, focal findings, and long-term behavioral problems are common.

Measles, mumps, varicella zoster, rubella, enteroviruses, and herpes viruses may cause encephalitis as a complication of the disease process. Human immunodeficiency virus infection may cause a subacute or chronic onset of encephalitis. In rare cases encephalitis may occur as a complication of a routine vaccination for smallpox, poliomyelitis, diphtheria, pertussis, or influenza. In recent years, 25% of cases of encephalitis reported to the CDC have been of indeterminate cause. The seasonal pattern of disease in the US indicates that the unidentified etiologic agents in most cases are enteroviruses (Cherry, 1992).

Pathophysiology

Acute viral encephalitis is an inflammatory process of the brain that produces altered functioning of the CNS. The encephalitis process is usually produced by the direct invasion of a virus into the CNS or by involvement of the CNS after a viral disease.

Encephalitis has a varied clinical course. Recovery may take days, weeks, or months. Some patients may die. Encephalitis in infants is associated with the most severe illness and sequelae. Residual effects of encephalitis may include developmental delays, seizure disorders, hydrocephalus, hemiparesis, hemiplegia, loss of hearing, and focal or sensory deficits. Herpes simplex type I encephalitis carries the worst prognosis, causing death or serious neurologic sequelae in more than 70% of patients.

History

The onset of the disease may be dramatic or insidious. There may be a history of headache, fever, nuchal rigidity, altered level of consciousness, seizure activity, ataxia, photophobia, diplopia, nausea, vomiting, or facial twitching. A careful history of the course of any recent viral infections or exposures should be ascertained. Table 26–6 summarizes clinical indicators of encephalitis.

TABLE 26–6. CLINICAL INDICATORS OF ENCEPHALITIS

Altered level of consciousness
Behavioral changes
Hallucinations
Seizures
Headache
Fever
Nuchal regidity
Neurologic deficits
Ataxia
Loss of bowel and bladder control

Physical Assessment

The patient's airway, breathing, and circulation should be carefully assessed and supported. A neurologic assessment should be performed including evaluation of cranial nerve function, level of consciousness, pupillary responses, and extraocular eye movements. The fontanelles in infants should be assessed for tenseness or bulging. Vital signs should be carefully monitored.

Laboratory Data

Lumbar Puncture. A lumbar puncture is performed to differentiate between encephalitis, meningitis, Reye syndrome, and an intracranial bleed. The CSF may be within normal limits, with normal to moderately elevated pressure and a normal glucose level. Five to a few hundred cells with a predominance of lymphocytes may be found. A viral culture of the CSF is necessary for identification of the causative organism; however, cultures of the CSF are most often sterile. Viruses of mumps, measles, and enteroviruses may be detected in the CSF. Arboviruses are rarely detected in the CSF or blood.

Cultures. Viral cultures of the blood, pharynx, urine, and stool may yield the infecting organism. Bacterial cultures of blood, urine, and pharynx should be obtained to rule out bacterial meningitis.

Blood Studies. A CBC with differential may help distinguish between bacterial meningitis and viral encephalitis. In encephalitis, the CBC usually shows a mild polymorphonuclear or mononuclear leukocytosis. Serum electrolytes should be obtained to rule out the SIADH, which may accompany encephalitis.

Urine. Urine electrolyte levels and osmolarity should be obtained to rule out the SIADH. A urinalysis and culture should be obtained.

T R I A G E
Encephalitis

Emergent ───────────────────────
Any infant or child in whom encephalitis is suspected should be rapidly assessed and treated immediately.

Nursing Diagnosis
Hyperthermia

Defining Characteristics

- Increase in body temperature
- Tachycardia
- Tachypnea

Nursing Interventions

- Administer antipyretics
- Use cooling blanket

Expected Outcomes

- Body temperature returns to normal
- Respiratory rate returns to normal
- Heart rate returns to normal

Nursing Diagnosis
Altered Cerebral Tissue Perfusion

Defining Characteristics

- Lethargy
- Altered level of consciousness

Nursing Interventions

- Monitor vital signs
- Monitor neurologic status
- Elevate head of bed
- Administer steroids as ordered

Expected Outcomes

- Child's level of consciousness improves
- Vital signs stabilize

Management

Treatment of nonherpetic viral encephalitis is primarily supportive. The patient's airway, breathing, and circulation should be continually assessed and supported. If present, acidosis should be corrected. Increased ICP should be carefully monitored and treated by hyperventilation if necessary. The head of the patient's bed should be elevated 30° with the patient's head in a midline position to prevent obstruction of cerebral venous return. Fluid intake should be carefully monitored and limited to two-thirds of maintenance. Electrolytes need to be carefully monitored. Osmotic diuretics may be administered. Urine output should be carefully monitored. If the child is critically ill, a urinary catheter should be inserted for accurate measurement of urinary output.

If the patient has a fever, antipyretic agents should be administered because hyperthermia compounds cerebral edema by increasing metabolism, which in turn causes an increase in cerebral blood flow (CBF). A cooling blanket may be necessary if the child's fever does not respond to antipyretics. Antibiotics are not administered, because they are of no value in viral infections. However, if a patient is thought to have herpes simplex type I encephalitis, antiviral therapy with acyclovir, 30 mg/kg/day q 8 hours IV, is administered pending results of a brain biopsy. Because patients with encephalitis are prone to seizures, precautions should be taken and anticonvulsants administered if the patient begins having a seizure in the ED. (See Chapter 29 for the management of seizure activity in the ED.) Children with encephalitis are usually admitted to the ICU.

Patient and Family Teaching and Psychosocial Support

A child with encephalitis has often become ill quite suddenly and his or her condition may deteriorate rapidly. Parents are frightened by the sudden seriousness of their child's condition and need reassurance that all that is possible is being done. All procedures and treatments should be carefully explained to the child and parents.

The parents should be encouraged to remain at the child's bedside as much as possible while in the ED. They need to be prepared for the hospitalization of their child and should be encouraged to remain with the child once the child is admitted to the hospital. Rehabilitation may be required after recovery from the acute illness.

REYE SYNDROME

Reye syndrome is a pediatric disease characterized by acute encephalopathy and fatty degeneration of the viscera, especially the liver. The first description of this entity was reported in 1963 by Australian pathologist HDK Reye and his colleagues. This distinct malady was identified with increasing frequency in the 1970s and 1980s. The incidence of Reye syndrome has decreased dramatically in the past decade due to public awareness of the contraindication of use of salicylates during childhood illnesses. The peak incidence of Reye syndrome occurred in 1980 (555 cases). Now, Reye syndrome is a relatively rare disease; approximately 30 confirmed cases are reported annually in the US (Boenning, 1992).

In the 1970s and 1980s the peak incidence occurred in children 6–11 years of age. However, cases involving patients 2 months–21 years of age have been documented. Currently, cases occur mainly among self-medicating adolescents who use aspirin. There is no preference for either sex.

Etiology

The etiology of Reye syndrome is still uncertain, but a clear link has been established between Reye syndrome and salicylate ingestion during viral infections. Since 1982, the American Academy of Pediatrics has recommended that aspirin products not be given to infants or children with symptoms of viral illnesses,

especially varicella (chicken pox) and influenza. The viral infections associated with Reye syndrome include influenza types A and B, varicella, coxsackie, adenovirus, echovirus, rubeola, and herpes simplex.

Pathophysiology

The pathophysiology of Reye syndrome includes disruption of the liver mitochondria or urea cycle, resulting in a build-up of fatty deposits in the liver due to inadequate lipid metabolism, which leads to metabolic encephalopathy. Electron microscopy reveals abnormally large and swollen mitochondria in the liver and brain cells. Hyperammonemia is caused by a reduction in the enzymes that convert ammonia to urea. Severe cerebral edema is present in fatal cases. Despite improvement in outcome with aggressive management, the mortality is 20–30% (Horowitz, 1992).

History

Early detection and intervention affect the course of the disease. Reye syndrome should be suspected in any infant, child, or adolescent who presents with an altered mental status and has recently appeared to recover from an URI or other viral illness, such as varicella (chicken pox). A careful history of any salicylate exposure should be obtained. It must be kept in mind that salicylates are present in many over-the-counter products other than aspirin. The history obtained from parents often includes intractable vomiting and CNS dysfunction, which may be manifested by seizures, alterations in breathing patterns, including apnea, and a decreased level of consciousness. In infants there may be a history of a high-pitched, abnormal crying.

The course of the illness has two phases. In the first phase, the child has a viral illness for 5–7 days with apparent recovery. In the second phase, the child has recurrent vomiting, followed by a progressive disturbance in level of consciousness, which can range from mild lethargy to coma.

Physical Assessment

Reye syndrome is characterized by fever, profoundly impaired consciousness, and liver dysfunction. The patient's airway, breathing, and circulatory status should be assessed continually. Acute respiratory failure and cardiac arrhythmias may occur. Therefore, a cardiac monitor should be used continuously while the patient is in the ED. Vital signs should be monitored carefully.

The patient's neurologic status should be continually assessed for changes in level of consciousness, disorientation, combativeness, pupil reactivity, posturing, rigidity, and seizure activity. Signs of increased ICP should be monitored carefully. Changes in respi-

TABLE 26–7. CLINICAL STAGING OF REYE SYNDROME

Stage	Level of Consciousness
0	Alert
I	Lethargic, sleepy
II	Delirious, combative
III	Unarousable, decorticate
IV	Unarousable, decerebrate
V	Comatose, unresponsive pupils, fixed dilated pupils, loss of deep tendon reflexes

ratory rate and depth are early indicators of increasing ICP. Hyperventilation may indicate the body's attempt to normalize ICP, since hypocarbia produces cerebral vasoconstriction, which decreases intravascular volume.

Clinical staging criteria that reflect deepening levels of stupor and coma (Table 26–7) have been developed by the CDC. The patient is evaluated upon diagnosis of Reye syndrome and a numerical grade of severity is assigned. The stage at time of diagnosis dictates the therapeutic interventions and the anticipated prognosis.

Laboratory and Diagnostic Tests

Venipuncture. Serum ammonia level is elevated (150–750 μg/dL) in early stages of the disease and often returns to normal within 48–72 hours. Elevation of ammonia levels is the product of initial virus-toxin interaction. The degree of elevation is thought to be correlated with the severity of the disease.

Liver function test results, including serum glutamic-oxaloacetic transaminase (SGOT), serum glutamic pyruvate transaminase (SGPT), and lactic dehydrogenase (LDH), are elevated. Prothrombin time and PT are twice the upper limit of normal. Blood urea nitrogen (BUN) and creatinine levels may show mild-to-moderate elevation.

Serum glucose levels may indicate hypoglycemia. Serum glucose levels may fall to below 50 mg/dL with reduced insulin levels and a diminished glucagon response.

Arterial Blood Gases. Arterial blood gases may reflect a blend of respiratory alkalosis with metabolic acidosis.

Lumbar Puncture. A lumbar puncture may be performed to rule out meningitis or encephalitis. In Reye syndrome the CSF is essentially normal, although the pressure may be elevated.

Liver Biopsy. A liver biopsy, the definitive diagnostic study for Reye syndrome, is frequently not performed because of the coagulopathy.

TRIAGE
Reye Syndrome

Emergent

An infant or child with signs and symptoms of Reye syndrome.

Nursing Diagnosis
Ineffective Breathing Pattern

Defining Characteristics
- Tachypnea
- Cyanosis

Nursing Interventions
- Administer oxygen
- Monitor vital signs
- Administer medications as ordered

Expected Outcomes
- Respiratory rate returns to normal
- Patient's color returns to normal

Nursing Diagnosis
Altered Tissue Perfusion (Cerebral)

Defining Characteristics
- Lethargy
- Unresponsiveness

Nursing Interventions
- Administer oxygen
- Monitor vital signs and ICP
- Limit fluid intake
- Administer medications as ordered
- Decrease stimulation

Expected Outcomes
- Level of consciousness returns to normal
- Vital signs and ICP return to normal

Management
Airway, breathing, and circulation should continually be assessed and supported. Children at the coma stage (Stage III and above) are electively intubated and placed on a respirator as a means of preventing cerebral ischemia.

Indications of increased ICP should be closely monitored and prevented. The head of the bed should be elevated to 30° with the child's head maintained in a midline, neutral position to prevent obstruction of cranial venous return. Body temperature should be maintained between 36.5°C and 37°C, since hyperthermia compounds cerebral edema by increasing cerebral metabolism, which in turn demands an increase in CBF. An ICP monitoring device may be indicated. Intracranial pressure should be controlled at levels below 20–25 mmHg with hyperventilation as necessary (Hazinski, 1992). A barbiturate may be administered to decrease cerebral metabolic demands, decrease CBF and cause cerebral vasoconstriction. Mannitol may be administered to elevate blood osmolality, which in turn causes fluid to move out of edematous brain tissue.

An arterial line may be inserted to monitor blood pressure and for direct access for blood gas studies. A CVP line may be inserted to monitor right ventricular pressure. Arterial oxygen tension levels maintained between 80 and 100 mmHG should provide adequate oxygen for brain cell metabolism despite decreased cerebral perfusion. The $PaCO_2$ is maintained between 22 and 27 mmHG to decrease cerebral blood volume and reduce ICP.

Fluid and electrolyte balance must be carefully maintained. Fluids are usually restricted to 50–75% of daily maintenance. Fluid intake and urine output with specific gravity are carefully monitored. A Foley catheter should be inserted for accurate urinary output. A minimum urine output of 0.5 ml/kg/hour is necessary to ensure kidney function. Serum electrolytes need to be carefully monitored.

Children with Reye syndrome are prone to hypoglycemia. Infants are particularly intolerant of hypoglycemia and may have seizures or a respiratory arrest. Untreated hypoglycemia leads to increased production of ammonia and fatty acidemia. An attempt is made to maintain a serum glucose level of 200–300 mg/dL with intravenous administration of hypertonic glucose solutions.

Vitamin K, 1–5 mg, may be administered to correct clotting abnormalities, which are the result of hepatic and cellular dysfunction and decreased production of clotting factors.

Patient and Family Teaching and Psychosocial Support

The child and family members need a great deal of emotional support because they are usually quite frightened by the suddenness and severity of the illness. Children in the early stages of the disease are often disoriented and confused. Therefore, they need simple, clear explanations they can comprehend along with calm reassurance from the emergency nurse. All procedures and laboratory data need to be carefully explained. Parents should be continually updated on their child's condition and be prepared for the child's admission to an ICU. All children believed to have Reye syndrome should be admitted to a pediatric ICU for close observation and supportive care. Families and professionals can obtain information on Reye syndrome from the National Reye's Syndrome Foundation, 426 North Lewis, Bryan OH 43506, (419) 636-2679.

KAWASAKI DISEASE

Kawasaki disease is an acute febrile systemic vasculitis of unknown etiology; it is seen predominantly in children younger than 9 years. It is also known as mucocutaneous lymph node syndrome. Although it can occur in children of all races and ethnic groups, Kawasaki disease is seen most often in children of Japanese background. It affects boys more frequently than girls. The peak incidence of Kawasaki disease occurs at about 1 year of age, and the disease is uncommon after mid-childhood. In the US, most cases occur during winter and spring. The disease is self-limiting; however, without treatment 20% of affected children may have cardiac sequelae (Melish, 1990). Kawasaki disease is now the most common cause of acquired heart disease in American children (Lux, 1991).

Etiology and Pathophysiology

Although the etiology is unknown, it is theorized that Kawasaki disease may be an infectious disease or possibly an immune response to an infectious agent. In several outbreaks, children with Kawasaki disease have had a higher incidence of antecedent respiratory illness than controls (Feigin, 1990). Environmental exposure may be a possible cause. There is no evidence that the syndrome is communicable.

During the acute phase of illness, progressive inflammation of the small blood vessels occurs. Within 12–25 days, the medium-sized arteries are affected. Aneurysms of the coronary artery or more rarely the cervical, iliac, or renal arteries may develop during this time. Eventually, the vessels heal, but thickening of the vessel walls may occur along with scarring and stenosis. Thrombi may form at the sites of stenosis, leading to myocardial ischemia or infarction. Infants and patients with prolonged fever are at greatest risk for developing cardiac complications.

Kawasaki disease presents in four phases. In the first phase, the child is markedly irritable and may have a very high fever. Cervical adenopathy is usually present but may disappear quickly. Within a few days, a rash and conjunctival injection occur.

The second phase usually begins around day 4 and is marked by a continued high fever that is unresponsive to antibiotics and usual doses of antipyretic agents. The child continues to be irritable and may have a "toxic" appearance. Photophobia may be present. There are three types of rash in Kawasaki disease. The rash may be morbilliform or scarletinaform, or it may consist of maculopapular erythematous plaques of varying sizes, which may coalesce. The child may have erythema and edema of the hands and feet, and a bright red "strawberry tongue" is common. Diarrhea frequently occurs. Joint pain often begins during this phase and may mimic acute juvenile rheumatoid arthritis. The second phase ends on about day 12, with the disappearance of the rash and remaining adenopathy.

The third phase is dominated by desquamation, which often begins a few days before the disappearance of fever. This is the hallmark of Kawasaki disease, and it may occur in varying patterns. Another constant feature during this phase is thrombocytosis, with platelet counts ranging from 500,000 to 3 million.

A fourth phase occurs in a few patients. It may progress from the other three phases, or it may arise clinically as a recurrence. During this phase all clinical signs of Kawasaki disease have resolved. Laboratory values, however, continue to indicate inflammation, with an elevation of white blood cell (WBC) count, C-reactive protein level, and erythrocyte sedimentation rate (ESR). This phase is resolved when all laboratory values return to normal.

The most serious consequences of Kawasaki diseases are cardiac complications, which may include aneurysms, coronary thrombosis, myocarditis, pericardial effusions, and arrythmias.

History
The clinical presentation of Kawasaki disease varies with the particular child; however, certain criteria are necessary for a diagnosis of Kawasaki disease (Table 26–8). Currently the disease is diagnosed solely on clinical grounds. Thus, knowledge of the clinical manifestations and the usual sequence of events is important.

The history should focus on the duration and extent of fever and on the child's general appearance and activity level. Irritability is a common complaint. The

TABLE 26–8. CRITERIA FOR DIAGNOSIS OF KAWASAKI DISEASE

Fever of at least 5 days' duration associated with at least four of the following five criteria:
1. Bilateral conjunctival injection
2. Changes in the oral mucosa, such as erythema, dry, fissured lips, or "strawberry tongue"
3. Changes in the extremities, such as peripheral edema, peripheral erythema, and periungual or generalized desquamation
4. Polymorphous rash, primarily truncal
5. Cervical lymphadenopathy

Modified from previously published criteria from the Centers for Disease Control.

parents should be asked about the development of any rash or erythema. A history of intake and output is important in assessing the child's level of hydration. The extent of diarrhea or vomiting should be elicited. Any history of joint pain or swelling should be noted. This tends to occur more often in older children.

Physical Assessment
A rapid overview of airway, breathing, and circulation should be made. Tachypnea and tachycardia may be present, especially if the child has a high fever. Cardiac monitoring should be undertaken after a thorough baseline cardiac assessment is made. Perfusion may be compromised because of cardiac involvement and high fever; warmth and color of and capillary refill time in the extremities should be carefully noted. The child's temperature should be carefully monitored and antipyretic agents given as needed.

Marked meningeal signs are uncommon, but the child may complain of a stiff or sore neck. In addition, irritability may appear to indicate CNS involvement. Palpation of the abdomen may reveal hepato- or splenomegaly. The extremities and skin should be carefully examined for edema, erythema, and the characteristic rash. The conjunctivae may be injected. Examination of the eyes with a bright light may be extremely uncomfortable for the child.

Laboratory and Diagnostic Tests

Blood Studies. In any child with a history of decreased intake, prolonged high fever, or diarrhea, serum electrolytes, BUN, and creatinine should be measured to assess hydration and electrolyte status. A CBC with platelet count should be assessed. The WBC count is elevated with a left shift; mild anemia may be noted. Thrombocytosis occurs during the third phase of the illness. C-reactive protein level and ESR are indices of an inflammatory process and are likely to be elevated in Kawasaki disease. Transaminase levels may be elevated. One or more blood cultures should be obtained to rule out bacteremia.

Electrocardiogram. Some authors (Nihill et al, 1987) have reported electrocardiographic abnormalities including tachycardia, PR and QT prolongation, and ST elevation or depression in patients with Kawasaki disease. Other cardiac studies (angiography or echocardiography) may be required to assess for cardiac complications.

X Rays. A chest x ray should be obtained to assess for heart size. Pulmonary infiltrates may be present.

Nursing Diagnosis
Decreased Cardiac Output

Defining Characteristic

- Changes in blood vessels
- Rhythm disturbances

Nursing Interventions

- Monitor cardiac rhythm
- Monitor vital signs and signs of cardiac perfusion
- Administer fluids cautiously
- Monitor intake and output

Expected Outcomes

- Heart rate, blood pressure remain within baseline range
- Signs of cardiac perfusion remain within baseline range

Nursing Diagnosis
Ineffective Thermoregulation

Defining Characteristics

- Increase in body temperature
- Increase in heart rate, respiratory rate

Nursing Interventions

- Administer antipyretics as needed
- Provide adequate oral or intravenous fluids
- Use cooling blanket or tepid sponging as indicated

Expected Outcome

- Body temperature, heart rate, and respiratory rate will return to normal

Nursing Diagnosis
Pain

Defining Characteristics

- Crying, inconsolability
- Lack of response to comfort measures

Nursing Interventions

- Provide quiet environment
- Darken room if possible
- Group nursing activities to provide breaks for patient

Expected Outcomes

- Crying decreases
- Patient is able to rest

Management

The treatment of Kawasaki disease is geared toward the prevention of complications. Although they have not been shown to be effective in limiting the course of the disease, antibiotics may be given before the diagnosis is certain. Steroids are not recommended and actually may be contraindicated.

High dose gamma globulin (2 g/kg) has been shown to be useful in reducing the risk of coronary artery disease when instituted early in the course of illness, although the mechanism of action is unknown (Morens and Melish, 1992). High doses of aspirin, 30–100 mg/kg/24 hours, are often given simultaneously. However, toxicity and GI hemorrhage have been associated with aspirin use in Kawasaki disease, so it should be used with caution (Nihill et al, 1987).

Beyond these measures, treatment is largely supportive. Intravenous fluids may be given to correct or prevent dehydration. Fluids should be administered with caution because of the possibility of cardiac compromise. Ideally, bedrest should be maintained for several weeks after the onset of fever because of the likelihood of myocarditis, but this may not be feasible with an active child who feels well.

Patient and Family Teaching and Psychosocial Support

Kawasaki disease is relatively uncommon, and parents need accurate information about the disease course and the importance of long-term follow-up care. The extremely high fever and concern over cardiac complications are especially anxiety-provoking for parents.

In terms of the clinical course, parents should be prepared for the likelihood of irritability persisting for as long as 2 months. Although the desquamation that occurs during the second and third weeks of the illness is painless, parents may be alarmed at the child's appearance and should be reassured during this time. Arthritis is likely to persist for several weeks; it may be relieved by passive range of motion performed in a warm tub of water. If the child is receiving salicylate therapy, the parents need to be aware of signs of aspirin toxicity—tinnitus, headache, dizziness, or confusion. The parents and the child may need to be prepared for the child's admission to the hospital and any diagnostic tests.

ACUTE RHEUMATIC FEVER

Rheumatic fever is an inflammatory disease that affects the connective tissue of the heart, joints, CNS, and subcutaneous tissue. The major sequela of rheumatic fever is heart damage in the form of scarring of the mitral valve, referred to as rheumatic heart disease. Rheumatic heart disease is the most common type of acquired heart disease in children.

After a steady decline in the 1960s and 1970s there was a resurgence of acute rheumatic fever in the US in the late 1980s. Acute rheumatic fever typically occurs in school-aged children and rarely occurs before the age of 3 years in children born in the US. However, it has been known to occur earlier than this in children from the Caribbean and the Far East.

Etiology
Group A beta-hemolytic streptococcus is the organism that leads to acute rheumatic fever. Group A beta-hemolytic streptococcal infection occurs 2–6 weeks before the onset of symptoms of rheumatic fever. However, in some cases, there may be a longer period between the acute streptococcal infection and the onset of rheumatic fever. Most often the preceding streptococcal infection is a pharyngitis or an URI. Prevention or prompt treatment of group A beta-hemolytic streptococcal infections can prevent rheumatic heart disease.

Pathophysiology
The pathophysiology of rheumatic fever is uncertain. It is generally thought to be an immune reaction to antigens of group A streptococcus. Changes in the heart include swelling, fragmentation, and alterations in the connective tissue. The structures most often affected are the mitral and aortic valves, which may become swollen and edematous. The pulmonic and tricuspid valves are rarely affected in children.

History
A history of a recent URI, especially pharyngitis, should be sought. The onset of symptoms, length of illness, presence of fever, and any medications taken should be elicited. The history may include weight loss, malaise, and joint and abdominal pain.

Physical Assessment
Careful assessment of airway, breathing, and circulation is important. Physical findings of acute rheumatic heart disease may include low-grade fever, tachycardia, carditis, subcutaneous nodules, chorea, and arthritis. The diagnosis of carditis is based on the presence of one or more of the following findings: abnormal murmurs, pericardial friction rub, cardiomegaly, and congestive heart failure. Changes in the conductivity of the heart as seen on an electrocardiogram (ECG) include prolonged PR interval and nonspecific ST or T wave changes.

Joints should be carefully examined for motion, tenderness, swelling, warmth, and redness. Joint involvement in rheumatic fever tends to localize in the larger joints of the extremities. The most frequently affected joints are the knees and ankles, followed by the wrists and elbows. The hands, feet, shoulder, and small joints are least frequently involved. If the only joints involved are the temporomandibular or vertebral joints, a cause for the arthritis other than rheumatic fever should be sought.

The skin should be carefully examined for subcutaneous nodules and erythema marginatum. Subcutaneous nodules are found over the extensor surfaces of joints. These nodules are firm, nontender, and movable. Erythema marginatum is normally found on the trunk and extremities. Chorea, an unusual finding in rheumatic fever, is characterized by involuntary and purposeless movements of the extremities and facial grimacing. Emotional lability may occur.

When there is evidence of a preceding streptococcal infection, the diagnosis of rheumatic fever is usually based on the presence of two major or one major and two minor manifestations from the revised Jones criteria for rheumatic fever (Table 26–9).

TABLE 26–9. REVISED JONES CRITERIA FOR MANIFESTATIONS OF RHEUMATIC FEVER

- MAJOR MANIFESTATIONS
  Carditis
  Polyarthritis
  Erythema marginatum
  Subcutaneous nodules
  Chorea

- MINOR MANIFESTATIONS
  Fever
  Polyarthralgia
  Elevated acute phase reactants (erythrocyte sedimentation rate, reactive protein)
  Prolonged PR interval on ECG
  Previous history of rheumatic fever

Laboratory and Diagnostic Tests

Blood Studies. A CBC with differential indicates leukocytosis and anemia. Erythrocyte sedimentation rate and C-reactive protein levels are elevated. An increased or rising antistreptolysin-O (ASO) titer is the most commonly used serologic test to detect previous group A streptococcal infection. The multiple antibody test can provide serologic confirmation of recent streptococcal infection.

Cultures. A throat culture should be obtained before antibiotic therapy is initiated. Blood cultures are obtained to rule out subacute bacterial endocarditis.

Electrocardiography. The ECG may indicate a prolonged PR interval and nonspecific ST or T wave changes.

X Rays. A chest x ray may reveal cardiomegaly or pulmonary edema.

T R I A G E
Acute Rheumatic Fever

Emergent
A child with signs of cardiac involvement.

Urgent
A child with suspected rheumatic fever; painful joints in absence of cardiac symptoms.

Nursing Diagnosis
Pain

Defining Characteristics

- Painful joints
- Crying

Nursing Interventions

- Administer analgesics as ordered
- Place child in comfortable position

Expected Outcomes

- Patient describes decrease in pain
- Child is calm

Nursing Diagnosis
Decreased Cardiac Output

Defining Characteristics

- Tachycardia
- Hypotension
- Rales
- Arrhythmias

Nursing Interventions

- Administer oxygen
- Administer digoxin as ordered
- Administer antidiuretics as ordered
- Administer steroids as ordered
- Monitor fluid intake and output

Expected Outcomes

- Vital signs return to normal.
- Breath sounds are clear.
- Electrocardiogram returns to normal.

Management
The emergency treatment of rheumatic heart disease involves eradication of the hemolytic streptococci, control of congestive heart failure, prevention of permanent cardiac damage, and prevention of recurrences of the disease. Penicillin is the drug of choice for combating the acute, underlying infection. Erythromycin may be used for patients allergic to penicillin. Prophylactic antibiotic therapy should be started as soon as treatment of the acute phase has been completed.

If carditis or congestive heart failure is present, steroids such as prednisone (1–2 mg/kg/day) should be administered to reduce the inflammatory process. Digoxin and diuretics may be used to treat congestive heart failure. Strict bed rest and respiratory isolation for all patients believed to have rheumatic fever should begin in the ED.

Arthritis is treated with bedrest and anti-inflammatory agents. Aspirin is often given in high doses (75–100 mg/kg/day divided into four doses) to produce a serum salicylate level in the range of 20–30 mg/dL.

If chorea is present, it is treated with haloperidol 0.01–0.03 mg/kg/day divided into four doses.

Patient and Family Teaching and Psychosocial Support
Upon stabilization in the ED, the patient should be admitted to a pediatric ICU or in-patient unit depending on his or her condition. The child and parent need emotional support and information regarding the disease and its treatment. Education geared toward prevention of recurrent attacks is crucial. Prophylaxis may continue for 10–15 years after the initial diag-

nosis. Some patients with rheumatic fever are treated for a lifetime.

TUBERCULOSIS

Despite a steady decline in incidence over the past several decades, tuberculosis (TB) remains an important cause of morbidity, mortality, and health care expenditure.

A steady increase in the reported number of new cases has occurred during the last several years. Approximately 1200–1600 new cases occur annually in children in the US (Starke, 1992). One barrier to the successful control of TB is complacency among the public and health care providers. As incidence decreased for the 25 years prior to 1985, some communities discontinued screening of school-aged children.

The incidence of TB is particularly high in minority groups. Incidence rates for Southeast Asian refugees have been reported to be 70 times higher than those for other persons living in the US (Starke, 1988). Childhood cases of TB also tend to cluster in cities with a large number of immigrants.

Etiology and Pathophysiology
Transmission of *Mycobacterium tuberculosis* generally occurs by infected airborne droplets. The duration of exposure required to transmit the infection depends on the infectiousness of the source case. Children with primary tuberculosis rarely infect other children. Tubercle bacilli are sparse in children's secretions, and children usually do not cough with sufficient force to effectively transmit droplets. Children are usually infected by an adult with active TB living in the same household. Day care centers and shelters can be a source of transmission. It is important to screen the adults accompanying the child to the ED for signs of or a history of TB. If anyone is at risk for having the disease and is untreated, he or she must be isolated while in the ED area to avoid transmission of TB.

An inflammatory reaction occurs at the focal site in the lung, with the accumulation of leukocytes, followed by localized bronchopneumonia. As epithelial cells proliferate in an attempt to wall off the invading organisms, the typical tubercle is formed. Some of the bacilli leave the focal area and are carried to the regional lymph nodes. At this point, the child develops a fever, and x rays may be abnormal. Extension of the primary lesion at the original site causes progressive tissue destruction as it spreads within the lung. Erosion of blood vessels by the disease process can cause widespread dissemination of the bacilli to sites within other areas of the body (miliary TB).

History
The diagnosis of TB in children is usually based on epidemiologic data: the best evidence of TB without a positive culture is recent exposure to an infected adult. Therefore, the history is extremely important. Information on the health of other family members, caregivers, and peers should be elicited from the parents, and all contacts should be examined. Children considered to be at risk for TB infection include immigrants, minorities, those with malnutrition or immunodeficiency (especially HIV), and those who are in institutions (American Academy of Pediatrics, 1991).

Most children have no symptoms when a TB test first turns positive. Occasionally, there may be history of fever, mild cough, weight loss, or night sweats. Infants may present with failure to thrive.

Physical Assessment
Clinical manifestations are extremely variable in children with TB. A broad range of symptoms may be noted, such as fever, malaise, or weight loss. More specific findings related to the site of infection may be noted. In lung disease, progressive infection causes tachypnea, diminished breath sounds, and crackles, along with dullness to percussion. Cough, chest pain, and hemoptysis may occur.

Laboratory and Diagnostic Tests
The most important diagnostic laboratory test is the mycobacterial culture done on sputum (older children) or gastric aspirate (infants). However, the organism is slow-growing, and recovery may take 1–10 weeks. The Mantoux skin test is more practical, but it is subject to error both in testing technique and interpretation. Host factors such as age, nutritional status, immune status, or viral infection can alter reactivity.

X Rays. The chest x ray often indicates a localized, nonspecific infiltrate. It usually occurs in one site but may be multifocal. The infection spreads to the lymph system early, leading to hilar adenitis, which can cause bronchial obstruction.

Blood Studies. Routine laboratory tests rarely aid in the diagnosis of TB, but they may reflect general health status. Transanimase levels may be elevated in miliary TB.

T R I A G E
Tuberculosis

Urgent ————————————————
Child with fever, tachypnea, retractions, and chest pain.

Non-urgent
Child who is afebrile with no respiratory distress.

Nursing Diagnosis
Ineffective Breathing Pattern

Defining Characteristics

- Tachypnea
- Retractions

Nursing Interventions

- Provide nasotracheal suction as necessary
- Place patient in position to facilitate respiratory effort
- Administer oxygen

Expected Outcomes

- Respiratory rate returns to normal
- Retractions lessen or disappear

Nursing Diagnosis
Noncompliance (Treatment of TB)

Defining Characteristics

- Lengthy course of therapy
- Limited access to health care system

Nursing Interventions

- Provide parents with information regarding normal course of illness, importance of prolonged therapy, and modes of transmission
- Provide referral to community nursing agencies, other public health resources

Expected Outcomes

- Patient and family comply with medical and nursing therapy and recommendations
- Patient and family perceive adequate support from health care system

Management
Tuberculosis does not present with life-threatening symptoms in children. Isolation is not normally necessary for an infected child, although infected adult caretakers may need to be isolated. The approach to treating tuberculosis has changed considerably over the past decade. Antimicrobial agents are available to cure most cases of TB, but the limiting factor is patient compliance. Until the 1980s, many TB regimens were 12–18 months long and were associated with a high rate of failure. Today, although the courses of drug therapy are substantially shorter (6–9 months), patients still require careful follow-up care to ensure compliance with the treatment.

Although they are less likely than adults to have a resistance to anti-TB drugs, children are also more likely to have extrapulmonary forms of the disease, especially meningitis and disseminated disease. Thus, it is important that drugs penetrate a variety of body tissues and fluids. Children also tolerate higher doses (per kilogram body weight) and tend to have fewer side effects than adults (Starke, 1992).

Multidrug therapy is generally used to decrease the emergence of resistance and to act against the varying populations of the tubercle bacilli that can exist in a given host. Thus, while different combinations may be given depending on the clinical status of the child, isoniazid, rifampin, and pyrazinamide are usually given for a period of 9 months. Durations of therapy shorter than this have been associated with an unacceptably high rate of relapse (Starke, 1988).

Corticosteroids may be of benefit when the inflammatory response contributes to tissue damage or impairs function. However, steroids should never be given without simultaneously administering anti-TB drugs.

Patients who are tuberculin-positive but who have no symptoms should be treated prophylactically to prevent the development of active disease. Treatment with isonicotinoylhydrazine (INH) does not alter the tuberculin reaction, but it has been shown to prevent the development of symptomatic TB for at least 30 years.

Who Should Receive Preventive Therapy for TB

- Children with a positive tuberculin test without clinical or x ray findings
- Children with a negative tuberculin test but known exposure to adults with infectious TB
- Previously treated children in whom immunosuppression develops, either from disease or from drug therapy
- Children who show recent conversion of the tuberculin skin test after exposure to an infectious person (Starke, 1990).

Patient and Family Teaching and Psychosocial Support
Tuberculosis has historically been regarded with fear. It is important to clarify any misconceptions the family may have regarding the disease, its transmission, or therapy. The success of treatment depends to a large part on acceptance and cooperation from the family. They require emotional support, factual information about the transmission of the disease, and referral to public health resources in the community.

A child with TB may return to school and activities when acute symptoms have disappeared and chemotherapy has been instituted. If the child is taking rifampin, the child and parents should be aware that the drug causes all body fluids to be stained orange (urine, tears) and that contact lenses may be stained. Nutrition should be discussed; optimal nutrition is an important adjunct to drug therapy.

MEASLES

Measles, or rubeola, was once considered to be well controlled in the US. The incidence began to rise in 1988 and was sustained through 1992. During early 1993, no new cases were reported to the CDC. During the marked increase in cases which occurred between 1988 and 1992, one-half of the cases occurred in unvaccinated preschoolers. Reasons for the resurgence include a low immunization rate for vulnerable preschoolers in certain areas of the country; a spread of the infection to unvaccinated infants younger than 15 months; and occurrence in vaccinated school-aged children, indicating vaccine failure (Adcock et al, 1992).

Measles is a highly contagious childhood illness; it is characterized by fever, respiratory symptoms, conjunctivitis, a maculopapular erythematous rash, and the pathognomic Koplik spots (tiny red spots with whitish blue centers that occur on the buccal mucosa). Before the development of the vaccine, outbreaks of measles were cyclical, occurring every 3–5 years. Boys and girls are affected equally; measles occurs most often in the winter and spring.

The complications of measles include otitis media, pneumonia, and encephalitis. When death occurs, it is usually linked to respiratory complications. Immunocompromised hosts may have a prolonged disease course with persistent excretion of the virus and increased rates of morbidity and mortality.

The first measles vaccine was licensed in 1963. Two types were used initially. Live attenuated vaccine was often given in combination with immune globulin to decrease side effects. The inactivated version of the vaccine failed to provide immunity and was subsequently taken off the market. The Moraten vaccine is currently used in the US. It has been associated with fewer severe reactions than previous vaccines, and provides 98% immunity. It can be given singly (monovalent) or in combination with mumps and rubella vaccine as the MMR (trivalent). The failure of the earlier vaccines is now linked to a resurgence of the disease among adolescents and college students.

Etiology and Pathophysiology

Measles is caused by a virus that is usually transmitted by contact with respiratory secretions or droplets. Its clinical course is divided into three stages. The usual incubation period is 10–12 days. During the prodromal stage, the child has a fever, rhinitis, and a cough. Conjunctivitis occurs along with photophobia and general malaise. Koplik spots appear on the buccal mucosa. The disease is contagious 1–2 days before these symptoms appear until 5 days after the rash appears.

After 3–5 days, the appearance of the maculopapular rash, which appears on the head and travels caudally, marks the beginning of the exanthem stage. During this phase the child typically has a high fever, lymphadenopathy, and pharyngitis. Diarrhea, abdominal pain, and leukopenia may occur.

History

A history of exposure to someone with active measles is important because the diagnosis is made chiefly on epidemiologic and clinical grounds. Immunization status, including date and type of vaccine given, should be elicited. A current risk factor in the development of measles is a recent visit to an ED. A recent study documented that patients with measles were about seven times more likely to have visited an ED than an uninfected patient (Adcock et al, 1992; Farizo, 1991).

A child with measles is likely to have high fever and upper respiratory symptoms. The parent or child may describe tearing, red or itching eyes, and photophobia. Gastrointestinal symptoms, such as vomiting, diarrhea, and abdominal pain, may be present.

Atypical measles may occur when the host has received killed measles virus before exposure. In this presentation, the onset of fever may be more abrupt and symptoms more severe than in ordinary measles.

Physical Assessment

The physical examination varies depending on when the patient seeks medical care. In the prodromal phase, the patient may have signs of an URI, with rhinitis, congestion, and injected pharynx. Shortly before development of the rash, Koplik spots usually appear. These lesions are initially about 1 mm in diameter but may coalesce into larger lesions. Initially there are only a few lesions, but within 12 hours they are usually numerous. The mucosal background is bright red and granular in appearance. Excessive lacrimation occurs in this phase, and corneal lesions may be seen with a slit-lamp examination.

In the exanthem phase the typical morbilliform rash is seen. The Koplik spots begin to disappear, and the rash begins behind the ears and on the forehead at the hair line. The exanthem is erythematous and maculopapular, coalescing most noticeably on the face. It begins to clear on the third or fourth day, again in a caudal direction. Adenopathy is common during this phase, as is splenomegaly.

TABLE 26–10. COMMON DISEASES PRESENTING WITH RASH

	Incubation Period	Common Age Group	Signs and Symptoms	Characteristic Rash	Management
Rubeola (Measles)	10–12 days	Preschoolers	High fever, cough, conjunctivitis, Koplik spots	Blotchy, erythematous maculopapular; spreads distally from hairline	Supportive; isolation; vaccination to prevent
Rubella (German Measles)	14–21 days	Toddlers, pre-schoolers	Low-grade fever, malaise, sore throat, headache	Fine, pinkish-red maculopapular; spreads distally from face; often pruritic	Supportive
Varicella (Chicken Pox)	10–21 days	Any age	Low-grade fever, symptoms of upper respiratory infection	Thin-walled vesicles with red halos	Supportive; calamine lotion; antipruritic
Fifth Disease (Erythema infection)	4–14 days; up to 20 days	Preschoolers, young school-aged	Occasional headache, nausea, myalgia	Bright red macular patches on cheeks followed by erythematous macular lacy rash on extremities	Supportive
Streptococcal Scarlet Fever	2–4 days	School-aged	Fevers, chills, malaise, sore throat, abdominal pain, headache	Sandpapery, erythematous; blanches on pressure	Supportive; antibiotics
Meningococcemia	1–10 days	Any age	Fever, irritability, toxicity	Pink macules, raised petechiae, purpura	Basic or advanced life support; antibiotics; anticonvulsants as indicated

Table 26–10 summarizes common childhood illnesses presenting with rashes.

Laboratory and Diagnostic Tests

Laboratory studies are rarely indicated in uncomplicated measles. An increase in antibody titers or the presence of antibody can confirm the diagnosis if necessary. During the prodromal and exanthem periods, the total leukocyte count is low. Lymphopenia may be especially pronounced.

TRIAGE
Measles

Urgent
Child with respiratory distress and fever.

Non-urgent
Child with rash who is afebrile.

Nursing Diagnosis

Alteration in comfort

Defining Characteristics

- Fever
- Photophobia, coryza, and cough

Nursing Interventions

- Provide antipyretics as needed
- Avoid chilling of patient
- Dim room lights
- Encourage fluids, provide cool mist

Expected Outcomes

- Patient's temperature returns to normal
- Patient is able to rest
- Patient verbalizes increase in comfort

Management

It is extremely important for the triage nurse to identify the patient with suspected measles so that proper respiratory precautions can be taken to prevent transmission. The treatment of a child with measles is supportive. It is important that the child maintain an adequate intake of fluids to prevent dehydration. Bedrest should be maintained during the acute phase; a darkened room may increase comfort for a patient with photophobia. Antitussives and acetaminophen can be used to decrease cough and fever. Hospitalization is rarely necessary, but may be required for a child with respiratory or CNS complications.

A single intramuscular dose of immunoglobulin G (IgG) (0.25 mg/kg) is recommended for the immunosuppressed patient or household contact who is exposed to measles. These children are at greater risk for complications, and shedding of the virus is prolonged. For other susceptible children, measles vaccine given within 72 hours of a single exposure affords protection (Adcock et al, 1992).

Patient and Family Teaching and Psychosocial Support

Other than providing instructions for symptomatic care, the most important aspect of teaching involves prevention of transmission to family members and friends. Respiratory transmission should be explained, and the dangers of measles to immunosuppressed patients should be discussed. This is also an appropriate time to inquire about the immunization status of other family members. The current recommendation of the American Academy of Pediatrics and the Advisory Council on Immunization Practices is a two-dose regimen, one given at 15 months and the second given on entering elementary or middle school (American Academy of Pediatrics, 1991).

INFECTIOUS MONONUCLEOSIS

Infectious mononucleosis is a clinical syndrome most often associated with a primary infection by Epstein-Barr virus (EBV). It may affect children of any age but is more common in adolescents and young adults than in infants. Although full recovery may take weeks, any complications are usually of short duration, without long-term sequelae.

Etiology and Pathophysiology

Most adult populations that have been studied have been found to have serologic reactivity to EBV, indicating that most adults carry the virus (Sumaya, 1992). The age at primary infection varies with socioeconomic setting. In developing countries, most children are exposed to the EBV early in life, most primary infections being subclinical or mildly symptomatic. In more developed countries, primary infection tends to occur in the adolescent or early adult years, usually manifesting as typical mononucleosis.

The cardinal clinical features of infectious mononucleosis are fever, sore throat, general malaise, and fatigue, accompanied by lymphadenopathy and pharyngitis. Young children may have diarrhea, otitis me-

dia, or pneumonia (Barkin and Rosen, 1990). Often a 2–5 day prodromal period, in which the child experiences malaise and fatigue, nausea, and vomiting, with or without fever, occurs before the full onset of symptoms. Splenomegaly or hepatomegaly is present in 30–50% of patients during the first 3 weeks. Pharyngitis may be severe and exudative, but it is rarely accompanied by streptococcal infection. An erythematous, maculopapular rash may occur, more often in young children than in older children. If ampicillin is given unintentionally, the rash may be more prominent (Niederman and Marcinak, 1993).

Complications may occur in the pulmonary, neurologic, or hematologic systems. Airway obstruction may be caused by intense inflammaton and hypertrophy of tonsillopharyngeal tissue. Thrombocytopenia, leading to bleeding disorders, may be related to splenic destruction, antiplatelet antibodies, or abnormal platelet function. Splenic rupture occurs rarely. Neurologic sequelae, including seizures, Guillain-Barré syndrome, or meningitis and encephalitis may present as a result of EBV invasion of the CNS.

Clinical recovery from infectious mononucleosis occurs gradually, after an acute phase lasting a few days to 3–4 weeks. Fever usually resolves within 2 weeks; a severe sense of fatigue may persist for several weeks to months. Splenomegaly may persist for 2 or 3 months.

History

The history in infectious mononucleosis may be quite nonspecific. The child may complain of fatigue or general malaise, or may present after several days of fever or sore throat. Other URI symptoms, such as cough, rhinitis, or abdominal pain may be part of the history. Comments about difficulty breathing or swallowing should be carefully noted. The parents should be asked about development of any rash.

Physical Assessment

A rapid assessment of airway, breathing, and circulation should be performed, noting any respiratory distress and signs of dehydration related to decreased intake or fever. The child's temperature should be monitored. The abdomen is palpated for evidence of hepato- or splenomegaly. The throat is visualized for signs of inflammation, and any palpable lymph nodes are noted.

Laboratory and Diagnostic Tests

Blood Studies. The diagnosis of infectious mononucleosis often can be made on the basis of a CBC with differential and substantiated by a test for heterophil antibodies. Patients typically show an absolute lymphocytosis (at least 50% lymphocytes) and prominent atypical lymphocytes (at least 10% of total leukocytes). However, children younger than 4 years frequently do not develop a detectable heterophil antibody response during EBV illness. An EBV titer may be obtained in this age group, although this is not often indicated.

Cultures. A throat culture for streptococcus may be obtained to rule out concomitant bacterial infection.

TRIAGE
Infectious Mononucleosis

Emergent ————————————————
A child with evidence of airway obstruction or respiratory distress.

Urgent ————————————————————
A child with prolonged or high fever; sore throat.

Nursing Diagnosis
Ineffective Airway Clearance

Defining Characteristics

- Increased respiratory and heart rates
- Retractions
- Stridorous respiratory sounds
- Desire to be positioned upright
- Look of distress or panic

Nursing Interventions

- Prepare intubation equipment
- Provide supplemental oxygen
- Elevate head of bed or have parent hold child in upright position

Expected Outcomes

- Respiratory and heart rates return to normal
- Stridor and retractions diminish

Nursing Diagnosis
High Risk for Altered Body Temperature

Defining Characteristics

- Increased body temperature
- Lethargy
- Complaints of general malaise

Nursing Interventions

- Administer antipyretic and analgesic agents as needed
- Encourage intake of cool fluids
- Provide for adequate rest and sleep

Expected Outcomes

- Body temperature returns to normal
- Patient verbalizes feeling better
- Patient is able to rest

Nursing Diagnosis
Diversional Activity Deficit

Defining Characteristics

- Disease with extended course, slow recovery
- Need for modified activity level, especially if splenomegaly present

Nursing Interventions

- Prepare parents for extended recovery period
- Suggest age-appropriate diversional activities
- Encourage visits from friends

Expected Outcomes

- Patient complies with activity restrictions
- Patient participates in constructive or fun activities

Management
The management of infectious mononucleosis is primarily supportive. Rest, fluids, and acetaminophen for pain or discomfort are recommended. Antiviral agents are not used in uncomplicated cases, but they may be prescribed for immunosuppressed patients. Short-term steroid therapy may prevent airway compromise and provide relief in patients with respiratory distress due to massively enlarged tonsils.

Patient and Family Teaching and Psychosocial Support
Patients and families should be advised of the often prolonged clinical course of infectious mononucleosis; up to 6 months may elapse before the child fully recovers. Patients should be cautioned against the child's participating in strenuous physical activity and contact sports during the period of organomegaly to minimize the risk of splenic rupture.

LYME DISEASE

Lyme disease is a systemic, tick-borne illness. It is usually associated with a pathognomic skin lesion, known as erythema chronicum migrans (ECM), which is present in 60–80% of patients (Rahn and Malawista, 1991). Although the disease responds well to early treatment, dissemination may occur in unidentified cases, often resulting in cardiac, neurologic, or joint manifestations.

Lyme disease is of increasing importance, because its scope of incidence, geographic distribution, and clinical spectrum have been expanding in recent years. It occurs in all ages and in both sexes. Data on the clinical course and treatment are still emerging, and many areas of uncertainty remain.

Etiology and Pathophysiology

Lyme disease is caused by the spirochete *Borrelia burgdorferi*. It is harbored by a tick of the variety *Ixodes daminii,* which lives primarily on white-tailed-deer and white-footed field mice. It is most common in states from Massachusetts to Maryland, Wisconsin, Minnesota, California, and Oregon, but it has been identified in 43 states (Rahn and Malawista, 1991). Its onset is generally between May 1 and November 30. Lyme disease is not spread person to person.

The multisystemic nature and slow evolution of the illness can make diagnosis difficult. There are three stages of Lyme disease. In the first, occurring 3–32 days after a tick bite, the characteristic ECM rash appears, followed by flu-like symptoms. In the second stage, which may follow by weeks or months, CNS impairment such as cranial neuritis, Bell palsy, iritis, and emotional or memory problems occur. Cardiovascular involvement, such as myocarditis or endocarditis, may appear at this time. The third, or chronic, phase begins several months into the disease and can last years. It is characterized by severe arthritic pain usually involving a knee joint. This is the most common late symptom, occurring in 50% of children with Lyme disease. The arthritis is characterized by spontaneous remissions and exacerbations, not always occurring in the same joints. Neurologic symptoms mimicking multiple sclerosis may occur. Bell palsy and aseptic meningitis are most common in children. Skin lesions or thickening of the dermis may be present.

History

In a child with suspected Lyme disease, a history of a tick bite or being in wooded areas is important. However, because of the small size of the tick, a patient may not have been aware of its presence. Complaints of general malaise or achiness, sore throat, fever may cause the parents to seek medical attention. Parents should be asked about the presence of any rash and its development.

In a child in the later stages of Lyme disease, the history may include complaints related to the neurologic, musculoskeletal, or cardiovascular systems. Complaints of headache, irritability, or stiff neck may occur. Any complaints of peripheral neuropathy, either pain or paresthesias, or confusion or loss of memory should be noted. Joint pain may be present. Fatigue, dizziness, or syncope could indicate cardiac involvement.

Physical Assessment

The clinical examination should focus on the areas of complaint and the skin, heart, CNS, and the musculoskeletal system. The child should be fully undressed to check for the presence of the characteristic rash. The lesion may first appear as a small papule typical of an insect bite. Within a few days, the initial redness expands to a plaque that may be 6–60 cm or more in diameter. Clearing begins to occur in the center, leaving a "bull's eye" type rash. The lesion may be described as burning and occasionally is pruritic. Many patients have multiple smaller secondary annular lesions without the indurated center.

A child with indications of disseminated disease should have a careful cardiovascular examination. Heart rate and rhythm should be assessed, along with quality of pulses and signs of perfusion. The neurologic examination should include assessment of cranial nerves and peripheral nerve function. The musculoskeletal examination should assess for range of joint motion, weakness, swelling, or favoring of an extremity.

Laboratory and Diagnostic Tests

Blood Studies. The definitive laboratory diagnosis of Lyme disease is difficult. The organism is technically difficult to culture; the scarcity of the organism makes tissue staining impractical; and antibody response tests are often inaccurate. Serologic testing by ELISA followed by a Western blot test is used most often. Immunoglobulin antibody usually develops within 2–4 weeks of the ECM rash, and IgG is usually elevated within 6–8 weeks of the onset. The WBC count may be elevated.

Lumbar Puncture. Antibodies to *Borrelia* may also be measured in CSF. In unconfirmed cases, neurologic symptoms may call for assessment of the CSF for meningitis.

Electrocardiogram. Varying degrees of atrioventricular (AV) block or ST-T segment irregularities may be noted.

Electromyography or Nerve Biopsy. These tests may be used to detect neuropathies.

Nursing Diagnosis
Pain

Defining Characteristics

- Complaints of pain
- Limited range of motion of joints
- Swelling of joints

Nursing Interventions

- Provide analgesics as indicated
- Apply heat to affected joints
- Provide or teach gentle range of motion exercises

Expected Outcomes

- Patient reports decreased pain
- Patient participates in activities

Nursing Diagnosis
Impaired Physical Mobility

Defining Characteristics

- Inability to bear weight without pain
- Bedrest prescribed for cardiac sequelae

Nursing Interventions

- Refer for physical therapy as indicated
- Have wheelchair available for patient's use
- Assist parents to anticipate implication of bedrest for child's developmental level and provide suggestions for diversionary activities

Expected Outcomes

- Patient moves about in wheelchair
- Patient returns to usual mobility status following period of prescribed bedrest

Nursing Diagnosis
Sensorineural Alterations

Defining Characteristics

- Sensory disturbances related to neuropathy
- Inability to feel, move parts of body (nerve palsies)
- Headaches, stiff neck

Nursing Interventions

- Limit unpleasant stimuli (eg, bright light, air movement)
- Assist patient and family in correct positioning of affected extremities
- Provide analgesics and other medications as appropriate

Expected Outcomes

- Patient reports increased comfort
- Musculoskeletal injuries and compromised function do not occur

Management
For children with early Lyme disease, doxycycline 100 mg bid (9 years or older) or ampicillin or amoxicillin 50 mg/kg/day (younger than 9 years) are generally prescribed. Doxycycline, amoxicillin, or erythromycin may be used (Kaslow, 1992). For disseminated disease, high-dose penicillin (400 mg/kg/day) is given. Isolation is not required; the patient may return to school and normal activity when symptoms allow.

Prevention of the disease involves awareness and taking precautions in wooded areas with long grass or brush. Protective clothing, such as long pants and long-sleeved shirts and hats, should be worn. The body should be checked for ticks after leaving an infested area. Insect repellants that contain diethyltoluomide (DEET) are effective against ticks and should be applied to the clothing.

Patient and Family Teaching and Psychosocial Support
Families with a child in the early stages of Lyme disease should be taught measures to prevent future occurrences. Symptoms that may indicate progression of the disease should be explained, and the importance of medical follow-up should be emphasized.

Lyme disease in the later stages can be frightening for the child and family. Information about diagnostic procedures, progression of the disease, and treatment plans may seem overwhelming and should be presented in small portions. The uncertainty of diagnosis can be extremely frustrating as new symptoms appear. The parents and child can be assured that information and results will be shared with them as they become available. Because Lyme disease may progress to a chronic illness, continuity personnel (nurses and social workers) should be assigned as soon as possible.

REFERENCES

Adams WG, Deaver KA, Cochi SL, et al (1993). Decline of childhood Haemophilus influenzae Type b (Hib) disease in the Hib vaccine era. *JAMA* 269:221–226

Adcock LM, Bissey JD, Feigin RD (1992). A new look at measles. *Infectious Disease Clinics of North America* 6:133–148

American Academy of Pediatrics, Committee on Infectious Diseases (1991). *Report of the Committee on Infectious Diseases* (22nd ed). Elk Grove Village, Il: American Academy of Pediatrics

Barkin RM (1992). Meningitis, bacterial. In Barkin RM (ed), *Pediatric emergency medicine.* St. Louis: Mosby, pp. 912–919

Behrman RM (1992). Neonatal sepsis. In Behrman RM (ed), *Textbook of pediatrics* (14th ed). Philadelphia: Saunders pp 501–504

Berry RK (1988). Home care of the child with AIDS. *Pediatric Nursing* 14:341–344

Boenning DA (1992). Reye syndrome. In Barkin RM (ed), *Pediatric emergency medicine.* St. Louis: Mosby, pp 777–779

Burroughs MH, Edelson PJ (1991). Medical care of the HIV-infected child. *Pediatric Clinics of North America* 38:45–65

Cherry JD (1992). Encephalitis. In Behrman RM (ed), *Textbook of pediatrics* (14th ed). Philadelphia: Saunders pp 666–669

Farizo KM, Stehr-Green PA, Simpson DM, et al (1991). Pediatric emergency room visits: A risk factor for acquiring measles. *Pediatrics* 87:74–79

Feigin RD (1990). Kawasaki disease. In Oski FA (ed), *Principles and practice of pediatrics.* Philadelphia: Lippincott, pp 1300–1304

Hazinski MF (1992). Reye's syndrome. In Hazinski MF (ed), *Nursing care of the critically ill child* (2nd ed). St. Louis: Mosby, pp 615–617

Hazinski MF, Barkin RM (1992). Shock. In Barkin RM (ed), *Pediatric emergency medicine.* St. Louis: Mosby, pp 84–111

Horowitz SJ (1992). Reye's syndrome. In Reece RM (ed), *Manual of emergency pediatrics* (4th ed). Philadelphia: Saunders, pp 111–112

Kaslow RA (1992). Current perspective on Lyme borreliosis. *JAMA* 267:1381–1383

Lang S (1993). Procedures involving the neurological system. In Bernardo LM, Bove M (eds), *Pediatric emergency procedures.* Boston: Jones and Bartlett, pp 143–161

Lux KM (1991). New hope for children with Kawasaki disease. *Journal of Pediatric Nursing* 6:159–165

Melish ME (1990). Kawasaki syndrome. In Gellis SS, Kagan BM (eds), *Current pediatric therapy.* Philadelphia: Saunders, pp 443–444

McKinney RE (1991). Antiviral therapy for human immunodeficiency virus infection in children. *Pediatric Clinics of North America* 38:133–151

Morens DM, Melish ME (1992). Kawasaki disease. In Feigin RD, Cherry JD (eds), *Textbook of pediatric infectious diseases.* Philadelphia: Saunders, pp 2137–2160

Niederman LG, Marcinak JF (1993). Sore throat. In Dershewitz RA (ed), *Ambulatory pediatric care.* Philadelphia: Lippincott, pp 315–319

Nihill MR, Felgin RD, Gruber R, Morens D (1987). Kawasaki disease. In Feigin RD, Cherry JD (eds). *Textbook of pediatric infectious diseases* (2nd ed). Philadelphia: Saunders

Novello AC, Wise PH, Willoughby A (1989). Final report of the United States Department of Health and Human Services Secretary's work group on pediatric human immunedeficiency virus infection and disease: Content and implications. *Pediatrics* 84:547–555

Rahn DW, Malawista SE (1991). Lyme disease: Recommendations for diagnosis and treatment. *Annals of Internal Medicine* 114:472–481

Starke JR (1988). Modern approach to the diagnosis and treatment of tuberculosis in children. *New Topics in Pediatric Infectious Disease* 35:441–459

Starke JR (1990). Tuberculosis. In Oski FA (ed). *Principles and practice of pediatrics.* Philadelphia: Lippincott, pp 1138–1149

Starke JR (1992). Current chemotherapy for tuberculosis in children. *Infectious Disease Clinics of North America* 6:215–235

Sumaya CV (1992). Epstein-Barr virus. In Feigin RD, Cherry JD (eds), *Textbook of pediatric infectious diseases* (3rd ed, vol II) Philadelphia: Saunders, pp 1547–1555

Thurber F, Berry B (1990). Children with AIDS: Issues and future directions. *Journal of Pediatric Nursing* 5:168–177

Ward-Wimmer D (1988). Nursing care of children with HIV infection. *Nursing Clinics of North America* 23:719–728

Wendell PM, Harris JS (1992). Meningitis. In Reece RM (ed), *Manual of emergency pediatrics* (4th ed) Philadelphia: Saunders, pp 72–76

SUGGESTED READING

AIDS
Caspe WB (1991). Guidelines for the care of children and adolescents with HIV infection. *Journal of Pediatrics* 119:S3

Karthas N (1990). When children have AIDS: How to support the family. *Nursing 90* 20:32C–32F

Quinn TC (1990). The epidemiology of the human immunodeficiency virus. *Annals of Emergency Medicine* 19:225–232

Kawasaki Disease
Burns JC (1989). Kawasaki disease. *Current Opinion in Pediatrics* 1:13–15

Kryzer TC, Derkay CS (1992). Kawasaki disease: A five-year experience at Children's National Medical Center. *International Journal of Pediatric Otorhinolaryngology* 23:211–220

McEnhill M, Vitale K (1989). Kawasaki disease: New challenges in care. *The American Journal of Maternal-Child Nursing* 14:406–410

Tuberculosis
Biddulph J (1990). Short-course chemotherapy for childhood tuberculosis. *Pediatric Infectious Disease Journal* 9:794

Girgis NI, Farid Z, Kilpatrick ME et al (1991). Dexamethasone as an adjunct to treatment of tuberculous meningitis. *Pediatric Infectious Disease Journal* 10:179

Measles

Cherry JD (1992). Measles. In Feigin RD, Cherry JD (eds), *Textbook of pediatric infectious diseases* (3rd ed). Philadelphia: Saunders, pp 1591–1605

Meeske K, Chamberlin D, Cipkala-Gaffin JA, Harlander C, Reed K (1991). Measles epidemic: Impact on pediatric oncology patients. *Journal of Pediatric Oncology Nursing* 8:151–158

Morbidity and Mortality Weekly Report (1992). Public sector vaccination efforts in response to the resurgence of measles among public school children—United States 1989–1991. 41:522–525

Taber LH (1990). Measles. In Oski FA (ed), *Principles and practice of pediatrics*. Philadelphia: Lippincott, pp 1227–1230

Infectious Mononucleosis

Sumaya CV (1992). Infectious mononucleosis and Epstein-Barr virus related syndromes. In Burg, FD, Ingelfinger JR, Wald ER (eds), *Gellis & Kagan's current pediatric therapy*. Philadelphia: Saunders, pp 608–609

Lyme Disease

Bresingham I (1990). Pediatric management problems: Lyme disease. *Pediatric Nursing* 16:280–281

Ostrov BE, Athreya BH (1990). Lyme disease: Difficulties in diagnosis and management. *Pediatric Clinics of North America* 38:535–549

Stechenberg BW (1990). Lyme disease. In Oski FA (ed), *Principles and practice of pediatrics*. Philadelphia: Lippincott, pp 1073–1074

CHAPTER 27

Gastrointestinal Emergencies

ARLENE M. SPERHAC
CATHERINE R. BENSON

INTRODUCTION

Gastrointestinal (GI) emergencies make up one of the largest categories of diseases in the pediatric population. Emergency department (ED) nurses must be prepared to deal with the physical and psychosocial needs of these children, and with the needs of their parents.

When children have abdominal discomfort, they are usually frightened. A calm, reassuring, supportive approach is needed by the nurse. If possible, the parents should be allowed to remain with the child when the assessment is done. In a frightening, strange environment it is helpful for the children to see their familiar, trusted family members as much as possible.

Privacy should be maintained when assessing the abdomen. To a school-aged child or young adolescent with a rapidly changing body, modesty can be a major concern. In addition, sights and sounds that are familiar to ED personnel can seem ominous to children and should be explained if the patient cannot be shielded from them.

Not only the child but also the family needs to be kept informed about what will be occurring. With a young child, the assurance that nurses give to the parents by keeping them informed is usually transmitted to the child. The staff's realistic assessment of the child's condition, as critical as it may be, is often less frightening than the parents' own perceptions of the situation. Therefore, the family should be kept as informed as possible.

The nurse's manner and her or his attention to comfort measures are important in gaining the confidence of the child. For example, warming the hands and stethoscope before placing them on a tender abdomen and a general responsiveness to the needs of the child and the family can do much to allay the child's fear (Sperhac, 1990). A frightened child in pain and his or her family must feel confident in the ED staff.

History

In children with GI diseases, a complete and careful history almost always points to the correct diagnosis (Crain et al, 1992). Questions that deal with the duration and onset of the problem, recent infections, medication, new foods, weight loss and associated symptoms, and level of activity should be asked. Prenatal and perinatal events, a complete dietary history, and a history of allergies or GI disease in other family members should be sought.

When obtaining the history of a child with a GI dysfunction, age is probably the most important factor. For children younger than 2 years, the parents interpret the cries as abdominal pain. Two- to five-year-old children can point a finger to the exact location. For older children the history is more reliable, and the symptoms are better described.

For each age group, different disease entities must be considered. Figure 27–1 provides a review of the anatomy of the GI tract in children. In an infant with an acute abdomen, a GI malformation, an incarcerated hernia, or torsion of the testis or the ovarian pedicle should be considered. In a pre-school-aged child, an acute abdomen is frequently related to an infection or an inflammatory process rather than a mechanical obstruction.

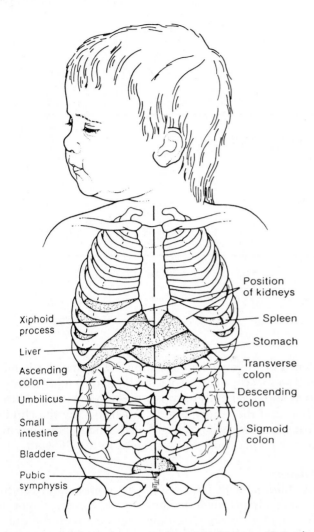

Figure 27–1. Abdominal structures. (From Mott SR, James SR, Sperhac AM [eds] [1990]. *Nursing care of children and families* [2nd ed]. Menlo Park, Calif: Addison-Wesley, p 381.)

process, but these symptoms give important information and must be noted.

Pain is the most useful of all subjective data. Numerous conditions cause abdominal pain in infants, children and adolescents (Tables 27–1, 27–2, and 27–3). A precise characterization of pain accurately differentiates inflammations from nongangrenous mechanical obstructions. An instantaneous onset or the sudden worsening of pain usually indicates an origin from a vascular accident or rupture of some hollow viscus, ie, a surgical condition. "Colicky" or intermittent pain usually develops when there has been an anatomic obstruction of the lumen of a peristaltic hollow conduit. Information regarding the onset, situation, nature, persistence, and radiation of the pain should be sought.

Bleeding usually causes a mildly inflammatory, painless reaction. Hemorrhage into the lumen of the GI tract is the single most impressive finding. If the bleeding is internal, acute anemia or hypovolemic shock may be the presenting feature.

Physiologic jaundice is more common in infancy than at any other time in life, and may be normal. Pathologic jaundice is relatively uncommon, but when present it is usually associated with diseases of the liver or biliary duct system.

Abdominal and pelvic injuries present special problems of diagnosis, since the extent of the trauma is often not immediately apparent. An accurate history must be obtained, and a careful record of all relevant information regarding the nature of the trauma sustained must be made as an aid to diagnosis.

In addition to age, sex needs to be considered. Some entities are more frequently encountered in boys than in girls. Growth parameters also need to be noted.

In most cases the history is obtained from the parents, though the children should also be questioned for validation and clarification, if possible. Close attention should be paid to the events preceding the problem.

Clinical Presentation

Children suffering from acute disease of an intra-abdominal organ can have pain, bleeding, jaundice, or some combination thereof. Other signs and symptoms may prove to be valuable aids in arriving at the correct diagnosis or in determining a course of management. For example, nausea and vomiting are often reflex phenomena and may not be related to the physiologic

TABLE 27–1. CAUSES OF ACUTE ABDOMINAL PAIN IN INFANTS AND CHILDREN YOUNGER THAN 2 YEARS

Intussusception
Intestinal malrotation
Fixed volvulus
Incarcerated inguinal hernia
Pyloric stenosis
Acute appendicitis
Trauma
Child abuse
Meckel diverticulum
Necrotizing enterocolitis
Hirschsprung disease (obstruction)
Toxins
Colic
Viral syndrome
Gastroenteritis
Sickling syndromes
Wilms tumor

(*From* Schwartz GR [ed] [1992]. *Principles and practice of emergency medicine* [vol 1]. *Philadelphia: Lea & Febiger, p 379*)

TABLE 27–2. CAUSES OF ACUTE ABDOMINAL PAIN IN CHILDREN OLDER THAN 2 YEARS

Nonspecific (61%)	Tumors
Acute appendicitis (32%)	Malrotation
Intussusception (1.3%)	Fixed volvulus
Trauma	Pancreatitis
Child Abuse	Acalculous cholecystitis
Toxins	Cholelithiasis
Incarcerated inguinal hernia	Urinary tract infection
Sepsis	Renal colic
Primary peritonitis	Testicular torsion
Enterocolitis	Ovarian cyst or mass
Diabetic ketoacidosis	Ovarian torsion
Hepatitis	Pneumonia
Peptic ulcer disease	Otitis media
Bacterial endocarditis	Tonsilitis
Leukemic ileocecal syndrome	Henoch-Schonlein purpura
Gastroenteritis	Cystic fibrosis
Functional abdominal pain	Rheumatic fever
Mesenteric adenitis	Porphyria
Foreign bodies	Uremia
Constipation	Hypercholesterolemia
Intestinal parasites	Collagen vascular disease
Lactose intolerance	Sickling syndromes
Meckel diverticulum	Ventriculoperitoneal shunt pseudocyst
Inflammatory bowel disease	Black widow spider bite

(*From Schwartz GR* [ed] [1992]. Principles and practice of emergency medicine [vol 1]. *Philadelphia: Lea & Febiger, p 380*)

PAIN WITH GASTROINTESTINAL EMERGENCIES

Inflammatory Conditions

Inflammatory disease within the peritoneal cavity is generally characterized by unremitting abdominal pain. Sudden onset of pain or the rapid worsening of symptoms usually indicates perforation of a hollow viscus. Gradual intensification of pain is associated with commonly encountered inflammatory conditions.

The location of the pain should be noted. Foregut diseases (stomach and duodenum) give symptoms that are epigastric in location; midgut problems (small intestine and right and transverse colons) generally are referred to the periumbilical region; hindgut inflammations (descending and sigmoid colons) are referred to the intraumbilical and suprapubic areas (Dieckmann, 1990).

In young children, localization of pain is usually inaccurate, because the child invariably points to the umbilical region irrespective of the site of the disease. Vague periumbilical pain is usually of little clinical significance in an older child, except in early appendicitis. Pain localized to one of the abdominal quadrants, however, suggests local organic disease.

TABLE 27–3. CAUSES OF ACUTE ABDOMINAL PAIN IN ADOLESCENTS

Trauma	Renal calculi
Acute appendicitis	Pelvic inflammatory disease
Ectopic pregnancy	Tubo-ovarian abscess
Toxic shock syndrome	Dysmenorrhea
Spermatic cord torsion	Mittelschmerz
Drug overdose	Ruptured ovarian cyst
Diabetic ketoacidosis	Ovarian cyst torsion
Gastroenteritis	Adenexal torsion
Mesenteric adenitis	Incomplete abortion
Inflammatory bowel disease	Displaced intrauterine device
Peptic ulcer disease	Epididymitis
Acalculous cholecystitis	Discitis
Cholelithiasis	Spondylitis
Choledochal cyst	Collagen vascular disease
Pancreatitis	Sickling syndromes
Hepatitis	Fitz-Hugh-Curtis syndrome
Constipation	Hyperlipemia
Urinary tract infection	Hypoglycemia

(*From Schwartz GR* [ed] [1992]. Principles and practice of emergency medicine [vol 1]. *Philadelphia: Lea & Febiger, p 380*)

Local abdominal tenderness confirms the existence of peritoneal irritation. With an anxious child with a low pain threshold, reaction to direct palpation can give little information. With adults and older children, rebound tenderness identifies the site of maximal irritation with much greater accuracy. With young children, however, rebound tenderness is a sign with limited clinical value.

Muscle spasm, also called guarding, is involuntary whenever the inflammatory process is intense, is located beneath the area palpated, and is maintained as a continuous muscular contraction. If the guarding is voluntary, a warm hand in contact with the abdominal wall for several minutes allows the examiner to distinguish between these two forms of muscle spasm.

Alimentary Tract Obstructions

The pain described with alimentary tract obstructions is characteristically intermittent, because it is associated with the major peristaltic wave. Young children frequently cannot communicate this pain verbally, but watching for intermittent facial grimacing or abdominal guarding may provide the information sought. Older children, upon specific questioning, may describe the pain as dull and cramping, rising slowly in a crescendo pattern and reaching a maximum that lasts about 30 seconds. Because, in older children, the major peristaltic wave in the small intestine occurs every 2–3 minutes, and in the colon every 15–20 minutes, this feature can be used to localize the site of the obstruction. Episodic pain is associated with intestinal peristalsis.

Because bowel sounds occur with peristalsis, cramping abdominal pain coexisting with high pitched, rushing, continuous bowel sounds, which are sounds characteristic of intestinal obstruction, is the foundation on which the diagnosis of mechanical obstruction can be made. There is a temporal relationship between the abdominal pain and the peristaltic wave.

Uncomplicated alimentary tract obstruction rarely results in anything other than mild tenderness to palpation. More severe tenderness usually indicates peritonitis. This is an important sign in a child with an obstruction; it means that a perforation has occurred or that gangrenous intestine is present. Intestinal necrosis necessitates prompt surgical intervention.

Other findings that may be helpful in diagnosis of alimentary tract obstruction include abdominal distention and a history of irregular bowel function. Abdominal distention is frequently a characteristic of obstruction, but it may also result from swallowing air with prolonged crying. The absence of distention, however, does not obviate the presence of an obstruction, since a high obstruction is not associated with abdominal distention. In lesions proximal to the upper jejunum, protracted and projectile vomiting can alleviate distention. As the obstruction progresses distally, vomiting becomes less prominent and more characteristic (such as the feculent vomitus of ileal contents), whereas abdominal distention becomes more prominent.

Irregular bowel function can be a feature of alimentary tract obstruction. If there is complete obstruction, passage of feces cannot occur. Intestinal content distal to the obstruction, however, can be evacuated. Likewise, the presence or absence of feces in the rectum on digital examination does not indicate the presence of an obstruction. Obstruction and continued fecal passage can coexist only in high-grade incomplete or partial intestinal obstruction.

Diagnosis

A combination of a complete history and a careful examination is essential in the diagnosis of inflammatory conditions and alimentary tract obstructions. The examination should include inspection of the fully exposed abdomen, palpation, auscultation, and a rectal or pelvic examination. The most important part, however, is a complete and detailed history. With information from the history and the physical examination, decisions regarding laboratory and radiographic studies can be made.

INFLAMMATORY CONDITIONS

Appendicitis

Appendicitis is the inflammation of the vermiform appendix, a blind sac at the end of the cecum. It is the most common reason for abdominal operations during childhood, the incidence increasing after the first year of life. Although rare in children younger than 2 years, appendicitis is associated with increased complications and mortality in this age group, mostly because the appendix perforates before appendicitis is diagnosed. Appendicitis in early childhood is characterized by a low incidence (1%), an overwhelming male predominance (8:1), a short history, and rapid progress. In the adolescent population the male-to-female ratio is closer to 1:1, and the progress of the disease is somewhat less rapid (Siegal et al, 1982).

Appendicitis is usually an acute conditon that, when undiagnosed, progresses to perforation and peritonitis. The estimated total incidence of appendicitis in the United States is 200,000 cases per year with 2000 deaths (Franken, 1982).

Etiology and Pathophysiology. Although the exact cause of appendicitis is poorly understood, obstruction seems to be a primary factor in the pathogenesis.

The obstruction may be secondary to inflammatory changes from blood-borne or enteric infections or may be mechanical from parasitic infestation, a fecalith, a foreign body, or stenosis. Decreased fiber and residue content in the diet may play a role as a factor in obstruction.

The progression of appendicitis in children has been described by Lillehei and Snyder (1989). Acute obstruction is followed by inflammation, since the local defense mechanisms are impaired sufficiently to allow invasion by the bacterial organisms in their lumen. The initial inflammation and then infection may then progress to perforation and peritonitis. Young children have a thinner appendiceal wall, hence progression is much more rapid. In addition, young children have an omentum that is not fully developed and is less efficient in walling off the inflammation, sealing perforated viscera, and confining an intraperitoneal disease. The proximity of abdominal and pelvic organs further favors the spread of peritonitis to other structures.

Assessment. Progression from simple to complicated appendicitis and peritonitis is more rapid in a child than in an adult. Upon arrival at the ED, therefore, a young child is frequently very ill.

It is important to remember, however, that the clinical course of appendicitis varies enormously, and the duration of symptoms has a wide range that is partly independent of the pathologic findings. Appendicitis must be excluded in every patient of any age with acute abdominal pain (Dieckmann, 1990).

One of the most difficult diagnoses in children is acute appendicitis. So many conditions mimic appendicitis and vice versa that frequently many diagnostic tests and a detailed history and physical examination are needed. Other diagnostic possibilities when appendicitis is being considered include Crohn disease, mesenteric adenitis, Meckel diverticulitis, acute rheumatic fever, diabetes mellitus, regional enteritis, abdominal epilepsy, ovarian lesions, intussusception, acute gastroenteritis, constipation, sickle cell crises, and infectious mononucleosis. In addition, there can be infection of the urinary tract, which may be ruled out with a urinalysis and an intravenous pyelogram, and pneumonia, in which case a chest x ray clarifies the diagnosis.

History. A history of persistent abdominal pain, insidious or abrupt in onset accompanied by persistent localized tenderness in the right lower quadrant, involuntary muscle spasm, and rigidity, is evidence of localized intraperitoneal irritation. Nausea and vomiting are frequently present, and a low-grade fever is more common than a high fever and chills at the onset of the disease.

Physical Assessment. It is important to distinguish between voluntary and involuntary muscle spasms, or guarding of the abdomen, in children. A young child frequently tenses the abdominal muscles with the touch of a cold hand or the sight of a unfamiliar person. So a gentle, unhurried approach that helps to reassure the child and allows him or her to relax, provides more reliable information. Narcotic analgesics should not be given, since they may mask the signs of intraperitoneal inflammation.

Classically, the most common signs and symptoms of appendicitis are abdominal pain, which begins as generalized and then shifts to the right lower quadrant; localized abdominal tenderness; and fever. The most intense site of pain may be McBurney point, which is approximately 3.75 cm above the anterior superior iliac crest along a straight line drawn from the umbilicus. Other important signs include rebound tenderness, hypoactive or absent bowel sounds, anorexia, nausea, and vomiting. Signs of peritonitis include sudden relief from pain after perforation. Then there is a subsequent increase in pain, which is diffuse and is accompanied by guarding of the abdomen, progressive abdominal distention, rapid shallow breathing (because abdominal muscles are not used), pallor, irritability, restlessness, and tachycardia. The temperature, after development of peritonitis, is usually elevated to 39.5°C or more (103°F–105°F). Active peristalsis can persist for some time with generalized peritonitis. The only sign of an inflamed retrocecal appendix, however, may be deep tenderness, and when the appendix is in the pelvic area, there may be no abdominal findings.

A rectal examination is the final step in the physical examination and further aids assessment. Peristalsis is generally decreased or absent in the presence of intraperitoneal infection, although in the early stages there may be hyperactivity. A positive psoas sign (a drawing up of the legs) is also suggestive of a right lower-quadrant inflammatory lesion.

Laboratory and Diagnostic Tests. The most important laboratory evaluation is a WBC count. The WBC count is usually elevated but is seldom higher than 15,000 to 20,000/mm^3 with a preponderance of immature polymorphonuclear cells (Lindzon and Mitchiner, 1989). Excessively high total leukocyte counts are suggestive of an abscess or peritonitis. In acute appendicitis, neutrophilia supports the diagnosis, and leukocytosis indicates the prognosis. In other words, the chance of infection appears to increase as the total leukocyte count rises above the upper normal limit, and a decreased neutrophil percentage suggests appendicitis. In some studies, however, patients with appendicitis had a normal WBC count (Eriksson et al, 1989).

The WBC should be only a small part of the overall assessment. Priority should be given to the physical findings, and the WBC and neutrophil precentage should be used to support or question these findings (Otu, 1989). A new technetium-99m-albumin colloid white blood cell scan has been useful when diagnosis is uncertain (Henneman et al, 1990).

Other laboratory studies are helpful in differentiating appendicitis from other conditions. In addition, studies such as a urinalysis help to provide an overall assessment of fluid loss. Erythrocyte sedimentation rate (ESR), electrolyte, glucose, blood urea nitrogen (BUN), amylase, serum glutamic-oxaloacetic transaminase (SGOT), and bilirubin levels should be ordered.

X rays may aid in the diagnosis of appendicitis. Abdominal x rays may show an appendiceal fecalith, which, although rare, clearly indicates the diagnosis of appendicitis. In many cases of appendicitis, however, abdominal x rays are normal (Franken, 1982). A barium enema study may increase the accuracy of diagnosis in difficult cases. The barium enema study may demonstrate nonfilling or partial filling of the appendix when there is appendicitis. The use of a barium enema study as an adjunct may be helpful if the findings are abnormal, but normal findings should not be relied upon to delay surgical treatment of a child with positive peritoneal signs in the right lower quadrant (Lillehei and Snyder, 1989).

TRIAGE
Appendicitis

Emergent
An infant or child with diffuse abdominal pain accompanied by guarding, a rigid, distended abdomen, tachypnea, shallow or grunting respirations, tachycardia, pallor, irritability, high fever, and decreased urine output.

Urgent
An infant or child with right lower quadrant abdominal pain; tense or tender abdomen; low-grade fever; hypoactive or absent bowel sounds; anorexia; nausea and vomiting.

Non-urgent
A older child with a history of mild diffuse abdominal pain; nausea; vomiting; low-grade fever.

Nursing Diagnosis
Pain

Defining Characteristics

- Complaints of abdominal pain
- Restlessness, irritability
- Insomnia
- Guarding behavior
- Crying, moaning
- Autonomic responses not seen in chronic stable pain (ie, diaphoresis, changes in blood pressure and pulse, pupillary dilatation, increased or decreased respiratory rate)

Nursing Interventions

- Identify and consistently use a pain assessment scale appropriate for the child's developmental age
- Encourage parental presence to facilitate pain assessment, provide support, and promote trust
- Promote security with honest explanations, opportunities for choice, and preparation for any painful procedures
- Make child as comfortable as possible
- Respond immediately to complaints of pain
- Administer analgesics as ordered
- Explain to the child how distraction techniques can help relieve pain, and teach a simple method of distraction (eg, counting, naming items in a picture, rhythmic breathing)
- Monitor the effectiveness of pain measures, changes in type, level, and location of pain

Expected Outcomes

- Pain assessment scale reliably measures the degree of the child's pain
- Child derives comfort from parents' presence
- Child communicates relief of pain
- Objective symptoms of pain decrease or are absent
- Child uses selected distraction techniques to manage the pain

Nursing Diagnosis
Anxiety

Defining Characteristics

- Autonomic symptoms (diaphoresis, increased blood pressure and pulse, pupillary dilation, increased respiratory rate)
- Restlessness
- Faintness, dizziness
- Nausea or vomiting
- Apprehension
- Crying
- Hyperattentiveness
- Withdrawal

Nursing Interventions

- Remove excess stimulation
- Encourage parental presence to provide emotional support
- Provide reassurance and comfort
- Speak slowly and calmly, using words suited to the child's age and developmental level
- Prepare the child for all procedures
- Encourage and allow time for ventilation of anxieties and fears
- Acknowledge the normalcy of anxiety and other feelings

Expected Outcomes

- Child communicates an increase in psychological comfort
- Objective symptoms of anxiety decrease or are absent
- Child uses effective coping mechanisms and parental support to manage anxiety
- Child expresses understanding of present illness

Nursing Diagnosis
High Risk for Fluid Volume Deficit

Defining Characteristics

- Decreased urine output
- Increased specific gravity
- Tachycardia
- Dry skin and mucous membranes
- Poor skin turgor
- Hemoconcentration

Nursing Interventions

- Monitor vital signs
- Assess for signs of dehydration
- Administer intravenous fluids as ordered
- Measure gastric output and check for the presence of blood

Expected Outcomes

- Urine output remains greater than 1 ml/kg/hour
- Urine specific gravity is maintained within normal range
- Symptoms of dehydration are improved or absent
- Adequate intake of fluids and electrolytes is maintained
- Vital signs are normal

Nursing Diagnosis
High Risk for Infection

Defining Characteristics

- Continuous or intermittent fever
- Elevated WBC count
- Increased abdominal pain
- Increased heart rate

Nursing Interventions

- Reduce the entry of organisms into the child by using meticulous handwashing and aseptic technique when indicated
- Assess for signs of localized or systemic infection
- Monitor presence, nature, and progression of abdominal pain
- Administer antibiotics as ordered

Expected Outcomes

- Vital signs are normal
- Abdominal pain decreases or is absent
- Child's risk of infection is reduced

Nursing Diagnosis
Knowledge Deficit (Lack of Understanding of Diagnosis or Acuity of Illness)

Defining Characteristics

- Requests for information regarding diagnosis or acuity of child's illness
- Inaccurate perception of child's health status
- Psychological alteration (eg, anxiety, anger) resulting from misinformation or lack of information

Nursing Interventions

- Assess child's and parent's understanding of the diagnosis, management, and outcome of the illness
- Encourage child and parent to ask questions
- Explain need for surgical intervention if medical intervention is ineffective
- Explain all procedures and treatments to child and parents as appropriate

Expected Outcomes

- Child and parent understand current illness, its management, and probable outcome
- Child and parent are prepared for operation if needed
- Child and parent understand all procedures and treatments
- Child and parent freely ask questions of health care personnel when lacking information

Management. Any question of the possibility of appendicitis should warrant as immediate a hospital ad-

TABLE 27–4. PRIORITIES IN NURSING MANAGEMENT OF APPENDICITIS IN A CHILD

Problem	Nursing Management
Hypovolemia	Begin intravenous infusion of Ringer lactate
	Monitor vital signs
	Monitor urine output
	Assess for signs of hypovolemia
	Insert nasogastric tube and measure gastric output
High risk infection	Wash hands and use aseptic technique
	Administer antibiotics as ordered
Pain	Use nonpharmacologic techniques to control pain
	Administer analgesics as ordered
	Monitor level of pain using a pain assessment scale
	Monitor the effectiveness of interventions to reduce pain
Anxiety	Explain all procedures to child and parents
	Provide reassurance
	Encourage parental presence
Preparation for appendectomy	Allow patient nothing by mouth
	Establish intravenous access
	Provide age-appropriate explanations

mission as if the diagnosis were certain. When appendicitis is suspected, the child must be given nothing by mouth. An intravenous infusion of Ringer lactate solution is frequently ordered in preparation for the operation. The urine concentration (specific gravity) and output per hour are generally used as guides for adequacy of fluid therapy. A nasogastric tube on low suction is also frequently ordered. Vital signs need to be monitored frequently. If the diagnosis of appendicitis is definitive, preoperative antibiotics such as cephalosporin or ampicillin are ordered. If perforation is believed to have occurred, an aminoglycoside antibiotic such as gentamicin or tobramycin is usually ordered. All efforts are directed toward the delivery of definitive therapy, which in appendicitis is a surgical procedure. An appendectomy is the only appropriate treatment of acute appendicitis. If there has been appendiceal perforation, antibiotics, transperitoneal drainage, and delayed wound closure may be used. There still remains controversy concerning skin closure and the duration of antibiotic therapy (Neilson, 1990). Table 27–4 presents priorities in the nursing management of appendicitis in a child.

Patient and Family Teaching and Psychosocial Support. During the preparation time an explanation geared to the age level of the child should be provided (Edwinson et al, 1988). This should be done in a calm, reassuring way. If the parents are available, they should also be kept informed and should be encouraged to help communicate to the child what can be expected.

Acute Gastroenteritis

Acute gastroenteritis is an illness in which vomiting or diarrhea predominates. (Mild vomiting and loose stools of slightly increased frequency can accompany most acute illnesses in childhood.) Vomiting involves the loss of gastric contents with loss of bile and pancreatic secretions by reverse peristalsis. Diarrhea involves increased peristalsis and decreased transit time with incomplete absorption and reabsorption of bile, pancreatic secretions, water, and electrolytes.

Etiology and Pathophysiology. Gastroenteritis can be attributed to a number of specific causes and predisposing factors. Some specific causes of gastroenteritis include an inflammatory process of bacterial or viral origin. The bacterial or viral organisms that cause gastroenteritis in children are varied. These include the *Shigella, Yersinia, Campylobacter,* and *Salmonella* groups of bacteria, as well as *Staphylococcus aureus* and *Escherichia coli,* which are normal flora but which cause problems under certain circumstances; pseudomonas, klebsiella, and proteus organisms are occasionally responsible (Bishop and Ulshen, 1988). The main virus responsible for most infectious gastroenteritis in children is the rotavirus (Bardhan et al, 1992).

The age of the child provides further clues as to the etiology. In the first year of life in bottle-fed infants, and later in breast-fed infants, *E. coli* is the usual disease agent. *Shigella* is the most common from the ages of 2 to 4 years, but the most severe form is apt to occur in the children older than 5 years. *Salmonella* and the viral causes are most prevalent in children younger than 2 years, although they can appear at any age.

If there are multiple cases of gastroenteritis in a household, the cause is frequently *Shigella.* A single case in a young child is more likely to be *E. coli,* a milk allergy, a new food, overfeeding, or starvation.

Intestinal parasites can be responsible for gastroenteritis. A toxic reaction to bacterial exotoxins, the ingestion of poisons or certain antibiotics, or dietary indiscretions are also causes. Allergies and intolerance to specific foods and episodes of nervous excitement or periods of emotional tension can be responsible.

Four main factors predispose a child to gastroenteritis. The first two factors are age and state of health. The younger the child and the more impaired his or her health, the more susceptible and more severe is the gastroenteritis. Climate is the third factor. Many of the causative organisms are more prevalent in warmer climates. The fourth factor is environment. Crowding, substandard sanitation, and poor facilities for preparation and refrigeration of food all tend to increase the likelihood of gastroenteritis. It has also been found that breast-fed infants are less susceptible and are better protected against reduced intake during gastroenteritis (Crain et al, 1992).

Assessment. The most serious and immediate physiologic disturbances of gastroenteritis are dehydration, acid-base derangements with acidosis, and shock, which occur when dehydration progresses to the point that circulatory status is seriously disturbed. When the diagnosis is not definite and the illness is severe, other factors need to be considered. Other entities in which gastroenteritis is one facet of the illness include Crohn disease, ulcerative colitis, immunodeficiencies, carbohydrate and fat malabsorption, intractable diarrhea of infancy, and Hirschsprung disease.

History. Since there are many causes of gastroenteritis, a history is important in diagnosing the cause. Occasionally the history may indicate the source and nature of the infection or the possibility of food poisoning, but in most instances the cause can be determined by bacteriologic and virologic studies of the stool, which are definitive.

The history should include questions on the onset, number, duration, type, and color of the diarrhea or stools, and the vomitus; the amount of fluid intake and the type of fluids that are taken; the diet and any recent medications or new foods that have been introduced; and recent infections. Information regarding weight loss, possible contact with contaminated foods, food allergies, and an estimation of recent urine output is helpful. In cases of overfeeding or starvation, the dietary history may provide the needed information. There have been instances of child abuse with the use of laxatives or poisons that have caused gastroenteritis; these possibilities may need to be considered.

Physical Assessment. The assessment is based on the history, particular attention being paid to the relative intake and output. The state of consciousness and general appearance of the child should be assessed. Urine output should be measured and specific gravity determined. The weight of the child should be compared with the weight before the illness. Vital signs should be taken and recorded. When counting respirations, it should be determined if there is a ketone smell on the breath. A fever or signs of shock necessitate immediate attention, as do severe dehydration and metabolic acidosis.

Assessment of mild, moderate, or severe dehydration should be based on the clinical presentation (Table 27–5). The metabolic acidosis that occurs from the increased bicarbonate losses from diarrhea is compensated for by the respiratory system through rapid deep breathing, which is referred to as Kussmaul or air hunger respirations. Signs of shock resulting from severe depletion of extracellular fluid volume include tachycardia, decreased blood pressure, cool, mottled skin, and dry mucous membranes.

TABLE 27–5. CLINICAL AND ANCILLARY FINDINGS BY DEGREE OF DEHYDRATION

Finding	Mild (<5%)	Moderate (10%)	Severe (15%)
Signs and symptoms			
Dry mucous membrane	±	+	+
Reduced skin turgor	−	±	+
Depressed anterior fontanelle	−	+	+
Sunken eyeballs	−	+	+
Hyperpnea	−	±	+
Hypotension (orthostatic)	−	±	+
Increased pulse	−	+	+
Ancillary data			
Urine			
Volume	Small[b]	Oliguria	Oliguria/anuria
Specific gravity[a]	≤1.020[b]	>1.030	>1.035
Blood			
BUN	WNL[b]	Elevated	Very high
pH (arterial)	7.40–7.30[b]	7.30–7.00	<7.10

+, present; −, absent; ±, variable; BUN, blood urea nitrogen; WNL, within normal limits.
[a]Specific gravity can provide evidence that confirms the physical assessment.
[b]Not usually indicated in mild dehydration.
(*From Barkin RM [ed] [1992]. Pediatric emergency medicine: Concepts and clinical practice. St. Louis: Mosby Year Book, p 135*)

Laboratory and Diagnostic Tests. In addition to a complete blood count (CBC) and a urinalysis, electrolyte, BUN, and venous blood gas levels should be measured, and an examination of the stool should be done. Many band forms in the differential WBC count are indicative of shigellosis. A dehydrated infant has an increased hematocrit as a result of fluid loss. The specific gravity of the urine, in general, gives a good indication of hydration, whereas the presence of ketones reflects increased ketoacid production as a result of increased fat metabolism due to caloric deprivation. Venous gases, which are obtained without a tourniquet to prevent lactate build-up, reflect the degree of bicarbonate loss, while the pCO_2 indicates the degree of compensation. In the measurement of electrolytes, the sodium level indicates if the dehydration is hypotonic, isotonic, or hypertonic. The serum potassium level does not necessarily reflect the total body potassium, because the cellular concentration is not measured. If there is question regarding potassium depletion, an electrocardiogram (ECG) can be done, which will show flattened T waves.

An elevated BUN level is found in reduced renal circulation, but is falsely low if the child has not ingested protein in the preceding 24 hours.

Examination of the stool is indicated in gastroenteritis. A stool examination with indicator paper for pH, a guiac test for occult blood, and a Clinitest tablet to detect stool containing carbohydrates rules out disaccharide intolerance. Bulky, fatty stools suggest malabsorption. Examination of the stool for leukocytes is important because no leukocytes are found in normal stools or if the disease-producing agent is a virus. Rectal swabs for culture are indicated if a bacterial agent is suspected.

TRIAGE
Acute Gastroenteritis

Emergent

An infant or child with bloody diarrhea; severe abdominal pain; severe dehydration; dry mucous membranes; tachycardia; decreased blood pressure; tachypnea; high fever (or hypothermia in young infants); oliguria or anuria and poor perfusion.

Urgent

An infant or child with diarrhea; vomiting; crampy abdominal pain; decreased oral intake; mild to moderate dehydration.

Non-urgent

An infant or child with a history of diarrhea, vomiting and crampy abdominal pain but no symptoms of dehydration.

Nursing Diagnosis
Diarrhea

Defining Characteristics

- Increased frequency of loose or liquid stools
- Cramping, abdominal pain
- Urgency
- Increased frequency of bowel sounds

Nursing Interventions

- Discontinue solid food intake initially to allow the intestine to rest
- Provide oral fluid and electrolyte replacements as ordered
- Provide intravenous replacement as ordered if oral intake is inadequate or contraindicated
- Practice meticulous handwashing when in contact with stool
- Monitor stools for amount, frequency, consistency, and color

Expected Outcomes

- Reduction in the frequency of stools occurs
- Vital signs are normal
- Intake exceeds output
- A normal urine specific gravity is maintained

Nursing Diagnosis
High Risk for Fluid Volume Deficit

Defining Characteristics

- Decreased urine output
- Increased specific gravity
- Tachycardia
- Dry skin and mucous membranes
- Poor skin turgor
- Hemoconcentration

Nursing Interventions

- Monitor vital signs
- Assess for signs of dehydration
- Administer intravenous fluids as ordered
- Measure gastric output and check for the presence of blood
- Monitor urine output

Expected Outcomes

- Urine output remains greater than 1 ml/kg/hour
- Urine specific gravity is maintained within normal range
- Symptoms of dehydration are improved or absent
- Adequate intake of fluids and electrolytes is maintained
- Vital signs are normal

Nursing Diagnosis
Pain

Defining Characteristics

- Complaints of abdominal pain
- Restlessness, irritability
- Insomnia
- Guarding behavior
- Crying, moaning
- Autonomic responses not seen in chronic stable pain (eg, diaphoresis, changes in blood pressure and pulse, pupillary dilation, increased or decreased respiratory rate)

Nursing Interventions

- Identify and consistently use a pain assessment scale appropriate for the child's developmental age

- Encourage parental presence to facilitate pain assessment, provide support, and promote trust
- Make child as comfortable as possible
- Respond immediately to complaints of pain
- Maintain position of comfort within the limits of ongoing treatment
- Encourage and teach alternative pain management methods (eg, distraction, counting, naming items in a picture, rhythmic breathing)
- Monitor the effectiveness of pain measures and changes in type, level, and location of pain

Expected Outcomes

- Pain assessment scale reliably measures the degree of the child's pain
- Child derives comfort from parents' presence
- Child communicates a tolerable level of pain
- Objective symptoms of pain decrease or are absent
- Child uses selected distraction techniques to manage the pain

Management. In most cases of gastroenteritis, antiemetics and antidiarrheal medications are not recommended (Crain et al, 1992). Antiemetics are rarely effective and tend to alter the level of consciousness. Antidiarrheal agents are also rarely effective and may be harmful; Kaopectate (attapulgite) may facilitate bacterial penetration, and the opiates and Lomotil (diphenoxylate) may encourage the proliferation of pathogens.

Antibiotic treatment is important in certain causes of bacterial gastroenteritis for clinical improvement and for eradication of the causative organism from the stools. The cause is seldom known, so the decision to initiate antibiotic therapy and the choice of the specific antimicrobial agents are made on a clinical basis before culture results are available (Ashkenazi and Cleary, 1991). Antibiotic treatment, however, is rarely indicated (Ghisolfi, 1992).

Mild Dehydration

Mild or moderate gastroenteritis, consisting of vomiting alone or vomiting with diarrhea, can usually be managed by oral rehydration therapy (ORT). In infants, Rehydralate (Ross Laboratories, Columbus, Ohio) is used for initial oral rehydration under close monitoring and supervision. Pedialyte (Ross Laboratories) and Ricelyte (Mead Johnson, Evanston, Illinois) can be used for maintenance. For children, clear liquids can be given starting with small amounts (1 tablespoon every 15 minutes) to minimize gastric distention. The amounts can be gradually increased, the frequency depending on the age of the child. If there is

diarrhea with no vomiting, clear liquids in large amounts every 3–4 hours should be given, since the lower frequency of feeding reduces activation of the gastrocolic reflex.

Several studies have advocated abrupt refeeding, rather than gradual refeeding, after a period of rehydration (Conway and Ireson, 1989; Fox et al, 1990). Isolauri et al (1989) found that oral rehydration and rapid feeding accelerated weight gain, shortened the duration of diarrhea, and reduced the requirement for intravenous fluid therapy. Oral rehydration and realimentation should be used more extensively in general practice.

If clear liquids are tolerated, soft foods such as gelatin desserts, soups (not creamed), bananas, applesauce, strained carrots, and toast can be given. For young children a hydrolyzed lactose-free formula may be used instead of milk.

In mild dehydration, if the parent seems to understand the instructions given regarding diet and risk for complications and appears to be cooperative, the child may be discharged home. If there is some question as to the care the child will receive or a question about the severity of the condition, especially with an infant, hospitalization is indicated. In moderately severe to severe dehydration, hospitalization is generally indicated. Table 27–6 presents the priorities in nursing management of dehydration in children.

Moderate to Severe Dehydration

Children suffering from moderate to severe dehydration may be admitted to the hospital if they are unable to tolerate oral fluids. Moineau and Newman (1990) reported that rapid intravenous rehydration is an effective treatment for children with moderate dehydration secondary to gastroenteritis.

In moderately severe to severe cases, appropriate treatment of the physiologic disturbances is the primary concern. Parenteral fluid therapy, comprehensive evaluation, and hospitalization are warranted. Fluid therapy in the ED is directed at restoring circu-

TABLE 27–6. PRIORITIES IN NURSING MANAGEMENT OF GASTROENTERITIS IN A CHILD

Problem	Nursing Management
Mild dehydration	Administer oral rehydration therapy
	Monitor intake and output
	Assess for signs of hypovolemia
Moderate to severe dehydration	Give intravenous fluids by rapid bolus administration
	Monitor vital signs
	Monitor skin perfusion and capillary refill
	Monitor intake and output accurately
	Measure specific gravity

lating volume. This phase of therapy may last 1–2 hours (Moineau and Newman, 1990). Rehydrating fluids may include 0.9 normal saline solution, lactated Ringer solution or 5% dextrose in normal saline solution. Fluid boluses of 20 mL/kg usually run over 20 minutes and must be closely monitored. In hypertonic dehydration with shock, plasma substitutes, such as a 5% albumin solution, are sometimes used. Measures to control fever and the administration of oxygen may be necessary in some patients. The child should be isolated to prevent possible spread of the infectious process to others. Accurate intake and output measurement is important. A urine collector is placed on the child to determine the volume of output and to measure specific gravity. Table 27–6 lists the priorities in the nursing management of moderate-to-severe dehydration in a child.

Patient and Family Teaching and Psychosocial Support. Instructions are given to parents regarding diet and signs and symptoms that may indicate a worsening of the condition, which would necessitate another ED visit. Parents should be given examples of the kinds of foods or fluids appropriate for the prescribed diet, for example, clear liquids could be fluids such as Pedialyte or Lytren for infants and ginger ale, cola, powdered soft drinks, gelatin, water, sports drinks, and Popsicles for older children. The parent should be further instructed that if the child develops signs of complications, such as deep breathing, listlessness, reduced urinary output, weight loss, or blood in the stools, the parent should return to the ED with the child.

Hiatal Hernia

A hiatal hernia is a congenital herniation through a diaphragmatic defect that allows the cardia of the stomach to slide or roll above the diaphragm and back into the abdomen. The muscular ring of the hiatus is not snug and allows the cardia to slide from the thorax to the abdomen. This sliding or rolling through the esophageal hiatus frequently causes inflammation of the distal esophagus because of the reflux of gastric contents into the esophagus with subsequent regurgitation. To distinguish this condition from the hiatal hernia that occurs in adults some pediatric gastroenterologists use the term *partial thoracic stomach.*

Etiology and Pathophysiology. The diaphragm forms between the eighth and tenth weeks of fetal life from four separate embryonic structures that fuse to form the partition separating the thoracic and abdominal cavities. Apertures through which the esophagus and great vessels traverse the diaphragm are normally found. A much larger esophageal aperture results in a hiatal hernia.

Assessment. Because there are other conditions that produce the return of stomach contents into the esophagus, a hiatal hernia must be differentiated from other causes of GI reflux. In newborns GI reflux is considered normal. Reflux is thought to result from delayed maturation of the lower esophageal neuromuscular function or impaired local hormonal control mechanisms. Infants with gastroesophogeal reflux with or without a hiatal hernia have normal gastric emptying (Jackson et al, 1989). Other causes of persistent vomiting are feeding problems (especially underfeeding), pyloric stenosis, and urinary tract infections.

History. The history is an important part of the diagnostic evaluation. Particular attention should be paid to the child's eating habits and the occurrence of symptoms, especially vomiting because it is the most common. Vomiting is sometimes so severe that there is a loss of calories sufficient to cause weight loss and failure to thrive.

Physical Assessment. Persistent vomiting is the principal complaint. Only occasionally is the onset of vomiting delayed until after 1 year of age. Vomiting is usually copious and is typically projectile. It occurs most frequently during or soon after feeding in early infancy; in late infancy the vomiting occurs at night. Repeated irritation of the esophageal lining with gastric acid can lead to esophagitis and consequently to bleeding. Occasional brown staining of the vomit from blood is a characteristic feature. Loss of blood may cause anemia. When questioning the parents it is important to refer to discoloration rather than to the presence of blood, since the brown discoloration of vomitus is frequently not equated with the presence of blood. Reflux of the stomach contents also predisposes to aspiration and the development of respiratory symptoms, especially pneumonia.

Gastric peristalsis may be seen and a "pyloric tumor" may be felt, leading to an incorrect diagnosis of pyloric stenosis. The "tumor" in hiatal hernia, however, tends to be softer than pyloric stenosis.

Because of loss of nourishment, these infants are hungry and take feedings eagerly. Most patients are underweight and may be dehydrated. Constipation is common. Heartburn may go unrecognized in infants but is a symptom in older children.

Laboratory and Diagnostic Tests. Several tests are available to evaluate the presence of a hiatal hernia. The initial test is a barium esophagram, in which the reflux of barium from the stomach to the esophagus can be seen by fluoroscopy.

TRIAGE
Hiatal Hernia

Emergent

An infant or child with hematemesis; severe dehydration; pallor; tachycardia; tachypnea; respiratory distress.

Urgent

An infant or child with a history of persistent vomiting and poor weight gain with mild dehydration.

Non-urgent

A child with history of persistent vomiting but no symptoms of dehydration.

Nursing Diagnosis

High Risk for Fluid Volume Deficit

Defining Characteristics

- Decreased urine output
- Increased specific gravity
- Tachycardia
- Dry skin and mucous membranes
- Poor skin turgor
- Hemoconcentration

Nursing Interventions

- Monitor vital signs
- Assess for signs of dehydration
- Administer intravenous fluids as ordered
- Measure gastric output and check for the presence of blood

Expected Outcomes

- Urine output remains grater than 1 ml/kg/hour
- Urine specific gravity is maintained within normal range
- Symptoms of dehydration are improved or absent
- Adequate intake of fluids and electrolytes is maintained
- Vital signs are normal

Nursing Diagnosis

Fear

Defining Characteristics

- Apprehension
- Muscle tightness

- Increased heart rate, respirations, and blood pressure
- Nausea, vomiting, diarrhea
- Sweating
- Irritability
- Dilated pupils
- Crying

Nursing Interventions

- Encourage parents to remain with the child as much as possible
- Orient the child and parent to the environment as needed
- When possible, allow the child to make choices
- Provide all information to the child and parent in understandable terms as often as possible
- Prepare the child for all procedures. (Gulanick et al, 1992)

Expected Outcomes

- The child and parents remain calm
- The child is comforted by the parents' presence
- Objective symptoms of fear are decreased or absent
- The child and parents relate an increase in psychological comfort

Nursing Diagnosis

High Risk for Aspiration

Defining Characteristics

- Difficulty swallowing
- Dyspnea, tachypnea, apnea
- Ineffective or asymmetric chest expansion
- Coughing, gagging, choking (Gulanick et al, 1992)

Nursing Interventions

- Perform suction as needed to maintain a clear, patent airway
- Administer oxygen therapy as needed
- Elevate the head of the bed
- Monitor respiratory function and effort (Gulanick et al, 1992)

Expected Outcomes

- Aspiration does not occur
- Breath sounds are clear and equal
- Respirations are unlabored

Management. Nursing interventions vary greatly depending on the condition of the child and on whether the hernia can be managed conservatively or surgically.

Conservative management consists of positioning the patient and starting a modified feeding regimen. These infants are placed in an upright posture at an angle of approximately 40°–60° to reduce GI reflux. This position facilitates clearance of regurgitated gastric juice from the terminal esophagus. This posture should be maintained consistently, particularly at night when gastric contents are neither buffered nor diluted by feedings. Thickened small-volume feedings have been used; however, some authors question this approach. Bailey et al (1987) reported that thickened feedings decreased reflux in one-third of the infants studied, had no effect on reflux in another one-third, and made reflux worse in another one-third; there was no way to predict which infants would benefit from thickened feedings.

Although there is usually a considerable reduction in the frequency of vomiting within 2–4 weeks of the start of treatment, it may take longer. By 6 weeks a normal physiologic barrier to reflux usually develops.

Once symptoms have been controlled for 4–6 weeks, therapy can be reduced in intensity. The reduction might consist of the child's being removed from the upright posture for a short period of time before the next feeding.

Surgical intervention is selected for children with severe complications, such as respiratory distress, esophagitis, or esophageal stricture. A commonly used surgical procedure is the Nissen fundoplication, which produces a valve mechanism by wrapping the fundus of the stomach around the distal esophagus (Allen et al, 1991).

An overall assessment of the infant needs to be made because he or she may range from healthy to critically ill. An infant with mild dehydration and a history of persistent vomiting may only require home care management of positioning and feeding. An infant who is very ill may have major fluid loss, anemia, and aspiration pneumonia from severe persistent vomiting. The fluid, electrolyte, and acid-base imbalances require hospitalization for parenteral correction and possible surgical intervention.

Patient and Family Teaching and Psychosocial Support. If conservative management is indicated, families require instruction regarding both the disorder and procedures such as positioning and feeding regimens. The anatomy of the stomach and esophagus is described to reinforce the necessity of positioning these children in an upright posture at an angle of approximately 40°–60°. Emphasis should be placed on maintaining this posture at night as well as during the day. Feeding regimens, such as small, frequent feedings or thickened formula should be explained thoroughly, and parents should be given the opportunity to prepare the feedings as they would at home. Instruction should include educating the parents regarding signs and symptoms of aspiration and respiratory distress and the importance of seeking immediate help if these symptoms occur. Both the child and parents should be prepared for any procedures they will encounter, as well as for hospitalization. Parents should be reassured that in most cases normal development in time reduces or terminates the disorder.

ALIMENTARY TRACT OBSTRUCTIONS

Intussusception

Intussusception is the invagination or telescoping of a segment of intestine into itself (Figure 27–2). The ileocecal region is most commonly involved. Intussusception is one of the most frequent causes of intestinal obstruction during infancy; half of the cases occur in the first year and the other half in the second year of life. The condition is three times more common in boys than in girls. Controversy exists regarding diagnosis (due to atypical presentations) and to treatment (barium enema versus surgical intervention) (Bisset and Kirks, 1988).

Etiology and Pathophysiology. Although the reasons for intussusception are uncertain, several theories have been suggested (Snyder and Walker, 1992). The greater disparity between the size of the ileum and

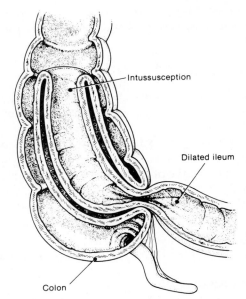

Figure 27–2. Telescoping bowel in the presence of intussusception. (From Scipien GM et al [eds]. *Comprehensive pediatric nursing* [3rd ed]. St Louis: Mosby, p 1071.)

that of the ileocecal valve in infants is believed to encourage telescoping at this point, where 95% of intussusceptions occur. In the other 5%, enlarged lymph nodes along the GI tract that occur with respiratory infections, cystic fibrosis, foreign bodies, GI polyps, or Meckel diverticulum appear to be the recognizable lead points (Lillehei and Snyder, 1989). Intussusception after an abdominal operation (Holcomb et al, 1991) and with Henoch-Schonlein purpura (Little and Danzl, 1991) has been reported.

Intussusception causes an interference with the vascular supply as well as an obstruction of the GI tract. Interference with lymphatic and venous drainage leads to edema, increased tissue pressure, and capillary and venule engorgement, which form a vicious circle. With increasing edema and eventual total venous obstruction, tissue pressure rises until arterial flow is stopped, which fosters necrosis. Goblet cells are stimulated to discharge mucus, which mixes with the blood to produce a currant jelly stool.

Assessment. Because other problems, such as polyps or Meckel diverticulum, may be a causative factor in intussusception, the child needs to be assessed as to the possible cause of the condition.

History. In general, intussusception occurs as an acute or subacute illness in previously healthy infants or children. A detailed history is an important aid in making the diagnosis. The typical history is of a well infant who screams and draws up his or her knees. Vomiting occurs soon after, and there are bouts of colicky pain at regular intervals. Gradually the child becomes apathetic, and when the diagnosis has been delayed, currant jelly stools are seen.

Physical Assessment. The assessment is based on the history. The classic signs and symptoms are intermittent abdominal pain, vomiting, blood and mucus in the stools, and a palpable tumor—a "sausage-shaped mass" in the upper epigastrium, although frequently one or several of these traits are missing. Accompanying features such as an upper respiratory infection, fever, and diarrhea may be misleading and may delay the diagnosis (Reijnen et al, 1990). Some children have no pain but are pale, listless, and apparently ill. If treatment has been postponed, the child appears acutely ill with fever, prostration, and signs of peritonitis.

An unhurried examination should be done during a pain-free interval. To identify the sausage-shaped characteristic mass, it is helpful to stand at the infant's head and attempt to roll the mass against the under surface of the liver. A rectal examination may allow for direct palpation of the intussusception itself and may reveal the characteristic bloody mucoid discharge.

Laboratory and Diagnostic Tests. Blood should be obtained for a baseline CBC and differential. A hemoglobin level, hematocrit, and type and crossmatch should be obtained. In a urinalysis attention should be paid to the specific gravity to assess hydration.

X rays of the abdomen show a scant amount of gas in the intestine and little or no intestinal content. Barium enema studies provide the definitive diagnosis of intussusception when the intussusception can be shown.

TRIAGE
Alimentary Tract Obstruction

Emergent
An infant or young child with marked abdominal distention and pain accompanied by guarding, a rigid abdomen, tachypnea, tachycardia, poor perfusion, and a high fever.

Urgent
An infant or young child with acute paroxysmal abdominal pain; mild dehydration; pallor; lethargy.

Non-urgent
An infant or young child with colicky abdominal pain or occasional vomiting with good hydration.

Nursing Diagnosis
Pain

Defining Characteristics
- Complaints of abdominal pain
- Restlessness, irritability
- Insomnia
- Guarding behavior
- Crying, moaning
- Autonomic responses not seen in chronic stable pain (eg, diaphoresis, changes in blood pressure and pulse, pupillary dilatation, increased or decreased respiratory rate)

Nursing Interventions
- Identify and consistently use a pain assessment scale or method appropriate for the child's developmental age
- Encourage parental presence to facilitate pain assessment, provide support, and promote trust
- Promote security with honest explanations, opportunities for choice and preparation for any painful procedures

- Make infant or child as comfortable as possible
- Respond immediately to complaints of pain
- Maintain position of comfort within limits of on-going treatment
- Administer analgesics as ordered
- Monitor the effectiveness of pain measures and changes in type, level and location of pain

Expected Outcomes

- Pain assessment scale or method reliably measures the degree of the infant or child's pain
- Infant or child derives comfort from parents' presence
- Objective symptoms of pain decrease or are absent
- Infant or child appears relaxed and comfortable

Nursing Diagnosis
High Risk for Fluid Volume Deficit

Defining Characteristics

- Decreased urine output
- Increased specific gravity
- Tachycardia
- Dry skin and mucous membranes
- Poor skin turgor
- Hemoconcentration

Nursing Interventions

- Monitor vital signs
- Assess for signs of dehydration
- Administer intravenous fluids and electrolytes as ordered
- Monitor the character and amount of stools
- Maintain child on nothing-by-mouth status
- Measure nasogastric output

Expected Outcomes

- Urine output remains greater than 1 ml/kg/hour
- Urine specific gravity is maintained within normal range
- Symptoms of dehydration are improved or absent
- Adequate intake of fluids and electrolytes is maintained
- Vital signs are normal

Nursing Diagnosis
Fear

Defining Characteristics

- Feelings of fright, apprehension
- Avoidance behaviors

- Increased heart rate, respirations, and blood pressure
- Attention deficits
- Hypervigilance and increased questioning
- Irritability
- Dilated pupils
- Crying

Nursing Interventions

- Acknowledge awareness of the child and parent's fear
- Stay with the child and parent if necessary
- Prepare the child and parent for all procedures
- Maintain a calm and tolerant manner while interacting with the child and parent
- Allow the child to make choices if possible
- Use simple language and brief statements geared to the child's developmental level when providing information or explanations
- Encourage the use of diversional activities (Gulanick et al, 1992)

Expected Outcomes

- The child and parent differentiate real from imagined situations
- Effective coping mechanisms are used
- Objective symptoms of fear are reduced or absent
- The child and parent express an increase in psychological comfort

Management. Initially a nasogastric tube should be inserted and connected to low suction, intravenous fluids should be started, and antibiotics should be given because edematous intestine is permeable to bacteria. The treatment of choice is nonsurgical hydrostatic reduction by barium enema (Barr et al, 1990; Hoffman et al, 1992; Skipper et al, 1990). The diagnostic enema is continued, and the intussusception is observed by fluoroscopy until the mass disappears in the ileum and several loops become filled with barium. This can take from a few minutes to half an hour and is successful 75% of the time. Failure of the barium enema to reduce the intussusception is an obvious indication for surgical treatment.

If the intussusception is reduced by barium enema, the child's condition is good, and the parents are reliable and can easily return to the hospital, the child may be sent home after a brief period of observation in the ED. If any of these factors is questioned or if the child needs surgical reduction, the child is admitted to the hospital.

Patient and Family Teaching and Psychosocial Support. Parents and young children need preparation before attempts to reduce the intussusception with a barium enema. The invasiveness of an enema can be particularly frightening for young children, and the presence of x ray machinery and unfamiliar personnel heighten their fears. Parents should be informed of the usual length of time required for barium enema reduction. In emergent situations, parents need considerable support. Parents also need to be informed of the need for surgical intervention should the barium enema fail to reduce the intussusception.

Pyloric Stenosis

Pyloric stenosis occurs when there is an obstruction of the pyloric sphincter by hypertrophy of the circular muscle of the pylorus. It is five times more common in boys than in girls with an incidence of 4–5 per 1000 live births.

Etiology and Pathophysiology. The most popular theory is one of hypertrophy of the circular smooth fibers of the pyloric sphincter secondary to spasm. Narrowing of the canal between the stomach and duodenum occurs until, over time, it progresses to a complete

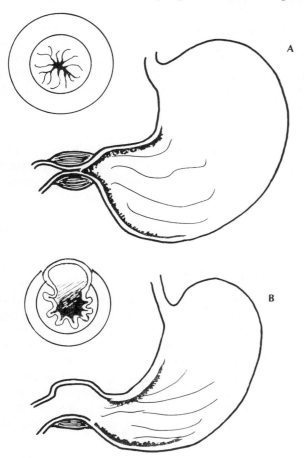

Figure 27–3. Hypertrophic pyloric stenosis. **A.** Enlarged muscular tumor nearly obliterates pyloric chanel. **B.** Longitudinal surgical division of muscle down to submucosa establishes adequate passageway. (From Whaley LF, Wong DL [eds]. *Nursing care of infants and children* [4th ed]. St Louis: Mosby, p 1513.)

obstruction. The muscle is thickened to as much as twice its normal size, and the stomach is dilated (Figure 27–3).

Assessment

History. A careful history should be obtained, since the diagnosis can be made with a high degree of accuracy for a patient who has a history of progressive, nonbilious vomiting that becomes projectile and may be blood-tinged (Bissonnette and Sullivan, 1991). A full-term infant typically manifests symptoms between the second and sixth weeks of life. The vomiting is at first intermittent then increases in frequency and severity until it follows every feeding and is projectile. The infant is hungry, and a second feeding after a vomiting episode produces vomitus of sour formula or clear gastric content. As less food and water make their way through the pylorus, the number of stools decreases and the urine becomes scanty. Weight loss is light or severe, depending on the duration and severity of symptoms.

Physical Assessment. A history of progressive vomiting, failure to gain weight, or weight loss indicates the need for an assessment for pyloric stenosis. The examination reveals a distended upper abdomen and gastric peristaltic waves that move from left to right across the epigastrium. An olive-shaped tumor, felt to the right of the umbilicus, is more readily palpable after the infant has vomited. The infant is active, irritable, and eager to feed. Dehydration, loss of skin turgor, fretfulness, and apathy may be present in severe cases of long duration.

Laboratory and Diagnostic Tests. In addition to the routine laboratory tests, electrolyte studies should be done, because the vomiting leads to metabolic alkalosis and sodium and potassium depletion. Accepted practice dictates diagnosis be made on clinical grounds. Ultrasonography and upper GI x ray series are reserved for patients with normal clinical examinations (Bowen, 1988; Forman et al, 1990). An upper GI series demonstrates elongation of the pylorus. Ultrasonography may show the thickened ring. Benign tumors may have symptoms similar to those of pyloric stenosis, but the age of onset and x ray findings are different.

T R I A G E
Pyloric Stenosis

Emergent ————————————————

An infant with vomiting; weight loss; abdominal distention; tachypnea; tachycardia; poor perfusion; unresponsiveness.

Urgent

An infant with vomiting; weight loss; symptoms of mild-to-moderate dehydration.

Non-urgent

An infant with vomiting; weight loss; good hydration.

Nursing Diagnosis
High Risk for Fluid Volume Deficit

Defining Characteristics

- Decreased urine output
- Increased specific gravity
- Tachycardia
- Dry skin and mucous membranes
- Poor skin turgor
- Hemoconcentration

Nursing Interventions

- Monitor vital signs
- Assess for signs of dehydration
- Administer intravenous fluids as ordered
- Measure gastric output
- Replace ongoing losses from the GI tract

Expected Outcomes

- Urine output remains greater than 1 mL/kg/hour
- Urine specific gravity is maintained within normal range
- Symptoms of dehydration are improved or absent
- Adequate intake of fluids and electrolytes is maintained
- Vital signs are normal

Management. Surgical relief of pyloric obstruction by pylorotomy is simple, safe, and effective. Before the operation can be done, however, the metabolic alkalosis needs to be corrected. An intravenous infusion is started with 5% dextrose in 0.45 normal saline solution with potassium added. Intake and output must be monitored closely.

In most cases of pyloric stenosis the child is admitted from the ED. Postponement of treatment worsens the condition because the child continues to vomit.

Patient and Family Teaching and Psychosocial Support. An explanation of the diagnosis and treatment needs to be given to the parents. The parents should be informed regarding treatments being undertaken to restore normal fluid and electrolyte balances. The parents should be prepared regarding the surgical corrective procedure, its relatively few risks, and its overall effectiveness. In addition, parents should be oriented to the hospital environment and routines they will encounter. The nurse providing instruction should encourage and allow time for the child and family to verbalize their fears, concerns, and questions.

Foreign Body
A foreign body in the alimentary tract is the result of a child's ingesting an article that cannot be digested. Foreign bodies include objects such as coins, marbles, buttons, thumbtacks, and bones. Rubber balloons are often swallowed and are the leading cause of choking deaths from children's products (Ryan et al, 1990). Most children with foreign bodies in the GI tract are 6 months–4 years of age. In older children the ingestion is usually accidental or is associated with psychiatric abnormalities.

Etiology and Pathophysiology. When a foreign object is swallowed, the common places for it to become lodged are the esophagus and the stomach. In general, any object that can be swallowed and that reaches the stomach passes through the intestine without difficulty 90% of the time.

A foreign body that remains in the esophagus needs immediate attention, since it may cause perforation. Foreign bodies are most frequently found in the cricopharyngeal area, which corresponds to the fourth cervical vertebrae. Children who have had operations for tracheoesophageal fistula are most prone to impaction with partially chewed meat because of narrowing of the lumen and dysmobility of the anastomosed esophagus.

Assessment

History. Ingestion of a foreign body may have been witnessed, or the child may have had a sudden onset of gagging, attempts at vomiting, hypersalivation, restrosternal pain, or respiratory distress. A history is needed to help determine what type of object the child may have swallowed. An approximate estimate of when the ingestion occurred is also important, since in the case of foreign bodies trapped in the esophagus, perforation and mediastinitis can occur soon after ingestion.

Assessment. The child's symptoms and the history are most important to the assessment. A child with an esophageal foreign body generally appears in distress with gagging, attempts at vomiting, hypersalivation, and respiratory distress. A child with a foreign body lower in the alimentary tract may complain of pain, but if the object has been lodged for a period of time, complications of hemorrhage and peritonitis may occur.

Laboratory and Diagnostic Tests. The routine laboratory tests are not remarkable unless bleeding and mediastinitis or peritonitis are present, which would be reflected in the hematocrit and the differential.

X rays of the area are done. Various diagnostic tools such as fluoroscopy and a chest x ray may be needed to accurately evaluate and treat these children (Laks and Barzilay, 1988). When there is ingestion of glass or wood, xeroradiography or ultrasonography may be used. Computed tomography (CT) is used when there is a deep foreign body or when a foreign body is suspected but cannot be seen (Flom and Ellis, 1992). If the object is opaque, as, fortunately, coins and many swallowed objects are, it can be readily visualized (Figure 27–4). If an object is nonopaque, an esophagram shows its size and location. Visualization of the foreign body by radiography provides a definite diagnosis. The child must be watched closely for complications.

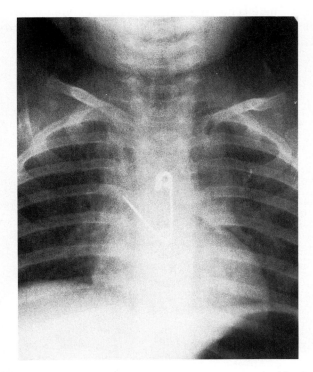

Figure 27–4. Safety pin in the esophagus of a 10-month-old infant. Note the presence of a perforation of the esophagus. (Courtesy of Kate A Feinstein, MD, and the Department of Radiology, Children's Memorial Medical Center, Chicago, Il.)

TRIAGE
Foreign Body

Emergent ⎯⎯⎯⎯⎯⎯⎯⎯⎯⎯⎯⎯⎯⎯⎯⎯⎯⎯
An infant or child with a sudden onset of dysphagia, hypersalivation, gagging, vomiting, and severe respiratory distress.

Urgent ⎯⎯⎯⎯⎯⎯⎯⎯⎯⎯⎯⎯⎯⎯⎯⎯⎯⎯⎯⎯
An infant or child with known foreign body ingestion without respiratory distress.

Nursing Diagnosis
Ineffective Breathing Pattern

Defining Characteristics

- Dyspnea, tachypnea, apnea
- Changes in heart rate, rhythm or quality
- Splinted, guarded respirations
- Orthopnea

Nursing Interventions

- Administer oxygen
- Suction secretions as needed to prevent aspiration
- Allow child to stay with parents and assume position of comfort to decrease anxiety
- Elevate the head of the bed to 30–45°
- Monitor respiratory status

Expected Outcomes

- Color is normal
- Vital signs are normal
- Airway remains patent
- Child remains calm
- Breath sounds are normal

Nursing Diagnosis
High Risk for Injury

Defining Characteristics

- Lack of knowledge of environmental hazards
- Lack of knowledge of safety precautions
- History of accidents

Nursing Interventions

- Discuss with parents the necessity of constant monitoring of small children
- Teach parents to buy age-appropriate, safe toys

and to avoid buying toys with sharp edges, easily breakable parts, or removable small parts

- Instruct parents about anticipated developmental changes in their children and to take necessary precautions to prevent common injuries
- Encourage parents to take a CPR or first aid class to know how to prevent and intervene in emergency situations

Expected Outcomes

- Parent identifies potentially hazardous factors in the environment
- Parent relates an intent to use safety measures to prevent injury

Management. If a smooth foreign object is in the proximal esophagus, the usual site of occurrence, removal can be accomplished with a Foley catheter. The tube is passed beyond the object, inflated, and withdrawn, bringing the foreign body with it. A mouth gag and forceps should be ready for use when the object nears the child's mouth. The procedure is carried out under fluoroscopic guidance. With sharp objects or objects lodged in the distal esophagus, removal is done using general anesthesia with an esophagoscope equipped with an appropriate forceps.

For foreign bodies that have reached the stomach, conservative management is in order. The progress of the foreign body can be followed by serial x rays. Surveillance of the digestive tract is necessary (Dabadie et al, 1989). Surgical removal is not considered unless 2–3 weeks have gone by without progress because if the object is left in place, ulceration, hemorrhage, pressure necrosis, complete obstruction, and perforation with peritonitis can occur.

A child who has had a foreign body in the esophagus that was removed with a catheter and has had no complications is likely to be discharged from the ED. If there is a question of trauma and subsequent swelling, hospitalization is advised. A child requiring general anesthesia for esophagoscopy is admitted to the hospital.

Hospitalization for retrieval of a coin from the stomach may be deferred for 4 weeks. Removal of an open safety pin caught in the duodenum may be delayed for no more than a few days.

Patient and Family Teaching and Psychosocial Support. Parents of children being discharged from the ED with orders for digestive tract surveillance must be instructed to examine all of the child's stools until the object swallowed has been recovered. The child may have a normal diet with extra roughage and should not be given a laxative. If there is severe abdominal pain, vomiting, or fever, the child should be brought to the ED. Parents of children who are being admitted to the hospital for esophagoscopy should be informed of the purpose and effectiveness of the procedure and of the risks of anesthesia. In emergent situations in particular, the nurse should be available to allay any concerns or fears the child or parent has and answer any questions. All parents should receive follow-up teaching regarding the prevention of accidental ingestions and aspirations. This teaching may be deferred until a clinic or well-child visit in those instances in which considerable parental guilt or anxiety exists regarding the current incident.

Hirschsprung Disease

Hirschsprung disease is a mechanical obstruction caused by inadequate motility in part of the intestine. It is four times more frequent in boys than in girls. In approximately 15% of affected children there is a family history of Hirschsprung disease (Schreiber, 1989).

Etiology and Pathophysiology. Abnormalities in the pelvic paraganglion system include the absence of ganglion cells from the distal colon, absence of peristalsis in the affected areas, and partial intestinal obstruction (Figure 27–5). This condition may be due to anoxia during development, which causes an arrest of the craniocaudal migration of neuroblasts (Schreiber, 1989). There is no association between an older maternal age and the occurrence of Hirschsprung disease (Ryan et al, 1992).

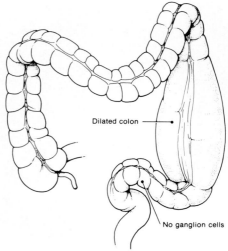

Dilated colon

No ganglion cells

Figure 27–5. The affected bowel in Hirschsprung disease. (From Scipien GM et al [eds]. *Comprehensive pediatric nursing* [3rd ed]. St. Louis: Mosby, p 1069.)

Assessment

History. Most of the infants are full term, appear normal at birth, and have symptoms within the first few weeks of life that are not always recognized. A history is usually given of an infant who failed to pass meconium spontaneously or passed it sparingly. Only 5% of these neonates are known to pass meconium during the first 24 hours. Information on the onset of constipation, the character of stools, and the frequency of bowel movements needs to be obtained. The child does not thrive and has constipation, abdominal distention, and episodes of diarrhea and vomiting.

Physical Assessment. The examination reveals an emaciated and dehydrated infant with a greatly distended abdomen. Abdominal distention and bilious vomiting are the usual symptoms. Dilated loops of small intestine are easily visualized and palpated in the abdomen. Fecal impaction in the colon feels like a ropy mass that extends down the left side of the abdomen and across the epigastrium. As the examiner withdraws a finger, a gush of flatus and foul-smelling stool follows. If the disorder is allowed to progress, other signs of intestinal obstruction, such as respiratory distress and shock, develop.

Laboratory and Diagnostic Tests. X ray studies using a barium enema frequently demonstrate the transition zone between the dilated proximal colon (megacolon) and the aganglionic distal segment. The typical megacolon and narrow segment, however, may not develop until 3–4 weeks or even months after birth in some children. The definitive method of diagnosis is a rectal biopsy done by suction or deep surgical wedge section. Manometric studies that show changes in motor response can be a helpful diagnostic aid.

TRIAGE
Hirschsprung Disease

Emergent
An infant or child with gross abdominal distention causing severe respiratory distress.

Urgent
An infant or child with gross abdominal distention causing tachypnea and mild-to-moderate respiratory distress.

Non-urgent
An infant or child with a long history of constipation; failure to thrive; episodes of vomiting and diarrhea; abdominal distention.

Nursing Diagnosis
Ineffective Breathing Pattern

Defining Characteristics

- Dyspnea, tachypnea, apnea
- Changes in heart rate, rhythm, or quality
- Splinted, guarded respirations
- Orthopnea

Nursing Interventions

- Administer oxygen
- Place patient in a position that facilitates lung expansion
- Elevate the head of the bed to 40–60°
- Insert a nasogastric tube as ordered for abdominal decompression
- Encourage the parents to stay with the child, and allow the child assume a position of comfort to decrease anxiety
- Assess respiratory status and effort

Expected Outcomes

- Color is normal
- Vital signs are normal
- Breath sounds are auscultated in all lung fields.
- Child remains calm

Nursing Diagnosis
Colonic Constipation

Defining Characteristics

- Straining or pain on defecation
- Passage of liquid fecal seepage
- Abdominal distention
- Hard, dry stools
- Decreased frequency of stools

Nursing Interventions

- Administer enemas or stool softeners as ordered
- Administer intravenous fluids as ordered
- Digitally relieve fecal impaction if possible

Expected Outcomes

- Abdominal distention is relieved
- Bowel elimination is improved

Nursing Diagnosis
Parental Role Conflict

Defining Characteristics

- Verbalization of concern about changes in parental role

- Verbalization of concern about effect of child's illness on family
- Verbalization of guilt about contributing to the child's illness through lack of knowledge or judgment
- Verbalization of feelings of guilt, anger, fear, anxiety, frustration

Nursing Interventions

- Allow parents to express their frustrations
- Foster open communication with parents, allowing time for questions, repetition of information, and honest answers
- Recognize parents as experts about their child
- Initiate referrals if needed.
- Provide information to empower parents to adapt to the chronic illness of their child

Expected Outcomes

- Parents identify chronic illness as the source of role conflict
- Parents participate in decision making regarding the child's health and illness
- Parents participate in the care of their child as they are able

Management. Initially there should be correction of fluid and electrolyte deficits with an intravenous infusion. Isotonic enemas may be needed to provide relief of the abdominal distention. A nasogastric tube is inserted. The only definitive treatment is removal of the aganglionic, nonfunctioning segment of intestine. A small infant is usually treated by a colostomy, which is reversed at 10 or more months of age (Foster et al, 1990). Surgical intervention, however, is usually postponed until the child is in a good nutritional state; it is not an emergency operation.

Occasionally a child has chronic but not severe symptoms of megacolon, in which case isotonic enemas, stool softeners, and a low residue diet that decrease the bulk of the stool may be ordered. In general, a child with Hirschsprung disease is admitted to the hospital initially to correct fluid and electrolyte levels before the operation is performed.

Patient and Family Teaching and Psychosocial Support. Parents require detailed information regarding the immediate and long-term treatment of their child. Initially, treatment is directed toward relieving the abdominal distention and correcting fluid and electrolyte deficits. Parents should be instructed that when their child has achieved a good nutritional state, surgical removal of the nonfunctioning portion of the intestine and possibly a colostomy must be performed. Parents

have a great deal of concern regarding surgical interventions, particularly if a colostomy is necessary. They require opportunities to express their fears and concerns and may experience feelings of grief related to the loss of their "ideal" child.

Inguinal Hernia

An inguinal hernia is a mass in the inguinal region that contains some part of the abdominal contents. Inguinal hernias account for approximately 80% of all hernias and are more common in boys than in girls. Such hernias are not usually evident until the child is 2–3 months of age. Advances in neonatal intensive care have resulted in the survival of many small premature infants, who have a high incidence of inguinal hernia (Grosfeld, 1989).

Etiology and Pathophysiology. An inguinal hernia is derived from the persistence of all or part of the processus vaginalis, the tube of peritoneum that precedes the testicle through the inguinal canal into the scrotum during the eighth month of gestation. When the upper portion fails to atrophy, abdominal contents can be forced into it, producing a palpable bulge or mass (Figure 27–6).

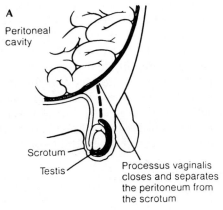

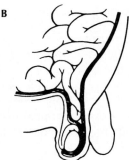

Figure 27–6. A The processus vaginalis precedes the testis into the scrotum during fetal development, then fuses, separating the peritoneal cavity from the scrotum. **B.** Herniation of the intestine into the inguinal canal as a result of incomplete fusion. (From Mott SR, James SR, Sperhac AM [eds] [1990]. *Nursing care of children and families* [2nd ed]. Menlo Park, Calif: Addison-Wesley, p 1402.)

Assessment. An inguinal hernia needs to be differentiated from lymph nodes, a hydrocele, an undescended testis, and torsion of the spermatic cord. With these conditions an increase in abdominal pressure, such as in crying, does not increase the size of the mass, and the mass is not reducible.

History. A good history is of value, because the mass is not always visualized by the examiner. Questions regarding the exact location of the mass, when it appeared, aggravating circumstances, and the reducibility of the mass should be asked. The hernia is usually manifested as a painless inguinal swelling that is absent when the child sleeps and that increases in size when there is coughing or straining.

Physical Assessment. Physical findings are often nonexistent, and one is forced to rely on parental observation of the hernia. Careful inspection of both sides of the groin indicates a small lump beneath a thick layer of adipose tissue. Slight pressure with the fingertips causes re-entry of the intestine into the abdominal cavity. Crying causes an increase in the size of the hernia.

Because of potential complications of a hernia, such as incarceration with intestinal obstruction and possible vascular compromise and intestinal necrosis, there is concern about the potential of the processus vaginalis to admit herniated intestine. When the contents of the hernial sac cannot be reduced, the hernia is said to be incarcerated. Partial or complete obstruction almost invariably follows incarceration. The symptoms of obstruction are tenderness and pain in that area, leading to intermittent or continuous crying, nausea, vomiting, and abdominal distention. Although inguinal hernias are less frequent in girls, incarceration and obstruction are more frequent in girls who have them, especially in the first 6 months of life (Kitchen et al, 1991).

Laboratory and Diagnostic Tests. In addition to the routine laboratory tests, which are not diagnositc, x rays may be ordered. In an uncomplicated inguinal hernia, plain x rays are of little value, although obstruction of the small intestine may be seen on plain x rays with incarceration (Franken, 1982). Inguinal herniography can be used to detect a unilateral inguinal hernia in children with contralateral patent processus vaginalis.

TRIAGE
Inguinal Hernia

Emergent

An infant or child with necrotic bulging in the area of the groin, scrotum or labia accompanied by pain, abdominal distention, no flatus, no stools, and vomiting.

Urgent

An infant or child with bulging in the area of the groin, scrotum or labia with redness, tenderness and pain, nausea and vomiting.

Non-urgent

An infant or child with an intermittent lump in the area of the groin, scrotum or labia, typically occurring with crying or straining.

Nursing Diagnosis
Altered Tissue Perfusion (Gastrointestinal)

Defining Characteristics

- Pale or cyanotic skin
- Changes in skin temperature
- Prolonged capillary refill
- Edema

Nursing Interventions

- Relieve external pressure by removing constrictive clothing
- Keep the child calm to avoid crying and a resultant increase in the size of the hernia
- Monitor skin color and temperature changes

Expected Outcomes

- Circulation to the herniated intestine is restored
- Child remains calm
- Inguinal area is pink and slightly warm

Nursing Diagnosis
Pain

Defining Characteristics

- Complaints of pain
- Restlessness, irritability
- Insomnia
- Guarding behavior
- Crying, moaning
- Autonomic responses not seen in chronic, stable pain (eg, diaphoresis, changes in blood pressure and pulse, pupillary dilation, increased or decreased respiratory rate)

Nursing Interventions

- Identify and consistently use a pain assessment scale appropriate for the child's developmental age
- Encourage parental presence to facilitate pain assessment, provide support and promote trust

- Promote security with honest explanations, opportunities for choice, and preparation for any painful procedures
- Make child as comfortable as possible
- Respond immediately to complaints of pain
- Maintain position of comfort within limits of ongoing treatment
- Administer analgesics as ordered
- Explain to the child how distraction techniques can help relieve pain, and teach a simple method of distraction (eg, counting, naming items in a picture, rhythmic breathing)
- Monitor the effectiveness of pain measures and changes in type, level and location of pain

Expected Outcomes

- Pain assessment scale reliably measures the degree of the child's pain
- Child derives comfort from parents' presence
- Child communicates relief of pain
- Objective symptoms of pain decrease or are absent
- Child uses selected distraction techniques to manage the pain
- Child appears relaxed and comfortable

Nursing Diagnosis
Anxiety

Defining Characteristics

- Autonomic symptoms (eg, diaphoresis, increased blood pressure and pulse, pupillary dilation, increased respiratory rate)
- Restlessness
- Faintness, dizziness
- Nausea or vomiting
- Apprehension
- Crying
- Hyperattentiveness
- Withdrawal

Nursing Interventions

- Remove excess stimulation
- Encourage parental presence to provide emotional support
- Orient the child and parent to the environment
- Speak slowly and calmly, using words suited to the child's age and developmental level
- Prepare the child for all procedures
- Encourage and allow time for expression of anxieties and fears
- Acknowledge the normalcy of anxiety and other feelings

Expected Outcomes

- Child communicates an increase in psychological comfort
- Objective symptoms of anxiety decrease or are absent
- Child uses effective coping mechanisms and parental support to manage anxiety

Management. The treatment of hernias is prompt, elective surgical repair. If the hernia is incarcerated it is best to reduce it immediately, before obstruction occurs, and to allow the injured tissues to recover before the operation is scheduled in 24–48 hours (Davies et al, 1990). If reduction is impossible, an operation should be performed without delay (Gyrtrup et al, 1990). For young infants, even those younger than 2 months, without incarceration, an aggressive approach with prompt surgical repair is recommended (Moss and Hatch, 1991).

Irreducible or strangulated hernias are treated by emergency exploration and herniotomy. In all inguinal hernias, the operation and follow-up care must be explained to the parents. A child with an uncomplicated inguinal hernia can be discharged home with arrangements as to when the elective surgical repair is to be done. A child with an incarcerated or strangulated hernia is admitted, and an emergency operation is done.

Patient and Family Teaching and Psychosocial Support. Preoperative teaching should be done with both the child and parents for all elective surgical repairs of inguinal hernias. In emergent situations in which the hernia is incarcerated, parents require information regarding the need for an emergency operation and all associated risks. Children should be given age appropriate explanations before procedures or surgical preparations. A great deal of anxiety exists for both parents and children in emergent situations, therefore the continuous presence of the nurse is helpful in allaying anxiety, providing reassurance, and addressing questions or concerns.

Umbilical Hernias
A hernia in the umbilical region is a very common defect. It is more common in premature infants and in black infants. A familial incidence is common.

Etiology and Pathophysiology. An umbilical hernia is caused by incomplete fascial closure of the umbilical ring, although the defect is entirely covered by skin and subcutaneous tissue. As the contents of the cord involute, the hernia becomes apparent. The size of the umbilical protrusion is variable. The underlying fascial defect can vary from 0.5–4.0 cm. Herniated small intestine is usually reducible.

Assessment. An umbilical hernia can be seen and allows a definite diagnosis. Because an umbilical hernia is sometimes a concomitant defect in Down syndrome, hypothyroidism, and Hurler syndrome, an additional assessment for these defects may be desirable.

History. Information should be gained regarding when the hernia was first noted, if there has been any increase or decrease in its size, and if it is affected by crying, coughing, or vomiting. Because the sight of the hernia is so disconcerting to parents, they need reassurance regarding its innocuous nature.

Physical Assessment. The hernia appears as a fullness in the umbilical region, which increases with crying or straining. It varies in size from that of a fingertip to that of an orange and frequently increases during the first months of life. The sac may contain only omentum, but when herniated intestine occupies it, the sac feels soft and silky, and the hernia is reduced with a gurgling sound. Incarceration and strangulation are very rare but require immediate surgical intervention.

Laboratory and Diagnostic Tests. In addition to the routine laboratory studies, if there is a large hernia a plain x ray of the abdomen may be ordered. The protruding hernial sac can be visualized.

T R I A G E
Umbilical Hernia

Emergent ─────────────────────
An infant or child with necrotic bulging in the umbilical region accompanied by pain, abdominal distention, and vomiting.

Urgent ─────────────────────
An infant or child with bulging in the umbilical region with redness, tenderness and pain, nausea and vomiting.

Non-urgent ─────────────────────
An infant or child with bulging in the umbilical region that increases with crying or straining.

Nursing Diagnosis
Anxiety

Defining Characteristics

- Autonomic symptoms (eg, diaphoresis, increased blood pressure and pulse, pupillary dilation, increased respiratory rate)
- Restlessness
- Faintness, dizziness
- Nausea or vomiting
- Apprehension
- Crying
- Hyperattentiveness
- Withdrawal

Nursing Interventions

- Remove excess stimulation
- Encourage parental presence to provide emotional support
- Provide reassurance and comfort
- Speak slowly and calmly, using words suited to the child's age and developmental level
- Prepare the child for all procedures
- Encourage and allow time for expression of anxieties and fears
- Acknowledge the normalcy of anxiety and other feelings

Expected Outcomes

- Child communicates an increase in psychological comfort
- Objective symptoms of anxiety decrease or are absent
- Child uses effective coping mechanisms and parental support to manage anxiety
- Child expresses understanding of present illness

Nursing Diagnosis
Altered Tissue Perfusion (Gastrointestinal)

Defining Characteristics

- Pale or cyanotic skin
- Skin temperature changes
- Prolonged capillary refill
- Edema

Nursing Interventions

- Relieve external pressure by removing constrictive clothing
- Keep the child calm to avoid crying and a resultant increase in the size of the hernia
- Monitor skin color and temperature changes

Expected Outcomes

- Circulation to the herniated intestine is restored
- Child remains calm
- Umbilical area is pink and slightly warm

Nursing Diagnosis

Pain

Defining Characteristics

- Complaints of pain
- Restlessness, irritability
- Insomnia
- Guarding behavior
- Crying, moaning
- Autonomic responses not seen in chronic, stable pain (eg, diaphoresis, changes in blood pressure and pulse, pupillary dilatation, increased or decreased respiratory rate)

Nursing Interventions

- Identify and consistently use a pain assessment scale appropriate for the child's developmental age
- Encourage parental presence to facilitate pain assessment, provide support, and promote trust
- Promote security with honest explanations, opportunities for choice, and preparation for any painful procedures
- Make child as comfortable as possible
- Respond immediately to complaints of pain
- Maintain position of comfort within limits of ongoing treatment
- Administer analgesics as ordered
- Explain to the child how distraction techniques can help relieve pain and teach a simple method of distraction (eg, counting, naming items in a picture, rhythmic breathing)
- Monitor the effectiveness of pain measures and changes in type, level and location of pain

Expected Outcomes

- Pain assessment scale reliably measures the degree of the child's pain
- Child derives comfort from parents' presence
- Child communicates relief of pain
- Objective symptoms of pain decrease or are absent
- Child uses selected distraction techniques to manage the pain
- Child appears relaxed and comfortable

Management. Usually umbilical hernias close spontaneously during the first year of life and should not be treated. Some investigators advocate taping the hernia, but there is no evidence that taping hastens closure of the defect, and it may lead to skin breakdown (Crain et al, 1992). Surgical treatment is advisable if the fascial defect exceeds 1.5 cm at 2 years of age. If the child is having abdominal pain or if the hernia persists until school age, it should be repaired. Most children with umbilical hernias are discharged home after the parents are reassured that there is nothing seriously wrong with the child.

Patient and Family Teaching and Psychosocial Support. Because most umbilical hernias close spontaneously and no treatment is needed, parents need to be reassured of the gradual normal closure and of the low probability of complications (Crain et al, 1992). Parents require specific instructions not to apply coins or tape over the hernia because these will not hasten its resolution and could cause skin irritation. For persistent umbilical hernias, both the child and the parents require preparation before the elective operation.

BLEEDING

Many lesions may cause bleeding within the GI tract. This complication manifests itself by hematemesis and passage of blood in the stool. Depending on the extent of blood loss, signs and symptoms of hypovolemia may be present.

Mixing of blood with acid in the stomach leads to the formation of acid hematin, which is the material responsible for the characteristic tarry or melanotic stools that are frequently seen. Bright red rectal bleeding is usually characteristic of lesions of the large intestine. Blood on the surface of the stool is characteristic of low rectal or anal bleeding.

Once the condition of a child with GI bleeding is stabilized with suitable fluids and blood, a complete history should be obtained. Assessment includes a complete physical examination and diagnostic laboratory tests. The tests frequently include gastroduodenal endoscopy, diagnostic angiography, and a GI barium study.

With fiberoptic gastroscopy, endoscopy has become increasingly popular for the evaluation of GI bleeding (Matloff, 1992; Mougenot, 1992). This study usually does not require general anesthesia and can be done in the ED. It allows identification of the lesion responsible for the hemorrhage in upper GI bleeds.

Celiac, superior mesenteric, and inferior mesenteric angiography are useful in the diagnosis of GI bleeding. Selection of the artery to be used is based on the clinical impression of the site of the bleeding. Bleeding in excess of 0.5–1.0 mL/minute usually can be detected in angiography as extravasation of contrast medium from the bleeding vessel. When endoscopy is inconclusive, angiography is performed. It is a good method for demonstrating bleeding sites in Meckel diverticulum, when there are bleeding sites in the small intestine, or in children with variceal bleeding. Barium studies are only occasionally used, because they cannot prove a visualized lesion to be a source of bleeding.

Meckel Diverticulum

Meckel diverticulum occurs when the omphalomesenteric duct, which connects the ileum to the yolk sac, fails to obliterate. The omphalomesenteric duct normally closes by the fifth or sixth week of fetal life, but if it persists in all or part of its courses, several types of malformations can result. These malformations can be cysts, fistulas, fibrotic cords, or, most commonly, Meckel diverticulum. Meckel diverticulum is the most common congenital malformation of the GI tract and is present in 2% of the population (St. Vil et al, 1991). The sexes are equally affected, but boys have a much higher incidence of complications of the lesion. It is estimated that about 15% of patients have complications. The most frequent complications are obstruction and diverticulitis (Ludtke et al, 1989). Most symptomatic Meckel diverticula are seen between 6 months and 2 years of age (Mitchiner, 1989). Meckel diverticulum is a great mimic and must be considered in all cases of intra-abdominal disease in which the cause is not readily apparent (Brown and Olshaker, 1988).

Etiology and Pathophysiology. Meckel diverticulum consists of an outpouching of the ileum that may vary in size from a small appendiceal process to a segment of intestine several inches long and wide. It may be connected to the umbilicus by a cord. It is a true diverticulum with a complete wall (Figure 27–7).

The mucosal lining of the diverticulum may be gastric and ileal, which is most frequent, or colonic and ileal. Sixty percent of clinically significant Meckel diverticula contain gastric mucosa capable of secretion of hydrochloric acid. The acid and pepsin production of the gastric mucosa causes ulceration of the adjacent ileal mucosa with resultant hemorrhage or perforation.

If a low intestinal obstruction develops, it is caused by intussusception or volvulus of the small intestine or by a diverticulum around the fibrous remnant of the obliterated omphalomesenteric duct. The diverticulum tends to invert and to cause intussusception more often in infancy than in later life.

Assessment

History. The diagnosis is usually based on the history. In more than half the cases of Meckel diverticulum in children younger than 2 years, the child has painless, profuse, rectal bleeding. The classic description of bleeding from a Meckel diverticulum in older children

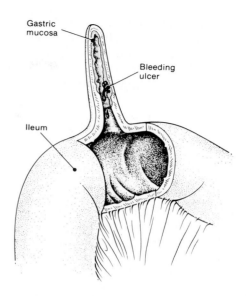

Figure 27–7. The outpouching of Meckel diverticulum. (From Scipien GM et al [eds] [1990]. *Comprehensive pediatric nursing* [3rd ed]. St Louis: Mosby, p 1086.)

is the alternate passage of dark and bright blood. Some patients have a history of occasional bouts of bright red blood in the stools and a few have a history of tarry stools.

Physical Assessment. Because the most frequent manifestation is GI bleeding, a child with Meckel diverticulum is frequently in a state of shock. There is profuse, painless, rectal bleeding. If diverticulitis develops, there are fever, leukocytosis, and tenderness and guarding in the right lower quadrant, all of which arouse suspicion of appendicitis. The pain is periumbilical early in the disease but may be to the right of the midline. Acute suppuration may lead to perforation in an infant. With perforation of the diverticulum, there is an increase in temperature and WBC count. The abdomen becomes rigid, and bowel sounds decrease or disappear.

Laboratory and Diagnostic Tests. Several diagnostic studies are routinely done if Meckel diverticulum is suspected. A technetium-99m-pertechnate scan is required for diagnosis (Rudolph, 1990). Rectosigmoidoscopy is performed first. Blood tests such as a CBC and screening tests for bleeding disorders are done. Abdominal angiography can be beneficial when the individual branch of the superior mesenteric artery leading to the diverticulum can be identified. An x ray diagnosis can seldom be made. Rarely do abdominal x rays that follow a barium enema show residual barium in the diverticulum.

Diagnostic studies are done to rule out other conditions. Rectosigmoidoscopy and a barium enema x ray are usually performed to eliminate other possible diagnoses, such as anal fissure, polyps, and intussusception without Meckel diverticulum. Blood studies are done to rule out bleeding disorders.

TRIAGE
Meckel Diverticulum

Emergent

An infant or child with painless, profuse rectal bleeding with signs and symptoms of shock, fever, abdominal rigidity and guarding, and decreased bowel sounds.

Urgent

An infant or child with painless rectal bleeding in mild to moderate amounts.

Non-urgent

An infant or child with occasional bouts of bright red bloody or tarry stools.

Nursing Diagnosis
High Risk for Fluid Volume Deficit

Defining Characteristics

- Decreased urine output
- Increased specific gravity
- Tachycardia
- Dry skin and mucous membranes
- Poor skin turgor
- Hemoconcentration

Nursing Interventions

- Monitor vital signs
- Assess for signs of dehydration
- Administer intravenous fluids as ordered
- Measure gastric output and check for the presence of blood
- Replace ongoing losses from the GI tract

Expected Outcomes

- Urine output remains greater than 1 ml/kg/hour
- Urine specific gravity is maintained within normal range
- Symptoms of dehydration are improved or absent

- Adequate intake of fluids and electrolytes is maintained
- Vital signs are normal

Nursing Diagnosis
Pain

Defining Characteristics

- Complaints of abdominal pain
- Restlessness, irritability
- Insomnia
- Guarding behavior
- Crying, moaning
- Autonomic responses not seen in chronic stable pain (eg, diaphoresis, changes in blood pressure and pulse, pupillary dilatation, increased or decreased respiratory rate)

Nursing Interventions

- Identify and consistently use a pain assessment scale appropriate for the child's developmental age
- Encourage parental presence to facilitate pain assessment, provide support, and promote trust
- Promote security with honest explanations, opportunities for choice, and preparation for any painful procedures
- Make child as comfortable as possible
- Respond immediately to complaints of pain
- Maintain position of comfort within limits of ongoing treatment
- Administer analgesics as ordered
- Explain to the child how distraction techniques can help relieve pain and teach a simple method of distraction (ie, counting, naming items in a picture, rhythmic breathing)
- Monitor the effectiveness of pain measures, and changes in type, level and location of pain

Expected Outcomes

- Pain assessment scale reliably measures the degree of the child's pain
- Child derives comfort from parents' presence
- Child verbalizes relief of pain
- Objective symptoms of pain decrease or are absent
- Child uses selected distraction techniques to manage pain
- Child appears relaxed and comfortable

Nursing Diagnosis
Fear Related to Change in Health Status and Bleeding

Defining Characteristics

- Feelings of fright, apprehension
- Avoidance behaviors
- Increased heart rate, respirations, and blood pressure
- Attention deficits
- Hypervigilance and increased questioning
- Irritability
- Dilated pupils
- Crying

Nursing Interventions (Gulanick et al, 1992)

- Acknowledge awareness of the child and parent's fear
- Stay with the child and parent if necessary
- Prepare the child and parent for all procedures
- Maintain a calm and tolerant manner while interacting with the child or parent
- Allow the child to make choices when possible
- Use simple language and brief statements geared to the child's developmental level when providing information or explanations
- Encourage the use of diversional activities

Expected Outcomes

- The child and parent differentiate real from imagined situations
- Effective coping mechanisms are used
- Objective symptoms of fear are reduced or absent
- The child and parent express an increase in psychological comfort

Nursing Diagnosis

Ineffective Breathing Pattern Related to Abdominal Pain and Distention

Defining Characteristics

- Dyspnea, tachypnea, apnea
- Changes in heart rate, rhythm or quality
- Splinted, guarded respirations
- Orthopnea

Nursing Interventions

- Administer oxygen
- Position to facilitate lung expansion
- Elevate the head of the bed 40 to 60 degrees
- Encourage the parents to stay with the child
- Allow the child to assume a comfortable position to decrease anxiety
- Assess respiratory status and effort

Expected Outcomes

- Color is normal
- Vital signs are normal
- Breath sounds are auscultated in all lung fields
- Child remains calm

Management. As with most acute abdominal conditions, the child receives nothing by mouth. A nasogastric tube is ordered and should be inserted, secured, and attached to low suction. To correct hypovolemic shock, blood is often started. Intravenous infusions to replace fluid loss are also often needed. All output (urine, nasogastric, and rectal) should be measured and recorded. For the infant with rectal bleeding, the diapers can be weighed and the blood loss estimated. The general rule for measurement is 1 mg = 1 mL. If an obstructive complication or inflammation is present, intravenous antibiotics may be ordered. In children with severe protracted bleeding, vasopressin, given intravenously, may be ordered.

Cimetidine also may be ordered to stop the bleeding before diverticulectomy is performed. As with all cases of bleeding, vital signs need to be monitored frequently and the child kept on bed rest.

Patient and Family Teaching and Psychosocial Support. Because the onset of rectal bleeding in Meckel's diverticulum is usually rapid and involves massive amounts of blood, much psychologic support is needed for both the child and the parents. It is important for the nurse to maintain a calm and reassuring attitude. The child who presents with massive rectal bleeding needs to be made ready for hospitalization.

Esophageal Varices

Esophageal varices are large dilated veins in the submucosal layer of the lower esophageal wall that develop as a result of portal hypertension. This is secondary to obstruction of the portal or splenic venous blood flow. The esophageal varices of portal hypertension are usually in the distal third of the esophagus.

Etiology and Pathophysiology. Bleeding from esophageal varices is a direct consequence of increased portal venous pressure and accounts for 5–8% of all cases of gastrointestinal bleeding in children. Increased resistance to portal flow leads to hemodynamic alterations that redirect the flow of blood away from the liver. As a result there is a reversal of venous blood flow that normally drains into the portal vein and the reopening of preexisting but nonfunctioning collateral circulation. This redirection of blood flow is responsible for the varices.

The causes of portal hypertension are varied. The most common include thrombosis, congenital malformation of the portal or splenic vein, and cirrhosis due to chronic liver disease. Portal vein thrombosis is now recognized as a complication of exchange transfusion and umbilical vein catheterization. It is frequently difficult to assess the cause of the esophageal varices, however.

Assessment

History. Massive hematemesis is the most frequent symptom. This usually does not occur in the child younger than 5 years. The bleeding episodes are often precipitated by a febrile illness. Some investigators suspect that aspirin is responsible rather than the illness. These children may have an early neonatal history of respiratory distress, omphalitis, or exchange transfusion. There is frequently a history of anemia and growth retardation. There may have been ascites that subsided as a result of recanalization of the thrombosis.

Physical Assessment. Examination of the child may reveal hepatomegaly and splenomegaly. If the liver is very cirrhotic, however, it is not palpable. On the abdomen, the caput medusae—a ring of dilated vessels about the umbilicus—may be seen. If ascites is present, the abdomen is dull to percussion and a fluid wave can be elicited. Sigmoidoscopy will reveal internal hemorrhoids or a blue to purple coloration of the rectal mucosa.

If the child is examined after a bleed, the portal system is decompressed and the spleen is no longer palpable. Examination must be repeated after the blood volume has been restored.

Laboratory and Diagnostic Tests. Routine laboratory tests include a complete blood count, platelet count, and urinalysis. Some additional immediate laboratory studies include tests of liver function and clotting, and ceruloplasmin concentration. Endoscopy is performed to visualize the site of bleeding after the child is stabilized.

Radiologic examination using a thick barium medium can demonstrate varices in up to 80% of cases. Splenoportography—visualization of the portal vein anatomy—is also used.

TRIAGE
Esophageal Varices

Emergent
Child with massive hematemesis, hypotension, tachycardia, diminished pulses, poor perfusion and respiratory distress.

Urgent
Child with reported hematemesis with mild to moderate signs and symptoms of respiratory distress.

Non-urgent
Child with blood-flecked emesis without signs and symptoms of shock or respiratory distress.

Nursing Diagnosis
High Risk for Aspiration Related to Esophageal Bleeding

Defining Characteristics (Gulanick et al, 1992)

- Dyspnea, tachypnea or apnea
- Abnormal ABGs
- Anxiety
- Irritability
- Coughing, gagging, choking
- Stridor

Nursing Interventions

- Suction orotrachea as needed
- Administer oxygen
- Position patient on side during vomiting episodes
- Elevate the head of the bed 30 degrees
- Monitor breath sounds and respiratory effort

Expected Outcomes

- Breath sounds are normal
- Secretions are managed adequately

Nursing Diagnosis
High Risk for Fluid Volume Deficit Related to Abnormal Fluid Loss

Defining Characteristics

- Decreased urine output
- Increased specific gravity
- Tachycardia
- Dry skin and mucous membranes
- Poor skin turgor
- Hemoconcentration

Nursing Interventions

- Monitor vital signs
- Maintain NPO
- Administer intravenous fluids with electrolytes as ordered
- Replace blood as ordered
- Maintain a nasogastric tube to intermittent suction or gravity drainage as ordered

- Maintain esophagogastric tube as ordered
- Administer gastric lavages via nasogastric tube as ordered
- Monitor character and amount of gastric drainage

Expected Outcomes

- Gastric drainage is clear or clearing
- Electrolytes are maintained within normal range
- Intake and output are balanced
- Vital signs are normal

Nursing Diagnosis

Fear Related to Blood Loss and Invasive Procedures

Defining Characteristics

- Feelings of fright, apprehension
- Avoidance behaviors
- Increased heart rate, respirations, and blood pressure
- Attention deficits
- Hypervigilance and increased questioning
- Irritability
- Dilated pupils
- Crying

Nursing Interventions (Gulanick et al, 1992)

- Acknowledge awareness of the child and parent's fears
- Stay with the child and parent if necessary
- Prepare the child and parent for all procedures
- Maintain a calm and tolerant manner while interacting with the child and parent
- Allow the child to make choices when possible
- Use simple language and brief statements geared to the child's developmental level when providing information or explanations
- Encourage the use of diversional activities

Expected Outcomes

- The child and parent differentiate real from imagined situations
- Effective coping mechanisms are used
- Objective symptoms of fear are reduced or absent
- The child and parent express an increase in psychological comfort

Management. Frequently, bleeding has stopped by the time the child reaches the hospital. Care for a child with esophageal varices is similar to that for a child with Meckel's diverticulum. Vital signs should be closely monitored, and serial hematocrit determinations should be made. Fresh blood is given to maintain the hematocrit between 30 and 35 percent. Small amounts of oral antacids help to coat the esophagus and to alkalinize any refluxed gastric contents. After the vital signs are stable, the child is admitted to the hospital for diagnostic work-up, and endoscopy is performed. The exact cause of the bleeding needs to be determined and measures taken to prevent recurrence.

If bleeding persists or recurs after blood replacement, injection sclerotherapy or endoscopic band ligation may be used (Matloff, 1992). If bleeding still continues, a total shunt is done (Langor et al, 1990).

Patient and Family Teaching and Psychosocial Support. Both the child and the family need a great deal of support since bleeding from esophageal varices often occurs without warning and is a frightening, life-threatening situation. The nurse needs to assess the child and parent's understanding of the cause of the gastrointestinal bleeding and provide information about the purpose of treatment measures. As many of the diagnostic treatments and procedures for bleeding esophageal varices are particularly unpleasant, explaining why they are necessary is of vital importance. These explanations may help to relieve the child and parent's anxiety, and may actually increase the effectiveness of the procedure; the child is calmer and more willing to cooperate.

JAUNDICE

Jaundice is frequently caused by diseases of the liver or biliary duct system. The most common causes of jaundice in the pediatric emergency patient are acute hepatitis and hepatic coma.

Hepatitis

Hepatitis is an inflammation of the liver. It is rapidly emerging as one of the major causes of morbidity in childhood and is a significant cause of mortality.

Etiology and Pathophysiology. Hepatitis of viral origin is caused by at least six types of viruses, Hepatitis A virus (HAV or infectious hepatitis); Hepatitis B virus (HBV or serum hepatitis); Hepatitis D virus (HDV); and at least three types of non-A and non-B viruses. Although each virus produces similar clinical manifestations, they are distinct in their epidemiologic and immunologic characteristics.

Type A mainly affects children under 15 years of age and has an average incubation period of 25 days. The period of communicability is unknown; the principal route of transmission is the oral-fecal route. Maternal-fetal transfer can occur from transplacental blood during the last trimester, but is most commonly transmitted during delivery. Type A is most common in low socio-economic groups where housing conditions are crowded. Epidemics have been attributed to poor sanitation, with shellfish providing a viral reservoir.

Type B, which affects all age groups, has an incubation period of 6 weeks to 6 months. The period of communicability varies; the principal route of transmission is parenteral, although fetal transfer can occur. Certain groups of people who are in contact with blood products or who require blood transfusions are especially at risk for contacting HBV, especially children with hemophilia, leukemia, or those requiring hemodialysis. In adolescents who use illicit parenteral drugs, 50–80% of acute active or prior HBV infection is found.

Hepatitis D virus is a defective RNA virus that requires a chronic HBV carrier state; it cannot replicate itself. It is uncommon in the United States.

In non-A and non-B hepatitis, no antigen or antibody has been identified, but viral particles can be seen in liver cells, and virus-like particles have been found in the circulation of apparently healthy blood donors. Infected serum may transmit the agent in 1–5 weeks.

In viral hepatitis, pathologic changes occur in the parenchymal cells of the liver. The initial changes involve swelling and degeneration, followed by autolysis. This results in impaired bile excretion, elevated transaminase and alkaline phosphatase levels, and decreased albumin synthesis. The disorder is usually self-limiting, with complete regeneration of cells occurring within 2–3 months.

Assessment. In infants with nonhemolytic jaundice, half will have viral hepatitis, and a quarter will have malformations of the bile duct. Before a diagnosis of acute hepatitis can be made in children, the following conditions need to be excluded: malformation of the bile duct; sepsis; syphilis; congenital rubella; toxoplasmosis; and cystic fibrosis. Hepatitis may also be a manifestation of disseminated viral infections, leptospirosis, or intoxications.

History. The manifestations of viral hepatitis are similar. No distinction can be made in the clinical course except for the incubation period. There is a rapid onset of type A, and a slower, more insidious onset in type B. Initially the child has nausea and vomiting, extreme anorexia, easy fatigability, and a slight to moderate fever, all of which are flu-like symptoms. There may be abdominal pain in the epigastrium or upper right quadrant.

Following this period, there is evidence of jaundice, which begins with darkening of the urine and light-colored stools, followed by yellowing of the sclera and skin. As the jaundice worsens, the child begins to feel better.

The caregiver should be questioned regarding illness in other family members or friends; sanitation practices such as impure drinking water or eating shellfish from contaminated water; recent immunizations or blood transfusions; ingestion of hepatotoxic drugs; parenteral administration of illicit drugs; and sexual contact with someone who uses illicit drugs.

Physical Assessment. Tender hepatomegaly may be the only important physical finding. The facial expression of the child should be observed as the liver is percussed. At times, tenderness is elicited on deep inspiration that permits the liver edge to flip over the examining fingers.

Early in the course of the illness, jaundice is not present, and splenomegaly may not be noted. Flu-like symptoms are the only complaints. Jaundice and a worsening of symptoms is a poor prognostic sign because most of these children develop fulminant or chronic, active hepatitis.

Laboratory and Diagnostic Tests. In routine tests, the complete blood count shows some leukopenia. Urinalysis shows proteinuria and some bilirubinuria early in the disease, before jaundice is evident. A liver profile, showing the severity of the disease, uses a screening panel that requires knowledge and understanding of the specificity and selectivity of the individual tests.

Common laboratory tests include sedimentation rate, which is normal with type B but elevated with type A; serum aminotransferase which is elevated; serum bilirubin, which is elevated; serum transaminases (SGOT and SGPT), which are elevated; and gamma glutamyl transpeptidase (GGT), which is elevated. The course of rising bilirubin and improved clinical signs is a good prognostic sign. No one test is specific for hepatitis. The specific tests for acute viral hepatitis A and B are detection of the hepatitis A antibody (anti-HAV) and the hepatitis surface antigen (HBsAg).

T R I A G E
Hepatitis

Emergent
Infant or child with jaundice, repeated vomiting, decreased level of consciousness, elevated temperature and hemorrhaging.

Urgent
Infant or child with jaundice, pruritus and right upper quadrant tenderness.

Non-urgent ————————————————
Infant or child with flu-like symptoms, malaise, fever, anorexia, gastrointestinal upset, fever, chills and headache.

Nursing Diagnosis
High Risk for Fluid Volume Deficit Related to Excessive Loss of Body Fluids

Defining Characteristics

- Decreased urine output
- Increased specific gravity
- Tachycardia
- Dry skin and mucous membranes
- Poor skin turgor
- Hemoconcentration

Nursing Interventions

- Monitor vital signs
- Assess for signs of dehydration
- Administer intravenous fluids as ordered
- Measure gastric and urine output

Expected Outcomes

- Urine output remains greater than 1 mL/kg/hour
- Urine specific gravity is maintained within normal range
- Symptoms of dehydration are improved or absent
- Adequate intake of fluids and electrolytes is maintained
- Vital signs are normal

Nursing Diagnosis
High Risk for Infection Transmission

Defining Characteristics

- Viral infection transmitted via feces and blood
- Use of suction equipment
- Use of invasive or drainage devices

Nursing Interventions

- Adhere to universal infection precautions
- Make referral to the public health department for follow-up regarding family exposure and cause of exposure
- Properly dispose of all items contaminated with blood or feces

Expected Outcomes

- Parents express understanding of need for isolation precautions until child is non-infectious
- Child and parents demonstrate meticulous hand-washing
- Parents describe mode of transmission of the disease
- Exposed individuals receive appropriate prophylaxis

Nursing Diagnosis
High Risk for Altered Protection Related to Coagulopathy

Defining Characteristic

- Altered clotting profiles

Nursing Interventions (Tucker et al, 1992)

- Assess for signs of bleeding around mucous membranes, injection sites, stools, and emesis
- Monitor coagulation studies
- Use small-gauge needles for injections and rotate sites
- Apply increased pressure for long periods to bleeding sites

Expected Outcomes (Tucker et al, 1992)

- Skin and mucous membranes are without bleeding
- No occult blood is in the urine, stools, or emesis
- Coagulation studies are normal

Management. There is no specific treatment for viral hepatitis. The most important concerns in the management of acute hepatitis are follow-up and prophylaxis of other exposed individuals (Rudolph, 1990). Management is based on palliative treatment of symptoms. Good hand washing and proper disposal of waste materials should be used in connection with these patients. An antiemetic drug may be ordered if vomiting is severe. Hemorrhage is a serious early complication of hepatitis, and requires immediate blood replacement.

In most cases, the child with hepatitis is not hospitalized. If the child has had severe vomiting and is dehydrated, hospitalization may be necessary to restore fluid balance.

Patient and Family Teaching and Psychosocial Support. It is vital that parents understand the importance of identifying all individuals who have been exposed to the infected child so that these individuals can receive prophylaxis. The child and parents should also be taught to recognize the signs and symptoms of hepatitis so they can watch for them in those individuals exposed to the child. Instruction should be given to the parents regarding home care, as hospitalization is rarely necessary. There is no solid evidence that bed rest, absolute or partial, influences the rate of recovery. The child therefore is allowed to regulate his or her own pace (Hupertz, 1992). The child is also allowed to choose the diet, within normal limits. Scrupulous hand washing after toileting and before eating is encouraged, and no drugs should be given unless prescribed because many drugs are excreted by the liver. Referral to a community health nurse may be helpful if further assessment of the family's understanding and use of preventive measures is indicated.

Hepatic Coma

Hepatic coma results from severe liver failure when the blood flow to the liver is decreased and ammonia cannot be detoxified.

Etiology and Pathophysiology. Hepatic coma occurs when the body's supply of protein, and consequently ammonia, is increased. The sources may be food, blood proteins, or the products that result from the breakdown of liver cells in fulminant hepatic necrosis. Central nervous system dysfunction is thought to result from ammonia toxicity. Other conditions precipitating hepatic coma include fluid and electrolyte imbalance, diuresis, progressive renal failure, and hypoxia. Hepatic necrosis may be drug- or poison-induced.

Assessment

History. Frequently the parent will have noticed behavioral changes. Questions regarding behavioral changes, which may include lethargy and confusion, should be asked. The occurrence of previous liver diseases, such as hepatitis, should be investigated.

Physical Assessment. The main clinical features are changes in the mental and neuromuscular state. A characteristic odor—fetor hepaticus which is similar to the smell of feces—is evident on the breath. Hepatic coma may be divided into four stages.

Stages of Hepatic Coma

- Stage I—normal level of consciousness interspersed with reduced mental alertness and periods of hypotonia
- Stage II—drowsiness; confusion; disorientation; swings in affect and mood
- Stage III—stupor and coma; fetor hepaticus; decerebrate posturing
- Stage IV—no response to pain; reflexes disappear; seizures; respiratory arrest

Mortality is at least 80% in children reaching stage IV hepatic coma.

The clinical features that affect mental and neuromuscular state are not difficult to recognize. They begin with confusion and incoordination with tremor, can progress to crying and agitation with roving eyes and muscle twitching, and can further progress to apathy and incontinence ending in coma.

Subtle changes in the respiratory pattern should be noted as an indicator of deepening coma. An increase in the effort of breathing is characterized by deeper inspiration and a more obvious phase of expiration. Fetor hepaticus is the most specific clinical sign of hepatic encephalopathy and occurs in stage III.

Laboratory and Diagnostic Tests. Specific laboratory tests for hepatic coma include a blood analysis of ammonia concentration, which is significantly elevated; blood urea nitrogen, which is initially low since urea is not formed by the liver and becomes elevated as renal function deteriorates; an elevated blood pH; and electrolyte disturbances. In pre-coma stages, an electroencephalogram, which shows slower brain wave activity, may be a useful diagnostic tool. The specific laboratory tests and history can provide a definite diagnosis of hepatic coma. It may be difficult, however, to identify the cause.

TRIAGE
Hepatic Coma

Emergent
Infant or child unresponsive to pain, without reflexes, seizing, or in respiratory arrest.

Urgent
Infant or child with mental confusion, increased respiratory effort, and fetor hepaticus.

Non-urgent
Infant or child with a history of malaise and mild tremors.

Nursing Diagnosis
Ineffective Breathing Pattern Related to Ascites and Central Nervous System Depression

Defining Characteristics
- Dyspnea, tachypnea, apnea
- Changes in heart rate, rhythm or quality
- Dysrhythmic respirations
- Orthopnea

Nursing Interventions

- Administer oxygen
- Position to facilitate lung expansion
- Monitor oxygen saturations and end-tidal CO_2
- Encourage the parents to stay with the child
- Allow the child to assume a comfortable position to decrease anxiety
- Assess respiratory status and effort

Expected Outcomes

- Color is normal
- Vital signs are normal
- Oxygen saturations and end-tidal CO_2 are normal
- Breath sounds are auscultated in all lung fields
- Respiratory rate and pattern are effective
- Gas exchange in the lungs is improved

Nursing Diagnosis

Altered Protection Related to Coagulopathy

Defining Characteristic

- Altered clotting profiles

Nursing Interventions (Tucker et al, 1992)

- Assess for signs of bleeding around mucous membranes, injection sites, stools, and emesis
- Monitor coagulation studies
- Use small-gauge needles for injections and rotate sites
- Apply increased pressure for long periods to bleeding sites

Expected Outcomes (Tucker et al, 1992)

- Skin and mucous membranes are without bleeding
- No occult blood is in the urine, stools, or emesis
- Coagulation studies are normal

Nursing Diagnosis

Sensory-Perceptual Alteration

Defining Characteristics

- Inaccurate interpretation of environmental stimuli
- Restlessness
- Disoriented about time, place, or people
- Altered behavior or communication pattern

Nursing Interventions (Tucker et al, 1992)

- Monitor for changes in neurologic status
- Reduce environmental stimuli
- Administer Lactulose as ordered to promote ammonia excretion
- Administer oral antibiotics as ordered to decrease nitrogen and ammonia-producing intestinal bacteria
- Monitor for toxic effects of all medications
- Provide a safe environment; keep siderails up

Expected Outcomes (Tucker et al, 1992)

- Serum ammonia, glucose, and BUN are within normal ranges
- Mental status is improving or normal
- No further injury is sustained

Nursing Diagnosis

High Risk for Infection

Defining Characteristics

- Continuous or intermittent fever
- Elevated WBC
- Increased heart rate

Nursing Interventions

- Reduce the entry of organisms into the child by using meticulous handwashing and aseptic technique when indicated
- Assess for signs of localized or systemic infection
- Administer antibiotics as ordered

Expected Outcomes

- Vital signs are normal
- Child's risk of infection is reduced

Management. There is no evidence that any known treatment aids the underlying liver disease. Attempts are thus made to reduce the levels of circulating toxins that are harmful to the brain. For the previously well child in whom a drug or poison induced hepatic necrosis is suspected as the cause, heroic measures are justified. Fluids are started; deranged clotting factors should be corrected with fresh frozen plasma. Frequent assessments of neurologic status and vital signs are performed and recorded. Endotracheal intubation and assisted ventilation may be necessary. Arterial and central lines are placed for frequent sampling of blood gases. Antibiotics and steroids may be ordered. Heroic measures can include two-volume blood exchange, peritoneal dialysis, hemodialysis, total body washout with hypothermia, hyperbaric oxygenation, and liver transplantation.

Patient and Family Teaching and Psychosocial Support. Parents require teaching about the disease process, prognosis and treatment plan. The nurse should reinforce any information given to the family by the physician regarding neurologic definitions and signs of progress. The family should be reassured that frequent assessments of neurologic status are necessary and do not necessarily indicate a worsening in the condition of the child. Changes in a child's behavior or level of consciousness are particularly frightening for parents; therefore a great deal of time should be allowed for explaining behavioral changes and providing emotional support.

REFERENCES

Allen B, Tompkins RK, Mulder DG (1991). Repair of large paraesophageal hernia with complete intrathoracic stomach. *American Surgeon* 57:642–647

Ashkenazi S, Cleary TG (1991). Antibiotic treatment of bacterial gastroenteritis. *Pediatric Infectious Disease Journal* 10: 140–148

Bailey DJ, Andres JM, Danek GD, Pineiro-Carrero VM (1987). Lack of efficacy of thickened feeding as a treatment for gastroesophageal reflux. *Journal of Pediatrics* 110:187–189

Bardhan PK, Salam MA, Molla AM (1992). Gastric emptying of liquid in children suffering from acute rotaviral gastroenteritis. *Gut* 33:26–29

Barr LL, Stansberry SD, Swischuk LE (1990). Significance of age, duration, obstruction and the dissection sign in intussusception. *Pediatric Radiology* 20:454–456

Bishop WP, Ulshen MH (1988). Bacterial gastroenteritis. *Pediatric Clinics of North America* 35:69–87

Bisset GS 3d, Kirks DR (1988). Intussusception in infants and children: diagnosis and therapy. *Radiology* 168:141–145

Bissonnette B, Sullivan PJ (1991). Pyloric stenosis. *Canadian Journal of Anaesthesia* 38:668–676

Bowen A (1988). The vomiting infant: Recent advances and unsettled issues in imaging [published erratum appears in Radiol Clin North Am 1988; 26:following ix]. *Radiologic Clinics of North America* 26:377–392

Brown CK, Olshaker JS (1988). Meckel's diverticulum. *American Journal of Emergency Medicine* 6:157–164

Conway SP, Ireson A (1989). Acute gastroenteritis in well nourished infants: Comparison of four feeding regimens. *Archives of Disease In Childhood* 64:87–91

Crain EF, Gershel JC, Gallagher EJ (1992). *Clinical manual of emergency pediatrics* (2nd ed). New York: McGraw-Hill, pp 151–153

Dabadie A, Roussey M, Betremieux P, Gambert C, Lefrancois C, Darnault P (1989). Acute pancreatitis from a duodenal foreign body in a child. *Journal of Pediatric Gastroenterology and Nutrition* 8:533–535

Davies N, Najmaldin A, Burge DM (1990). Irreducible inguinal hernia in children below two years of age. *British Journal of Surgery* 77:1291–1292

Dieckmann RA (1990). Abdominal pain. In Grossman M, Dieckmann RA (eds), *Pediatric emergency medicine: A clinician's reference.* Philadelphia: Lippincott, pp 196–202

Edwinson M, Arnbjornsson E, Ekman R (1988). Psychologic preparation program for children undergoing acute appendectomy. *Pediatrics* 82:30–36

Eriksson S, Granstrom L, Bark S (1989). Laboratory tests in patients with suspected acute appendicitis. *Acta Chirurgica Scandinavica* 155:117–120

Flom LL, Ellis GL (1992). Radiologic evaluation of foreign bodies. *Emergency Medicine Clinics of North America* 10:163–177

Forman HP, Leonidas JC, Kronfeld GD (1990). A rational approach to the diagnosis of hypertrophic pyloric stenosis: Do the results match the claims? *Journal of Pediatric Surgery* 25:262–266

Foster P, Cowan G, Wrenn EL Jr (1990). Twenty-five years' experience with Hirschsprung's disease. *Journal of Pediatric Surgery* 25:531–534

Fox R, Leen CL, Dunbar EM, Ellis ME, Mandal BK (1990). Acute gastroenteritis in infants under 6 months old. *Archives of Disease in Childhood* 65:936–938

Franken EA (1982). *Gastrointestinal imaging in pediatrics* (2nd ed). New York: Harper & Row, pp 319–323

Ghisolfi J (1992). Acute diarrhoea and severe prolonged diarrhoea. In Navarro J, Schmitz J (eds), *Paediatric gastroenterology* New York: Oxford University Press, pp 182–188

Grosfeld JL (1989). Current concepts in inguinal hernia in infants and children. *World Journal of Surgery* 13:506–515

Gulanick M, Puzas MK, Wilson CR (1992). *Nursing care plans for newborns and children.* St. Louis: Mosby, pp 221–273

Gyrtrup HJ, Mejdahl S, Kvist E, Skeie E (1990). Emergency presentation of inguinal hernia in childhood—treatment strategy: A follow-up study. *Annales Chirurgiae et Gynaecologiae* 79:97–100

Henneman PL, Marcus CS, Inkelis SH, Butler JA, Baumgartner FJ (1990). Evaluation of children with possible appendicitis using technetium 99m leukocyte scan. *Pediatrics* 85:838–843

Hoffman RD, Levine HA, Baram S, Tiberin E, Soroker D (1992). Painless intussusception: Giving conservative treatment another chance. *Postgraduate Medicine* 91:283–284

Holcomb GW 3d, Ross AJ 3d, O'Neill JA Jr (1991). Postoperative intussusception: Increasing frequency or increasing awareness? *Southern Medical Journal* 84:1334–1339

Hupertz VF (1992). Hepatitis. In Reece RM (ed), *Manual of emergency pediatrics* (4th ed). Philadelphia: Saunders, pp 45–46

Isolauri E, Jalonen T, Maki M (1989). Acute gastroenteritis: Changing pattern of clinical features and management. *Acta Paediatrica Scandinavica* 78:685–691

Jackson PT, Glasgow JF, Thomas PS, Carre IJ (1989). Children with gastroesophageal reflux with or without partial thoracic stomach (hiatal hernia) have normal gastric emptying. *Journal of Pediatric Gastroenterology and Nutrition* 8: 37–40

Kitchen WH, Doyle LW, Ford GW (1991). Inguinal hernia in very low birthweight children: A continuing risk to age 8 years. *Journal of Paediatrics and Child Health* 27:300–301

Laks Y, Barzilay Z (1988). Foreign body aspiration in childhood. *Pediatric Emergency Care* 4:102–106

Langer BF, Greig PD, Taylor BR (1990). Emergency surgical treatment of variceal hemorrhage. *Surgical Clinics of North America* 70:307–317

Lillehei CW, Snyder JD (1989). Acute appendicitis. In Snyder JD and Walker WA (eds), *Common problems in pediatric gastroenterology and nutrition.* Chicago: Year Book, pp 125–130

Lindzon RD, Mitchiner JC (1989). Conditions requiring surgery. In Barkin RM, Rosen P (eds), *Emergency pediatrics: A guide to ambulatory care* (3rd ed). St. Louis: Mosby, pp 528–531

Little KJ, Danzl DF (1991). Intussusception associated with Henoch-Schonlein purpura. *Journal of Emergency Medicine* 9 [Suppl] 1:29–32

Ludtke FE, Mende V, Kohler H, Lepsien G (1989). Incidence and frequency or complications and management of Meckel's diverticulum. *Surgery, Gynecology and Obstetrics* 169:537–542

Matloff DS (1992). Treatment of acute variceal bleeding. *Gastroenterology Clinics of North America* 21:103–118

Mitchiner JC (1989). Meckel's diverticulum. In Barkin RM, Rosen P (eds), *Emergency pediatrics: A guide to ambulatory care* (3rd ed). St. Louis: Mosby, pp 534–536

Moineau G, Newman J (1990). Rapid intravenous rehydration in the pediatric emergency department. *Pediatric Emergency Care* 6:186–188

Moss RL, Hatch EI Jr (1991). Inguinal hernia repair in early infancy. *American Journal of Surgery* 161:596–599

Mougenot JF (1992). Gastric haemorrhage. In Navarro J, Schmitz J (eds), *Paediatric gastroenterology.* New York: Oxford University Press, pp 446–457

Neilson IR, Laberge JM, Nguyen LT, et al (1990). Appendicitis in children: Current therapeutic recommendations. *Journal of Pediatric Surgery* 25:1113–1116

Otu AA (1989). Tropical surgical abdominal emergencies: Acute appendicitis. *Tropical and Geographical Medicine* 41:118–122

Reijnen JA, Festen C, Joosten JH, van Wieringen PM (1990). Atypical characteristics of a group of children with intussusception. *Acta Paediatrica Scandinavica* 79:675–679

Rudolph CD (1990). Gastrointestinal bleeding. In Grossman M, Dieckman RA (eds), *Pediatric emergency medicine: A clinician's reference* Philadelphia: Lippincott, pp 167–171

Ryan CA, Yacoub W, Paton T, Avard D (1990). Childhood deaths from toy balloons. *American Journal of Diseases of Children* 144:1221–1224

Ryan ET, Ecker JL, Christakis NA, Folkman J (1992). Hirschsprung's disease: Associated abnormalities and demography. *Journal of Pediatric Surgery* 27:76–81

Schreiber RA (1989). Hirschsprung disease. In Snyder JD, Walker WA (eds), *Common problems in pediatric gastroenterology and nutrition* Chicago: Year Book, pp 186–192

Siegal B, Hyman E, Lahat E, Oland U (1982). Acute appendicitis in early childhood. *Helvetica Paediatrica Acta* 37:215–219

Skipper RP, Boeckman CR, Klein RL (1990). Childhood intussusception. *Surgery, Gynecology and Obstetrics* 171:151–153

Sperhac AM (1990). Physical assessment. In Mott S, James S, Sperhac AM (eds), *Nursing care of children and families.* Redwood City, Calif: Addison-Wesley, pp 343–400

St-Vil D, Brandt ML, Panic S, Bensoussan AL, Blanchard H (1991). Meckel's diverticulum in children: A 20-year review. *Journal of Pediatric Surgery* 26:1289–1292

Tucker SM, Canobbio MM, Paquette EV, Wells MF (1992). *Patient care standards: Nursing process, diagnosis, and outcomes* (5th ed.). St. Louis: Mosby, pp 240–307

SUGGESTED READING

Carpenito LJ (1989). *Nursing diagnosis: Application to clinical practice* (3rd ed). Philadelphia: Lippincott

Carpenito LJ (1991). *Handbook of nursing diagnosis* (4th ed). Philadelphia: Lippincott

CHAPTER 28

Genitourinary Emergencies and Disorders

SUSAN J. KELLEY

■ DISORDERS OF THE FEMALE GENITALIA

VAGINAL BLEEDING

Types of Bleeding

Prepubertal Vaginal Bleeding. Vaginal bleeding in an infant or prepubescent child can be a frightening event for the child and parents. The presence of scant amounts of vaginal bleeding is common in the neonate and is due to withdrawal of maternal estrogen. Bleeding commonly occurs at 3–5 days of age and generally requires no treatment (Fontanaros and Hellman, 1991). Vaginal bleeding related to menarche can occur normally at any time between 9 and 16 years. When vaginal bleeding occurs after the first few weeks of life, and before menarche, it is abnormal and associated with a variety of conditions. In a prepubertal child it can be a sign of injury, foreign body, or serious disease indicating a local genital tract disorder or endocrinologic or hematologic disease.

Vaginal bleeding in infants and children can be caused by a variety of conditions including trauma, a foreign body, infection, hormone imbalance, or genital tumors. The possibility of sexual abuse should always be considered in the differential diagnosis. Table 28–1 summarizes possible causes of vaginal bleeding in a prepubescent girl.

Vaginal bleeding due to *trauma* is a potential emergency. A penetrating injury to the vagina can cause damage to the rectum, bladder, or abdominal viscera. A vaginal laceration may cause only minimal bleeding and may not necessarily reflect the seriousness of the injury.

There are several *hormonal causes* of vaginal bleeding in prepubescent females. Vaginal bleeding in the first 3 weeks of life is usually caused by hormonal fluctuations. This is due to exposure to high levels of circulating maternal hormones before birth that stimulate growth of the uterine endometrium as well as an increase in breast tissue. Soon after birth the endometrium sloughs, resulting in a few days of light vaginal bleeding. The bleeding stops spontaneously and requires no treatment. Parents need a great amount of reassurance that the bleeding is normal and will subside without intervention.

Hormonal stimulation that produces vaginal bleeding in an older infant or child may be associated with precocious puberty. It is usually accompanied by an increase in breast tissue or growth of pubic hair. When this occurs in children younger than 8 years, the child should be referred to an endocrinologist for further evaluation.

Vulvovaginitis is a common cause of bleeding in prepubertal children and may be the result of pruritus and scratching due to pinworms. Perineal excoriations

TABLE 28–1. ETIOLOGY OF PREPUBERTAL VAGINAL BLEEDING

Neonatal physiologic bleeding due to
   withdrawal of maternal hormones
Trauma
Foreign body
Urethral prolapse
Vulvovaginitis
Tumors
Precocious puberty
Lichen sclerosis

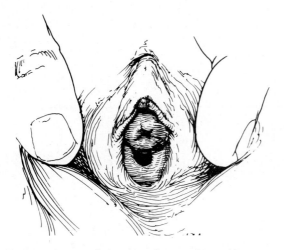

Figure 28–1. The smooth doughnut shape and central lumen are characteristic features of a urethral prolapse, which, if large or swollen, often conceals the vagina below it. (From Fleischer GR, Ludwig S [eds] [1993]. *Textbook of pediatric emergency medicine* [3rd ed]. Baltimore: Williams & Wilkins, p 920)

can be caused by rectal *Enterobius vermicularis* infection (pinworms) that produce intense itching and scratching, especially at night. Other organisms associated with vaginal bleeding include group A beta-hemolytic streptococci and *Shigella* (see section on Vulvovaginitis).

Trauma to the vulva can include lacerations, hematomas, or ecchymoses. Vaginal or rectal injuries should be considered whenever trauma to the vulva is noted.

Urethral prolapse is a common cause of apparent vaginal bleeding in children. Urethral prolapse is identified by the characteristic doughnut shape, with a swollen, dark red protruding urethral mucosa and central lumen (Figure 28–1). Often, the vaginal orifice is concealed by the prolapse. Most urethral prolapses occur in girls between the ages of 2 and 10 years. Painless vaginal bleeding is often the presenting complaint. The bleeding comes from ischemic mucosa and may be accompanied by dysuria or urinary frequency. Straight catheterization of the bladder may be performed to confirm patency. If it appears healthy, the prolapsed mucosa may be treated by instructing the parents to apply warm compresses or sitz baths for 10–14 days. If the prolapsed tissue appears necrotic, surgical intervention may be needed. This operation is often performed within a few days of diagnosis on an elective, outpatient basis.

Bleeding at Onset of Menses. Occasionally, parents bring their daughter to the ED because she is experiencing her first menstrual period. If the child's age and degree of pubertal development are appropriate for her age, no further evaluation is necessary. The child and family require reassurance and teaching regarding the normal menstrual cycle and other physical changes that occur at time of puberty.

Postpubertal Bleeding. Dysfunctional uterine bleeding, or irregular and excessive vaginal bleeding, is a common cause of postpubertal vaginal bleeding. Breakthrough bleeding can occur when one is taking oral contraceptives. Most other causes of vaginal bleeding in adolescents are more serious and include ectopic pregnancy, placenta previa, spontaneous abortions, endometriosis, trauma, and bleeding dyscrasias.

History

For a prepubescent child with vaginal bleeding, a careful history should be elicited as to the amount, frequency, and duration of the bleeding. A history of any recent trauma or possibility of sexual abuse needs to be carefully ascertained (see Chapter 9). Any recent or chronic illness should be determined. A recent history of pinworm infection in family members should be explored. A careful history of onset of menses and any secondary sex characteristics should be elicited.

When vaginal bleeding occurs after menarche, a comprehensive history from the adolescent assists in determining the source of bleeding. A careful history regarding sexual activity (in the absence of parents), last menstrual cycle, possibility of pregnancy, use of contraceptives, and any previous pregnancies and their outcomes should be ascertained. The patient's mother should be asked if she was exposed to estrogen therapy during pregnancy.

Physical Assessment

Whenever trauma to the vagina is suspected, the child's abdomen should be carefully evaluated. If an intra-abdominal injury is present, lower quadrant tenderness may be noted. A surgical consultation is indicated, and the child may need a careful examination of the vagina under sedation or anesthesia.

Foreign bodies may cause vaginal bleeding. If the foreign body has been in the vagina for more than several days, a foul smelling discharge usually is present. If the foreign object cannot be easily visualized and removed, it may be necessary to gently irrigate the vaginal cavity with 50 mL of normal saline solution using a urethral catheter attached to a 25-mL syringe. If this procedure fails to dislodge and remove the foreign body, an examination using anesthesia is indicated.

If the patient is pregnant, uterine bleeding during the first 20 weeks indicates either spontaneous abortion or ectopic pregnancy. If bleeding is profuse, administration of intravenous fluids is necessary. A pelvic examination is performed to determine the cause of bleeding.

If the patient is in the second or third trimester of pregnancy, placenta previa and abruptio placentae are possible. Because it may trigger a sudden hemorrhage, a pelvic examination should be delayed until the patient's condition is stabilized and an obstetrician has been consulted.

Gynecologic Examination

The gynecologic examination of a pediatric patient requires sensitivity, patience, and a specialized approach. A careful explanation by the nurse before and during the examination is crucial. The nurse and physician may choose to examine the child together to avoid having the child examined more than once. The mother or other family member should be allowed to be present, if so desired by the patient.

The approach to the examination usually depends on the age of the child. Examination of the external genitalia can usually be accomplished with the younger child on the mother's lap leaning back with her legs held apart by the mother, in a frog-like position. The older child should be placed on the examining table in a supine, frog-leg position with the hips flexed and the soles of the feet touching. The examiner may gently depress the perineum downward and laterally with both hands to visualize the hymenal ring and vagina. If old enough, the child may choose to assist the examiner by holding her labia majora apart. This gives the child some sense of control over the examination.

A school-aged girl may choose to be placed in the knee-chest position to allow visualization of the vagina. This is usually accomplished by requesting the child to get up on her hands and knees on the examining table, bringing her knees close to her chest with her buttocks in the air. She should be instructed to rest her head on her folded arms facing her mother or nurse for comfort and support. The child should be instructed to cough or exhale to relax her abdominal muscles while the examiner gently separates the labia and buttocks. This allows the vaginal opening to fall open for visualization with light from an otoscope. The nurse can do breathing exercises with the child or adolescent to decrease anxiety and increase relaxation.

An internal examination with a vaginal speculum is usually not necessary in the examination of a prepubescent girl. However, when it is necessary to use an instrument, a pediatric vaginal speculum or small nasal speculum may be used to examine the vagina. Any discharge, bleeding, hematomas, contusions, or foreign bodies should be noted. Afterward, the child should be returned to the supine position for the collection of specimens. When a child is too frightened, uncomfortable, or uncooperative for a speculum examination, or if bleeding is profuse, then a decision may be made to examine the child using anesthesia.

Under no circumstances should a frightened child be physically restrained for a vaginal examination.

An adolescent can be examined in the traditional lithotomy position. The emergency department (ED) is a less than ideal place for the first pelvic examination; therefore, when the patient's condition allows, the examination should be deferred to a more relaxed outpatient setting.

In all age groups, the labia minora, introitus, hymen, urethral meatus, and clitoris should be visualized and inspected for signs of trauma, infection, bleeding, or anatomic abnormality.

Laboratory and Diagnostic Tests

When there is a history of bleeding, but no abnormalities or bleeding are noted on examination, urine and stool specimens should be analyzed for blood. A urine culture and urinalysis should be obtained to rule out a urinary tract infection (UTI). Whenever severe trauma to the vagina is suspected, a baseline hemoglobin level should be obtained. Hematuria may indicate injury to the urethra or bladder. If trauma to the urethra is suspected, a cystogram may be necessary. A vaginal culture should be obtained because *Shigella* vaginitis can cause vaginal bleeding that is often more noticeable than the associated discharge.

Abdominal or pelvic ultrasonography may be ordered when a mass is suspected.

A hematocrit, hemoglobin level, and pregnancy test should be obtained when there are findings suggestive of pregnancy.

T R I A G E
Vaginal Bleeding

Emergent —————————————————
A child or adolescent with profuse vaginal bleeding; pregnancy with acute onset of bleeding; unstable vital signs.

Urgent —————————————————
A child with controlled and minimal bleeding; mild to moderate pain.

Non-urgent —————————————————
A child with history of vaginal bleeding that has stopped; no discomfort; stable vital signs.

Nursing Diagnosis
Pain

Defining Characteristics

- Verbalization of pain
- Crying or facial expression of pain

Nursing Intervention

- Administer analgesic

Expected Outcomes

- Child verbalizes that pain has decreased
- Nonverbal cues indicate child is more comfortable

Nursing Diagnosis

Knowledge Deficit (Vaginal Bleeding)

Defining Characteristic

- Inadequate knowledge related to vaginal bleeding

Nursing Interventions

- Carefully explain all procedures and treatments
- Inform parents of any needs the child may have on discharge from the ED

Expected Outcome

- Patient and family members verbalize understanding of patient's condition and treatment

Management

In cases of profuse bleeding, efforts are initially directed toward controlling the bleeding and supporting airway, breathing and circulation. At least one intravenous line should be started immediately. If severe bleeding is due to trauma, the child often is taken to the operating room for examination and surgical intervention using anesthesia.

Vaginal bleeding in a neonate due to fluctuation in hormonal levels requires no intervention other than reassurance. Prepubescent children with vaginal bleeding believed to be due to hormonal stimulation should be referred to an endocrinologist for further evaluation and treatment. Vaginal bleeding due to the onset of menses requires reassurance and education regarding menstruation.

Patient and Family Teaching and Psychosocial Support

Vaginal bleeding can be a frightening experience for a child and her parents. Much reassurance is necessary, even when the cause of bleeding is found to be normal, as in physiologic bleeding in the newborn and bleeding at the onset of menses. Adolescents and their family members who seek emergency care for the onset of menses may require more information and support than it may be possible to provide in the ED. These patients should be referred to an adolescent clinic where their educational needs can be met in an unrushed setting with a health care provider with whom they can develop an ongoing relationship. Printed educational materials on menstruation and other bodily changes related to puberty should be made available in the ED.

VULVOVAGINITIS

Vulvovaginitis, the most common gynecologic problem in children, is the inflammation of both the vulva and the vagina. Vulvovaginitis usually begins with vulvitis and vaginitis then occurs secondarily. Vaginal discharge is one of the most common symptoms of vulvovaginitis. It is important to note that a normal physiologic discharge occurs in the first 2–3 weeks of life and 6–12 months before menarche.

Etiology

Occasionally, simple vulvitis may be observed. In these patients, the inflammation of the labia may be caused by an infection, trauma, or allergic reaction. Common causes of allergic vulvitis include soaps, bubble bath, and close-fitting synthetic undergarments.

Predisposing factors that make prepubescent girls susceptible to vulvovaginitis include lack of estrogen, which causes the vaginal lining to be thin and dry and have a neutral to alkaline pH. These conditions are ideal for bacterial growth. Poor perineal hygiene, particularly the improper habit of wiping from the back to the front after defecation, results in fecal contamination of the genitalia and contributes to vulvovaginitis. The labia minora and majora are smaller in a child than in an adult, allowing less protection of the vagina from invasion by microorganisms.

The types, causes, clinical presentation, and treatment of nonsexually transmitted vulvovaginitis in children are summarized in Table 28–2. The clinical presentation, diagnostic tests, and treatment of sexually transmitted diseases (STDs) in adolescents are presented in Table 28–3. The treatment of STDs in children is discussed in Chapter 9.

History

The child with vulvovaginitis may give a history of dysuria, vaginal discharge, or pruritus. The parents may have noticed discomfort in the child manifested by gait disturbance and rubbing or scratching of the genitalia.

Physical Assessment

Examination of the perineum may reveal an erythematous labia majora and a slight vaginal discharge, or

TABLE 28-2. VULVOVAGINITIS IN CHILDREN

Type	Cause	Presentation	Treatment
Bacterial			
■ NONSPECIFIC			
Mixed flora	Poor hygiene	Red, swollen vulva	Proper perineal hygiene
	Improper "back to front" wiping	Dysuria	Sitz baths
	Transmission of infecting organism from respiratory tract to genitals by contaminated fingers	Pruritus	Estrogen cream
		Brown or green malodorous discharge	
	Foreign body		
■ SPECIFIC			
Group A beta-hemolytic streptococci	Same as above	Discharge	Penicillin or cephalosporin
Gardnerella vaginalis	Same as above	Discharge	Metronidazole
Shigella flexneri	Fecal contamination	Diarrhea	Trimethoprim and sulfamethoxazole
		Fever	
Protozoal			
Candida	Tight undergarments	White discharge	Topical nystatin
Trichomonas	Acquired during delivery in 0–3-month-olds	Bubbly discharge	Metronidazole
Pinworm (Enterobius vermicularis)	Pinworms migrate from rectum	Perianal itching	Mebendazole
		Excoriation of vulva	Treat all family members

leukorrhea. It is important to note that a white discharge may be noted in the newborn period and that this occurrence is normal and not due to infection, but rather is the result of maternal estrogen in the residual circulation. This condition is self-limiting and requires no intervention except reassurance of the parents. Pubescent girls also may experience a mucoid discharge. The color, odor, and thickness of the vaginal discharge should be noted.

Laboratory and Diagnostic Tests
A vaginal culture identifies the infecting organism and the organism's sensitivity to antibiotics. A microscopic examination of the discharge may determine the infecting organism in many cases and determine the treatment regimen until culture results are available.

> **TRIAGE**
> **Vulvovaginitis**
>
> *Non-urgent* ─────────────
> Child with localized infection, no signs of trauma

Nursing Diagnosis
Knowledge Deficit (Vulvovaginitis)

Defining Characteristic
- Verbalization of inadequate knowledge

Nursing Interventions
- Carefully explain all procedures and treatments
- Inform parents of any further needs the child may have

Expected Outcome
- Patient and family members verbalize increased knowledge related to patient's condition and treatment

Management
The treatment for a child with vulvovaginitis is summarized in Table 28–2.

■ DISORDERS OF MALE GENITALIA

TESTICULAR TORSION

Testicular torsion, the most serious cause of acute painful scrotal swelling, is caused by twisting of the spermatic cord leading to venous and arterial obstruction (Figure 28–2). Testicular torsion should be the pri-

TABLE 28–3. SEXUALLY TRANSMITTED DISEASES (STDs) IN ADOLESCENTS

STD	Presentation	Laboratory Tests	Treatment
Gonorrhea	Penile discharge Vaginal discharge Rectal inflammation, discharge Pharyngitis Dysuria, frequency Pelvic pain Asymptomatic	Pharyngeal, rectal, vaginal, and urethral (male) cultures	Ceftriaxone, 250 mg IM followed by oral doxycycline 100 mg bid × 7 days If allergic to penicillin: Spectinomycin 2 gm IM in place of ceftriaxone If pregnant: Oral erythromycin 500 mg × 7 days in place of doxycycline
Syphilis	Primary syphilis: Chancres may appear on penis, vulva, cervix, rectum, mouth Secondary syphilis: Fever, pharyngitis; rash on trunk, upper extremities, palms, and soles of feet; lymphadenopathy; splenomegaly Late syphilis: Vasculitis; neurologic and cardiac involvement	VDRL or RPR serologic tests Microscopic exam of lesion; scrapings reveal spirochete	Benzathine penicillin G 2.4 million U IM In nonpregnant, penicillin-allergic patients: Oral doxycycline 100 mg bid × 14 days
Chlamydia	May be asymptomatic Discharge Dysuria Pelvic pain Urinary frequency	ELISA antibody test Monoclonal antibody test	Doxycycline 100 mg bid × 7 days If allergic to doxycycline or pregnant: Oral erythromycin 500 mg qid × 7 days
Herpes genitalis	Dysuria Vulvar pruritis and burning Painful lesions on vulva, perianal area, vagina, cervix Occasional fever	Microscopic exam of cells from lesion Viral culture	Analgesics Antipruritics In primary herpes, oral acyclovir 200 mg 5 times/day × 7–10 days[a] For recurrent episodes: Oral acyclovir 200 mg 5 times/day × 5 days[a] Sitz baths
Condylomata acuminata	Nontender lesions (warts) on genitals or perirectal area	Biopsy	Liquid nitrogen Trichloroacetic acid Podophyllin
Trichomoniasis	Vaginitis; discharge Asymptomatic in boys	Saline wet prep to identify protozoa	Oral metronidazole 2 g as single dose

VDRL, Veneral Disease Research Laboratories; RPR, rapid plasma reagin; ELISA, enzyme-linked immunosorbent assay.
[a]Acyclovir is contraindicated in pregnancy.

mary consideration in any case of scrotal pain or swelling (Fontanarosa and Hellman, 1991). The frequency of testicular torsion has been estimated at 1 in 4000 males younger than 25 years. Although torsion can occur at any age, approximately two-thirds of all cases occur in boys between 12 and 18 years of age (Tonetti and Tonetti, 1990).

All suspected cases of testicular torsion should be evaluated immediately, because testicular survival depends on the duration of ischemia. The risk of permanent testicular damage depends on the duration of torsion and the severity of rotation of the testis and spermatic cord. Therefore, prompt triage is critical, and a urologist or surgeon must be notified immediately.

History

A patient with testicular torsion typically arrives at the ED with acute testicular pain, which at times radiates to the groin and lower abdominal quadrants. The duration of pain is usually less than 24 hours. Some patients describe a history of similar severe testicular pain that resolved spontaneously (Tonetti and Tonetti,

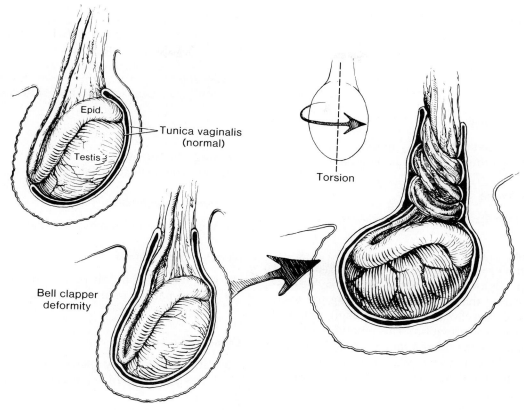

Figure 28–2. Torsion of the testis. Abnormality of testicular fixation—bell-clapper deformity—allows torsion of spermatic vessels with subsequent infarction of the gonad. Epid., epididymis. (From Fleischer GR, Ludwig S [eds] [1993] *Textbook of pediatric emergency medicine* [3rd ed]. Baltimore: Williams & Wilkins, p 283)

1990). The patient may also complain of nausea and vomiting. Although there may be a recent history of trauma to the genitals or strenuous exercise, a testicular torsion can occur at rest or while a patient is asleep.

Physical Assessment
The involved testis lies higher in the scrotum than the other testis, with a horizontal rather than vertical orientation. Scrotal edema is present. The patient's blood pressure may be elevated because of pain and anxiety; fever is rarely present. Depending on the duration of the symptoms, there are variable amounts of scrotal swelling and redness. If the testis can be delineated, it is firmer than normal and exquisitely tender (Tonetti and Tonetti, 1990).

Laboratory and Diagnostic Test
In testicular torsion the scrotum does not transilluminate. The diagnosis is based on a Doppler ultrasonographic examination of the testicles that reveals an absence of blood flow to the affected testis. Computed tomography (CT) or a nucleotide scan may be performed. Urinalysis is important to rule out an infectious cause for the testicular pain and swelling.

TRIAGE
Testicular Torsion

Emergent
A child in whom testicular torsion is suspected.

Nursing Diagnosis
Pain

Defining Characteristics
- Verbalization of pain
- Facial expression of pain

Nursing Intervention
- Administer analgesic

Expected Outcomes
- Patient verbalizes that pain has decreased
- Nonverbal cues indicate patient is more comfortable

Nursing Diagnosis
Anxiety

Defining Characteristic
- Verbalization of worry, fear

Nursing Interventions
- Reassure patient and family members
- Allow for as much privacy as possible

Expected Outcome
- Patient verbalizes less worry and fear

Management
If the duration of the torsion has been less than 3 or 4 hours, manual detorsion by the physician may be possible by elevating the scrotum and rotating the testis in an outward direction toward the thigh followed by prompt surgical attention. The emergency nurse should ensure that the patient take nothing by mouth while in the ED. Often an analgesic is administered while the patient awaits transport to the operating room.

Patient and Family Teaching and Psychosocial Support
The emergency nurse should make the patient as comfortable as possible while awaiting evaluation and surgical treatment. Pain, examination, and an operation on the genitals are embarrassing for the patient and provoke great anxiety. Young children may fear castration. Adolescents may have concerns regarding their sexuality after the operation. Therefore, emotional support and accurate information are extremely important. The patient and family need to be prepared for the child's admission to the hospital after the operation.

BALANITIS

Balanitis is an inflammation of the glans of the penis. It is a form of cellulitis from infection due to a break in the penile skin. Balanitis occurs more frequently in uncircumcised boys and may be associated with trauma or poor hygiene.

Assessment
The foreskin may appear crusted, swollen, and reddened. It is often accompanied by a deep rash over the scrotum, pubis, and buttocks and by dysuria.

T R I A G E
Balanitis

Non-urgent —————————————————————
A child with localized infection; no signs of trauma.

Nursing Diagnosis
Knowledge Deficit (Balanitis)

Defining Characteristic
- Verbalization of inadequate knowledge

Nursing Interventions
- Carefully explain all procedures and treatments
- Inform parents of any further needs the child may have

Expected Outcomes
- Patient and family members verbalize increased knowledge related to patient's condition and treatment

Management
The area should be carefully cleansed with soap and warm water and allowed to dry completely. An ointment such as petroleum jelly or bacitracin should be applied sparingly. The child may be given amoxicillin or a cephalosporin for 10 days.

If the foreskin produces total obstruction, there may be acute urinary retention. In this event, a physician inserts the tip of a mosquito forceps into the orifice of the foreskin and stretches the skin. Any collected pus is removed. Circumcision is performed only after the inflammation has subsided.

Parents should be instructed to cleanse and dry the area and to change diapers frequently. They may also be instructed to expose the inflamed area to air as much as possible. If there is crusting of the foreskin, warm soaks may be applied three times daily, 20 minutes at a time.

PARAPHIMOSIS

Paraphimosis is a condition in which the foreskin in an uncircumcised boy has been retracted proximally over the glans and cannot be drawn back into its normal position over the glans. Immediate treatment is necessary because there is rapid increased swelling, pain, and potential compromise of circulation to the glans.

This condition is frequently caused by an infection. Poor hygiene and collection of smegma under the foreskin can lead to chronic inflammation.

Assessment

The child is usually brought to the ED with a history of swelling of the glans, pain, and an inability to return the foreskin over the glans.

TRIAGE
Paraphimosis

Urgent ————————————————————
A child with localized infection; swelling of the glans

Nursing Diagnosis

Knowledge Deficit (Paraphimosis)

Defining Characteristic

- Verbalization of inadequate knowledge

Nursing Interventions

- Carefully explain all procedures and treatments
- Inform parents of any further needs the child may have

Expected Outcome

- Patient and family members verbalize increased knowledge related to patient's condition and treatment

Nursing Diagnosis

Pain

Defining Characteristics

- Verbalization of pain
- Facial expression of pain

Nursing Intervention

- Administer analgesic

Expected Outcomes

- Patient verbalizes pain has decreased
- Nonverbal cues indicate patient is more comfortable

Nursing Diagnosis

Anxiety

Defining Characteristic

- Verbalization of worry, fear

Nursing Interventions

- Reassure patient and family members
- Allow for as much privacy as possible

Expected Outcome

- Patient verbalizes less worry and fear

Management

Cool compresses should be applied to the penis and an analgesic administered. A local dorsal penile nerve block with 1% lidocaine (without epinephrine) may be given. Manual reduction of the foreskin is then attempted by the physician during which the glans is gently pushed proximally through the obstruction while traction is maintained on the swollen preputial tissue "like turning a sock inside out" (McDonald, 1992). If manual reduction fails, referral is made immediately to a urologist or surgeon for a dorsal slit procedure to relieve the obstruction (McDonald, 1992).

The child can be discharged home from the ED once he has demonstrated an ability to void. Proper cleansing of the uncircumcised penis should be taught to the child and parents. Parents are advised to seek a follow-up appointment with a surgeon to arrange for circumcision once the swelling has subsided.

EPIDIDYMITIS

Epididymitis is an inflammation of the epididymis. It is an uncommon cause of scrotal swelling in prepubertal boys and often is associated with an anatomic abnormality. Epididymitis may be the complication of gonorrhea, urethritis, prostatitis, or instrumentation of the urethra. It is often accompanied by orchitis.

Assessment

There is often a history of pain and swelling of the scrotum accompanied by fever and dysuria. The pain of epididymitis is usually described as dull and aching, whereas with orchitis the pain is more severe and the testes are enlarged.

A urinalysis and urine culture should be obtained to rule out a UTI. If a urethral discharge is present, cultures should be obtained for gonorrhea and chlamydia.

An examination shows the epididymis to be enlarged, hard, and tender. Often the scrotal skin overlying the epididymis is thickly edematous, whereas the testicle may be normal (Tonetti and Tonetti, 1990).

TRIAGE
Epididymitis

Urgent ―――――――――――――――――――
A child with localized infection; swelling of the glans.

Nursing Diagnosis
Knowledge Deficit (Epididymitis)

Defining Characteristic
- Verbalization of inadequate knowledge

Nursing Interventions
- Carefully explain all procedures and treatments
- Inform parents of any further needs the child may have

Expected Outcome
- Patient and family members verbalize increased knowledge related to patient's condition and treatment

Nursing Diagnosis
Pain

Defining Characteristics
- Verbalization of pain
- Facial expression of pain

Nursing Intervention
- Administer analgesic

Expected Outcomes
- Patient verbalizes that pain has decreased
- Nonverbal cues indicate patient is more comfortable

Management
Treatment includes scrotal support, analgesia, and application of ice. In nonsexually transmitted epididymitis, appropriate initial therapy is oral trimethoprim-sulfamethoxazole (TMP/SMX) 10 mg/ kg/24 hours. If the patient is allergic to sulfa drugs, alternative an-

tibiotics include ampicillin or a first-generation cephalosporin (Combest, 1992). If epididymitis is caused by a STD, the treatment for children older than 9 years is ceftriaxone 250 mg IM, followed by oral doxycycline 100 mg bid for 10 days. In children younger than 9 years, ceftriaxone 250 mg IM is given along with oral erythromycin 50 mg/kg/24 hours (Combest, 1992).

Hospitalization may be required if the patient is acutely ill with a UTI, fever, dehydration, and nausea and vomiting (Combest, 1992).

SEXUALLY TRANSMITTED DISEASES

Sexually transmitted diseases have become of increased concern and incidence in the adolescent population. The term STD refers to a group of diseases that are usually transmitted from one person to another during sexual activity.

With prepubertal children, unless a STD has been transmitted from a mother to her newborn, it has most likely been acquired through sexual abuse. Sexually transmitted diseases in infancy that can be perinatally transmitted include herpes simplex virus type II, condyloma acuminata, gonorrhea, chlamydia, and syphilis. When a STD is present after infancy, it should be considered to have been acquired through sexual abuse until proven otherwise. Chapter 9 provides information on the recognition and management of STDs in children.

TRIAGE
Sexually Transmitted Diseases

Urgent ―――――――――――――――――――
A child with suspected sexual abuse. An adolescent female girl with abdominal pain; fever.

Non-urgent ―――――――――――――――――
An adolescent with vaginal or penile discharge.

Nursing Diagnosis
Knowledge Deficit (Sexually Transmitted Diseases)

Defining Characteristic
- Verbalization of inadequate knowledge

Nursing Interventions
- Carefully explain all procedures and treatments

- Inform patient about medication administration
- Teach adolescent STD prevention.

Expected Outcome

- Patient verbalizes increased knowledge related to condition and treatment.

Management

Table 28–3 summarizes the presentation and treatment of the STDs commonly found in adolescents. The presence of one STD should alert the clinician to the possibility of other STDs in the same adolescent and his or her sexual partners. Each time an adolescent is treated in the ED for a STD the nurse should emphasize prevention of STDs, including prevention of infection with the human immunodeficiency virus (HIV). All adolescents should be strongly encouraged to seek follow-up care, as well as routine health care, in an adolescent clinic or other health care setting.

■ URINARY TRACT DISEASE

URINARY TRACT INFECTION

Urinary tract infections in childhood are defined as clinically significant bacterial growth in urine obtained by bladder catheterization, suprapubic aspiration, or clean voided specimens (Feld, 1991). A UTI is the second most common form of bacterial infection in children next to upper respiratory tract infection. In infants and children, UTIs may be easily overlooked because of nonspecific symptoms (Feld, 1991). Between 1 and 2% of infants and children have bacteriuria at any given time. During infancy boys are at increased risk for UTIs because of the higher incidence of anatomic defects in boys. After infancy, the prevalence is much higher for girls than for boys. A major reason for this higher incidence in girls past infancy is the short urethra of the girls and the proximity of the rectum to the urethra. Five percent of all girls have a UTI before puberty compared with 1% of boys. The peak incidence of UTI occurs between 2 and 6 years of age.

Etiology

Virtually all UTIs occur by the ascending route. *Escherichia coli* is the most common causative pathogen and is responsible in 70–90% of cases. Other common pathogens include *Klebsiella pneumoniae*, *Proteus* species, *Enterobacter aerogenes*, enterococci, and *Staphylococcus epidermidis*.

Pathophysiology

Poor perineal hygiene, the short urethra of girls, infrequent voiding, sexual activity, and circumcision in-

TABLE 28–4. CLINICAL MANIFESTATIONS OF URINARY TRACT INFECTIONS BY AGE GROUP

■ INFANTS
Lethargy
Poor appetite
Irritability
Fever
Vomiting
Diarrhea
Jaundice
Poor feeding
Cloudy or malodorous urine
Severe diaper rash
Failure to thrive
■ CHILDREN
Fever
Frequency
Urgency
Dysuria
Cloudy or malodorous urine
Hematuria
Enuresis
Abdominal pain

crease the risk of a UTI. The acute, uncomplicated infection is usually confined to the bladder. The inflammatory changes of the bladder and urethral mucosa are responsible for the symptoms of frequency, urgency, and dysuria (Hertz, 1992). Complications of recurrent urinary tract infections include chronic renal failure, bacteremia, perinephric abscess, and urolithiasis (Hertz, 1992).

History

Infants and children with UTIs often present to the ED with complaints that are vague and suggestive of a variety of clinical entities. In fact, nearly 40% of children with UTIs have no symptoms (McCracken, 1989). Neonates may have very general symptoms, such as those seen in septicemia, including irritability, poor appetite, and lethargy. The clinical indicators of UTIs in infants are more often gastrointestinal than genitourinary in character and include jaundice, vomiting, diarrhea, irritability, malodorous diapers, and a history of poor feeding. Fever may or may not be present. The history in older children may include abdominal pain, vomiting, dysuria, frequency, and fever. Previously toilet trained children may have episodes of enuresis. Any past history of UTIs should be elicited as should the use of bubble bath or other irritants. Table 28–4 summarizes the clinical manifestations of UTIs in infants and children.

Physical Assessment

The patient should be assessed for abdominal pain, jaundice, pinworms, and irritation or trauma to the

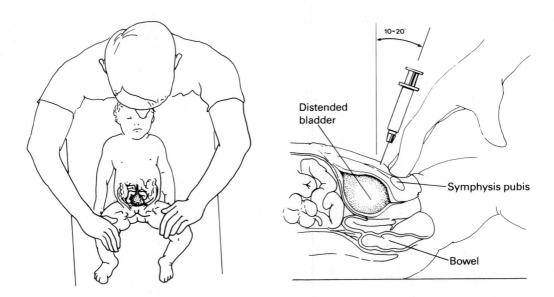

Figure 28–3. Suprapubic bladder aspiration. The infant should be held firmly in a supine position with the legs in a frog-leg position (left). The suprapubic bladder tap is performed by inserting a 22-gauge needle (attached to a 3-mL syringe) into the bladder and aspirating urine as the syringe is gradually withdrawn (right).

perineum, which could cause dysuria. An abdominal examination may reveal suprapubic tenderness. Infants should be assessed for signs of septicemia (see Chapter 26).

Laboratory and Diagnostic Tests

The diagnosis of a UTI is based on the presence of bacteriuria, or organisms in the urine. Therefore, proper collection of urine cultures is essential to the accurate diagnosis of a UTI. However, obtaining uncontaminated urine specimens in infants and children is a challenge.

A suprapubic bladder aspiration, performed by a physician, is the most effective method of collecting urine from a young infant (Figure 28–3). Urine obtained by this method is generally free of bacterial contaminants. Because the infant's bladder should be full for this procedure it is best to wait until 45 minutes after the last void to conduct the bladder tap.

In many instances, a straight urethral catheterization at the bladder is performed to obtain a sterile specimen. Although less reliable, a sterile urine collection bag can be applied to the perineum after the area has been thoroughly cleansed. This method has an increased risk of contamination of the urine with vaginal and fecal flora because of the difficulty of thoroughly cleansing the perinuem (Hertz, 1992). In older children, after proper cleansing, a midstream clean-catch urine specimen can be obtained in a sterile receptacle by the nurse or the patient's mother after the first portion of urine has passed into the toilet. However, specimens obtained by this method are also frequently contaminated by perineal bacteria. A first morning void is preferred but rarely available in the ED. A first morning void can, however, be obtained at home when follow-up urine cultures are necessary.

The urine specimen should be cultured within 30 minutes or placed in a refrigerator to prevent the colony count from being unreliably elevated. The diagnosis of a UTI is based on a urine culture indicating a colony count of more than 100,000 organisms/mL. Growth of several different organisms is an indication that the specimen was contaminated, in which case the culture should be repeated.

Uncentrifuged urine can be Gram stained and examined with high-power fields to determine the presence of bacteria. In the presence of a UTI, routine urinalysis may reveal red blood cells, white blood cells (WBC), protein, and bacteria.

The assessment of infants and children with UTIs, may involve renal ultrasonography and a voiding cystourethrogram because of the high frequency of anatomic abnormalities, particularly vesicoureteral reflux (Feld, 1991).

Nursing Diagnosis
Anxiety

Defining Characteristic

- Verbalization of worry, fear

Nursing Interventions

- Reassure patient and family members
- Allow for as much privacy as possible

Expected Outcome

- Patient verbalizes less worry and fear

Nursing Diagnosis
Knowledge Deficit (Urinary Tract Infection)

Defining Characteristic

- Verbalization of inadequate knowledge

Nursing Interventions

- Carefully explain all procedures and treatments
- Inform parents of any further needs the child may have.

Expected Outcome

- Patient and family members verbalize increased knowledge related to patient's condition and treatment

Nursing Diagnosis
Pain

Defining Characteristics

- Verbalization of pain
- Facial expression of pain

Nursing Intervention

- Administer analgesic

Expected Outcomes

- Patient verbalizes that pain has decreased
- Nonverbal cues indicate patient is more comfortable

Management

The goal of treatment is directed toward eradication of the infecting microorganism and prevention of recurrence. Antibiotic treatment is initiated before cultures are available if the UTI is symptomatic and the urinalysis and Gram stain are suggestive of a UTI.

Newborns with UTIs should be admitted to the hospital for intravenous administration of gentamicin. Older infants and children with uncomplicated UTIs may be treated on an outpatient basis with ampicillin, 100 mg/kg/day given orally in four divided doses, or TMP/SMX, 8/40 mg/kg/day in two divided oral doses, pending culture results. Dagan et al (1992) found that once-daily oral cefixime (8 mg/kg/day) is as effective in the treatment of uncomplicated acute UTIs in children 6 months–13 years of age as TMP/SMX given twice daily.

Patient and Family Teaching and Psychosocial Support

Parents need to be instructed in the administration of medication, increased fluid intake, and use of sitz baths to relieve discomfort. Parents should be advised to return to the ED or their primary health care provider if the child is unable to retain the medication because of persistent vomiting or if oliguria, high fever, lethargy, or signs of dehydration occur. Regardless of how the child is progressing clinically, another urine culture should be obtained and found to be negative after 48 hours of antibiotic therapy. If the repeat culture is positive, a different antibiotic should be prescribed according to the sensitivity report. The child needs to have another culture after another 24–48 hours. Because recurrence is common, the child needs to be followed carefully on completion of the antibiotic therapy.

The importance of keeping appointments for follow-up radiological tests should be emphasized because they can detect any renal damage and treatable anatomic and functional abnormalities. With appropriate interventions, such as antimicrobial prophylaxis for vesicoureteral reflux or surgical treatment of obstructive lesions, subsequent renal damage can be averted and recurrent infections eliminated or decreased (Shapiro, 1992).

Parents should be taught proper perineal care of their children, such as wiping from front to back after toileting to prevent subsequent UTIs. They should also be told to avoid the use of bubble baths or feminine sprays. If old enough, the child should take showers instead of baths. Some children are infrequent voiders and need to be encouraged to void at frequent intervals because overdistension of the bladder can decrease blood flow and lead to infection (Wilson and Killion, 1989).

ACUTE GLOMERULONEPHRITIS

Acute glomerulonephritis (AGN), an immune complex disease, is the most common noninfectious renal disease in childhood. Poststreptococcal glomerulonephritis is the most common form of glomerulonephritis in children. Most cases are related to a previous infection with nephritogenic strains of group A beta-hemolytic streptococci. Acute glomerulonephritis may follow a cutaneous infection such as impetigo. There is a latent period of 10–14 days between the streptococcal infection and the onset of clinical manifestations. Acute glomerulonephritis occurs most frequently in children 3–12 years of age, with a peak incidence at 7 years. Children younger than 2 years are rarely affected; boys are affected more often than girls.

Epidemiology
In the northern sections of the United States, the initial streptococcal infections usually involve pharyngitis and an upper respiratory infection, whereas impetigo, infected insect bites, and scabies are the leading causes in the southern states. Although most cases are related to a previous infection with nephritogenic strains of group A beta-hemolytic streptococci, other bacterial infections, as well as viral and parasitic diseases, have been associated with AGN.

Pathophysiology
The renal involvement is thought to result from an antigen-antibody response that is stimulated by the initial streptococcal infection, followed by an immune-complex reaction. These immune complexes become trapped in the glomerular capillary loop.

The kidneys are normal to moderately enlarged during the initial phase. A microscopic examination reveals a diffuse proliferative exudative process. The glomerular capillary loops become obliterated by edema and the filtration rate is reduced. This results in a reduced capacity to form filtrate from plasma flow. This decreased plasma filtration results in excessive retention of sodium and water, followed by expanded plasma and interstitial fluid volumes, which may cause circulatory congestion and edema. Children with AGN usually recover completely, and recurrence is unusual.

History
Within the 2 weeks preceding the ED visit there may be a history of pharyngitis, skin infection such as impetigo, headache, hematuria, dysuria, edema, and weight gain. With increasing degrees of renal failure, there may be a history of nausea, vomiting, and abdominal pain.

Physical Assessment
The child's airway, breathing, and circulation should be carefully assessed and supported. The child may be found to have edema, hypertension, and, in some severe cases, signs of congestive heart failure. The edema may be noted primarily in the face in the morning, but then spreads to the extremities and abdomen during the day. Congestive heart failure results from fluid retention that leads to vascular overload. The child may appear pale, lethargic, and irritable. In some severe cases the patient may present with seizure activity secondary to hypertension or cerebral ischemia, or with oliguria or anuria, the result of acute renal failure (ARF).

Laboratory and Diagnostic Tests

Urinalysis. The results of urinalysis usually include a high specific gravity, a protein level, and increased numbers of red blood cells, WBCs, epithelial cells, and casts, but no bacteria.

Cultures. A positive throat culture is useful in establishing the diagnosis. However, in most patients, the throat culture is negative. Throat cultures should be obtained from all household members and other close contacts. A urine culture should also be obtained.

Serologic Tests. A complete blood count (CBC), serum antistreptolysin-O (ASO), and streptozyme titers, serum complement levels C3 and C4, and serum creatinine and blood urea nitrogen (BUN) levels should be obtained. The serum ASO and immunoglobulin G levels are elevated. The BUN level is elevated disproportionately to the creatinine level. Hyponatremia and hyperkalemia may be present and are specifically related to the degree of oliguria (Knepper, 1992).

Electrocardiography. An electrocardiogram (ECG) may reveal elevation or depression of the ST segment, prolonged QRS and ST segments, lengthening of the PR interval, and flattened or inverted T waves.

X Rays. A chest x ray may show cardiac enlargement, pulmonary congestion, and plural effusion during the acute phase.

Emergent —————————————————————
A child with severe hypertension; edema; oliguria.

Urgent ——————————————————————
A child with mild hypertension; urine output > 1.0 mL/kg/hour; no signs of cardiac involvement.

Nursing Diagnosis
Fluid Volume Excess

Defining Characteristics

- Edema
- Hypertension
- Oliguria

Nursing Interventions

- Limit fluid intake
- Closely monitor blood pressure
- Administer antihypertensives if ordered
- Administer diuretics if ordered

Expected Outcomes

- Edema decreases
- Patient is normotensive
- Urine output is normal

Nursing Diagnosis
Knowledge Deficit (Acute Glomerulonephritis)

Defining Characteristic

- Verbalization of inadequate knowledge

Nursing Interventions

- Carefully explain all interventions
- Provide discharge instructions

Expected Outcome

- Patient and family members verbalize increased knowledge related to patient's condition and treatment

Management
The management of AGN is generally supportive. Fluid and sodium intake (oral and intravenous) should be restricted. This therapy usually improves mild hypertension. Intake and output should be carefully measured and recorded. Electrolyte balance should be carefully maintained.

If severe hypertension is present, hydralazine 0.15 mg/kg IM is usually effective in lowering blood pressure within 15–60 minutes. Reduction in the vascular circulatory volume may be necessary to lower blood pressure. This can be achieved through administration of a diuretic such as furosemide, 1 mg/kg IV. Decreased sodium intake limits the reaccumulation of fluid and recurrence of hypertension.

If ARF with marked oliguria is present, severe restriction of sodium, potassium, protein, and fluid intake is necessary. Occasionally, peritoneal dialysis or hemodialysis is necessary.

Patients with AGN who are hypertensive should be admitted to the hospital for close observation. Children with mild cases of AGN who are not hypertensive can be followed on an outpatient basis.

Patient and Family Teaching and Psychosocial Support
The child and parents often are anxious and need much reassurance while in the ED. All procedures should be carefully explained. When appropriate, the patient and family members should be prepared for the child's admission to the hospital. If the child is to be treated on an outpatient basis, the medication regimen and need for follow-up care should be reinforced.

ACUTE RENAL FAILURE

Acute renal failure is a sudden decrease in glomerular filtration rate (GFR) to a level where the kidneys are unable to perform the functions of fluid balance, blood pressure control, acid-base balance, and solute excretion (Knepper, 1992). Acute renal failure occurs when there is an abrupt loss of renal excretory function due to impaired blood flow. The kidneys are unable to regulate the volume and composition of urine. Acute renal failure is uncommon in children, but the mortality is high in this age group. The prognosis depends on the etiology and prompt identification and treatment. Acute renal failure is categorized by changes in creatinine clearance.

Etiology
The causes of ARF include renal trauma, shock, toxic agents, and dehydration. The causes of ARF are usually classified as prerenal (decreased renal perfusion), renal (intrinsic parenchymal damage), and postrenal (obstructive). Prerenal causes are the most common cause of ARF in children and are related to reduction

of renal perfusion to a normal kidney. Dehydration secondary to gastroenteritis, hypovolemic shock, distributive shock, an operation, trauma, burns, diabetic ketoacidosis, congestive heart failure, and sepsis are common causes. Postrenal causes, uncommon in children older than 1 year, include upper urinary tract obstruction, bladder neck obstruction, and trauma. Renal causes include diseases such as glomerulonephritis, pyelonephritis, malignant tumors, and nephrotoxic agents that damage the glomeruli, tubules, or renal vasculature.

Pathophysiology

Acute renal failure is characterized by a severe reduction in GFR, an elevated serum urea nitrogen level, and decreased tubular reabsorption of sodium from the proximal tubule, with an increased concentration of sodium in the distal tubule. Glomerular filtration is reduced, preventing urinary losses of sodium.

History

An infant or child with renal failure may present with a history of oliguria (urine flow less than 0.5 mL/kg/hour), symptoms related to AGN, or a history of exposure to nephrotoxic substances, such as carbon tetrachloride, heavy metals, or prescribed medications, such as sulfonamides, neomycin, or kanamycin. In most cases, the child initially presents with signs and symptoms of a precipitating disorder such as shock, burns, near drowning, AGN, or dehydration. In such cases the risk of ARF should be anticipated and carefully monitored.

TABLE 28–5. LABORATORY VALUES ASSOCIATED WITH ACUTE RENAL FAILURE (ARF)

Determination	Findings in ARF	Normal Values
Potassium	Hyperkalemia	Newborn 5.0–7.7 mEq/L Infant 4.1–5.3 mEq/L Child 3.5–4.7 mEq/L
Sodium	Hyponatremia	Newborn 139–162 mEq/L Infant 139–146 mEq/L Child 138–145 mEq/L
Calcium	Hypocalcemia	Newborn 3.7–7.0 mEq/L Infant 5.2–6.0 mEq/L Child 5.0–5.7 mEq/L
Creatinine serum	Elevated	0.3–1.1 mg/dL
Blood urea nitrogen	Elevated	Newborn/Infant 5–15 mg/dL Child 10–20 mg/dL
Arterial blood gases	Metabolic acidosis	pO_2 Newborn 60–70 mmHg Child 80–90 mmHg pCO_2 35–45 mmHg pH 7.35–7.45

Physical Assessment

The airway, breathing, and circulation should be assessed continually. Signs of volume overload, such as edema, rales, tachycardia, and cardiac gallop, may be present. Hypertension, seizures, lethargy, coma, anorexia, nausea, and fever may be present. Whenever an acutely ill child becomes oliguric, ARF should be suspected (Kennedy, 1992). Fluid intake and output and vital signs should be monitored carefully.

Laboratory and Diagnostic Tests

Urine electrolytes and urinalysis with specific gravity should be obtained. A CBC, serum electrolytes, BUN, creatinine, and arterial blood gas levels should also be obtained. An ECG should also be performed. Table 28–5 outlines the abnormal laboratory values associated with ARF.

T R I A G E
Acute Renal Failure

Emergent
A child with hypertension; oliguria; edema; tachycardia; altered level of consciousness.

Urgent
A child with normal urine output but at risk for acute renal failure.

Nursing Diagnosis
Fluid Volume Excess

Defining Characteristics

- Edema
- Hypertension
- Oliguria

Nursing Interventions

- Restrict fluid intake
- Closely monitor blood pressure
- Administer antihypertensive drugs if ordered
- Administer diuretics if ordered

Expected Outcomes

- Edema decreases
- Patient is normotensive
- Urine output is normal

Nursing Diagnosis
Anxiety

Defining Characteristic

- Verbalization of distress, worry, fear

Nursing Interventions

- Reassure child and family members
- Allow parents to remain at bedside as much as possible

Expected Outcome

- Patient and family verbalize less worry and fear

Nursing Diagnosis

Knowledge Deficit (Acute Renal Failure)

Defining Characteristic

- Verbalization of inadequate knowledge

Nursing Interventions

- Carefully explain all interventions
- Prepare child and family members for hospitalization

Expected Outcome

- Patient and family members verbalize increased knowledge related to patient's condition and treatment

Management

Treatment of ARF is directed toward the etiology, management of any complications, and supportive therapy. An important part of treatment of ARF is early detection so that fluid overload can be prevented and drug and potassium accumulation can be minimized (Kennedy, 1992). If dehydration exists and has caused inadequate perfusion, volume replacement by intravenous therapy is essential. A Foley catheter should be inserted immediately upon diagnosis to collect urine for analysis and to accurately measure output. Urine output should be measured hourly. If oliguria exists in the presence of adequate hydration, a rapid-acting diuretic may be administered while the patient is still in the ED.

Hyperkalemia, the most life-threatening condition in ARF, must be corrected immediately if concentrations are in excess of 7.0 mEq/L. Careful cardiac monitoring is necessary because of the risk of arrhythmias associated with hyperkalemia. A prolonged QRS complex, depressed ST segment, high-peaked T waves, bradycardia, or heart block may occur with hyperkalemia.

In patients with a normal ECG, the effects of hyperkalemia may need to be corrected with sodium polystyrene sulfonate, 1 g resin/kg dose every 4–6 hours orally or rectally, to bind potassium and remove it from the body. A patient with an abnormal ECG should receive calcium chloride 10%, 10–25 mg/kg/dose (maximum 500 mg) intravenously over 10 minutes, while being monitored for bradycardia.

Nursing care for an infant or child with ARF includes precise measurement of intake and output and careful monitoring of all vital signs. Hypertension may occur in ARF because of overexpansion of extracellular fluid volume. An antihypertensive agent such as hydralazine may be ordered. Fluids and sodium are restricted in patients with hypertension. Children with ARF require dialysis when there is severe fluid overload that does not respond to diuretic therapy. The patient must be observed continuously for signs of congestive heart failure. The child's neurologic status should be closely monitored for changes in mental status or seizure activity.

Patient and Family Teaching and Psychosocial Support

The child and parents need a great deal of support. All diagnostic procedures and treatments should be explained carefully. The parents need to be kept informed of the child's condition and should be allowed to be at the child's bedside as much as possible. The child and family need preparation for admission to a pediatric intensive care unit for close monitoring.

REFERENCES

Combest FE (1992). Epididymitis. In Barkin RM (ed), *Pediatric emergency medicine.* St. Louis: Mosby, pp 1050–1051

Dagan R, Einhorn M, Lang R, et al (1992). Once daily cefixime compared with twice daily trimethoprim/sulfamethoxazole for treatment of urinary tract infection in infants and children. *Pediatric Infectious Diseases Journal* 11:198–203

Feld LG (1991). Urinary tract infections in childhood: Definition, pathogenesis, diagnosis, and management. *Pharmacotherapy* 11:326

Fontanarosa PM, Hellman J (1991). Pediatric genitourinary emergencies. *Topics in Emergency Medicine* 13:84–92

Hertz AL (1992). Urinary tract infection. In Barkin RM (ed), *Pediatric emergency medicine.* St. Louis: Mosby, pp 1070–1074

Kennedy J (1992). Renal disorders. In Hazinski MF (ed.), *Nursing care of the critically ill child* (2nd ed). St. Louis: Mosby, pp 629–713

Knepper JG (1992). Poststreptococcal glomerulonephritis, acute. In Barkin RM (ed), *Pediatric emergency medicine.* St. Louis: Mosby, pp 1068–1069

McCracken G (1989). Options in antimicrobial management of urinary tract infections in infants and children. *Pediatric Infectious Disease Journal* 8:522–555

McDonald FW (1992). Paraphimosis. In Reece RM (ed), *Manual of emergency pediatrics* (3rd ed). Philadelphia: Saunders, pp 1058–1059

Shapiro ED (1992). Infections of the urinary tract. *Pediatric Infectious Diseases Journal* 11:165–168

Tonetti JA, Tonetti FW (1990). Testicular torsion or acute epididymitis? Diagnosis and treatment. *Journal of Emergency Nursing* 16:96–98

Wilson D, and Killion D (1989). Urinary tract infections in the pediatric patient. *Nurse Practitioner* 14:38–42

CHAPTER 29

Seizure Emergencies and Disorders

SUSAN J. KELLEY

INTRODUCTION

Seizure disorders are among the most frequently encountered neurologic emergencies in childhood. About 1 child in 15 has at least one seizure in the first 7 years of life (Oppenheimer and Rosman, 1992). Seizures can occur in a wide variety of conditions involving the central nervous system (CNS) and are a symptom of an underlying CNS disorder.

A seizure is a paroxysmal involuntary disturbance of brain function that may be manifested as an impairment of or loss of consciousness, abnormal motor activity, behavioral abnormalities, sensory disturbances, or autonomic dysfunction (Haslam, 1992).

Etiology

Seizure disorders have numerous and varied causes. Seizure disorders are diagnosed as idiopathic if the cause is unknown and as organic or symptomatic if the cause was acquired and therefore identifiable. Most seizure disorders are idiopathic. Idiopathic epilepsy is usually familial, with possible genetic factors that lower the seizure threshold. A seizure disorder also may be acquired as a result of perinatal injuries, birth trauma, head trauma, hypoxia, CNS infections, acute cerebral edema, occupying lesions in the brain, metabolic disorders, endogenous or exogenous toxins, and a variety of other causes. Substances that can cause seizures include amphetamines, cyclic antidepressants, overdosed anticonvulsants, carbon monoxide, cocaine, cyanide, insulin, lead, nicotine, and theophyline (Tunik and Young, 1992). Table 29–1 summarizes the specific causes of seizures by age of onset.

Pathophysiology

Seizures result from abnormal electrical discharges initiated by a group of hyperexcitable cells that may arise from central areas in the brain that affect consciousness immediately; may be restricted to one area of the cerebral cortex, producing manifestations characteristic of the particular anatomic focus; or may begin in a localized area of the cortex and spread to other positions of the brain, which may produce generalized neurologic manifestations. During a seizure there is an increase of oxygen and glucose consumption, cerebral blood flow (CBF), and carbon dioxide, lactic acid, and pyruvate production.

TYPES OF SEIZURES

Children are brought to the ED with many types of seizures. Seizures are classified into two categories: partial (focal or local) and generalized. Generalized seizures, which involve all parts or large parts of the cerebral cortex, include tonic-clonic (grand mal), petit mal, atonic, and myoclonic seizures.

Partial seizures, which arise in one part of the brain, include motor, sensory, autonomic, and psychomotor seizures. Partial seizures are further classified into simple (no loss of consciousness) and complex (an impairment of consciousness). Partial seizures can evolve into generalized seizures, especially in patients not taking anticonvulsant medications.

Other types of seizures seen in the ED include neonatal seizures and febrile seizures.

Rapid identification of the cause and type of sei-

TABLE 29–1. SEIZURES: CAUSE BY AGE OF ONSET

- ■ **FIRST MONTH OF LIFE**

    - ■ FIRST DAY
        Hypoxia
        Drugs
        Trauma
        Infection
        Hyperglycemia
        Hypoglycemia
        Pyridoxine deficiency

    - ■ DAYS 2–3
        Infection
        Drug withdrawal
        Hypoglycemia
        Hypocalcemia
        Developmental malformation
        Intracranial hemorrhage
        Inborn error of metabolism
        Hyponatremia or hypernatremia

    - ■ DAY 4 AND BEYOND
        Infection
        Hypocalcemia
        Hyperphosphatemia
        Hyponatremia
        Developmental malformation
        Drug withdrawal
        Inborn error of metabolism

- ■ **1–6 MONTHS**
    As above

- ■ **6 MONTHS–3 YEARS**
    Febrile seizures
    Birth injury
    Infection
    Toxin
    Trauma
    Metabolic disorder
    Cerebral degenerative disease

- ■ **OLDER THAN 3 YEARS**
    Idiopathic
    Infection
    Trauma
    Cerebral degenerative disease

(From Fuchs S [1992]. Seizures. In Barkin RM [ed], Pediatric emergency medicine. St. Louis: Mosby, p 925)

zure activity is critical to immediate and appropriate intervention. Brief seizures rarely produce lasting neurologic damage. Prolonged and serial seizures, however, especially statis epilepticus, can be life-threatening and may be associated with permanent neurologic damage.

Generalized Seizures

Tonic-Clonic Seizures. Generalized tonic-clonic (grand mal) seizures can occur at any age and may be focal or generalized. A patient with focal seizures is usually conscious, whereas a patient with generalized seizures is unconscious. These are the most common and dramatic of all seizure manifestations in children. Generalized tonic-clonic seizures often occur without warning; however, 20–30% of children may experience a sensory or motor aura. This type of seizure may involve an immediate loss of consciousness, falling to the ground, dilated pupils, eye deviation upward or outward, and a tonic phase lasting 10–30 seconds. The tonic rigidity is then followed by a clonic phase with violent jerking movements of the extremities. It is often associated with incontinence of urine or stool. This phase may last anywhere from 30 seconds to 30 minutes, followed by a postictal state in which the child may remain semiconscious or unconscious for anywhere from a few minutes to several hours. On awakening from the postictal state, the child may be disoriented, with ataxia and impaired speech. The child usually has no recollection of the seizure.

Absence Seizures. Absence (petit mal) seizures are associated with very brief losses of consciousness, which may or may not be accompanied by minor motor manifestations, such as staring or blinking, and often go unrecognized. No postictal state follows the seizure. The age of onset of absence seizures is abrupt, usually between 5 and 9 years. There may be associated automatisms, such as lip smacking, twitching of the face, and blinking of eyelids, or slight hand movements. Absence seizures are often mistaken for inattentiveness or day-dreaming and may lead to behavioral or learning difficulties.

Atonic Seizures. Atonic, or akinetic, seizures are manifested as a sudden, momentary loss of muscle tone and posture control causing the child to collapse or drop to the floor. For children who are sitting, a seizure is manifested by a sudden dropping forward of the head. These seizures may occur at any age but are unusual before 18 months of age.

Infantile Spasms. Infantile spasms occur most commonly between 4 and 8 months of age. In one-third of patients no cause can be identified. In the other two-thirds the seizures are the result of a definable brain disease. Perinatal causes are most common. Infantile spasms usually consist of a series of sudden, brief, symmetric contractions during which the head is flexed, the arms and legs are extended, and the hips are flexed. The eyes may roll upward or inward. The seizure is often preceded by a cry. There may or may not be loss of consciousness and change in color. These seizures tend to occur in a series and as often as several hundred times a day.

Infants who come to the ED with a history consistent with infantile spasms but who have not had their disorder diagnosed are usually admitted for a complete neurologic evaluation. Long-term treatment of infantile spasms includes intramuscular corticotropin (ACTH) or oral steroids. In the ED, immediate control is best achieved by intravenous diazepam (Oppenheimer and Rosman, 1992).

The prognosis for normal intellectual development is poor. Many patients with infantile spasms ultimately are mentally deficient, and about 50% have another form of seizure, most frequently generalized tonic-clonic seizures.

Partial Seizures

Complex Partial Seizures. Complex partial (psychomotor) seizures usually manifest as semipurposeful but inappropriate repetitive movements. Complex partial seizures are often associated with an altered state of consciousness and automatisms. The automatisms may include lip smacking, eye blinking, and purposeless hand or body movements. Complex partial seizures are often preceded by an aura that is sensory (visual, auditory, or olfactory). Although the child does not lose consciousness during the seizure, he or she does not remember the seizure. Postictal confusion or sleep may follow the seizure. Complex partial seizures are associated with focal lesions of the temporal lobe and are therefore often referred to as temporal lobe seizures.

Neonatal Seizures. Neonatal seizures occur during the first month of life, most occurring in the first 2 days. Neonatal seizures may be caused by perinatal anoxia or trauma, metabolic disorders, acute infectious processes, or drug withdrawal. Seizures in neonates often are subtle, and therefore are difficult to recognize (Ballweg, 1991). Subtle seizure activity in neonates may include repeated blinking or fluttering of the eyelids, staring episodes, clonic movements of the chin, tonic horizontal eye deviations, vertical deviation of the eyes, repetitive sucking or puckering, tongue protrusion, drooling, and tonic posturing of a single limb (Ballweg, 1991).

Febrile Seizures. Febrile seizures are divided into two categories: simple and complex. Simple febrile seizures are brief, lasting from 10–15 minutes, and are generalized. Complex febrile seizures are prolonged and may have focal features.

Simple febrile seizures usually occur between the ages of 3 months and 5 years in previously well children and within the first 24 hours of a febrile illness. There is often a positive family history for febrile seizures and a negative family history for other types of seizure disorders. Approximately 5% of all children experience a febrile seizure by the age of 5 years. In most cases the seizure occurred at home and has ceased on arrival in the ED. The child usually presents in a postictal state that lessens during the stay in the ED.

Febrile seizures are associated with an acute, benign febrile illness. Children with one simple febrile seizure have a 30% chance of having a second febrile seizure. The rate of recurrence appears to depend on the age at the time of the first febrile seizure. The younger the patient at the time of the first febrile seizure the greater is the chance for recurrence. Fifty percent of recurrences take place within the first year. Children normally have a convulsive threshold that is high enough to suppress excessive neuronal discharges. Febrile seizures occur when a febrile illness lowers the convulsive threshold temporarily.

If a child continues to have seizures in the ED, intravenous diazepam is usually given.

Clinical Entities Simulating Seizures

Numerous clinical entities must be differentiated from seizures. A careful history differentiates among seizure-like episodes (Fuchs, 1992). In children, seizure-like episodes include breathholding spells, night tremors and terrors, migraine headaches, and tics (Fuchs, 1992). In adolescents, clinical entities that may simulate seizures include hyperventilation, hysteria, syncope, pseudoseizures, and orthostatic hypotension (Fuchs, 1992).

Status Epilepticus

In most brief, self-limiting seizures, the seizure activity has ceased before the patient arrives in the ED, since, by definition, these seizures last less than 15 minutes. A child having an active seizure in the ED is usually in a state of prolonged or serial seizure activity.

Status epilepticus is a state of continual seizure activity lasting more than 30 minutes or a series of shorter seizures occurring repetitively, so that recovery between seizures is incomplete. It is estimated that 3–10% of children with seizure disorders experience at least one episode of status epilepticus (Oppenheimer and Rosman, 1992).

Status epilepticus may be caused by inadequate anticonvulsant therapy that occurs with a rapid or sudden withdrawal of anticonvulsants; CNS infections, head trauma; metabolic disturbances; or ingestion of a toxic substance. The precipitant must be identified early in the course of treatment. A careful history and evaluation are critical.

A patient in status epilepticus presents with continual seizure activity that is usually generalized and bilaterally symmetric or, occasionally, unilateral. The patient is generally unresponsive and has increased secretions and depressed respirations. Status epilepticus is followed by a postictal state of relative mental and motor impairment.

ASSESSMENT

History

A rapid but thorough history should be obtained from the parents or caretaker. A history of a known seizure disorder, febrile illness, ingestion of a toxic substance, lead poisoning, or recent head trauma should be sought. If a past history of a seizure disorder exists, a careful medication history should be obtained. Many parents are reluctant to admit that they discontinued anticonvulsant therapy against their physician's orders, missed doses, or ran out of medication. This information should be carefully elicited. Parents should be asked to describe the child's activity before the onset of the seizure. A careful description of the onset, type, and duration of seizure activity should be obtained. Other important information to be obtained includes any problems in the prenatal or perinatal period and any history of developmental delay. A family history of seizure disorders should be ascertained.

If the seizure has stopped before arrival in the ED, the following information should be obtained from the parents: child's activity before the onset of the seizure; child's color; eye movements; description of movements of the extremities; history of incontinence; length and pattern of seizure activity; and child's level of responsiveness during and immediately after the seizure.

When obtaining the history from the parents, the nurse must keep in mind how frightening it may have been for them to witness this seizure. Parents often overestimate the duration of the seizure because of their fear and anxiety at the time of occurrence. A careful history and assessment help differentiate between a simple febrile seizure, a generalized seizure with increased temperature due to increased muscle activity, meningitis, and encephalitis. Identification of infants with meningitis or encephalitis can be most difficult. A infant with meningitis or encephalitis may have a recent history of irritability, a high-pitched cry, poor feeding, fever, and vomiting. With children 1–5 years of age with meningitis or encephalitis, there may be a preceding history of headache, nuchal rigidity, and vomiting. Lethargy observed in the ED can be the result of a postictal state or the presence of meningitis or encephalitis.

Physical Assessment

The patient's airway, breathing, and circulation (ABCs) should be rapidly and continually assessed. The respi-

rations of a patient who is having an active seizure are irregular, and their rate is lower than normal. The respirations of a patient in the postictal state are often shallow.

Vital signs should be carefully monitored. Blood pressure and heart rate may increase during a seizure. Anticonvulsant therapy can cause hypotension, cardiac arrhythmias, and apnea. A cardiac monitor and oxygen saturation monitor should be placed on all patients in status epilepticus. The patient's temperature should be carefully monitored throughout the seizure. Increased muscle activity during a prolonged seizure may cause an increase in body temperature.

All seizure characteristics should be carefully observed and recorded. Movements of the extremities, trunk, head, face, and eyes should be described. The length of all seizures should be timed carefully. The patient's level of consciousness, pupillary response, and purposeful movements should be assessed continually, and signs of increased intracranial pressure (ICP) should be monitored.

Level of consciousness and purposeful movements of the extremities should be observed. Pupil size and reaction to light should be noted. The child should be carefully examined for evidence of head trauma, even in the absence of a history of trauma. The skin should be examined for petechiae or purpura, which is often seen in meningitis or septicemia, and for the hypopigmented macules seen in tuberous sclerosis. The anterior and posterior fontanelles in infants should be evaluated for fullness or bulging. The termination of the seizure should be described, as should the postictal level of consciousness and any purposeful movements. The length and depth of postictal sleep should be recorded. The nurse should check to see if the patient is wearing a medical alert bracelet or has a medical identification card. Needle marks could indicate the patient has diabetes or, if an adolescent, uses intravenous drugs.

Laboratory and Diagnostic Tests

Some or all of these tests may be indicated on the basis of the history, previously diagnosed seizure disorder, and physical findings.

Lumbar Puncture. A lumbar puncture should be performed as soon as possible on all infants and children who present with a first-time history of a seizure to rule out the presence of meningitis or encephalitis, increased ICP, or intracranial bleeding.

Complete Blood Count. A complete blood count (CBC) should be done to rule out an acute bacterial infection or sepsis. An increase in leukocytes (more than 10,000/mm³) may be found as a response to the stress of the seizure and does not necessarily imply the presence of an infection. Anemia may be seen with lead poisoning, sickle cell anemia, and leukemia, each of which may be associated with seizures.

Blood Culture. A blood culture should be obtained to rule out sepsis or bacteremia.

Urine Culture and Urinalysis. Urinary tract infections are a common cause of hyperthermia in children. A suprapubic bladder tap may be performed to obtain a sterile urine culture in infants.

Toxic Screen. Toxic screens (serum, gastric contents, and urine) should be done to rule out the possibility of an ingestion or lead poisoning in a child without a previously diagnosed seizure disorder.

Anticonvulsant Levels. If the child has a known seizure disorder and is receiving medication, levels of anticonvulsant medications should be measured.

Serum Electrolytes. Serum glucose, sodium, potassium, calcium, phosphorus, magnesium, and blood urea nitrogen (BUN) levels should be obtained. A reagent strip provides a rapid glucose value.

Radiography. X rays of the skull may be indicated if a history of trauma is suspected. Evidence of a chronically raised ICP may be seen. Computed tomography (CT) may be performed to assess an acutely ill child.

TRIAGE
Seizures

Emergent
A child with active seizures; history of head trauma; suspected meningitis; decreased level of consciousness.

Urgent
A child with known seizure disorder but alert and stable; fever; previous history of febrile seizure but alert and stable.

Nursing Diagnosis
Ineffective Airway Clearance

Defining Characteristics

- Abnormal breath sounds
- Increased secretions

Nursing Interventions

- Continually assess and support child's airway
- Insert oropharyngeal airway in unconscious child
- Suction oropharyngeal cavity to clear secretions
- Remove or loosen any clothing around child's neck

Expected Outcome

- Airway remains patent

Nursing Diagnosis
Altered Tissue Perfusion (Cerebral)

Defining Characteristics

- Decreased level of consciousness
- Pupils nonreactive or slow to react to light

Nursing Interventions

- Continually assess child's neurologic status
- Administer humidified oxygen
- Hyperventilate patient if there is evidence of increased ICP
- Insert intravenous line
- Administer anticonvulsant as ordered
- Restrict intravenous fluid volume to prevent increased ICP

Expected Outcomes

- Seizure activity ceases
- Child's pupils remain reactive and are of a normal size
- Child regains consciousness after seizure and postictal period
- Fluid intake and output are carefully measured and recorded

Nursing Diagnosis
Impaired Gas Exchange

Defining Characteristics

- Hypoxia
- Irritability

Nursing Interventions

- Assess child's color and capillary refill
- Administer humidified oxygen through face mask
- Assist in endotracheal intubation if necessary
- Provide artificial ventilations if necessary
- Continually assess vital signs

Expected Outcomes

- Arterial blood gases remain within normal range

- Child's color remains normal
- Capillary refill is normal
- Vital signs remain stable

Nursing Diagnosis
High Risk for Injury

Defining Characteristics

- Involuntary muscle activity
- Altered consciousness

Nursing Intervention

- Prevent child from striking head or extremities during seizure activity by placing padding around side rails

Expected Outcome

- Child remains free from injury during seizure

Nursing Diagnosis
Knowledge Deficit (Parental)

Defining Characteristics

- Inadequate follow-through on anticonvulsant therapy
- Verbalization of inadequate knowledge

Nursing Interventions

- Continually inform parents of child's condition and all procedures
- Instruct parents on how to care for their child during a seizure
- Instruct parents on proper administration of medication
- Teach parents methods for fever control
- Emphasize to parents the importance of regular visits to the child's primary care provider or neurologist for ongoing management of the seizure disorder

Expected Outcomes

- Parents demonstrate understanding of child's condition and all procedures
- Parents demonstrate an understanding of safety precautions to be taken during a seizure
- Parents administer medications properly
- Parents demonstrate awareness of fever control
- Parents attend regular visits to primary care provider

Management

ABCs. The airway, breathing, and circulation should be assessed rapidly and supported. Table 29–2 sum-

TABLE 29–2. PRIORITIES IN THE EMERGENCY NURSING CARE OF A CHILD IN STATUS EPILEPTICUS

Establish patent airway
    Suction judiciously
    Position to open airway
Support breathing
    Administer 100% oxygen by face mask
    Use bag valve-mask for assisted ventilation
    Prepare for intubation
Monitor circulation
    Take frequent vital signs
    Perform pulse oximetry
    Use cardiorespiratory monitor
Establish vascular access
    Start intravenous lines
    Start intraosseous access
    Start central venous access
Insert nasogastric tube
Administer anticonvulsants
Monitor neurologic status
Provide thermoregulation

marizes the nurse's priorities in care of the child in status epilepticus. A patent airway and adequate ventilation are established and maintained. An oropharyngeal airway should be inserted, and secretions should be suctioned judiciously. Clothing around the neck should be loosened. Oxygen (100% by face mask) should be administered to prevent hypoxic damage to the CNS. Apnea or depressed respirations may occur. Assisted ventilation by bag-valve-mask or endotracheal intubation may be necessary. Equipment for intubation should be readily available at the bedside. A cardiorespiratory monitor, pulse oximeter, and end tidal CO_2 monitor should be used.

The child should be placed in a semiprone position, and a nasogastric tube should be inserted to decompress the stomach and minimize the danger of aspiration.

Protecting the Patient. All body parts, particularly the head, should be carefully protected during a seizure. The extremities should never be restrained or held down because a fracture could result. All side rails of the bed should be padded.

Thermoregulation. The patient's temperature is taken every 15 minutes. Acetaminophen is administered orally only if the patient is totally alert; it is given rectally if the patient is having a seizure or is in the postictal state. All clothing should be removed immediately to allow release of body heat through the skin. A tepid sponge bath should be given if the patient's condition is stable. Alcohol should never be used in sponge baths because it is rapidly absorbed through the skin and can be toxic and even cause death.

TABLE 29–3. ANTICONVULSANT DRUGS USED TO TREAT STATUS EPILEPTICUS

Drug	Dosage	Administration	Special Nursing Concerns	Advantages	Disadvantages
Phenobarbital	15–20 mg/kg Maximum: 300 mg	30–100 mg/minute IV or IM	May produce sedation, respiratory, and cardiovascular depression. Vital signs must be closely monitored	Produces prolonged anticonvulsant effect due to long half-life (40–80 hours)	Effective brain concentrations are achieved slowly (20–60 minutes)
Diazepam	0.2–0.5 mg/kg Maximum: 2–4 mg for infants; 5–10 mg for older children May be repeated in 15–30 minutes × 3 Do not dilute in intravenous solution	At a rate of 1 mg/minute IV	May cause respiratory depression or arrest. Ambu bag and facial mask should be readily available Pulse oximeter should be used to monitor oxygen saturation	Very effective in status epilepticus. Can stop seizure activity in seconds	Anticonvulsant effect is poorly sustained because of short half-life (30–60 minutes). A second longer-acting anticonvulsant is usually required
Phenytoin	18–20 mg/kg Maximum: 1 g Begin maintenance in 12 hours	25–50 mg/minute IV; line must be flushed with normal saline solution before and after injection, or precipitation of drug will occur	May cause cardiac arrythmias. Cardiac monitor must be used. Observe for allergic reactions	Effective in about 80% of patients with status epilepticus; penetrates the brain rapidly and stops the seizures in 5–30 minutes	Can precipitate cardiac arrhythmias
Paraldehyde	0.1–0.25 ml/kg Maximum: 7 ml/dose May be repeated in 1 hour and then every 2–4 hours	Usually given per rectum through rectal tube. May be given through nasogastric tube, IM, or IV	Use glass syringe. Must be mixed with equal amounts of mineral oil when given rectally. Rectal tube should be clamped and buttocks held together past administration so patient will retain medication	Generally safe	Slow onset of action
Valporic acid	20–30 mg/kg	Per rectum in retention enema	The 250 mg/mL syrup is mixed with equal amounts of water	Generally safe	Slow absorption rate Mild gastrointestinal disturbances Liver toxicity

Intravenous Therapy. An intravenous line should be inserted as soon as possible to establish a route for anticonvulsant therapy and fluid administration. If intravenous access cannot be established, intraosseous access may be initiated. Fluid intake and output should be monitored carefully. Fluid intake should be restricted until cerebral edema has been ruled out.

Anticonvulsant Therapy. The goal of anticonvulsant therapy in status epilepticus and other forms of seizure activity is the prompt cessation of seizure activity without respiratory or cardiovascular depression. Children should be connected to a cardiac monitor and oxygen saturation monitor before anticonvulsant drugs are administered. A number of anticonvulsant drugs are currently used for status epilepticus, each with its own advantages and disadvantages. These drugs and their proper dosages, routes, advantages, disadvantages, and special nursing concerns are listed in Table 29–3. Intravenous anticonvulsants should not be given as a continuous intravenous infusion and should be diluted with normal saline (Thomas, 1991). Anticonvulsant therapies for other types of seizure disorders are listed in Table 29–4. Monotherapy, or treatment

TABLE 29–4. ANTICONVULSANT THERAPY FOR VARIOUS TYPES OF SEIZURES

Type of Seizure	Drug	Acute Treatment	Administration	Special Nursing Concerns
Neonatal Seizures				
Metabolic cause	Glucose 10%	2 ml/kg	IV	Measure blood glucose level before and after administration
	Calcium gluconate 5%	4 ml/kg	IV	May cause bradycardia and hypotension
	Magnesium sulfate 50%	0.2 ml/kg	IM	May cause respiratory and cardiovascular depression
Varied cause	Phenobarbital	20 mg/kg	IV	May produce respiratory and cardiovascular depression
	Phenytoin	20 mg/kg	IV slow push	May cause cardiac arrhythmias. Cardiac monitor necessary
	Diazepam	0.2–0.3 mg/kg	IV slow push, rectal	May cause respiratory depression or arrest
	Lorazepam	0.05–0.1 mg/kg	IV	
Absence seizures	Ethosuximide	20 mg/kg/24 hours	po	May cause abdominal discomfort, rash
Complex partial seizures	Phenobarbital	2–5 mg/kg/24 hours	IV slow push, IM, or po	May produce cardiovascular or respiratory depression when given IV; lethargy
Atonic and myoclonic seizures	Clonazepam	0.01–0.2 mg/kg/24 hours	po	May cause respiratory depression or arrest
	Valproate	15–60 mg/kg/24 hours	po	May cause drowsiness, hepatoxicity
Generalized tonic-clonic seizures (grand mal)	Phenobarbital or	3–5 mg/kg	IV slow push or IM	May produce cardiovascular or respiratory depression *Never give diazepam and phenobarbital together*
	Diazepam or	0.2–0.3 mg/kg	IV slow push	Can cause drowsiness, blurred vision, rashes, blood dyscrasias
	Carbamazepine	10–30 mg/kg/day	po	

with a single drug, should be used on an outpatient basis when possible to increase compliance and decrease adverse effects and drug interactions (Sagraves, 1990).

Barbituate Coma. If status epilepticus is unresponsive to the drug treatment described in Table 29–3, the patient may be admitted to an intensive care unit for control of status epilepticus by administration of barbituates such as phenobarbitol or thiopental sodium to induce coma (Hazinski, 1992).

Disposition. Whether the patient is admitted to the hospital or discharged home depends on the patient's history, laboratory findings, and physical findings. Children with first-time febrile seizures are often admitted to the hospital for further observation and diagnostic testing. Children with previously undiagnosed afebrile generalized seizures are often admitted for further evaluation and anticonvulsant therapy. Children with previously diagnosed seizure disorders whose condition has stabilized are often discharged home with a referral to their neurologist.

Patient and Family Teaching and Psychosocial Support

Parents are often extremely distressed by the occurrence of a seizure in their child, especially a first-time seizure. They often fear their child is dying and feel helpless. Parents of a child with seizures should be informed that it is rare for a child to die during a seizure (Killam, 1992). Parents need to be instructed to never leave their child unattended in the bathtub or while swimming. Older children can be encouraged to take showers (Killam, 1992). Parents should be taught never to attempt giving medicine orally to a child who is having a seizure or is unconscious.

Parents should be taught to observe their child carefully during seizures so that they can accurately describe the seizure activity to the nurse and physician. Parents can be instructed to look at a watch or clock as soon as possible after a seizure starts so they can time it accurately and have a clearer idea of whether or not they should seek emergency treatment (Killam, 1992). Parents should seek emergency care if a seizure lasts more than 5–10 minutes.

Parents should be informed that generalized

tonic-clonic seizures are painless and that because of loss of consciousness at the onset of the seizure, children often have no memory of the seizure (Killam, 1992). Parents should be taught that a change in the respiratory pattern or a brief cessation of respirations is considered a normal part of a generalized tonic-clonic seizure (Killam, 1992). If respirations do not resume after a seizure, it could indicate the presence of a foreign body.

Teaching should include proper administration of medication and signs of drug reactions or toxicity. Parents need to be cautioned of the dangers of abrupt discontinuation of medicine. Protecting the child, especially his or her head, during subsequent seizures should be emphasized. Parents need to be told that it is impossible to "swallow a tongue." They should be instructed never to place an object or fingers into a child's mouth during a seizure. Instead they should be instructed to place the child in a side-lying position with the child's head turned to the side to prevent aspiration. If a fever is associated with the onset of seizures, fever control should be taught.

REFERENCES

Ballweg DD (1991). Neonatal seizures: An overview. *Neonatal Network* 10:15–21

Fuchs S (1992). Seizures. In Barkin RM (ed), *Pediatric emergency medicine.* St. Louis: Mosby, pp 923–930

Haslam RHA (1992). Seizures in childhood. In Behrman RE (ed), *Textbook of pediatrics* (14th ed). Philadelphia: Saunders, pp 1491–1506

Hazinski MF (1992). *Neurologic disorders.* In Hazinski MF (ed), *Nursing care of the critically ill child* (2nd ed). St. Louis: Mosby, pp 521–628

Killam P (1992). Childhood epilepsy: Myth vs. reality. *American Journal of Nursing* 92:77–82

Oppenheimer EY, Rosman NP (1992). Recurring seizures. In Reece RM (ed), *Manual of emergency pediatrics* (4th ed). Philadelphia: Saunders, pp 105–111

Sagraves R (1990). Antiepileptic drug therapy for pediatric generalized tonic-clonic seizures. *Journal of Pediatric Health Care* 4:314–319

Thomas DO (1991). Seizures. In Thomas DO (ed), *Handbook of pediatric emergency nursing.* Gaithersburg, Md: Aspen, pp 153–159

Tunik MG, Young GM (1992). Status epilepticus in children: The acute management. *Pediatric Clinics of North America* 39:1007–1030

CHAPTER 30

Care of the Pediatric Organ Transplant Recipient

LISA MARIE BERNARDO
MARIANNE BOVE

INTRODUCTION

Organ transplantation is an accepted treatment for children suffering from end-stage organ disease. The most commonly transplanted organs in children are the heart, liver, and kidney. Heart-lung, heart-liver, intestinal, and multivisceral transplants have been performed. Nearly 350 children receive liver transplants each year in the US (Whitington et al, 1993); approximately 100 children receive heart transplants (Kriett and Kaye, 1990); and approximately 400 children receive kidneys (McEnery et al, 1992).

With the advent of immunosuppressive agents such as cyclosporine A and FK 506 more children are surviving the transplant experience and are returning to their homes. Therefore, it is likely that these children will present to emergency departments (EDs) for treatment that may or may not be related to their transplanted organ. This chapter outlines the indications for organ transplantation, the operative procedures, and the emergency nursing care of a child with an organ transplant.

INDICATIONS FOR ORGAN TRANSPLANTATION

The two most common indications for liver transplantation in children are biliary atresia and metabolic liver disease, the most common being alpha-1-antitrypsin deficiency (Whitington et al, 1993). End stage renal disease is the indication for renal transplantation, congenital renal disease (renal hypoplasia, renal dysplasia and obstructive uropathy) being seen most commonly in children younger than 5 years (Castillo, 1992). Among older children, hereditary, metabolic, or acquired renal diseases occur most frequently (Castillo, 1992). Candidates for renal transplants must have adequate urologic functioning. Pretransplant preparatory operations may be needed to correct any underlying abnormalities (Perez-Woods et al, 1991).

Two indications for heart transplantation are dilated cardiomyopathy and congenital heart disease not amenable to conventional treatment (Perez-Woods et al, 1991). These children become candidates for transplantation if death is expected in 6–12 months and if no other medical or surgical modalities are appropriate (Perez-Woods et al, 1991). Although infants born with hypoplastic left heart syndrome do receive palliative surgical correction, transplantation may afford an improved outcome and less morbidity (Perez-Woods et al, 1991).

SURGICAL CONSIDERATIONS

Understanding how organs are transplanted assists emergency nurses in interpreting a child's physical findings. The surgical procedure for orthotopic (placing the organ in its correct anatomic position) liver transplantation is performed through bilateral subcostal incisions with midline extension and removal of the xiphoid process (Staschak and Zamberlan, 1990). The recipient's liver is removed, and the donor liver is transplanted and anastomosed to the hepatic artery, portal vein and supra- and infrahepatic vena cavae. In

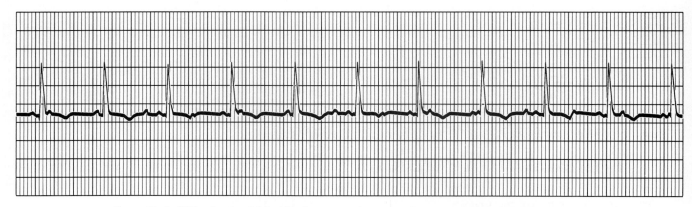

Figure 30–1. ECG strip of a child with a heart transplant. Note the presence of the two P waves.

a child with biliary artresia, in which the bile ducts are absent, the donor common bile duct is anastomosed to a Roux-en-Y limb of jejunum (Staschak and Zamberlan, 1990). A cholecystectomy is performed on the donor liver (Corbo-Richert and Zamberlan, 1992).

For orthotopic heart transplantation, a sternotomy is performed, and the recipient is placed on cardiac bypass. The heart is removed except for part of the right atrium, to which the donor heart is attached (Lynn Cipriani, personal communication, 1993). The donor heart is then anastomosed to the pulmonary vessels and aorta.

Because the native right atrium retains its sinoatrial (SA) node, the child's electrocardiogram (ECG) demonstrates two P waves (Figure 30–1). Furthermore, because the donor heart is denervated, these recipients may never or rarely experience angina pectoris, even if severe occlusive coronary artery disease is present (Gao et al, 1989). Before transplantation, a child with cardiomyopathy may have a heart the size of a cantaloupe; after transplantation, the extra space around the normal-sized donor heart allows the lungs to inflate properly in the chest cavity (Lynn Cipriani, personal communication, 1993).

Renal transplants differ from liver and heart transplants in three respects: a live, related donor may be used; the transplant may not be orthotopic; and the native kidneys are not removed. The native kidneys are usually not removed because they may continue to produce urine, and the anemia associated with chronic renal failure is more severe after bilateral nephrectomies (Ramos et al, 1991). For renal transplantation, a large flank-abdominal incision is made. Two approaches to transplantation are possible. The first approach, in which the donor kidney is attached to the iliac vessels, is used when the donor kidney fits into

the iliac fossa (Perez-Woods et al, 1991). The second approach—graft implantation onto the recipient's aorta and vena cava—is undertaken when the donor kidney is from an adult or large child (Perez-Woods et al, 1991).

The donor kidney may be palpated in the upper outer abdominal quadrants, where it is afforded little protection. This placement makes it vulnerable to injury. In kidney and liver recipients, incidental appendectomies are not usually performed; therefore, it is possible for the child to have appendicitis at some point in time (Corbo-Richert and Zamberlan, 1992).

IMMUNOSUPPRESSION

After the donor organ is successfully transplanted, the child is closely monitored for organ function and organ rejection. To prevent the body's rejection of the donor organ, immunosuppressive agents are administered. These agents prevent the T cells from destroying the organ.

The most common immunosuppressive agents are cyclosporine A, azathioprine, and corticosteroids. FK 506, an experimental drug, recently approved by the FDA, is also gaining popularity in pediatrics. The action, dosage, side effects and interactions of each medication are listed in Table 30–1. Other medications that these children may take include trimethoprim-sulfamethoxazole (TMP/SMX) to prevent *Pneumocyctis carinii* pneumonia (PCP), acyclovir for prophyaxis of cytomegalovirus (CMV) and Epstein-Barr virus (EBV), fluodrocortisone to prevent hyperkalemia associated with FK 506, nystatin to prevent oral fungal infections (usually seen with prednisone), and an antacid to prevent the gastric irritation associated with prednisone.

TABLE 30–1. COMMON IMMUNOSUPPRESSIVE THERAPIES

Medication	Action	Dosage	Side Effects	Interactions
Cyclosporine	Inhibits effect of inter-leukin-2 on T lympho-cytes	5–10 mg/kg per day, IV or by mouth	Nausea, vomiting, an-orexia, leukopenia, thrombocytopenia, headache, seizures	Drugs that increase cyclosporine levels: steroids, cimetidine, erythromycin; drugs that de-crease cyclosporine levels: phenytoin, phenobarbital, rifampin
Azathioprine	Inhibits RNA and DNA synthesis	1–3 mg/kg per day IV or by mouth	Bone marrow suppres-sion, megaloblastic anemia, hepatic dys-function, hair loss	Bone marrow toxicity and im-munosuppression with allo-purinol
Corticosteroids (prednisone)	Inhibit T-cell migration to sites of antigen depos-its; block lymphocyte proliferation and inter-action between mono-cytes and lymphocytes	10–15 mg/day, IV or by mouth	Increased blood pressure; cushingoid features; poor wound healing; sodium and water re-tention	—
FK 506	Suppresses T-cell medi-ated immunity	0.15 mg/kg/day, IV or by mouth	Headache, nausea, vom-iting, flushing	Increased cyclosporine concen-tration; potential for inhibition of metabolism of other drugs

Data from:

Weiskittel PD (1991). Immunosuppressive therapy. In Gaedeke Norris MK, House MA (eds), *Organ and tissue transplantation: Nursing care from procurement through rehabilitation.* Philadelphia: F. A. Davis, pp 199–221

Goto T, Kino T, Halanaka H, et al (1987). Discovery of FK 506, a novel immunosuppressant isolated from *Streptomycetes tsubaensis. Transplant Proceedings* 19[Suppl 6]:4–8

Jain AB, Fung JJ, Venkataramanan R, Todo S, Alessiani M, Starzl TE (1990). FK 506 dosage in human organ transplantation. *Transplant Proceedings* 22[Suppl 1]:23–24

Shapiro R, Fung J, Jain AB, Parks P, Todo S, Starzl TE (1990). The side effects of FK 506 in humans. *Transplant Proceedings* 22:35–36

Venkataramanan R, Jain A, Cardoff E, et al (1990). Pharmacokinetics of FK 506: Preclinical and clinical studies. *Transplant Proceedings* 22[Suppl 1]:52–56

(*From Zamberlan K, Bernardo LM, Bove M [1992]. Tips on nursing care of the pediatric organ recipient in the emergency department. Journal of Emergency Nursing 18:74–77*)

Long-term use of immunosuppressive therapy can cause hypertension and lymphoproliferative dis-ease (LPD). Hypertension is associated with cyclo-sporine. This association is unclear but is thought to be related to renal vasoconstriction induced by the cyclo-sporine (Fricker et al, 1990). Hypertension occurs in more than 70% of kidney recipients, which unfor-tunately accelerates deterioration of the donor kidney (Castillo, 1992). Captopril or nifedipine may be ad-ministered to control hypertension and may be dis-continued by 6 months after transplantation (Corbo-Richert and Zamberlan, 1992). Hypertension is not observed, however, among children taking FK 506 (Lynn Cipriani, personal communication, 1993). Be-cause of the risk of hypertension, parents are taught to measure and record their child's blood pressure at least twice daily.

Immunosuppression allows the EBV to cause lymphocytic proliferation, which can become a true lymphoma (Zitelli et al, 1991). Signs of LPD include lymphadenopathy, fever, asymmetric or marked tonsil-loadenoidal hypertrophy, and intestinal obstruction

(Zitelli et al, 1991). The diagnosis is confirmed by a lymph node biopsy (Corbo-Richert and Zamberlan, 1992). Treatment usually involves a reduction or discon-tinuation of the immunosuppressive regimen (Corbo-Richert and Zamberlan, 1992; Zitelli et al, 1991) and a 14-day course of acyclovir.

SPECIFIC EMERGENCIES RELATED TO ORGAN TRANSPLANTATION

Transplant recipients and their families may live close to the transplant center for anywhere from 2 weeks to 6 months after the operation. During this time, the child's health is monitored by the transplant center. After this time, the child and family return to their home, which may be a great distance from the trans-plant center. The child's primary health care provider may be unsure of how to treat the child should a prob-lem arise. Therefore, the child may be referred to the ED for evaluation.

In one study of pediatric and adult heart and

heart-lung recipients who presented to an ED for treatment, the most common presenting complaint was fever, followed by dyspnea, nausea, vomiting, and diarrhea, and chest pain (Sternbach et al, 1992). The final diagnoses were rule-out sepsis and rule-out rejection (Sternbach et al, 1992). These findings should alert emergency nurses to the high index of suspicion for rejection or infection in organ recipients, both of which can prove fatal.

Rejection

The child may present to the ED with organ rejection. The signs of rejection vary with the transplanted organ (Table 30–2). Specific management strategies for a child in rejection are described in the Management section.

Infection

Because of the child's immunosuppressed state, he or she is susceptible to a variety of viral, bacterial, fungal, and protozoal infections. Bacterial infections most often occur in the postoperative period. The most common viral infection is CMV. Signs of CMV are pneumonia in heart recipients and gastrointestinal symptoms (vomiting and diarrhea) in liver recipients. Other viral infections include adenovirus and EBV (Corbo-Richert and Zamberlan, 1991). Cytomegalovirus infection occurs in 60% of children who receive kidneys

TABLE 30–2. SIGNS OF REJECTION IN PEDIATRIC ORGAN RECIPIENTS

- **HEART OR HEART-LUNG RECIPIENTS**
  Fever
  Tiredness
  Decreased appetite
  Nausea
  Sudden increase in weight
  Irregular heart beat

- **LIVER RECIPIENTS**
  Fever
  Increased abdominal size
  Ascites
  Jaundice
  Clay-colored stools
  Dark urine
  Decreased appetite

- **KIDNEY RECIPIENTS**
  Fever
  Weakness
  Edema
  Decreased urine output
  Graft tenderness
  Increased blood pressure
  Irritability
  Decreased appetite

within the first year of transplantation (Castillo, 1992). Common fungal infections are by *Candida* species (Corbo-Richert and Zamberlan, 1991), whereas protozoal infections are by *Pneumocystis*. Among heart and heart-lung recipients, sinusitis, otitis, and urinary tract infections with common organisms and herpetic gingivostomatitis have been reported without serious sequelae (Fricker et al, 1990).

The signs of infection are similar to those of rejection; they include fever and malaise. Fever is a low-grade temperature of 100°F for more than 24 hours or a sudden temperature of 101°F or higher. The fever is believed to be a sign of a new infection instead of a reactivation of a prior infection (Sternbach et al, 1992). Treatment of infection is discussed in the Management section.

Children receiving maintenance doses of immunosuppressive agents should be able to ward off a common cold. However, exposure to such childhood illnesses as measles and varicella compromise the child's health (Corbo-Richert and Zamberlan, 1991). The treatment of varicella exposure is discussed in the Management section.

ASSESSMENT

History

A careful history of the child's health condition alerts the emergency nurse to the transplant recipient's needs. The emergency nurse assesses each of the following aspects of the child's health history.

History of the Current Problem. The reason for the child's ED visit is ascertained. The child may have been brought in because of a temperature spike or on the recommendation of the primary health care provider. The child's current symptoms and their duration should be assessed. This information includes the temperature reading; the amount, consistency, color and frequency of stools; and the amount and frequency of vomiting. The child's exposure to other children who may have varicella or other contagious diseases should be obtained.

Past Health History. The nurse should ascertain which organ was transplanted, when the transplant was done, and at which transplant center the operation was performed. She or he ascertain why the transplant was needed, as for a congenital or an acquired condition. The presence of a medical alert bracelet or necklace should be determined.

Current Medications. The nurse needs to determine which immunosuppressive agents the child is currently taking; they will probably be cyclosporine and prednisone. Cyclosporine is mixed with juice or milk to improve the taste and to increase absorption; it is administered twice a day, doses 12 hours apart, usually at meal or snack times. Prednisone is usually crushed and given with food or milk to decrease its irritating effect on the child's stomach (Lawrence, 1986). FK 506 is administered in capsule form and is taken twice a day by either swallowing the capsule or sprinkling the powder onto a spoonful of food. The nurse should determine if the child is taking any other medications. The medication schedule should be elicited, and the nurse should determine if any doses were missed because of vomiting. Any food or drug allergies should be noted. The parents should be asked if the child was given acetaminophen, because the child is allowed to take acetaminophen for fever or minor pain relief. Non-prescription drugs, such as aspirin, antacids, cough medicines, cold pills, and laxatives are not allowed because they can interact adversely with the immunosuppressive medications (Lawrence, 1986) or mask signs of infection.

Immunization Status. The child's immunization status is assessed. Because of the child's poor health status before transplantation, the child may not have received a complete immunization schedule. Within 3 months of transplantation, the child is usually able to resume an immunization schedule provided that minimal immunosuppression has occurred (Corbo-Richert and Zamberlan, 1992).

Immunizations may be administered to organ recipients with some modifications. Inactivated vaccines, such as diphtheria-tetanus-pertussis (DTP) and *Hemophilus influenza* type b conjugates, may be administered to appropriately-aged children (Corbo-Richert and Zamberlan, 1992; Zitelli et al, 1991). The inactivated polio vaccine (IPV), developed by Salk, is administered instead of the Sabin vaccine (Corbo-Richert and Zamberlan, 1992; Zitelli et al, 1991). The child cannot receive live-virus vaccines, such as trivalent oral polio vaccine (Sabin vaccine) and measles, mumps and rubella (MMR), because vaccine-provoked disease could occur because of the child's immunosuppressed status (Lawrence, 1986). However, MMR has been administered without adverse effects to organ recipients who live in endemic areas (Corbo-Richert and Zamberlan, 1992). Organ recipients and their families should receive yearly influenza vaccinations.

Current Health Care Provider. To assure continuity of care, the nurse should ascertain the names of the child's primary care provider and the transplant coordinator. The transplant center should be contacted to obtain specific information unique to the child, such as recent immunosuppressive drug levels. Recommendations for assessment and intervention strategies can be obtained from the transplant center.

Physical Examination

Airway. Airway patency is provided.

Breathing. Respiratory rate and rhythm are assessed. The patient is observed for chest symmetry and expansion. Any retractions or nasal flaring is noted. The anterior and posterior chest are auscultated for equality of breath sounds and for the presence of adventitious sounds. The presence of a sternal scar or chest tube scars is noted.

Circulation. An apical heart rate is obtained, and its rhythm, the presence of murmurs, and the crispness of heart sounds are noted. Capillary refill and the equality and strength of peripheral pulses are assessed. Skin color and temperature are noted. Blood pressure is measured and compared with the blood pressure measured by the parents at home. The nurse ascertains if the blood pressure is within the child's usual range.

Nervous System. The child's orientation to person, place and time, as age appropriate, are assessed. The size and equality of the pupils are noted.

Head, Eyes, Ear, Nose, Throat. The presence of facial hair is noted. The mouth is inspected for gum hyperplasia and bleeding. Any mouth ulcerations are noted. The patient is observed for otic, nasal, and eye drainage. Ear pain is assessed.

Neck. The submandibular, neck, and posterior lymph nodes are palpated, and any swelling is noted. Jugular vein distention is noted.

Abdomen. The abdomen is auscultated for bowel sounds and palpated for pain or discomfort. The margin of the liver and whether or not a transplanted kidney is palpable are noted. The patient is observed for ascites and subcostal or flank/abdominal scars. The child is asked if he or she has any difficulty voiding.

Musculoskeletal System. Weakness or tenderness is assessed.

Integumentary System. Rashes, lesions, lack of skin integrity or fragility, and hirsutism are noted. A temperature reading is obtained.

TABLE 30–3. LABORATORY AND DIAGNOSTIC TESTS

- ■ ALL RECIPIENTS
  Culture and sensitivity of blood, urine, and sputum
  Viral cultures of blood, urine, and sputum
  Viral titers
  CBC with differential and platelet count
  Electrolytes, BUN, creatinine, calcium, and glucose
  Immunosuppressive drug levels
  Venous or arterial blood gases

- ■ HEART OR HEART AND LUNG RECIPIENTS
  Cardiac enzymes
  12-lead ECG

- ■ LIVER RECIPIENTS
  Liver enzymes
  PT and PTT

- ■ KIDNEY RECIPIENTS
  Phosphate, CO_2
  Urinalysis

CBC, complete blood count; BUN, blood urea nitrogen; ECG, electrocardiogram; PT, prothrombin time; PTT, partial thromboplastin time.

Additional Assessment

After the body systems are assessed, the child is weighed. The parent is asked if the current weight is within the child's usual range. The child's and family's emotional status is assessed. Do they appear calm, distressed, anxious? Because they are used to the transplant center's methods of treatment, they may be unsure of the organization of the ED. The nurse must explain to the child and family how the particular ED operates. The patient and family should be encouraged to ask questions and to ask for assistance as needed.

Laboratory and Diagnostic Tests

Laboratory tests are listed in Table 30–3. Diagnostic tests include x rays of the chest or abdomen or both. A lumbar puncture may be indicated if the source of the fever is not found. If rejection is suspected, the diagnosis can only be made with a biopsy. The child is admitted to the hospital for the biopsy.

TRIAGE
Rejection

Emergent

A child with cardiopulmonary arrest; seizure activity; major trauma.

Urgent

A child with fever; infection; rejection; minor trauma.

Nursing Diagnosis
High Risk for Infection

Defining Characteristic

- Fever

Nursing Interventions

- Administer medications and intravenous fluids as ordered
- Obtain laboratory tests
- Monitor vital signs
- Prepare for possible admission

Expected Outcomes

- Patient's comfort increases
- Fever is controlled or lowered

Nursing Diagnosis
Noncompliance (Medication)

Defining Characteristics

- Nontherapeutic medication levels
- Verbalization of not following medication regime
- Signs of organ rejection

Nursing Interventions

- Obtain laboratory tests; assist with diagnostic testing
- Seek counseling for patient as to reasons for noncompliance
- Prepare for possible admission to hospital
- Administer medications as ordered

Expected Outcomes

- Patient will verbalize an understanding of the need for medication regimen
- Patient will verbalize an understanding of the treatment process

Management

The emergency treatment of an organ transplant recipient experiencing a condition such as cardiac or trauma arrest is treated by advanced cardiac or trauma life support measures. Some emergency care professionals may be hesitant to administer medications for fear of harming the transplanted organ. However, medications, fluids, and oxygen do not harm a transplanted organ when administered in weight-appropriate dosages (Zamberlan et al, 1992).

If the child has oral trauma that requires invasive treatment, penicillin or cephalexin may be administered. The transplant center should be contacted for specific recommendations.

Fever. A fever in an organ recipient more than 3 months after transplantation may indicate a common childhood illness (Corbo-Richert and Zamberlan, 1992). Among heart and heart-lung recipients, fever is most commonly caused by infections, usually pulmonary (Sternbach et al, 1992).

The child is taken to a treatment area for further evaluation. The appropriate laboratory tests are performed. Finding a vein for cannulation may be difficult because of the child's repeated phlebotomies during hospitalization.

Because vomiting and diarrhea can decrease absorption of cyclosporine and FK 506, the child may require intravenous hydration. If the laboratory findings show a nontherapeutic cyclosporine or FK 506 level, the child may need to be admitted to the hospital to receive the medication. Hospital admission for further testing and observation is warranted for transplant recipients whose fever source cannot be identified.

Exposure to Varicella. An organ recipient may have been exposed to varicella. Exposure means that the recipient has been in a room for 1 hour with a child who either has broken out with chicken pox or who has the lesions develop within 24 hours. These children should receive human varicella-zoster immune globulin (VZIG) within 72 hours after their exposure if they do not have a history positive for varicella (Corbo-Richert and Zamberlan, 1992; Perez-Woods et al, 1991). If varicella develops despite the VZIG, acyclovir should be administered intravenously within 24 hours of the eruption of lesions and continued for 7–10 days (McGregor et al, 1989). The immunosuppressive therapy may need to be reduced (Perez-Woods et al, 1991). The dosage of VZIG is weight-based, and the vaccine is administered intramuscularly.

Rejection. Organ rejection has been identified as one of the major concerns facing the families of organ recipients. The parents recognize the child's prior symptoms of organ rejection and may be very distraught. The child and family fear facing another bout of hospitalization and, possibly, another organ transplant.

The child is taken to a treatment area and appropriate diagnostic and laboratory tests are obtained. If rejection is suspected, the transplant center is consulted. The child may require admission to the hospital in preparation for a biopsy. The child may need a bolus of corticosteroids to treat a rejection episode. Large doses of corticosteroids are administered slowly by intravenous infusion through an infusion pump for 20–60 minutes. The child is observed for episodes of hypertension (Children's Hospital of Pittsburgh Drug Reference Manual).

Patient and Family Teaching and Psychosocial Support

For the most part, the parents are able to measure accurately the child's blood pressure and temperature. They are able to administer the immunosuppressive medications as prescribed. Furthermore, they know the signs of infection and organ rejection and the side effects of immunosuppression. The parents are usually adept at not exposing their child to ill or contagious children. The emergency nurse can ask the family if any assistance is needed in home care or if they have any questions about the care they received in the ED. If the child received a cast or sutures, follow-up care with the appropriate health professionals is arranged.

Families of organ transplant recipients are well-versed in the health care their children receive. These families may appear overbearing and may seem to direct their child's emergency care (Zamberlan et al, 1992). The organ recipient and family have been through a very emotionally trying time, which may have started at the child's birth. The child and family have worked hard to achieve a "normal" life; therefore, the following nursing interventions may make the ED visit less stressful for the child, family, and professional staff.

First, the child and family should be encouraged to talk about the child's transplant experience. Acknowledging this experience demonstrates the emergency nurse's respect for the uniqueness of the child and family. Second, the child and family should be encouraged to participate in the child's care. For example, the child should be asked about the location of the best phlebotomy site or the preferred fluid for mixing with oral cyclosporine. Pharmacologic and nonpharmacologic means of pain control are used as appropriate. The family is encouraged to ask questions, especially about the treatment process in the ED, such as laboratory waiting times. The telephone number of the transplant coordinator should be obtained from the parent in case a consultation is made. The parent is asked if he or she would like to talk with the coordinator.

Finally, the organ transplant recipient should be treated as any other child. These children have fears and hopes just like other children. They can usually resume an active lifestyle, with the exception of contact sports; they attend school and participate in extracurricular activities. Procedures should be explained at the child's level of understanding, and any fears should be acknowledged. Rejection, not only of the transplanted organ but by friends and peers, is a common feeling experienced by adolescent heart transplant recipients (Fricker and Lawrence, 1991). Their parents also fear the adolescent's organ rejection; they also worry about financial concerns and long-term postoperative care (Fricker and Lawrence, 1991). Furthermore, heart recipients cannot receive life insurance coverage (Fricker and Lawrence, 1991).

Noncompliance with the immunosuppressive therapy may become a problem for older children and adolescents who do not want to be "different" from their peers. Contraceptive choices for sexually active recipients are limited because of the medication regimen and risk of infection (Perez-Woods et al, 1991). This noncompliance can lead to organ rejection and eventually the need for retransplantation. Counseling from a health professional who understands chronically ill children and their families is warranted.

CONCLUSION

Organ transplantation and immunosuppressive therapy make it possible for children with end-stage organ disease to have a second chance at life. Although longitudinal data are not comprehensive, the short-term reported survival rates look promising. Long-term survival rates for liver recipients range from 60 to 85% (Zitelli et al, 1991). Among 30 children and adolescents who underwent heart, heart-liver, or heart-lung transplanation, 10 lived longer than 1 year after the transplant (Fricker et al, 1990). Among 754 children who underwent renal transplants, the 1-year graft survival rate was 88% for those receiving organs from living, related donors and 71% for those receiving cadaveric grafts (Castillo, 1992).

Although the child's life is saved, the quality of that child's life comes into question. While 20 school-aged children described their quality of life as good to excellent after liver transplantation, they had negative feelings about their appearance and peer relationships; they also reported feeling insecure and lonely (Zamberlan, 1988). Adolescents who received heart transplants reported feeling hopeful about their futures; they also report thinking frequently about the donors whose organs saved their lives (Fricker and Lawrence, 1991). The future for pediatric organ recipients looks promising and rewarding.

REFERENCES

Castillo J (1992). Urinary and renal disorders. In Barkin RM (ed), *Pediatric emergency medicine*. St. Louis: Mosby Year Book, pp 1034–1080

Children's Hospital of Pittsburg (1990). *Drug Reference Manual* (unpublished handbook)

Corbo-Richert B, Zamberlan KE (1992). Organ transplants. In Ludder-Jackson P, Vessey J (eds), *Primary care of the child with a chronic condition*. St. Louis: Mosby Year Book, pp 389–407.

Fricker FJ, Lawrence KS (1991). Adolescent issues in heart transplantation. *The Journal of Heart and Lung Transplantation* 10:853–855

Fricker FJ, Trento A, Griffith B, et al (1990). Experience with heart transplantation in children at the University of Pittsburgh and Children's Hospital. In Dunn JM, Donner RM (eds), *Heart transplantation in children*. Mount Kisco, NY: Futura, pp 233–241

Gao SZ, Schroeder JS, Hunt SA (1989). Acute myocardial infarction in cardiac-transplant recipients. *American Journal of Cardiology* 64:1093–1097

Kriett JM, Kaye MP (1990). The registry of the international society for heart transplantation: Seventh official report—1990. *The Journal of Heart Transplantation* 9:323–330

Lawrence K (ed) (1986). *Pediatric heart and heart/lung transplant home care booklet*. Pittsburgh: Children's Hospital of Pittsburgh

McEnery PT, Stablein DM, Arbus G, Tejani A (1992). Renal transplantation in children. *New England Journal of Medicine* 326:1727–1732

McGregor RS, Zitelli BJ, Urbach AH (1989). Varicella in pediatric orthotopic liver transplant recipients. *Pediatrics* 83:256–260

Perez-Woods R, Hedenkamp EA, Ulfig K, Newman D, Fioravante VL (1991). In Williams BA, Grady KL, Sandiford-Guttenbeil DM (eds), *Organ transplantation: A manual for nurses*. New York: Springer, pp 249–274

Ramos EL, Tilney NL, Ravenscraft MD (1991). Clinical aspects of renal transplantation. In Brenner BM, Rector FC (eds), *The kidney* (volume II, 4th ed). Philadelphia: Saunders, pp 2361–2407

Starze TE (1993). FK506 versus cyclosporin. *Transplantation Proceedings* 25:511–512

Staschak S, Zamberlan K (1990). Liver transplantation: Nursing diagnoses and management. In Sigardson-Poor KM, Haggerty LM (eds), *Nursing care of the transplant recipient*. Philadelphia: Saunders, pp 140–181

Sternbach GL, Varon J, Hunt SA (1992). Emergency department presentation and care of heart and heart/lung transplant recipients. *Annals of Emergency Medicine* 21:1140–1144

Whitington PF, Alonso EM, Piper J (1993). Liver transplantation for inborn errors of metabolism. *International Pediatrics* 8:30–39

Zamberlan K (1988). Quality of life in school-age children following liver transplantation. *Dissertation Abstracts International* 50:150–05b

Zamberlan K, Bernardo LM, Bove M (1992). Tips on nursing care of the pediatric organ recipient in the emergency department. *Journal of Emergency Nursing* 18:74–77

Zitelli BJ, Gartner JC, Malatack JJ, Urbach AH, Zamberlan K (1991). Liver transplantation in children: A pediatrician's perspective. *Pediatric Annals* 20:691

APPENDIX A

Instructions to Parents

INSTRUCTIONS TO PARENTS OF A CHILD WITH A FEVER

When your child has a fever you can do several things to decrease the fever and to make your child more comfortable. Always remember that a fever is a sign that your child is ill. You should contact your doctor if your child's fever is high (greater than 102°F or 38.9°C) or persists for several days, if your child is younger than 6 months, or if your child appears ill to you.

To decrease your child's fever you should:

1. Remove any heavy clothing while indoors. Light clothing allows heat to escape through the skin. Avoid wrapping the child in heavy blankets.
2. Give your child plenty of fluids. Drinking fluids is more important than eating when a child is ill. If your child also has vomiting or diarrhea, avoid fluids that are heavy, such as milk.
3. If your child's temperature is over 101°F (or 38.3°C) you may give your child *one* of the following:
   Acetaminophen (Tylenol) 10 mg per kg of body weight.
   Your child's dose is _____ mg every 4 hours.

   or

   If your child is older than 6 months of age, you can give ibuprofen (Advil or Pediaprofen) 15 mg per kg of body weight.
   Your child's dose is _____ mg every 6 hours.
4. *Do not* give aspirin for fever control in children.
5. If your child's temperature remains high, you may give your child a bath or sponge bath with lukewarm water for 10 to 15 minutes. Never use cold water or rubbing alcohol. Placing alcohol on your child's skin or in the bath water is dangerous, because the alcohol may be absorbed through the skin.

Call your primary care provider or return to the emergency department if:

1. An infant younger than 6 months has a fever greater than 101°F (38.3°C).
2. The fever persists for more than 48 hours.
3. Your child becomes lethargic, irritable; sleeps a lot; or refuses to eat or drink.
4. Your child has a rash, ear pain, seizures, breathing difficulty, stiff neck, vomiting, or diarrhea.
5. You have any concerns or questions.

INSTRUCTIONS TO PARENTS OF A CHILD WITH CROUP

Your child has a virus that causes swelling of the voice box and other parts of the airway. This is called croup, and the swelling causes that harsh, barking cough. Because croup is a virus, there is no antibiotic for it. But there are some important things you can do at home to make your child's breathing easier and to help him or her rest.

1. Give lots of cold fluids, such as ice water, cold sodas, fruit juices, sherbet, Popsicles, or Jell-O.
2. Make a mist tent: using a cool mist vaporizer, point the mist at the child's crib. Add only water to the vaporizer. Attach a sheet across the top of the crib and let it hang down to cover the side opposite the vaporizer. This cool, damp air soothes the throat and keeps mucus loose. Use this day and night.
3. Use fever control if your child's temperature goes above 101°F (38.3°C). See fever control sheet.
4. A steroid medicine may be given at home to reduce swelling in the airway. Follow the directions for the oral medication carefully and give with food.

Watch for other signs that mean the croup is getting worse:

1. Breathing becomes faster, noisier, or both.
2. A paleness or bluish color appears around the mouth, nose, eyes, or ears.
3. Coughing becomes more frequent, and the child is not able to rest well.
4. Your child will not take liquids or is drooling much more than usual.
5. The dents above the breast bone, below the breast bone, or in between the ribs become deeper.

If any of these things happen, call your primary care provider or bring your child back to the emergency department.

Prepared by Anne Phelan.

INSTRUCTIONS TO PARENTS
OF A CHILD WITH A COLD

Your child has an upper respiratory tract infection, or cold. The cold is caused by a virus and must run its course. There is no specific medicine to cure a cold, but there are several things you can do to make your child more comfortable.

1. **Fever control**—Follow the instructions on the fever control sheet. Acetaminophen or ibuprofen will also help the aches and pains.
2. **Rest**—Encourage quiet activities and frequent naps.
3. **Fluids**—Extra liquids help to thin out the mucus, keep fever down, and replace lost water.
4. A cool mist vaporizer may help to keep the mucus loose.
5. Babies may need salt water nose drops and bulb suctioning to pull out mucus from the nose.
6. Cough syrups should usually not be given to children because the cough is the body's way of loosening mucus in the lungs.

Call your primary care provider if the fever is high (over 102°F or 38.9°C rectally) and does not decrease with fever control, if the cough interferes with rest or drinking fluids, or if the child seems to get worse instead of better.

Prepared by Anne Phelan.

INSTRUCTIONS TO PARENTS
OF A CHILD WITH ASTHMA

Your child has a breathing problem called asthma. This usually happens in children who have allergies or when there has been asthma in other family members. During an asthma attack, the small breathing tubes in the lungs are squeezed tight, and extra mucus is made. This causes the child to have fast or noisy breathing. Older children may seem nervous and may be able to tell you that they can't breathe right. Asthma attacks can be caused by many different things: for example, exposure to something the child is allergic to such as cigarette smoke, pollen, dust, or animal dander; a cold or pneumonia; or an emotional upset. In children the most frequent cause is an allergy. If your child is over 4 years old, he or she should be tested to see what things he or she is allergic to.

You will most likely be given a prescription for a liquid, pills, inhaler, or nebulizer, for your child to take at home. Please be sure that the nurse or primary care provider has explained when and how to give the medicines. One of the important things to remember about asthma medications is that they only stay in the blood stream for a certain length of time. If too much time passes before the medicine is given again, the wheezing can return.

Give your child plenty of fluids to drink. Milk and other thick liquids should be avoided. Clear liquids are best until the asthma attack has subsided.

Call your primary care provider or return to the emergency department if:

1. Your child begins to have wheezing when he or she has taken the asthma medicine.
2. Your child has persistent vomiting and is unable to keep the medicine down.
3. Your child is breathing fast or is using extra muscles to breathe (dents between ribs or above or below the breast bone).
4. Your child's lips or skin turn blue or gray.
5. Your child has chest pain or a frequent cough that interferes with his or her ability to breathe.

Prepared by Anne Phelan.

INSTRUCTIONS FOR PARENTS OF A CHILD WITH BRONCHIOLITIS

Your child has a virus called bronchiolitis. This is why the baby's breathing is noisy (wheezing) and difficult. Because this is a virus, there is no antibiotic that will make your child better. Bronchiolitis usually clears up very quickly, about 3 days after the breathing trouble began. Even though there is no quick "cure," there are some important things you can do to help the baby breathe easier:

1. Give the baby lots of clear liquids. When children are sick they often do not feel like eating, and even milk may be heavy for them. Offer your baby lots of juices, water, soup, broth, flat sodas, or Jell-O water. Young babies should drink some Pedialyte or Lytren, a special mineral water.
2. Use a cool mist vaporizer. Add only water, and point it directly at the baby's crib. For extra relief you may turn on the warm water of the shower and let the bathroom fill with steam, then sit in the room with the child.
3. Raise the top part of your baby's mattress slightly so that the head of the bed will be higher.
4. Keep the baby's nose clear. You can clean the nostrils with a cotton swab or use a suction bulb to pull out the mucus.
5. Use fever control if the baby's temperature reaches 101°F (38.3°C) or higher rectally.
6. If Albuterol is prescribed, be sure to give the doses at the recommended times.

There are also some things to watch for that mean the baby is having more trouble breathing:

1. Breathing is faster or noisier.
2. Small dents appear above, below, or in between the ribs when the baby breathes in.
3. There is a paleness or bluish-gray color around the nose and mouth.
4. The baby seems unable to relax or sleep well.
5. The baby refuses or chokes on liquids.

If any of theses things start to happen, call the primary care provider who saw your baby for this illness or bring your baby back to the emergency department.

Prepared by Anne Phelan.

INSTRUCTIONS TO PARENTS OF A CHILD WITH PNEUMONIA

Your child has been found to have pneumonia. This means that a small part of one of the lungs has become congested with mucus. Many times medicines such as antibiotics are prescribed. If your primary care provider has given you a prescription, please make sure you understand how to use the medicine so that it will work most effectively.

There are other important things for you to do to help your child feel comfortable and to get better faster:

1. Give lots of fluids. Sick children often do not feel like eating solid foods, and milk products may also be heavy on their stomachs. Fluids like fruit juices, soup, broths, water, sodas, Jell-O, and Popsicles help to thin out the mucus and move it out of the lung.
2. Use a cool mist vaporizer. Add only water to the vaporizer, and point it toward the head of the child's bed.
3. Perform chest physical therapy. Position the child on his or her stomach with the shoulders a little lower than the waist. Make a cup with the palms of your hand and clap the child's back in the direction of the shoulder blades. Make sure your child's nurse has shown you this, as well as different positions for draining different sections of the lung. With small children it is sometimes helpful to call this a coughing game to cough up and spit out the mucus. This should be done about every 4 hours while the child is awake.
4. Use fever control if your child's temperature goes over 101°F (or 38.3°C) rectally or orally.

There are also some signs to watch for that mean the child's breathing is getting more difficult:

1. Breathing becomes faster, noisier, or both.
2. You notice a bluish or grayish color around the nose or mouth.
3. You can see dents above or below the breast bone or in between the ribs when your child breathes in.
4. The fever remains above 103°F (or 39.4°C) rectally, even after fever control.
5. Your child won't drink fluids or starts to choke on liquids.
6. Vomiting occurs so often that your child cannot keep the medicine down.

If one or more of these things start to happen, call your primary care provider or bring your child back to the emergency department.

Prepared by Anne Phelan.

INSTRUCTIONS TO PARENTS REGARDING ACCIDENTAL POISONINGS

Accidental poisoning is one of the leading causes of death in infants and small children. Many things that are used in the home can injure or even kill a child if they are swallowed.

These common household substances are poisonous and should be kept locked away:

- Ammonia, bleach, detergents
- Drain and oven cleaners
- Furniture polish
- Soaps, shampoos
- Paints, paint thinner, turpentine
- Pesticides or rat poisons
- Cosmetics (including nail polish, removers, perfumes, permanent wave solutions)
- Alcoholic beverages
- Moth balls
- Medicines of all kinds, including over-the-counter drugs, vitamins, and cough syrups

Poisoning can be prevented. Here are some things that you can do to protect your child:

1. Store all nonfood items in their original containers. Store them high in a locked cabinet or medicine chest, separated from food.
2. When your child must take medicine, never call it "candy."
3. Buy brands of products that have safety caps. Even if they have safety caps, lock them away in a safe place.

4. Be careful, when visiting friends or family, that your child does not have access to any of their medicines or household products.

Keep a bottle of ipecac syrup in the house. It is the safest way to make a person vomit. It is also a poison, however, and should be used only when the poison control center or a medical person tells you to give it to your child.

Should a poisoning occur, take the following actions:

1. Try to determine what substance was swallowed.
2. Immediately call the Poison Control Center or your primary care provider for advice.
3. Save the poison container and a sample of the vomit, if any. During vomiting, turn your child's head to the side.

Vomiting should *not* be induced if:

1. A corrosive such as lye or a strong acid has been swallowed.
2. The child is drowsy, unconscious, or convulsing.

A child who has swallowed a poison is likely to attempt the same thing again within a year. Practice poison prevention.

Prepared by Elena Hopkins-Lotz.

INSTRUCTIONS TO PARENTS OF A CHILD WITH MINOR HEAD INJURY

After a minor head injury you should watch your child closely for 24 to 48 hours. Most children do not have problems after a minor head injury, but if you should see any of these symptoms listed below, contact your child's primary care provider immediately.

Call your primary care provider if your child shows:

1. Decreased level of consciousness:
   Becomes drowsy or cannot be awakened.
   Does not recognize you or familiar objects.
   Has confused speech or does not know where he is.
2. Irritability—is more fussy than usual and cannot be comforted.
3. Vomiting—cannot keep food or fluids down.
4. Weakness of either arm or leg—stumbles or falls more than usual.
5. Headache or a stiff neck lasting longer than 24 hours.
6. Convulsions (fits or seizures).
7. Complains of blurred vision or you notice the child's pupils are different sizes.

8. Bleeding or clear fluid dripping from ears or nose.

Most children can return to normal activities after a minor head injury. If your child should not do some activities, your doctor will write them down for you. Children may be tired for a day or two after a minor head injury and may require frequent rest periods. Usually there are no restrictions on activity, other than those you and your child feel are too tiring. Your child should be able to return to normal activities, including school, within 2 days.

Activity Restriction:

_____

_____

_____, MD

_____

Used with permission of the Children's Hospital Medical Center of Cincinnati.

APPENDIX B

Normal Pediatric Laboratory Values

HEMATOLOGY

Age	2 weeks	1 month	3 months	6 months	1 year	2–6 years	7–12 years	Adult female	Adult male
Hemoglobin (g/dL)	13–20	14–16	9.5–14.5	10.5–14	10.5–14	10.5–14	11.0–16.0	12.0–16.0	14.0–18.0
Hematocrit (%)	42–66	53	31–41	33–42	33–42	33–40	33–40	37–47	42–52
White blood cells per mm³	5000–20,000	6000–18,000	6000–17,000	6000–16,000	6000–15,000	7000–13,000	5000–13,500	5000–10,000	5000–10,000
Polymorphonuclear leukocytes (%)	40	30	30	45	45	45	55	55	55
Lymphocytes (%)	48	63	63	48	48	48	38	35	35
Eosinophils (%)	3	2	2	2	2	2	2	3	3
Monocytes (%)	9	5	5	5	5	5	5	7	7
Platelet Count	150,000–200,000	250,000	300,000	300,000	300,000	300,000	300,000	300,000	300,000

SERUM AND BLOOD CHEMISTRY

Test	Normal Values	Test	Normal Values
Albumin (g/dL)	3.8–5.0	Glucose (mg/dL)	Infants: 60–80
Alkaline phosphatase (BU)	Infants: 8–12		Children: 90–125
	Children: 4–10	Lead (μg/100 mL WB)	<20
Amylase (U)	<150 units	Phosphorus (mg/dL)	3.5–4.5
Bilirubin (mg/dL)	Direct <0.4	Potassium (mEq/L)	3.5–4.5
	Total <1.0	Protein, total (g/dL)	6–8
BUN (mg/dL)	Birth–2 years: 5–15	Prothrombin time (seconds)	12–15 (depends on control)
	> 2 years: 10–20	SGOT (OD units)	8–36 OD
Calcium (mg/dL)	9–11	SGPT (OD units)	6–35 OD
Chloride, serum (mEq/L)	95–110	Sodium (mEq/L)	135–148
Cholesterol (mg/dL)	150–250	Uric acid (mg/dL)	3–5
Creatinine, serum (mg/dL)	1–5 years: 0.3–0.5		
	5–10 years: 0.5–0.8		

BU, Bodansky units; BUN, blood urea nitrogen; SGOT, serum glutamic-oxaloacetic transaminase; SGPT, serum glutamic pyruvate transaminase.

BLOOD GASES

	Arterial		Venous	
pO$_2$	Newborns 60–70 mmHg		pO$_2$	10–25 mmHg
	Older children and adults 80–90 mmHG			
pCO$_2$	35–45 mmHg		pCO$_2$	41–51mmHG
pH	7.35–7.45		pH	7.32–7.42

URINALYSIS

Test	Age	Normal Values	Test	Age	Normal Values
Microscopic			pH	Newborn	5–7
White blood cells	All ages	0–4/high-power field		Infants and children	4.8–7.8
Red blood cells	All ages	Rare/high-power field	Specific gravity	Newborn/infant	1.001–1.020
Casts	All ages	Rare/high-power field		Children	1.002–1.030
Osmolality	Premature and newborn	100–600 mosm/L			
	Infants and children	50–1400 mosm/L			

APPENDIX C

Immunization Schedules

IMMUNIZATION SCHEDULE RECOMMENDED BY THE AMERICAN ACADEMY OF PEDIATRICS

	DTP[a]	Polio[b]	MMR	Hepatitis B[c]	*Haemophilus*[a]	Tetanus-Diphtheria
Birth				X		
1–2 months				X		
2 months	X	X			X[d]	
4 months	X	X			X[d]	
6 months	X				X[d]	
6–18 months				X		
12–15 months					X[d]	
15 months			X			
15–18 months	X[e]	X				
4–6 years	X[e]	X				
11–12 years			X[f]	X[g]		
14–16 years				X[g]		X

[a]The HbOC-DTP combination vaccine may be substituted for separate vaccinations for *Haemophilus* and DTP.
[b]Children in close contact with immunosuppressed individuals should receive inactivated polio vaccine.
[c]Infants of mothers who tested seropositive for hepatitis B surface antigen (HBsAg+) should receive hepatitis B immune globulin (HBIG) at or shortly after the first dose. These infants will also require a second hepatitis B vaccine dose at 1 month and a third hepatitis B vaccine injection at 6 months of age.
[d]Depends on which *Haemophilus influenza* type B vaccine was given previously.
[e]For the fourth and fifth dose, the acellular (DTaP) pertussis vaccine may be substituted for the DTP vaccine.
[f]Except where public health authorities require otherwise.
[g]Where resources permit, the hepatitis B vaccine series of three immunizations should be given to previously unimmunized preadolescents or adolescents.
Copyright © 1993 by the American Academy of Pediatrics.

APPENDIX D

Anthropometric Charts

Anthropometric (growth) charts are important tools for determining if a child's height, weight, and head circumference are within the normal range for the child's age. Growth measurements are related to both genetic and environmental factors. Information on the parents' stature and weight is important when assessing a child's growth because heredity plays an important role in the child's growth pattern. Environmental factors that influence a child's growth include psychosocial problems, feeding disorders, and undernutrition. Some chronic illnesses interfere with normal growth and development.

For children 36 months old and younger, the child's length, weight, and head circumference are obtained and each is plotted according to age on the chart of the correct gender. For children older than 3 years, height and weight are plotted. The percentiles obtained for each measurement should be documented in the child's medical record.

Changes over time in percentile ranks are important clinical indicators. Height and weight measurements below the 10th percentile may be related to undernutrition, and the child should be referred to his or her primary care provider for evaluation. Children with weights below the third percentile are often admitted to the hospital for evaluation. A head circumference that is found to be in a significantly higher or lower percentile than other measurements may indicate a neurologic disorder and warrants an evaluation. Nonorganic failure-to-thrive is characterized by measurements in which weight is at a lower percentile rank than length and length is at a lower percentile rank than head circumference.

GIRLS: BIRTH TO 36 MONTHS PHYSICAL GROWTH NATIONAL CENTER FOR HEALTH STATISTICS PERCENTILES (LENGTH)

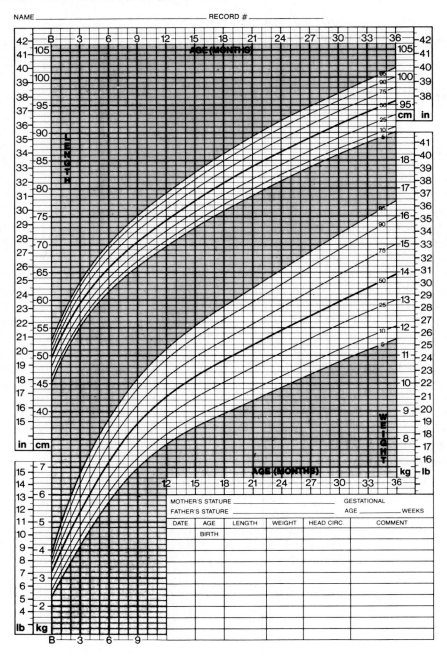

(Adapted from Hammill PVV, Drizd TA, Johnson CL, et al [1979]. Physical growth: National Center for Health Statistics percentiles. *American Journal of Clinical Nutrition* 32:607–609. Data from the Fels Longitudinal Study, Wright State University School of Medicine, Yellow Springs, Ohio. Courtesy of Ross Laboratories)

BOYS: BIRTH TO 36 MONTHS PHYSICAL GROWTH NATIONAL CENTER FOR HEALTH STATISTICS PERCENTILES (LENGTH)

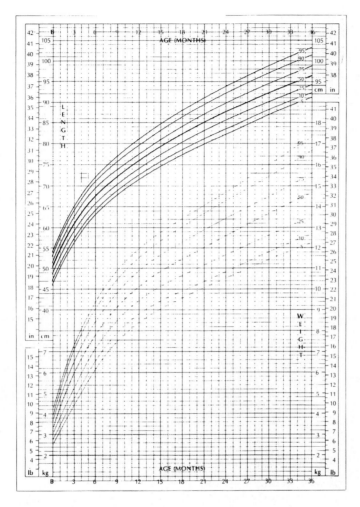

DATE	AGE	LENGTH	WEIGHT	HEAD CIRC	COMMENT

(Adapted from Hammill PVV, Drizd TA, Johnson CL, et al [1979]. Physical growth: National Center for Health Statistics percentiles. *American Journal of Clinical Nutrition* 32:607–609. Data from the Fels Longitudinal Study, Wright State University School of Medicine, Yellow Springs, Ohio. Courtesy of Ross Laboratories)

GIRLS: BIRTH TO 36 MONTHS PHYSICAL GROWTH NATIONAL CENTER FOR HEALTH STATISTICS PERCENTILES (HEAD CIRCUMFERENCE)

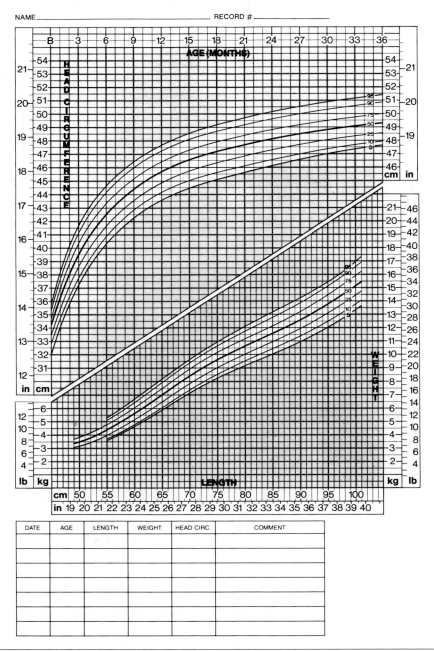

(Adapted from Hammill PVV, Drizd TA, Johnson CL, et al [1979]. Physical growth: National Center for Health Statistics percentiles. *American Journal of Clinical Nutrition* 32:607–609. Data from the Fels Longitudinal Study, Wright State University School of Medicine, Yellow Springs, Ohio. Courtesy of Ross Laboratories)

BOYS: BIRTH TO 36 MONTHS PHYSICAL GROWTH NATIONAL CENTER FOR HEALTH STATISTICS PERCENTILES (HEAD CIRCUMFERENCE)

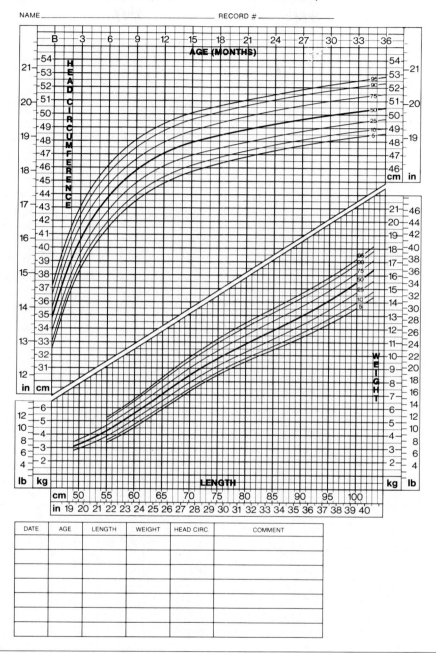

(Adapted from Hammill PVV, Drizd TA, Johnson CL, et al [1979]. Physical growth: National Center for Health Statistics percentiles. *American Journal of Clinical Nutrition* 32:607–609. Data from the Fels Longitudinal Study, Wright State University School of Medicine, Yellow Springs, Ohio. Courtesy of Ross Laboratories)

GIRLS: 2 TO 18 YEARS PHYSICAL GROWTH NATIONAL CENTER
FOR HEALTH STATISTICS PERCENTILES

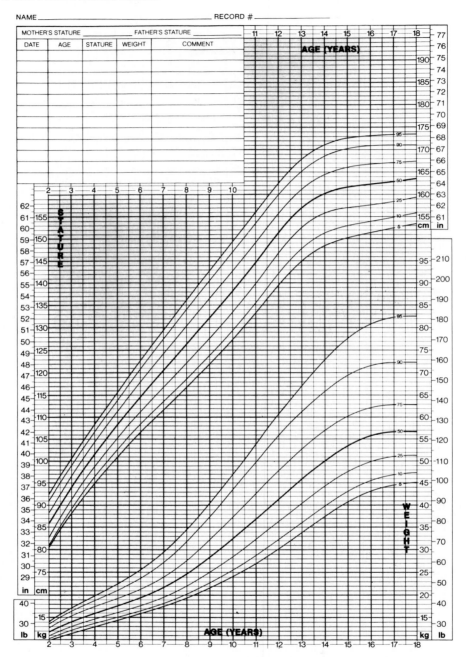

(Adapted from Hammill PVV, Drizd TA, Johnson CL, et al [1979]. Physical growth: National Center for Health Statistics percentiles. *American Journal of Clinical Nutrition* 32:607–609. Data from the National Center for Health Statistics, Hyattsville, Md. Courtesy of Ross Laboratories)

BOYS: 2 TO 18 YEARS PHYSICAL GROWTH NATIONAL CENTER FOR HEALTH STATISTICS PERCENTILES

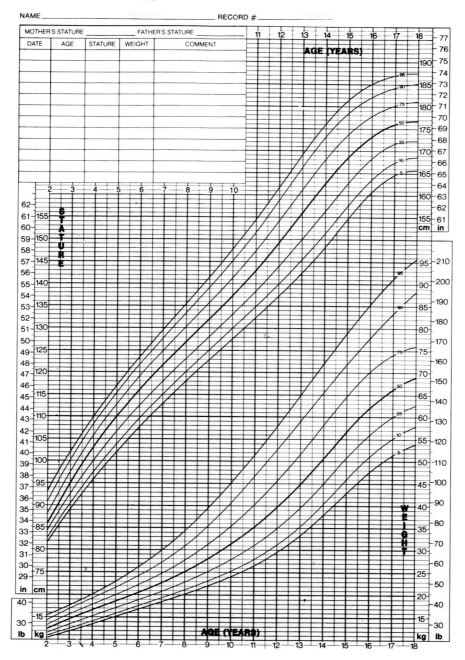

(Adapted from Hammill PVV, Drizd TA, Johnson CL, et al [1979]. Physical growth: National Center for Health Statistics percentiles. *American Journal of Clinical Nutrition* 32:607–609. Data from the National Center for Health Statistics, Hyattsville, Md. Courtesy of Ross Laboratories)

GIRLS: PREPUBESCENT PHYSICAL GROWTH NATIONAL CENTER FOR HEALTH STATISTICS PERCENTILES

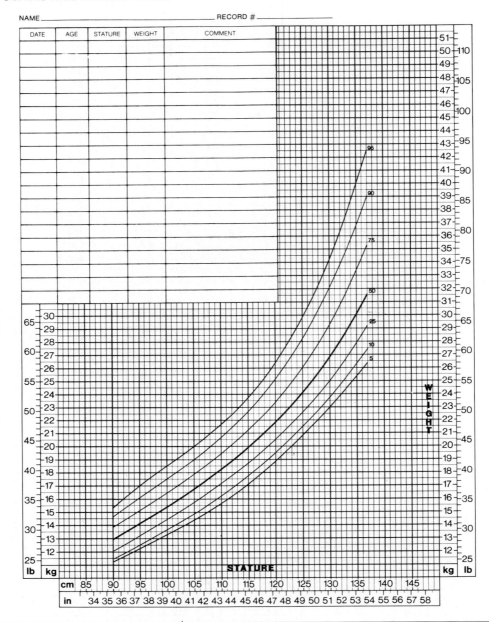

(Adapted from Hammill PVV, Drizd TA, Johnson CL, et al [1979]. Physical growth: National Center for Health Statistics percentiles. *American Journal of Clinical Nutrition* 32:607–609. Data from the National Center for Health Statistics, Hyattsville, Md. Courtesy of Ross Laboratories)

BOYS: PREPUBESCENT PHYSICAL GROWTH NATIONAL CENTER
FOR HEALTH STATISTICS PERCENTILES

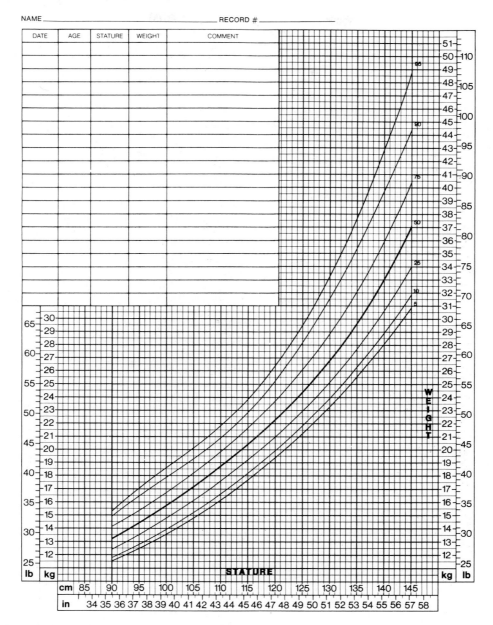

(Adapted from Hammill PVV, Drizd TA, Johnson CL, et al: Physical growth: National Center for Health Statistics percentiles. *American Journal of Clinical Nutrition* 32:607–609. Data from the National Center for Health Statistics, Hyattsville, Md. Courtesy of Ross Laboratories)

Index